Managing Infections in Patients With Hematological Malignancies

CONTEMPORARY HEMATOLOGY

Judith E. Karp, MD, Series Editor

For other titles published in the series, go to
www.springer.com/series/7681

Managing Infections in Patients With Hematological Malignancies

Edited by

Michael Kleinberg, MD, PhD
University of Maryland
School of Medicine
Baltimore, MD

Humana Press

Editor
Michael Kleinberg, MD, PhD
Section of Infectious Diseases
Marlene and Stewart Greenebaum Cancer Center
University of Maryland School of Medicine
Baltimore, MD
mkleinbe@umaryland.edu

Series Editor
Judith E. Karp, MD
The Sidney Kimmel Comprehensive Cancer
Center at Johns Hopkins
Division of Hematologic Malignancies
Baltimore, MD

ISBN 978-1-58829-986-4 e-ISBN 978-1-59745-415-5
DOI 10.1007/978-1-59745-415-5
Springer New York Dordrecht Heidelberg London

Library of Congress Control Number: 2009937445

Printed on acid-free paper

Springer is part of Springer Science+Business Media (www.springer.com)

Preface

Managing infections that complicate care of neutropenic patients with leukemia and hematopoietic stem cell recipients has become a distinct specialty. So much so, that an otherwise veteran infectious diseases specialist would be uncomfortable for the first time applying his or her general expertise to the neutropenic patient. There is no shortage of review articles, expert opinions, consensus guidelines, and books to guide both hematology and infectious diseases practitioners. Expert reviews are valuable in educating and informing clinicians about the myriad of pathogens that can cause infections in immunocompromised patients. Their practical usefulness is limited to some extent because most expert reviews presuppose knowing the identity of the pathogen. Clinical medicine is not practiced looking backwards. In this volume, we therefore attempted to write an owners manual rather than a collection of reviews.

The audience for this book is the practicing hematologist who treats neutropenic patients with leukemia and stem cell transplant recipients. This targeted hematologist has experience treating infections but not the formal background of the infectious diseases specialist. This book is not a substitute for formal training in infectious diseases. However, we hope that it will provide a working insight into infections and cancer; enough information to promote understanding of the principles that are the basis for the approach to neutropenic fever and other infections in patients with hematological malignancies. This book is divided into three sections. The first section consists of three chapters reviewing viral, bacterial, and fungal pathogens. The emphasis has been on usefulness with brief descriptions of the microbes and diseases they cause in patients with hematological malignancies, diagnostic methods, and treatments. These three chapters have extensive tables to improve quick access to information. The second section consists of chapters devoted to management of infections in patients with the different underlying hematological malignancies. The emphasis in these chapters is not a comprehensive review of all possible infections. Instead, the authors have focused on their approaches to diagnosing potential pathogens in their infected patients. The authors of these chapters draw on their extensive expertise in providing a roadmap for hematologists to manage efficiently the complexities of infections in their patients. The third section consists of several important topics that are often ignored in most books about infections and hematological malignancies. Treating the population of patients seen in a large cancer center entails several considerations beyond finding the germ and prescribing the right drug.

We hope that clinicians "in the trenches" will find this book useful not just in treating individual patients, but also in building strong infectious diseases programs within their respective cancer centers. History tells us that the future will continue to change with new pathogens, new treatments for hematological malignancies, and other new challenges.

Baltimore, MD

Michael Kleinberg, MD, PhD

Contents

Contributors

George Alangaden, M.D.
Section of Infectious Diseases, Barbara Ann Karmanos Cancer Institute,
Wayne State University, Detroit, MI, USA

Nikolaos G. Almyroudis, M.D.
Department of Medicine, Division of Infectious Diseases,
Roswell Park Cancer Institute, and Department of Medicine,
School of Medicine and Biomedical Sciences,
University at Buffalo, Buffalo, NY, USA

Elias J. Anaissie, M.D.
Myeloma Institute for Research and Therapy,
University of Arkansas for Medical Sciences, Little Rock, AR, USA

Minoo Battiwalla, M.D.
Department of Medicine, Roswell Park Cancer Institute, Buffalo, NY, USA

E.J. Bow, M.D.
Health Sciences Centre, Winnipeg, MB, Canada

Pranatharthi H. Chandrasekar, M.D.
Section of Infectious Diseases, Barbara Ann Karmanos Cancer Institute,
Wayne State University, and Harper University Hospital, Detroit, MI, USA

Alan Cross, M.D.
Center for Vaccine Development, University of Maryland
School of Medicine, Baltimore, MD, USA

Ben E. de Pauw, M.D.
Department of Blood Transfusion and Transplant Immunology,
University Medical Center St Radboud, Nijmegen, The Netherlands

Jay A. Fishman, M.D.
Associate Director, MGH Transplantation Center, Director, Transplant
Infectious Disease & Compromised Host Program, Massachusetts General
Hospital, Associate Professor of Medicine, Harvard Medical School
Boston, MA, USA

Graeme N. Forrest, M.D.
Division of Infectious Diseases, Oregon Health and Science University, Portland Veterans Affairs Medical Center, 3701 SW US Veterans Hospital Road P3ID, 97239, Portland, Oregon, USA

Alexandra Herbers, M.D.
Department of Haematology, Radboud University Nijmegen Medical Center, Nijmegen, The Netherlands

Michael Kleinberg, M.D., Ph.D.
Section of Infectious Diseases, Marlene and Stewart Greenebaum Cancer Center, University of Maryland School of Medicine, Baltimore, MD, USA

Stanley I. Martin, M.D.
Transplant Infectious Diseases Service, Division of Infectious Diseases, Ohio State University Medical Center, Columbus, OH, USA

Gloria Mattiuzzi, M.D.
Leader, Hematologic Malignancies Supportive Care Program, Department of Leukemia, M.D. Anderson Cancer Center, Houston, TX, USA

Marcio Nucci, M.D.
Department of Internal Medicine, Hematology and Bone Marrow Transplant Unit, and Mycology Lab, University Hospital, Federal University of Rio de Janeiro, Rio de Janeiro, Brazil

Luis Ostrosky-Zeichner, M.D., F.A.C.P., F.I.D.S.A.
Department of Medicine and Epidemiology, Division of Infectious Diseases, University of Texas Medical School at Houston, Houston, TX, USA

Mary-Claire Roghmann, M.D., M.S.
Division of Epidemiology and Preventive Medicine, Department of Medicine, University of Maryland School of Medicine, Baltimore, MD, USA

Kenneth V. I. Rolston, M.D.
Department of Infectious Diseases, Infection Control and Employee Health, The University of Texas, M.D. Anderson Cancer Center, Houston, TX, USA

Brahm H. Segal, M.D.
Department of Medicine, Division of Infectious Diseases, Roswell Park Cancer Institute, Buffalo, NY, USA

Kerri Thom, M.D., M.S.
Division of Epidemiology and Preventive Medicine, Department of Medicine, University of Maryland School of Medicine, Baltimore, MD, USA

John R. Wingard, M.D.
Department of Medicine, Department of Pediatrics, Blood and Bone Marrow Transplant Program, University of Florida Shands Cancer Center, Gainesville, FL, USA

Chapter 1

Introduction: Approach to the Patient

Michael Kleinberg and E.J. Bow

Abstract The empirical treatment of febrile neutropenic patients with suspected infections is one of the true success stories in the supportive care of patients with hematological malignancies. The essence of the febrile neutropenia paradigm is the shift of focus from microbial pathogens to the immune deficiencies of the host: immune deficiencies intrinsic to the underlying malignancies themselves and to the therapies employed to treat them. The impact of immune dysfunction can be best understood in terms of assessments of risks and likelihoods: the risks of acquiring a particular infection and the likelihoods of achieving a successful outcome if infected. The risks of prolonged neutropenia associated with treatment of acute leukemia are probably the best known to hematologists and infectious diseases specialists because of a long record of groundbreaking studies published over the last 50 years. The lessons learned have been applied to other patients with different immune defects, such as recipients of allogeneic stem cell transplants. There have been many reviews, chapters, position papers from professional societies, etc. over the years, promoting various guidelines for the general approach to managing infections in patients with hematological malignancies. However, experienced clinicians know that these guidelines, irrespective of their origins, are merely stepping stones to the initial approach to the potentially infected patient. There is no substitute for standing at the patient's bedside. The goal should be to individualize therapy based on the generic paradigm, taking into account unique features in any patient's situation that might optimize the condition for success and diminish the risks of failure.

1. Introduction

Dramatic improvements in the outcomes of neutropenic patients with serious infections represent one of the most significant advances in the treatment of hematological malignancies. The expected mortality rate was greater than 60% for the bacteremic neutropenic patient treated for acute leukemia in the 1960s [1]. Forty years later, the mortality rate has dropped to less than 5%

From: *Managing Infections in Patients With Hematological Malignancies*: Contemporary Hematology, Edited by: M. Kleinberg, DOI 10.1007/978-1-59745-415-5_1,

[2], outcomes even better in many cases compared to bacteremias in patients without neutropenia. Success in treating neutropenic infections comes despite extension of therapy for acute leukemia to older patients with greater debilities who would never have been considered as candidates for myeloablative chemotherapy in earlier decades. The improved outcomes can be traced to the improved general supportive care for patients with leukemia, the development of more potent anti-infectives with broader spectrum, and the development of the febrile neutropenia paradigm for managing the infected neutropenic patient. The latter is nothing more than a structured approach to the empirical administration of anti-infectives to the potentially infected neutropenia patient while awaiting the results of diagnostic tests such as cultures. Today, this empirical approach is a universally established standard of care for patients with acute leukemia. However, it should be noted that this was not the case in the 1960s and 1970s when the febrile neutropenia paradigm was a sharp break from infection diseases orthodoxy. More recently, variations of the febrile neutropenia approach have been adapted to non-neutropenic immunocompromised patients, such as stem cell transplant recipients with suspected infections.

2. Treatment of Infections in Neutropenic Patients: A Brief History

Fever and infection represent the most important complications of myeloablative cytotoxic therapy that results in severe mucositis and prolonged neutropenia. More than 90% of patients undergoing intensive cytotoxic therapy for acute leukemia (AL) or myeloablative conditioning for allogeneic hematopoietic stem cell transplantation (HSCT) will develop a febrile neutropenic episode suspicious for infection [3, 4]. The differential diagnosis must consider both infectious and non-infectious causes, and vary over the course of the bone marrow reconstitution/engraftment.

It was more than 40 years ago that the relationship between the circulating neutrophil count and the risk of pyogenic infection was established through the observations of Bodey et al. [5, 6]. During the 1950s, infectious diseases physicians adhered to the then accepted principles of infectious diseases practice by not prescribing antibacterial therapy until a source of infection and/or a specific pathogen had been identified. The infection-related mortality among febrile neutropenic patients with acute leukemia was very high during that period [7]. It was not until the early 1960s that the first randomized clinical trial on empirical antibiotic therapy in leukemia patients permitted the investigators, Curtin and Marshall, to conclude that "in some patients, therapy must be started before bacteriological data become available" [8]. The most common cause of infection during that period was penicillin-resistant *Staphylococcus aureus*. The principle of early administration of empirical antibacterial therapy did not become well accepted until Schimpff and colleagues from the University of Maryland Cancer Center published their observations on the importance of prompt initiation of broad-spectrum combination antibacterial therapy with carbenicillin and gentamicin, broadening the spectrum of antimicrobial activity against gram-negative bacteria [9]. Moreover, the seminal observations by this group describing the relationship between mucosal colonization by healthcare facility-acquired bacterial pathogens and invasive infection in patients with acute myeloid leukemia provided a foundation for our understanding of the pathogenesis of these infections [10] and for the introduction of preventative strategies [11].

The introduction of new antibiotics led to the successful treatment of targeted pathogens which were soon replaced by other bacteria with some resistance to the newly introduced antibacterials. After the introduction of methicillin in the early 1960s targeting *Staphylococcus aureus*, gram-negative enteric bacilli such as *Escherichia coli* and *Klebsiella pneumoniae* emerged as the predominant pathogens. Introduction of the first generation cephalosporin, cephalothin, effective against enteric bacteria, led to improved outcomes when combined often with an aminoglycoside. Predictable in hindsight, *Pseudomonas aeruginosa*, resistant to cephalothin and poorly responsive to aminoglycosides, emerged as a prominent pathogen associated with mortality rates of more than 75%, especially among patients who failed to recover myeloid function [7]. Subsequently, the introduction of the first anti-pseudomonal carboxypenicillin, carbenicillin, had a significant impact upon survival for leukemia patients with *P. aeruginosa* bacteremia. Compared to treatment with other monotherapies available at that time, such as polymyxin or gentamicin where survival rates for *Pseudomonas* bacteremias were only 20–40%, carbenicillin treatment was associated with improved survivals in excess of 75%. In the 1980s, the introduction of more potent anti-pseudomonal penicillins and third generation cephalosporins, such as ceftazidime, with broad anti-gram negative bacterial coverage replaced the older antibacterial agents.

The duration of antibacterial therapy once initiated was examined by Pizzo and his colleagues at the National Cancer Institute [12]. These investigators observed recrudescence rates of 41% among neutropenic patients in whom the initial empirical antibiotic regimen had been discontinued at the time of defervescence. Based upon these observations, guidelines have generally recommended that the initial antibacterial regimen be continued until myeloid recovery defined by an increase in the circulating absolute neutrophil count to at least 0.5×10^9/L over two successive days [13].

Every advance in infection management of neutropenic patients led to the revelation of new problems. With more and more effective antibacterial agents targeting bacterial infections, it became clear in the 1980s that the problem of life-threatening infections had not been solved in many neutropenic patients. The question of how to manage patients with persistent neutropenic fever despite broad-spectrum antibacterial therapy was addressed first by Pizzo and colleagues in the early 1980s [14] and later by the European Organization for Research and Treatment of Cancer (EORTC) [15]. Pizzo demonstrated that the persistent pyrexia was associated with systemic fungal infections in a high proportion of patients and that the empirical addition of a systemic antifungal agent, amphotericin B deoxycholate improved outcomes. Since those seminal observations, empirical anti-fungal therapy has become a standard practice world-wide [13, 16–22]. The role of other antibacterial approaches specifically targeting gram-positive infections among patients with the persistent neutropenic fever syndrome has also been studied [23].

And so, after almost 50 years of evolving treatment strategies, there is a consensus approach to managing infections in patients with hematological malignancies practiced in broad outlines by virtually all hematologists and infectious diseases practitioners. The consensus approach to febrile neutropenia is undeniably effective as will be detailed in the chapters that follow. The remainder of this chapter will discuss some general concepts on how the findings from the large body of published studies can be applied at the patient's bedside.

3. Centrality of the Host and Immune Deficiency

In general, people with normal immune function are infected by professional pathogens such as *Streptococcus pneumoniae, Staphylococcus aureus*, influenza, and other bacteria, viruses, and parasites that have evolved to survive the innate and adaptive immune defenses. Commensal GI and skin flora, fungal spores, and environmental microbes ingested, inhaled and contacted daily do not cause disease in the absence of injury, overwhelming exposure, or some other event that heightens infectivity. In contrast, these otherwise innocuous microbes cause the majority of infections in neutropenic patients and in hematopoietic stem cell recipients. Pathogens and the infections they cause will be discussed extensively in the chapters that follow. However, it is the immune defects in the patient with hematological malignancies that permit infections by these otherwise harmless germs. Not surprisingly, the phenotypes of infections will be modulated heavily across the spectrum of immune deficiencies of patients with hematological malignancies.

One of the most important concepts in the approach to infections in the febrile neutropenic patient is the recognition of risk [24–29]. Risk can be defined in two ways. First, risk may be defined in terms of the probability for developing a febrile neutropenic infection; and second, it may be defined in terms of the likelihood for significantly poor outcomes due to that infection. An understanding of the risks in the latter case may be used to define the approaches to management; for instance, in-patient versus out-patient treatment strategies and administration of intravenous versus oral formulations of antimicrobial therapy. These considerations have significant economic and quality of life ramifications. These two aspects of risk will be expanded upon in several of the chapters that follow.

The centrality of the host is illustrated in the brief history of febrile neutropenia mentioned above. The neutropenic patient can never be rendered free of all infections as long as the neutropenia persists. It is not possible to sterilize the neutropenic patient. Rather, the recurring story is that of conquering a troublesome pathogen by improvements in the approach to infection management or the introduction of new anti-infectives, followed soon after by the appearance of a new opportunistic germ. As long as the patient's immune system remains crippled, there will always be a microbe, resistant to previous anti-infectives, capable of causing a life-threatening infection. This concept is at the heart of the management of infections in patients with hematological malignancies. This is also the most difficult concept to apply at the bedside of an individual patient.

4. Expectations

The immune dysfunction of the patient with a hematological malignancy determines the risk for acquiring a serious infection (modulated in part by the toxicity of chemotherapy and GVHD, co-morbid medical conditions, etc.).

The core concept of the febrile neutropenia paradigm is anticipation; that is, the prediction of likely pathogens in the potentially infected neutropenic patient and the probability that the pathogen will be treated successfully with the chosen course of anti-infectives. Positive blood cultures are not meant to diagnose a bacterial infection, but rather to confirm the correctness of the initial pathogen diagnosis and the appropriateness of the original antibiotic prescription. For this anticipatory strategy to be effective, the clinician must estimate correctly the probability that the febrile patient is truly infected, consider the likely pathogens, and predict the susceptibilities of these pathogens to anti-infectives. Much of this information is well-described from febrile neutropenia trials and in hospital-specific antibiotic susceptibility profiles for bacterial infections in the neutropenic patient with acute leukemia. Similar information for viral and fungal infections is not well understood and limits the estimates of risk for these kinds of infections.

It is important to recognize that infection incidence rates from febrile neutropenia trials and even hospital-specific antibiotic susceptibility profiles reflect results from a population of patients. The challenge to the clinician is in applying this information at the bedside of the individual patient. The clinician cannot consider all patients with febrile neutropenia to be identical to each other or to the "average" patient composite characterized by the mean and median of the study populations. Most neutropenic patients with fevers and suspected infections will be managed successfully with generic protocol antimicrobial strategies. However, experienced clinicians recognize when trial-based estimates of infection risk, potential pathogens, and antimicrobial susceptibilities must be modified by individual patient considerations. For instance, the presence of cellulitis surrounding an indwelling catheter exit site may merit the addition of vancomycin. Or, a broad spectrum antibiotic with anaerobic activity may be preferred in a patient with abdominal pain and tenderness and suspected neutropenic enterocolitis. Less obvious, broader spectrum coverage should be considered for a patient hospitalized, even briefly, in a ward such as an intensive care unit, endemic with multiple-drug resistant bacteria. This process of generating an estimate of risk for the individual patient with febrile neutropenia may seem daunting, especially to the non-infectious diseases specialist. However, the complexity of this process can be reduced by a systematic focus on potential infections rather than just fever and neutropenia and by predicting likely pathogens and their susceptibilities to antimicrobials. Developing a disciplined approach will be discussed in more detail in later chapters.

The large number of studies of bacterial infections in febrile neutropenia in patients with acute leukemia serves as an excellent illustration of the concepts of risk and expectations. In general, acute leukemia febrile neutropenia trials are single or multiple institution studies that compare the efficacies of two antibiotic regimens through randomized allocation of neutropenic patients into two treatment arms. While the particulars of individual trials do vary, there are considerable similarities between virtually all studies owing to the homogeneity of the depth and duration of neutropenia produced by the chemotherapies used to treat acute leukemia. The incidence of microbiologically and clinically documented bacterial infections varies between 20 and 40% [30–34]. These high rates of bacterial infections justify the empirical approach of treating all febrile neutropenic patients with antibiotics. It is remarkable that the infectious mortality associated with the initial febrile neutropenia event is 0–2%, especially considering the high frequency of bacteremias. In fact, today the clinician can stand at the bedside of a patient with newly diagnosed acute leukemia and answer with confidence that the risk of death from infection associated with that first fever is less than the risk of death from bacteremias in many other non-cancer patients without neutropenia. This low rate of infectious mortality also explains the proliferation of so many permutations on the basic paradigm, so much so that it seems that no two institutions use the same febrile neutropenia protocols [35]. All protocols will appear effective to their advocates. In fact, using the clinically appropriate infectious mortality outcome endpoint, there is no standard comparative trial design with sufficient statistical power to differentiate between two variations of standard febrile neutropenia protocols. Therefore, it is not surprising to find that many physicians feel most comfortable using the febrile neutropenia protocols they learned at the institutions where they trained, and they are sometimes resistant to adopting the specifically established guidelines at other hospitals.

It is important to recognize that there is potential danger even when the attributable mortality rate associated with the initial febrile neutropenia event is so low. For example, suppose that an institution adopts new antibiotic guidelines that lead to a doubling of the baseline mortality rate for initial febrile neutropenia from 1 to 2%. It is doubtful that treating physicians or even a database tracking patient outcomes would be capable of identifying this "spike" in the mortality rate because adverse outcomes are so rare. This example illustrates the potential problems in dealing with serious future issues such as the increasing rates of antibacterial resistance in both Gram positive and Gram negative bacteria. Even a serious problem with resistance, one that doubles the mortality rates for the initial febrile neutropenia event, may get lost in the noise of statistical fluctuations and may not be detectable in standard clinical trial designs. Therefore, it is imperative that institutions design their own febrile neutropenia protocols with this in mind. Cancer centers should focus considerably on adherence to the best practices in much the same way that airlines, surgeons, and critical care specialists developed quality assurance checklists and procedures to further reduce the already low rates of airline accidents, surgical deaths [36], and blood stream infections [37], respectively. To maintain low mortality rates for infections associated with the initial neutropenic fever, cancer centers should all have standard procedures for a periodic review of the appropriateness of protocol empirical antibiotics in light of changing bacterial resistance patterns, mechanisms to quickly identify the initial fever in the neutropenic patient, administration of antibiotic within 15–30 min of prescription, and a robust quality control system. This critically important topic will be discussed further in Chap. 13.

Most often, infectious mortality in patients with hematological malignancies is not due to infections associated with the initial neutropenic fever [38–41]. These later infections are often referred to as secondary infections or superinfections and will be discussed in detail in Chap. 5. Unfortunately, estimating the risk for developing these subsequent infections is not as straightforward as for the risks of febrile neutropenia. For neutropenic patients, the cumulative risk for later infections appears to be time-dependent, that is, there is a fixed risk per day of neutropenia developing an infection. Over time, patients with the longest periods of neutropenia will have the highest cumulative risks of developing later infections [5]. The risks for developing infections in allogeneic stem cell recipients are significantly more complicated and will be discussed in Chap. 8.

5. Attributable Success and Attributable Failure

The second element of risk is the likelihood of achieving a successful response in an immunocompromised patient with a hematological malignancy in whom a specific infection is treated with the appropriate anti-infectives. In general, a successful outcome depends on three factors; the potency of the anti-infective against the pathogen, the correct identification of all the causative infections and pathogens, and the degree and duration of the immune dysfunction. For an example of the latter, a patient with newly diagnosed acute leukemia or an autologous stem cell recipient is likely to recover near complete immune function with the resolution of neutropenia. These patients are likely to have better outcomes for any infections compared to patients with refractory leukemia and persistent neutropenia or allogeneic stem cell recipients with slow engraftment or ongoing GVHD and resultant unresolved immune dysfunction. Therefore, achieving a successful outcome depends on more than just prescribing the correct anti-infective.

The task of estimating the chances for successful outcomes is complicated by one fundamental problem. For many infections, physicians are unable to assess conclusively whether a patient's lack of response to an anti-infective is due to failure of the drug or to failure of the host. An example of the latter is a patient with refractory leukemia and chronic neutropenia. This patient is not expected to have a long life span; in fact, it is predictable that the patient may succumb to one infection or another at some point in an uncertain future. The perpetually neutropenic patient may survive one or more life-threatening infections. For these successes, most would agree that the prescribed anti-infectives functioned successfully, especially because there was no assistance from immune system. However, at some point, the crippled immune system will fail, despite the best efforts with anti-infectives known to be effective in identical infections in patients whose neutropenia has resolved. Attribution of the cause in these anti-infective treatment failures is difficult and controversial. For instance, in a multicenter trial of unrelated allogeneic HSCT, there were sharp disagreements between the local site investigators and the central expert panel in attributing the causes of death of study participants [42]. The expert panel changed 56% of the local cause-of-death determinations, many of which reclassified infection-related causes to progression of malignancies or advanced GVHD. An infection may have been the "final nail in the coffin," but it was the malignancy-related failures and treatment toxicities that were the principal causes of the deaths. Because of this uncertainty, all-cause mortality is more widely accepted as a trial endpoint than mortality attributed to infection because determining whether death has occurred is less controversial than determining why the death occurred. Use of the all-cause mortality endpoint is probably reasonable when a majority of deaths are infection related. However, use of the all-cause mortality endpoint is suspect when non-infectious mortality rates exceed infection-related rates.

Attribution of success and failure is central to the interpretation of trials of anti-infectives in infections in patients with hematological malignancies.

Unfortunately, the design of trials examining outcomes for infections in patients with hematological malignancies largely ignores this difficult issue. Most influential studies are randomized trials, often with blinding, that compare two anti-infectives against defined pathogen(s) in patients with hematological malignancies. Sometimes, there is enrollment stratification for known pre-existing risks to prevent confounding results by skewed assignment to the two treatment arms. Other heterogeneities that cannot be foreseen at enrollment, such as bone marrow recovery after chemotherapy or occurrence of severe GVHD, are assumed to be balanced between the two arms through randomization. The endpoints of many of these trials are often complex, usually as concessions to sample size limitations and feasibilities of trial design. For example, side effects and breakthrough infections with pathogens resistant to the study anti-infectives are considered treatment failures in febrile neutropenia trials even if the patient's infection was successfully treated by bedside clinical criteria [30, 32, 34, 43]. Disregarding these complexities, trial results are designed to show that either the two agents are equivalent (or non-inferior), or in some cases, superior or inferior within the bounds of statistical uncertainty. However, these trials are not designed statistically to be a clinically relevant measure of anti-infective efficacy, despite comments to the contrary in the discussion sections of publications. Several of these pivotal trials will be discussed in the chapters that follow.

Examining a trial comparing voriconazole and amphotericin B deoxycholate for treatment of aspergillosis in patients with acute leukemia and stem cell recipients illustrates how difficult it is to predict individual patient responses because of problems in attributing bad outcomes to anti-infective failure [44]. In this trial (to be discussed more fully in the Chap. 4), patients with aspergillosis were randomized to receive either voriconazole or amphotericin B deoxycholate for 12 weeks. Analysis showed that patients treated with voriconazole had a 53% rate of success by trial defined criteria which was 21% better than the success-rate for the amphotericin B-treated patients. This difference met the statistical criteria for superiority, and the results of this trial led to the licensing of voriconazole around the world for treatment of aspergillosis. While this study clearly showed that voriconazole should be preferred over amphotericin B deoxycholate in treating aspergillosis, the trial-defined success rate of 53% hardly inspires confidence of a successful outcome in the voriconazole-treated individual patient. However, a closer examination of all the outcomes in this trial show that only 28% of the voriconazole-treated patients failed because of aspergillosis that was unresponsive to voriconazole [44]. The other 25% were judged failures by trial-defined criteria, and included patients lost to follow-up, deaths unrelated to aspergillosis, and patients alive after 12 weeks but with responses to treatment less satisfactory than the preset defined criteria for success. There is an inherent uncertainty in attributing outcomes to infection versus noninfectious causes and it is likely to be impossible to resolve this uncertainty. In the real world, the physician at the bedside must be satisfied with an educated best estimate, rather than being able to predict treatment success with absolute certainty. For example, the clinician caring for a neutropenic patient with aspergillosis should expect a successful clinical response with voriconazole much better than the stated 53% in the trial report. In fact, clinical responses for *Aspergillus* pneumonia treated with voriconazole are consistent with the outcomes for serious bacterial pneumonias treated with antibiotics generally regarded as highly effective.

As discussed in the preceding paragraphs, it is difficult with so many infections to know accurately just how effectively an anti-infective performs, even when the pathogens and infections are reasonably well-understood. In many cases, a treating physician may not even know with certainty the identity of the infecting pathogen. Patients with hematological malignancies are notorious for being multiply infected with more than one pathogen at a time, or for developing serial infections, including the sudden onset of a life-threatening superinfection. Unfortunately, this leads frequently to successive cycles of empirical anti-infective prescription in an attempt to stay ahead of new clinically diagnosed infections for which no pathogens have yet been identified. The danger in this situation is that the estimates made by any clinician in these situations may be erroneous, especially when they result from a string of serial assumptions.

The third consideration for estimating the likelihood of achieving a successful response in the immunocompromised patient with a hematological malignancy is determining how the nature and extent of immune dysfunction contribute to the outcomes. This important topic will be discussed extensively in several of the chapters that follow. In the face of a serious infection, many physicians will attempt to reverse the immune suppression. There is little published data suggesting that this intuitively attractive approach is helpful. The effects of some measures, such as administering G-CSF to hasten granulocyte recovery or stopping marrow suppressive agents, may be seen in a few days and should be pursued. Reducing the doses of some immunosuppressants such as corticosteroids is unlikely to have any benefit in the short or even intermediate term. The immune suppression induced by other agents such as alemtuzumab or anti-thymocyte globulin is probably irreversible on the time scale of an infection. Unfortunately, patients with the greatest degree of immune dysfunction have the highest likelihoods of developing infection, especially with fungal and viral pathogens, and they are also likely to have the poorest outcomes.

6. Approach to the Patient

The treating physician should not be daunted by the complexity of treating infections in patients with hematological malignancies. Chapters 2–4 in this book provide the information necessary to choose the best anti-infectives to treat specific pathogens. Chapters 5–8 focus on the host and the specific immune deficiencies that influence the outcomes of infections. The remaining chapters discuss important issues that detail the institutional component of an effective infectious diseases program.

The following comments should be kept in mind

1. The importance of the careful construction of institution-specific infectious diseases protocols as described in Chap. 13 cannot be overemphasized. A common approach to treating infections leads to institutional memory and experience which is the foundation for a wise evolution of the protocols over time.
2. Having said that, an institutional protocol is only a guide that provides a common starting point for managing infections. This protocol should not

be a sacred text etched in stone. The clinician should strive to develop sufficient expertise to recognize the outlier patient whose infection deviates from the norm.

3. Even though empirical treatment is rampant (and often necessary) in patients with hematological malignancies, the proper management of infections must always be grounded in a thorough understanding of the potential pathogens, the pharmacokinetics and pharmacodynamics of anti-infectives used to treat these infections, the expected course of the treated infections, and the impact of the underlying malignancies and immune dysfunction on outcomes. There should always be in place the necessary expertise to construct a reasoned approach, grounded in the fundamentals of infectious diseases, to diagnosis and to treat even in the most difficult situations.
4. Infections do not respond instantaneously after anti-infectives are started. Persistence of fever for 3–4 days is to be expected in the patient successfully treated for febrile neutropenia (see Chap. 5). The patient with aspergillosis may worsen clinically after starting antifungals, and the chest CT may worsen for 14 days even with ultimately successful treatment (Chap. 4). Persistence of fever should not supersede other clinical indicators of patient improvement. A persistent fever should not be an automatic invitation to modify an otherwise appropriate anti-infective regimen.

There will, undoubtedly, be major changes in the future for the management of infections in patients with hematological malignancies. These changes will be driven by new pathogens, increased resistance to existing anti-infectives, and evolution in practice of oncology, in particular for allogeneic stem cell transplants. Sadly, changes we are less likely to see will be continuation with the anti-infective pipeline which has, in the past regularly produced new agents to attack new problems. As drug resistance in both Gram positive and Gram negative bacteria spreads, monotherapy for febrile neutropenia will likely become the first casualty to this inexorable onslaught. This tsunami of resistant bacteria will not wash over all the institutions at once; rather, hospitals with high rates of *Pseudomonas, Acinetobacter*, and *Klebsiella*, resistant to all beta-lactam antibiotics and *Staphylococcus aureus* and *Enterococcus*, increasingly resistant to vancomycin, will be in the forefront of development of novel empirical treatment regimens.

References

1. McCabe WR, Jackson GG (1962) Gram-negative bacteremia: II. Clinical, laboratory, and therapeutic observations. Arch Intern Med 110:856–864
2. Schimpff SC, Gaya H, Klastersky J et al (1978) Three antibiotic regimens in the treatment of infection in febrile granulocytopenic patients with cancer: the EORTC international antimicrobial therapy project group. J Infect Dis 137:14–29
3. Bow EJ (2003) Infectious complications in patients receiving cytotoxic therapy for acute leukemia: history, background and approaches to management. In: Wingard JR, Bowden RA (eds) Management of Infection in Oncology Patients. Martin Dunitz, London, pp 71–104
4. (2000) Guidelines for preventing opportunistic infections among hematopoietic stem cell transplant recipients. Biol Blood Marrow Transplant 6:659–713
5. Bodey GP, Buckley M, Sathe YS, Freireich EJ (1966) Quantitative relationships between circulating leukocytes and infection in patients with acute leukemia. Ann Intern Med 64:328–40

6. Bodey GP, Rodriguez V, Chang HY, Narboni G (1978) Fever and infection in leukemic patients: a study of 494 consecutive patients. Cancer 41:1610–22
7. Bodey GP (1997) The treatment of febrile neutropenia: from the Dark Ages to the present. Support Care Cancer 5:351–7
8. Curtin JA, Marshall BD Jr (1962) Use of antibiotics in cancer and leukemia. J Chronic Dis 15:713–8
9. Schimpff SC, Satterlee W, Young VM, Serpick A (1971) Empiric therapy with carbenicillin and gentamicin for febrile patients with cancer and granulocytopenia. N Engl J Med 284:1061–5
10. Schimpff SC, Young VM, Greene WH, Vermeulen GD, Moody MR, Wiernik PH (1972) Origin of infection in acute nonlymphocytic leukemia. Significance of hospital acquisition of potential pathogens. Ann Intern Med 77:707–14
11. Bow EJ (2005) Management of the febrile neutropenic cancer patient: lessons from 40 years of study. Clin Microbiol Infect 11(Suppl 5):24–9
12. Pizzo PA, Robichaud KJ, Gill FA, Witebsky FG, Levine AS, Deisseroth AB et al (1979) Duration of empiric antibiotic therapy in granulocytopenic patients with cancer. Am J Med 67:194–200
13. Hughes WT, Armstrong D, Bodey GP, Bow EJ, Brown AE, Calandra T et al (2002) 2002 guidelines for the use of antimicrobial agents in neutropenic patients with cancer. Clin Infect Dis 34:730–51
14. Pizzo PA, Robichaud KJ, Gill FA, Witebsky FG (1982) Empiric antibiotic and antifungal therapy for cancer patients with prolonged fever and granulocytopenia. Am J Med 72:101–11
15. EORTC International Antimicrobial Therapy Project Group (1989). Empiric antifungal therapy in febrile granulocytopenic patients. EORTC International Antimicrobial Therapy Cooperative Group. Am J Med 86:668–672
16. Link H, Bohme A, Cornely OA, Hoffken K, Kellner O, Kern WV et al (2003) Antimicrobial therapy of unexplained fever in neutropenic patients – guidelines of the Infectious Diseases Working Party (AGIHO) of the German Society of Hematology and Oncology (DGHO), Study Group Interventional Therapy of Unexplained Fever, Arbeitsgemeinschaft Supportivmassnahmen in der Onkologie (ASO) of the Deutsche Krebsgesellschaft (DKG-German Cancer Society). Ann Hematol 82(Suppl 2):S105–S117
17. Freifeld AG, Baden LR, Brown AE, Elting L, Gelfand M, Greene JN et al (2004) Fever and neutropenia. J Natl Compr Canc Netw 2:390–432
18. Santolaya ME, Rabagliati R, Bidart T, Paya E, Guzman AM, Morales R et al (2005) Consensus: rational approach towards the patient with cancer, fever and neutropenia. Rev Chilena Infectol 22(Suppl 2):S79–113
19. Garcia-Rodriguez JA, Gobernado M, Gomis M, Mensa J, Picazo J, Prieto J et al (2001) Clinical guide for the evaluation and treatment of patients with neutropenia and fever. Rev Esp Quimioter 14:75–83
20. Guidelines for the use of antimicrobial agents in patients with febrile neutropenia in Taiwan (2005). J Microbiol Immunol Infect 38:455–457
21. Masaoka T (2000) Febrile neutropenia – guideline in Japan. Gan To Kagaku Ryoho 27:161–5
22. Masaoka T (2004) Evidence-based recommendations for antimicrobial use in febrile neutropenia in Japan: executive summary. Clin Infect Dis 39(Suppl 1):S49–S52
23. Wade JC, Glasmacher A (2004) Vancomycin does not benefit persistently febrile neutropenic people with cancer. Cancer Treat Rev 30:119–26
24. Kern WV (2001) Risk assessment and risk-based therapeutic strategies in febrile neutropenia. Curr Opin Infect Dis 14:415–22
25. Rolston KV (1998) Risk assessment and risk-based therapy in febrile neutropenic patients. Eur J Clin Microbiol Infect Dis 17:461–3
26. Klastersky J, Paesmans M, Rubenstein EB, Boyer M, Elting L, Feld R et al (2000) The Multinational Association for Supportive Care in Cancer risk index: a

multinational scoring system for identifying low-risk febrile neutropenic cancer patients. J Clin Oncol 18:3038–51
27. Klastersky J, Paesmans M, Georgala A, Muanza F, Plehiers B, Dubreucq L et al (2006) Outpatient oral antibiotics for febrile neutropenic cancer patients using a score predictive for complications. J Clin Oncol 24:4129–34
28. Talcott JA, Siegel RD, Finberg R, Goldman L (1992) Risk assessment in cancer patients with fever and neutropenia: a prospective, two-center validation of a prediction rule. J Clin Oncol 10:316–22
29. Talcott JA, Siegal RD, Finberg R, Goldman L (1988) The medical course of cancer patients with fever and neutropenia: clinical identification of a low-risk subgroup at presentation. Arch Intern Med 108:2561
30. Cordonnier C, Herbrecht R, Pico JL, Gardembas M et al (1997) Cefepime/amikacin versus ceftazidime/amikacin as empirical therapy for febrile episodes in neutropenic patients: a comparative study. Clin Infect Dis 24:41–51
31. Peacock JE, Herrington DA, Wade JC, Lazarus HM et al (2002) Ciprofloxacin plus piperacillin compared with tobramycin plus piperacillin as empirical therapy in febrile neutropenic patients. Ann Intern Med 137:77–86
32. Sanz MA, Lopez J, Lahuerta JJ, Rovira M et al (2002) Cefepime plus amikacin versus piperacillin-tazobactam plus amikacin for initial antibiotic therapy in haematology patients with febrile neutropenia: results of an open, randomized, multicentre trial. J Antimicrob Chemother 50:79–88
33. Pizzo PA, Hathorn JW, Hiemenz J, Browne M et al (1986) A randomized trial comparing ceftazidime alone with combination antibiotic therapy in cancer patients with fever and neutropenia. N Engl J Med 315:552–558
34. Cometta A, Zinner S, de Bock R, Calandra T et al (1995) Piperacillin-tazobactam plus amikacin versus ceftazidime plus amikacin as empiric therapy for fever in granulocytopenic patients with cancer. Antimicrob Agents Chemother 39: 445–452
35. Phillips B, Selwood K, Lane SM, Skinner R et al (2007) Variation in policies for the management of febrile neutropenia in United Kingdom Children's Cancer Study Group centres. Arch Dis Child 92:495–498
36. Haynes AB, Weiser TG, Berry WR, Lipsitz SR et al (2009) A surgical safety checklist to reduce morbidity and mortality in a global population. N Engl J Med 360:491–499
37. Provonost P, Needham D, Berenholz S, Sinopoli D et al (2006) An intervention to decrease catheter-related bloodstream infections in the ICU. New Engl J Med 355:2725–2732
38. Akova M, Paesmans M, Calandra T, Viscoli C (2005) A European Organization for Research and Treatment of Cancer-international antimicrobial therapy group study of secondary infections in febrile, neutropenic patients with cancer. Clin Infect Dis 40:239–245
39. Nucci M, Spector N, Bueno AP, Solza C et al (1997) Risk factors and attributable mortality associated with superinfection in neutropenic patients with cancer. Clin Infect Dis 24:575–579
40. Brown AE (1984) Neutropenia, fever, and infection. Am J Med 76:421–426
41. Elting LS, Rubenstein EB, Rolston KVI, Bodey GP (1997) Outcomes of bacteremia in patients with cancer and neutropenia: observations from two decades of epidemiological and clinical trials. Clin Infect Dis 25:247–259
42. Copelan E, Casper JT, Carter SL, van Burik JH et al (2007) A scheme for defining cause of death and its application in the T cell depletion trial. Biol Blood Marrow Trans 13:1469–1476
43. Bennett JE, Powers J, Walsh T, Viscoli C et al (2003) Forum report: issues in clinical trials of empirical antifungal therapy in treating febrile neutropenic patients. Clin Infect Dis 36(Suppl 3):S117–122
44. Herbrecht R, Denning DW, Patterson TF, Bennett JE et al (2002) Voriconazole versus amphotericin B for primary therapy of invasive aspergillosis. N Engl J Med 347:408–415

Pathogens

Chapter 2

Viruses

Stanley I. Martin and Jay A. Fishman

Abstract Viral infections are an important and often unrecognized component of disease in immunocompromised patients. The diagnosis and management of viral infections have expanded largely because of new quantitative molecular diagnostic assays. Well-recognized pathogens such as herpes simplex virus (HSV), cytomegalovirus (CMV), and respiratory viruses have been joined by newly recognized pathogens such as BK virus, human herpesvirus-6 (HHV-6), and human metapneumovirus in this highly susceptible patient population. The role of Epstein-Barr virus (EBV) and Human herpesvirus-8 (HHV-8) in lymphoproliferative diseases also continue to be clarified. As a result, the management of viral infections in patients with hematologic malignancies continues to be a growing challenge for the clinician.

Keywords Antivirals • Cytomegalovirus • Herpes viruses • Hematological malignancy • Respiratory viruses • Epstein-Barr virus • Polyoma virus • Adenovirus • Viral infections

1. Herpesviruses

The herpesviruses are large, enveloped double-stranded DNA viruses that produce a lifelong infection within the host. The ability to establish latency makes these viruses a common and potentially life-threatening challenge in patients with hematologic malignancies or in those who have undergone hematopoietic stem cell transplantation (HSCT). Herpesvirus infection should be considered a dynamic interaction between latent virus and the immune system of the individual patient. In the immunocompromised host, latent infection reactivates leading to invasive disease, immune-mediated complications or, Epstein-Barr virus (EBV) and human herpesvirus-8 (HHV-8), malignancy.

There are eight known human herpesviruses that are traditionally divided into three subfamilies based on genomic organization, homology, and location of latency (Table 2-1).

From: *Managing Infections in Patients With Hematological Malignancies*: Contemporary Hematology, Edited by: M. Kleinberg, DOI 10.1007/978-1-59745-415-5_2,

Table 2-1. Classification of the herpesviruses.

Virus	Subfamily	Location of latency
Herpes simplex virus, type 1	α	Dorsal root ganglia
Herpes simplex virus, type 2	α	Dorsal root ganglia
Varicella-zoster virus	α	Dorsal root ganglia
Cytomegalovirus	β	Bone marrow myeloprogenitor cells
Human herpesvirus-6	β	Bone marrow myeloprogenitor cells
Human herpesvirus-7	β	Bone marrow myeloprogenitor cells
Epstein-Barr virus	γ	B lymphocytes
Human herpesvirus-8 (Kasposi's sarcoma herpesvirus)	γ	B lymphocytes

2. Herpes Simplex Virus, Type 1 and 2

Herpes simplex viruses, type 1 and 2 (HSV-1 and HSV-2), are transmitted through intimate or mucocutaneous contact including the oral mucosa, genitalia, ocular epithelium, anal mucosa, respiratory tract, and bloodstream. HSV-1 is classically associated with herpes labialis, infection of the oral mucosa. HSV-2 is classically associated with herpes genitalis, infection of the genital tract. Both are common throughout the United States. Previous studies have suggested that as many as 62% of healthy adults have serologic evidence of previous infection with HSV-1, and 21% with HSV-2 [1]. Recent trends suggest an overall decrease in the incidence of HSV-2, though HSV-1 may be becoming a more common cause of genital herpes infection [2]. Clinically, the two viruses are indistinguishable.

2.1. Clinical Syndromes

Localized reactivation of HSV-1 or -2 can lead to cutaneous herpes lesions or keratoconjunctivitis through distribution of the involved nerve fibers from the dorsal root ganglia where the virus remains latent. With the loss of cellular immunity in the setting of hematologic malignancy, disseminated disease has been reported [3]. Diffuse cutaneous eruptions covering multiple dermatomes may occur, or may involve other organs with or without concomitant cutaneous lesions (Table 2-2).

Tonsillar abscess formation due to HSV has also been reported in a patient with a history of chronic myelogenous leukemia who underwent HSCT [9]. In patients with chronic lymphocytic leukemia, a syndrome of generalized lymphadenopathy has been attributed to HSV alone [10] and with coinfection of HSV-1, HSV-2, and EBV [11]. Localized lymphadenopathy due to HSV may be seen in individuals with oral or genital infections that may be asymptomatic in the severely compromised host. Necrotizing spinal myelopathy has been reported in a patient with T-cell leukemia, confirmed with immunohistochemical staining [12]. These presentations are uncommon.

Table 2-2. HSV-1 and HSV-2 syndromes.

Anatomic location/syndrome	Symptoms/presentation
Mucocutaneous	
Oral/peri-oral Genital Disseminated	Vesicle formation with or without ulceration in affected skin areas, usually followed by crusting of the visible lesions
Esophagitis	Odynophagia, dysphagia, retrosternal chest pain [4]
Hepatitis	Fever, abdominal pain, leucopenia, nausea/vomiting, with or without cutaneous lesions [5]
Pneumonitis	Dyspnea, cough, fever [6]
Central/Peripheral Nervous System	
Meningitis	Fever, headache, nausea/vomiting, photophobia, stiff neck
Encephalitis	Fever, headache, impaired consciousness, seizures, other focal neurologic deficits
Radiculopathy (myelitis)	Autonomic dysfunction [7], radiculopathy, possibly transverse melts [8]
Ocular	
Keratoconjunctivitis	Pain, decreased vision, characteristic dendritic corneal lesions
Chorioretinitis	Decreased vision, acute retinal necrosis with blindness
Immunologic	
Erythema multiforme	Distinctive eruption on affected skin with characteristic histology (T-cell infiltration)

HSV Herpes simplex virus

2.2. Diagnosis

The diagnosis of HSV can often be made clinically for limited oral, peri-oral, or genital infections with characteristic vesicles or ulcerations. The use of the classic Tzanck smear looking for viral cytopathic effect can be useful although the study is limited by lack of specificity and the need for expert interpretation. Molecular techniques and immunostaining provide increased speed, sensitivity, and specificity and are gaining wider use (Table 2-3).

Mucocutaneous disease is often diagnosed with fluorescent immunostaining of cell scrapings taken from the lesions. This allows testing for other herpesviruses that may cause a similar clinical picture (e.g., varicella-zoster virus), and to exclude HSV involvement in the evaluation of oral lesions that could result from other causes such as drug toxicity. Esophagitis, pneumonitis and hepatitis are also frequently best diagnosed through the use of immunohistochemical staining for HSV-specific antigens on biopsy specimens. In these settings, HSV may be a part of a dual infection (e.g., with *Candida* species, other viruses). Cultures are of little value in disease involving organs beyond the mucocutaneous barrier. Cultures from respiratory specimens, in particular, can be misleading if positive, given the frequency of asymptomatic shedding of the virus from the oropharynx in immunocompromised individuals. Disease involving the central nervous system (CNS) is frequently diagnosed by molecular amplification assays such as polymerase chain reaction (PCR)

Table 2-3. HSV-1 and -2 Diagnostics.

Diagnostic test	Description	Comments
Serology	Evaluation of the serum for presence of HSV-1 and HSV-2-specific IgG and IgM antibodies	Can be negative in acute infection or in patients with hypogammaglobulinemia; indicates only past infection
Culture	Swabs taken from the lesions or biopsies from tissue samples grow HSV in cell culture media; results in 24–48 h depending on viral titer	Dependent on proper processing of specimen (viral culture media and transport and storage at 4°C); sensitivity decreases if lesions are over 48 h old; may give false positive results from respiratory specimens
PCR	Molecular gene amplification specific for HSV; commonly used on CSF, tissue lesions or vitreous fluid	Assay not standardized, but high sensitivity and specificity
Routine pathological examination	Histopathology of biopsies with routine H&E staining or from Tzanck smears reveal giant multinucleated cells, cytopathic effect or intranuclear inclusions	Cellular changes from tissue can be seen with other herpesviruses (VZV, CMV, etc.); dependent on quality of sample and local expertise
Fluorescent or immunohistochemical staining	Slides of cells prepared from scrapings of lesions or tissue biopsies; HSV-specific monoclonal antibodies with indirect fluorescence or direct immunostaining	Proper cell handling technique required

HSV Herpes simplex virus; *PCR* Polymerase chain reaction; *CSF* Cerebrospinal fluid; *H&E* Hematoxylin and eosin; *VZV* Varicella-zoster virus; *CMV* Cytomegalovirus

of cerebrospinal fluid (CSF) samples. The sensitivity and specificity of HSV PCR from CSF is thought to be close to 95% [13], though specimens taken early or late in the clinical course may be more likely to be falsely negative [14]. Brain biopsy with immunohistochemical staining remains definitive for HSV encephalitis if PCR is unrevealing and diagnosis is essential. Ocular disease is often made on clinical examination, though PCR of cell scrapings in keratoconjunctivitis or vitreous fluid in the case of retinal disease may also play a role [15].

2.3. Therapy

Treatment should be considered in all patients with active HSV infection and underlying hematologic malignancy or HSCT. Immunocompromised hosts are at a greater risk for severe disease and dissemination. Minor herpes labialis infections can spread rapidly to the pharynx, the esophagus, and via the bloodstream to multiple organs and cutaneous dermatomes. The most widely available agents for treatment of HSV infections are nucleoside analogues that inhibit the synthesis of HSV viral DNA. The most frequently used agent by far is acyclovir, though valacyclovir, famciclovir, vidarabine, and foscarnet can be used depending on the clinical scenario (Table 2-4). Intravenous therapy should be considered as initial therapy for progressive or disseminated infection in immunocompromised hosts.

Valacyclovir is an L-valine ester prodrug of acyclovir. After absorption, it is metabolized into acyclovir by the liver. This prodrug form of acyclovir can achieve higher plasma levels than equivalent doses of oral acyclovir, and thus less frequent dosing can be used for similar therapeutic levels of drug (bid vs. 5/day).

Table 2-4. HSV therapeutics.

Syndrome	Therapeutic options
Mucocutaneous HSV	Acyclovir 400 mg po 5x/day Acyclovir 5 mg/kg IV q 8 h Valacyclovir 500 mg to 1 g po bid Famciclovir 500 mg po bid
Disseminated HSV	Acyclovir 10 mg/kg IV q 8 h
Esophagitis	Acyclovir 5 mg/kg IV q 8 h
Hepatitis	Acyclovir 5–10 mg/kg IV q 8 h
Pneumonitis	Acyclovir 5–10 mg/kg IV q 8 h
Encephalitis/meningitis	Acyclovir 10 mg/kg IV q 8 h
Keratoconjunctivitis	Topical therapy with either: 3% acyclovir gel 3% vidarabine ointment 1% trifluorothymidine drops
Chorioretinitis or acute retinal necrosis	Acyclovir 10 mg/kg IV q 8 h
Erythema multiforme	Treat as localized mucocutaneous disease

HSV Herpes simplex virus

Famciclovir is the diacetyl ester prodrug of penciclovir and is rapidly converted by the body. Vidarabine was the first antiherpesvirus drug to be of proven value, but is rarely used in clinical practice due to inferiority in clinical trials to acyclovir and significant toxicities, including neurotoxicity with parasthesias, ataxia, seizures, and rarely coma [16, 17]. Foscarnet is a direct noncompetitive inhibitor of herpesvirus DNA polymerase and has in vitro activity against all herpesviruses. Foscarnet undergoes little intracellular metabolism, and is not dependent on the herpetic thymidine kinase (required to phosphorylate acyclovir to the active state) and therefore may be used in the treatment of acyclovir-resistant strains of HSV that arise due to mutations in the viral thymidine kinase. The utility of foscarnet is limited by nephrotoxicity, symptomatic hypocalcemia, and other electrolyte (magnesium, potassium) losses that require co-infusion with a large amount of fluid.

With the exception of the topical ocular antiviral agents, dosages of all agents listed in Table 2-4 are modified in the setting of renal insufficiency. Length of therapy is usually for 7–14 days, with the exception of disease involving the CNS, wherein therapy is often extended to a total of 14–21 days because of risk for recurrence [18, 19]. For acyclovir resistance, foscarnet is generally used at doses of 40 mg/kg IV every 8 h for 14–21 days, depending on clinical response [20].

Patients with hematologic malignancies have a higher incidence of HSV shedding in their saliva, are at increased risk for reactivation of HSV with intensified immunosuppression, and are at increased risk of atypical manifestations and dissemination of disease. In the setting of HSCT, HSV-seropositive individuals may have a reactivation rate of 65–90% [21]. Thus, the routine implementation of prophylaxis has been advocated in any patient who has evidence of prior infection with HSV (HSV-1 or -2 seropositive) with hematologic malignancy undergoing chemotherapy or HSCT. Suppression can be in the form of acyclovir 400 mg po bid or higher, valacyclovir 500 mg po qd or bid, or famciclovir 250 mg po bid beginning on the day of conditioning or induction and continuing until resolution of neutropenia or 6 weeks, whichever is longer. If patients cannot tolerate oral therapy, then IV acyclovir 250 mg/m^2 IV every 12 h is also effective [22].

3. Varicella-Zoster Virus

Varicella-zoster virus (VZV) is the third member of the α-subfamily of human herpesviruses. Classically, VZV is associated with two clinical syndromes: varicella, known as chickenpox, and herpes zoster, known as shingles. As with HSV, the patient with an underlying lymphoproliferative disorder or HSCT is at higher risk for dissemination of disease and systemic involvement, blurring the clinical entities. Although frequently considered a benign childhood illness in the immunocompetent population, VZV carries an overall case fatality rate of 2–4 deaths per 100,000, with greatest risk among older adults and infants [23]. Older estimates before the era of effective antiviral therapy and zoster immunoglobulin put the mortality in those children with acute lymphocytic leukemia who developed primary VZV at 7% [24]. Compared to HSV, however, infection is even more ubiquitous, with over 90% of people in temperate climates infected before adolescence [25]. Infection is typically spread via the respiratory tract during acquisition of primary infection, or by physical contact with mucocutaneous lesions. Due to the great infectivity of VZV, attack rates can be as high as 100% in the susceptible host [26].

3.1. Clinical Syndromes

Primary infection, or varicella, presents with fever and often the simultaneous development of a characteristic cutaneous vesicular rash that can involve mucosal surfaces (oropharynx, conjunctiva, genitourinary tract, etc.). It begins with small macular erythematous lesions that progress to a vesicular stage before crusting-over during a 1-2 day period. The lesions evolve at different times so that some lesions may be healing while fresh lesions emerge.

Primary infection in patients with leukemia or in patients who have undergone HSCT occurs most often in children and can lead to dissemination with involvement of multiple organs, including the CNS as meningitis, encephalitis, or vasculitis of the intracranial vessels. In the immunocompromised or immunologically naïve host, infection produces skin lesions that persist for longer periods, and may be associated with hepatitis, cholangitis, pneumonitis, uveitis, or cause a sepsis-like syndrome with disseminated intravascular coagulation [24]. Bacterial superinfection of skin lesions can occur with organisms including *Staphylococcus aureus*, leading to cellulitis, deeper soft-tissue involvement, and sepsis [27].

3.2. Diagnosis

Often, the diagnosis of routine varicella or zoster can be made based on physical examination when a characteristic rash and distribution is observed or when exposure in the case of primary infection is present. The differential includes other viral infections such as HSV or enteroviruses, both of which can have atypical presentations in the immunocompromised host. Again, as with HSV, the Tzanck smear of cell scrapings from a cutaneous lesion may be useful, but lacks sensitivity and specificity. Use of specific molecular techniques is common for diagnosis of VZV (Table 2-5).

There is some serological cross-reactivity between VZV and HSV-1 due to similarities in the viral glycoprotein B [28]. Multiple methods exist to measure antibodies to VZV, including fluorescent antibody to membrane antigen (FAMA) methods, enzyme-linked immunosorbent assays (EIA), latex agglutination methods, complement fixation assays, and other immunofluorescent assays. Individual laboratories may vary in their approach. Overall, serologic tests are not as clinically useful in rapidly diagnosing VZV as PCR and antigen detection. Most cases of VZV in the immunocompromised occur as a result of viral reactivation; serologic testing to determine those at risk for primary infection is not 100% reliable in these hosts [29]. Though the exact sensitivity and specificity of PCR from CSF for VZV is unclear, PCR is becoming relied upon by more and more physicians for diagnosing CNS infections due to herpesviruses in general. The VZV PCR assay is likely most useful earlier in the patient's clinical course, particularly if primary infection is suspected and seroconversion may be delayed [30, 31]. PCR can also be used to distinguish infection between wild-type VZV and that of the vaccine strain [32].

Table 2-5. VZV diagnostics.

Diagnostic test	Description	Comments
Serology	Evaluation of the serum for presence of VZV-specific IgG and IgM antibodies	Can be negative in acute infection or in patients with hypogammaglobulinemia; indicates past infection
Culture	Swabs from mucocutaneous lesions or biopsies can grow VZV in cell cultures in 3–5 days	Dependent on proper processing of specimen (requires transport and storage at 4°C); difficult to isolate from nasopharynx
PCR	Molecular gene amplification specific for VZV; used on CSF, tissues or skin lesions	Sensitive and specific, but not universally available
Routine pathological examination	Pathological examination from biopsies with routine H&E staining or from Tzanck smears can reveal giant multinucleated cells, cytopathic effect or intranuclear inclusions	Most cellular changes also seen with other herpesviruses (HSV, CMV, etc.); dependent on quality of sample, local expertise
Fluorescent or immunohistochemical staining	Slides of cells from scrapings of lesions or biopsies; VZV-specific monoclonal antibodies for indirect fluorescence or immunostaining	Proper cell handling technique required

VZV Varicella-zoster virus; *PCR* Polymerase chain reaction; *CSF* Cerebrospinal fluid; *H&E* Hematoxylin and eosin; *HSV* Herpes simplex virus; *CMV* Cytomegalovirus

3.3. Therapy

In the non-immunocompromised population, primary infection with VZV is self-limited and usually treated with symptomatic intervention only. Antiviral therapy is indicated for reactivation disease such as shingles, or for diffuse disease in immunocompromised individuals. Intravenous acyclovir (10 mg/kg every 8 h) is considered first-line therapy for any patient with a hematologic malignancy or HSCT who develops primary infection or reactivation of VZV. Patients improving on this regimen may be converted to oral therapy with either acyclovir at 800 mg po 5x/day or valacyclovir 1 g po tid to complete the course. Famciclovir at a dose of 500 mg po tid may also be of value in this setting. The latter agents (famciclovir and valacyclovir) have better oral bioavailability than acyclovir. Most experts recommend extending therapy for at least 2 days beyond crusting of all lesions. Resistance is rare, reported most often in patients with underlying HIV infection [26]. Foscarnet may be an alternative agent when resistance develops. All of these medications require dose reduction with renal insufficiency.

Patients with hematologic malignancies or HSCT, regardless of serostatus, should avoid exposure to persons with active VZV infections [29]. Use of VZV immunoglobulin (VZIG) should be considered in the prevention of infection in seronegative patients and as a means to possibly reduce the risk for severe disease in patients with hematologic malignancies exposed to VZV. Vaccination with the live VZV vaccine should be considered in advance of immune suppression but cannot be used in immunocompromised hosts. In VZV-seronegative patients, administration of VZIG as soon as possible within 96 h after exposure is indicated [33]. Some experts also report using those VZIG in HSCT patients with a significant exposure who are already known to be seropositive, but are often hypogammaglobulinemic. Significant exposures include contacts with individuals with chicken pox or who received the live VZV vaccine and subsequently developed a varicella-like rash with the risk of transmitting the vaccine-related strain of VZV [33]. Dosing of VZIG is 125 international units per 10 kg of body weight with a maximum dose of 625 units and a minimum dose of 125 units given intramuscularly. Administration after 96 h from the exposure is of unclear value.

In order to prevent the spread of VZV infection to other immunocompromised individuals or VZV-seronegative individuals in the hospital setting, patients with VZV disease should be placed under airborne and contact precautions [34]. Although intravenous acyclovir over several months and oral acyclovir dosed at 800 mg po bid for up to 1 year have been shown to prevent VZV in patients undergoing HSCT [35], long-term acyclovir prophylaxis to prevent VZV is not routinely recommended [33]. Prevention in most immunocompetent individuals is now through the use of the live, attenuated VZV vaccine. Though different formulations exist, all vaccines use the Oka strain of VZV isolated from a healthy child with varicella and then attenuated through sequential passage in cell culture [26]. Currently, live vaccine is contraindicated for use among HSCT recipients and other immunocompromised individuals. Further research is needed to determine the efficacy and safety of the VZV vaccine in this population. Ideally, however, all healthcare workers, family members of patients, or other household contacts who are VZV-seronegative should be immunized as soon as the decision is made to perform HSCT.

Completion of the vaccine should be done 4 or more weeks before the conditioning regimen begins [33]. An inactivated vaccine is under development.

4. Cytomegalovirus

Cytomegalovirus (CMV) is a member of the β-subfamily of herpesviruses. Infection in the United States population is common, with an age-adjusted estimate of 58.9% [36]. Risk increases steadily throughout an individual's lifetime, and lower socioeconomic status as well as ethnic background may play a role in the risk of infection. Spread of the virus is usually through mucocutaneous or intimate contact, as well as through congenital acquisition or transplantation of organs and transfusion of blood products. In the immunocompromised patient population, coinfection with multiple strains have been reported [37]. CMV is one of the most important viruses in immunocompromised patients. Primary infection acquired through HSCT or blood products, or reactivation of latent virus can lead to significant morbidity.

4.1. Clinical Syndromes

Primary infection of CMV is classically associated with a mononucleosis-like syndrome that results in fever, lymphadenopathy, and leucopenia, often with a relative lymphocytosis similar to primary infection with EBV. In the case of CMV, the frequently used heterophile agglutinin test in EBV will be negative, however. In the immunocompromised patient, or in the patient with underlying inflammatory disorder, CMV viral replication can lead to invasive tissue or end-organ disease (Table 2-6).

Virtually, all organ systems can be affected by invasive CMV infection. Aside from the syndromes listed in Table 2-6, CMV has also been blamed for causing a hemorrhagic cystitis in patients after HSCT [42, 43]. T-cell function is the primary determinant for control of CMV infection. Aggressive chemotherapy and use of T-cell depleting agents such as alemtuzumab increase the risk for CMV disease in patients with hematologic malignancy. Alemtuzumab in particular has been associated with rates of CMV viremia in patients with lymphoproliferative disorders of 15–44% [44–46].

4.2. Diagnosis

The development of sensitive molecular techniques to diagnose active CMV infection has revolutionized the approach to CMV management in the immunosuppressed population. Identifying patients at risk who will require preemptive or prophylactic therapy is becoming a more prominent approach to HSCT care in particular. Quantitative assays to measure the viral load in the blood have impacted management of infection (Table 2-7).

Serologics are most useful in determining past exposure and in identifying patients at risk for reactive disease when immunosuppressed. If negative, the patient may be at high risk for acquiring CMV infection if transplanted from a CMV seropositive donor. Cell culture techniques using human fibroblast cell lines are time-consuming, with results in 10 days to as long as 4–6 weeks in order to detect the cytopathic changes indicative of a positive assay. Shell vial cultures allow detection of CMV antigens prior to the development of

Table 2-6. CMV syndromesa.

Anatomic location/syndrome	Symptoms/presentation
Mononucleosis	Fever, lymphadenopathy, leucopenia with relative lymphocytosis
Pneumonitis	Most severe complication of CMV infection with cough, dyspnea, interstitial infiltrates on chest radiography superinfection [38]
Gastrointestinal	
Esophagitis/gastritis	Odynophagia, dysphagia, retrosternal chest pain, anorexia, nausea, vomiting
Enteritis/colitis	Fever, watery diarrhea (occasionally bloody), plaque-like pseudomembranes, erosive or ulcerative disease
Hepatitis/cholangitis	Fever, abdominal pain, leucopenia, nausea/vomiting, elevated transaminases (bacterial co-infection)
Pancreatitis	Fever, abdominal pain, and peritonitis, infection of the biliary tract [39]
Myocarditis	Congestive heart failure
Central/Peripheral Nervous System	
Meningoencephalitis	Vasculitis with fever, headache, nausea/vomiting, photophobia, impaired consciousness, seizures, focal neurologic deficits
Polyradiculopathy	Hyporeflexia, limb weakness, parasthesias and possibly sensory loss, myelitis [40]
Guillain–Barré syndrome	Progressive ascending paresis [41]
Ocular	
Retinitis	Decreased vision, acute retinal necrosis with blindness
Hematologic	
Disseminated intravascular coagulation	Consumptive coagulopathy with thrombocytopenia and hemolytic anemia usually in the setting of fever and sepsis-like syndrome

CMV Cytomegalovirus
[a]Non-exclusive syndromes

cytopathic changes. The overall sensitivity and specificity are limited by the frequency of asymptomatic shedding in immunocompromised hosts in respiratory, urinary, and gastrointestinal sites [47]. Molecular-based techniques such as antigenemia assays, nucleic acid amplification, and hybrid capture assays are commonly used in the diagnosis of active CMV disease. The antigenemia assay is limited in the setting of profound neutropenia because of the lack of circulating granulocytes. Though exact predictive values of these tests may vary depending on what study is referenced, all appear to have a high sensitivity and specificity in immunocompromised patients [48–50] and in patients who have undergone allogeneic HSCT [51]. PCR from whole blood tends to be a more sensitive assay than the others, but less specific than plasma when used for molecular amplification. The pp65 antigenemia assay, when not limited by neutropenia, may be the most specific in terms of predicting active disease [51]. PCR, the hybrid capture assay, and the antigenemia assay are all likely useful in monitoring a patient's response to therapy. Viral loads may take several weeks to become undetectable on therapy, however [52, 53], and retesting a patient less than 1 week after initiation of treatment is generally not advised.

Table 2-7. CMV diagnostics.

Diagnostic test	Description	Comments
Serology	Evaluation of the serum for presence of CMV-specific IgG and IgM antibodies	Determines risk for latent CMV reactivation, past infection; may be negative in acute infection and with hypogammaglobulinemia or immunosuppression
Culture	Shell vial culture of CMV with human fibroblasts for detection of immediate early antigens	Shell vial technique can be positive in 2–3 days; lacks specificity for detecting active CMV disease
Antigenemia assay	Rapid detection of CMV-specific proteins (pp65) in peripheral blood leukocytes, correlates with total viremia	Semi-quantitative; requires circulating peripheral blood polymorphonuclear cells
Hybrid capture assay	Signal amplification with RNA probe for CMV DNA; detection with antibodies specific for RNA:DNA hybrids	Semi-quantitative; range of ~1,400–600,000 copies of CMV/mL
Nucleic acid amplification	PCR of DNA with gene amplification specific for CMV; nucleic acid sequence-based amplification (NASBA) for immediate-early and late gene expression	Few data on immunocompetent hosts; various assays are not comparable; highly sensitive with detection level ~500 copies/mL or less
Pathologic inspection with or without immunohistochemical staining	H&E stain can reveal "owl's eye" intranuclear inclusions; sensitivity can be increased with staining for CMV-specific proteins	Proper cell handling technique required

CMV Cytomegalovirus; *PCR* Polymerase chain reaction; *H&E* Hematoxylin and eosin

4.3. Therapy

Although the nucleoside analogue acyclovir has some activity against CMV in vitro, the related purine analogue ganciclovir has become the gold standard for management of CMV disease. Acyclovir has been used in prophylaxis, but lacks the potency required for treatment of established CMV disease [54]. Other antivirals that have clinical utility for the treatment of CMV include valganciclovir, which is the prodrug of ganciclovir, foscarnet, and cidofovir. The latter two are generally reserved for infections caused by ganciclovir-resistant strains of CMV because they can cause significant nephrotoxicity and other side effects. Other agents are less well-studied; use of ancillary agents may have benefit in certain clinical scenarios (Table 2-8).

Both valganciclovir and ganciclovir are capable of inducing hematologic abnormalities including neutropenia, anemia, and thrombocytopenia. Valganciclovir is the L-valyl ester prodrug of ganciclovir, and as such has a 1.7-fold greater bioavailability than oral ganciclovir. A 900 mg dose of valganciclovir is able to achieve a systemic exposure of IV ganciclovir dosed at 5 mg/kg [57], and has now replaced oral ganciclovir in clinical practice [54]. Ganciclovir resistance among CMV isolates is frequently due to a mutation of the phosphatase UL 97 gene, or less commonly the DNA polymerase UL 54 gene [58]. New resistance mutations are under study. In cases of resistance, either documented or presumed due to no decrease in viral load after up to 3 weeks of therapy,

Table 2-8. CMV therapeutics.

Agent	Dose	Comments
Ganciclovir	5 mg/kg IV every 12 h for 7–14 days, followed by 5 mg/kg IV once daily	Induction therapy used initially followed by maintenance; length of therapy varies (treat to negative assay)
	1–1.5 g po tid	Oral formulation generally avoided as initial therapy for active CMV disease due to poor bioavailability
Valganciclovir	900 mg po bid for initial therapy, followed by 900 mg po qd or 450 mg po bid	Data are limited on use as initial therapy for active CMV disease; some failures in GI disease
Foscarnet	40–60 mg/kg IV every 8–12 h, or 90 mg/kg IV every 12 h	Dosing and duration of therapy less well-studied; given with saline hydration and electrolyte (Mg, K) replacement (renal toxicity)
Cidofovir	5 mg/kg IV once weekly	Given with saline hydration and probenecid (renal toxicity)
Other agents		
CMV immune globulin	150 mg/kg IV	Clinical utility likely limited to HSCT patients with CMV pneumonitis [55] or hypogammaglobulinemia
Fomivirsen	330 μg intravitreally	Used for the treatment of CMV retinitis only
Maribavir	Under study (orphan drug)	Novel anti-CMV agent currently undergoing active investigation
Leflunomide	100–200 mg po qd for up to 7 days, followed by 20–60 mg po qd (not approved for this indication); ideal dosing parameters unclear [56]	Immunosuppressive agent; induction therapy followed by maintenance; monitor serum levels (goal 60–80 mcg/mL) to avoid toxicity (liver); experimental use with failure of other antiviral agents; clinical benefit for active CMV disease unclear

CMV Cytomegalovirus; *IVIG* Intravenous immunoglobulin; *HSCT* Hematopoietic stem cell transplant

foscarnet or cidofovir or combination therapy is recommended. All of these antiviral agents require dose reduction in the setting of renal insufficiency. Foscarnet and cidofovir may provoke significant renal toxicity.

Although the use of CMV-negative and leukocyte-depleted blood products can help prevent CMV infection in seronegative patients, the risk is never reduced to zero. Prophylaxis and preemptive treatment have reduced the significant morbidity and mortality associated with CMV disease in this population. Late CMV disease post-HSCT remains a significant risk for mortality and likely reflects ongoing immune dysfunction and ineffective T-cell control of viral replication [59]. Risk factors include ongoing pharmacological immunosuppression such as high-dose corticosteroids, graft versus host disease (GVHD), need for donor lymphocyte infusions, and previous CMV disease. Prophylaxis with IV ganciclovir for up to 100 days post-transplant has been effective in preventing reactive CMV infection in seropositive HSCT recipients [60], as has use of oral acyclovir and valacyclovir [61, 62]. Many centers, however, advocate the preemptive approach in order to avoid unnecessary toxicity from prolonged antiviral drug use. Testing the blood of at-risk patients on a regular basis using molecular amplification or antigen detection techniques can often uncover low-level asymptomatic viremia that may be amenable to antiviral therapy before symptomatic CMV disease can evolve. IV ganciclovir and valganciclovir have been used, though there are no large randomized, comparative studies completed in the HSCT population regarding valganciclovir for this purpose [63].

5. Human Herpesvirus-6 and -7

The role of the β-herpesviruses, human herpesvirus-6 (HHV-6) and human herpesvirus-7 (HHV-7), in causing disease among immunosuppressed patients remains unclear; prospective studies are needed to define the effects of reactive infections in patients with hematologic malignancies. Both viruses infect most individuals at a young age, occasionally causing a self-limited childhood febrile illness with or without skin rash. Primary infection in adults is rare, though a mononucleosis-like syndrome caused by HHV-6 has been described in a few case reports [64, 65]. Among HSCT recipients, HHV-6 has also been associated with a syndrome of pneumonitis, hepatitis, encephalitis, bone marrow suppression, as well as asymptomatic viremia of unclear significance [66–73]. HHV-7 has been associated with meningitis and encephalitis and other neurologic dysfunction [74–76] with a possible role in bone marrow suppression uncertain [77].

Diagnostic assays for HHV-6 and -7 are evolving. All, unfortunately, still have limitations in differentiating active disease from latent virus (Table 2-9).

Serology can be performed using a variety of assays such as EIA, radioimmunoassays, or indirect fluorescence assays. Because most adults are seropositive, only paired sera showing a ≥ 4-fold rise in titers can be considered diagnostic. IgM antibodies in HHV-6 may be limited by the presence of false positives in the general population [78]. Older HHV-7 serology assays are also limited by cross-reactivity with HHV-6 [79]. These tests are not widely available and have little clinical utility. PCR assays have been performed on serum, plasma, whole blood, CSF, and tissue. Cell-free samples such as serum,

Table 2-9. HHV-6 and HHV-7 diagnostics.

Diagnostic test	Description	Comments
Serology	HHV-6 or HHV-7-specific IgG and IgM antibodies	Indicates presence of past infection; may be negative in acute infection or with hypogammaglobulinemia; paired samples for diagnosis
PCR	Quantitative amplification of HHV-6 or HHV-7-specific DNA from tissue or body fluid	PCR may not distinguish latent virus from active infection
Immunohistochemical antigen staining	Staining of tissues with monoclonal antibodies to HHV-6 or HHV-7 antigens	Proper cell handling technique required

HHV-6 Human herpesvirus-6; *HHV-7* Human herpesvirus-7; *PCR* Polymerase chain reaction plasma, or CSF may be better at differentiating active infection from the presence of latent virus [80]. Immunohistochemical staining of tissue samples for HHV-6 or HHV-7 can also be limited, and does not necessarily separate active from latent virus. PCR and antigen staining assays for HHV-7 have not been found to have much clinical utility to date and are frequently unavailable for routine testing outside of the research setting.

The need for, and the activity of, antiviral therapy in HHV-6 and, in particular HHV-7, remain unclear. Both ganciclovir and foscarnet have been used in the treatment of presumed HHV-6 infections [69, 70]. In vitro reports of resistance to ganciclovir among HHV-6 isolates have been reported [81]. There are no prospective studies to guide management with these agents. As of yet, there are no convincing clinical scenarios in which therapy of HHV-7 infection is warranted [82]. In vitro, both foscarnet and ganciclovir inhibit HHV-7 replication [83].

6. Epstein-Barr Virus

Epstein, Achong, and Barr first described the infectious agent isolated from the cells of Burkitt's lymphoma in 1964 [84]. The relationship between EBV and heterophile-positive infectious mononucleosis is well-established. The relationship between EBV and malignancies such as Burkitt's lymphoma, nasopharyngeal carcinoma, post-transplant lymphoproliferative disorder (PTLD), Hodgkin's disease, and others is an area of active investigation. Seroprevalence studies indicate EBV infection to be present in greater than 90% of adults in most populations.

6.1. Clinical Syndromes

Primary infection with EBV in childhood is often asymptomatic. In adolescence or adulthood, it can frequently result in infectious mononucleosis, causing fever, lymphadenopathy, and pharyngitis. Virtually, every organ system may be affected by active EBV infection. The role of EBV in the pathogenesis of malignancies and lymphoproliferative disorders is particularly challenging in patients with hematological disorders (Table 2-10).

In the setting of infectious mononucleosis, diverse complications have been reported, including the classic association of splenic rupture and hematologic dysfunction. Hemolytic anemia, thrombocytopenia, and disseminated intravascular coagulation have all been reported. Oral hairy leukoplakia is an uncommon benign lesion most frequently associated with human immunodeficiency virus (HIV) infection. Although reported in the setting of HSCT, it is exceptionally rare [90]. The development of post-transplant lymphoproliferative disorder (PTLD) is the most often encountered and most feared complication of EBV infection after HSCT. Risk is greatest among those who are EBV-seronegative prior to transplant.

6.2. Diagnosis

Infectious mononucleosis can be a clinical diagnosis in an immunocompetent patient in the right clinical setting. Supportive evidence in the form of atypical lymphocytes seen on peripheral blood smear and the presence of heterophile antibodies are sometimes employed. In the immunocompromised individual, serology may not be detectable, particularly in acute infection.

Table 2-10. EBV clinical syndromes.

Anatomic location/syndrome	Symptoms/presentation
Infectious mononucleosis	Fever, lymphadenopathy, pharyngitis, splenomegaly
Neurologic syndromes	
Meningitis/encephalitis	Fever, confusion, headache, and cerebral edema [85]
Transverse myelitis	Back pain, sensory loss, areflexia, ataxia, and difficulty with bowel and bladder function [86]
Optic neuritis	Visual loss, possibly in combination with other neurologic deficits [87]
Pneumonitis	Lymphocytic interstitial pneumonitis commonly with pediatric HIV/AIDS [88]
Myocarditis	Congestive heart failure [89]
Nephritis	Reports of tubulointerstitial nephritis, membranous nephropathy, and glomerulonephritis
Rash	Diffuse morbilliform rash associated with administration of penicillins in the setting of primary infection
Oral hairy leukoplakia	White linear plaques usually on lateral surface of the tongue
Lymphoproliferative disorders	
Hemophagocytic lymphohistiocytosis	Unusual syndrome of fever, lymphadenopathy, hepatosplenomegaly, hepatitis, pancytopenia, coagulopathy and T-cell, and histiocyte proliferation with hemophagocytosis in bone marrow, spleen and lymph nodes
X-linked lymphoproliferative disorder	An inherited mutation of the X chromosome that leads to fulminant infectious mononucleosis after EBV infection with high mortality
Post-transplant lymphoproliferative disorder	Largely B-cell proliferation after solid organ or HSCT with extranodal presentations and risk for malignant B-cell lymphomas; T-, NK-, and null cell tumors – role of EBV variable
Malignancies	
Burkitt's lymphoma	Lymphoma typically arising in the jaw; most frequently in Africa; both malaria and EBV may be cofactors
Nasopharyngeal carcinoma	Tumor strongly associated with EBV, most frequently in southern China
Hodgkin's disease	EBV gene expression has been consistently detected in Reed-Sternberg cells associated with Hodgkin's disease; exact rates/role of EBV varies by region
Non-Hodgkin's lymphoma	EBV may be related to non-Hodgkin's lymphomas of HIV-infected population, as well as the post-transplant patient
Leiomyomas/sarcomas	EBV associated with smooth muscle tumors in patients with HIV, children

HIV Human immunodeficiency virus; *AIDS* Acquired immunodeficiency syndrome; *EBV* Epstein-Barr virus; *HSCT* Hematopoietic stem cell transplant

The myriad complications of EBV infection in this patient population and their atypical presentations have made use of molecular diagnostics essential for the diagnosis and management of active EBV infections (Table 2-11).

Serologic assays for heterophile antibodies, anti-viral capsid antigen IgM, IgG, early antigen IgG, and nuclear antigen IgG can be performed independently through indirect immunofluorescence, EIA, or in combination simultaneously with a multiplexed bead assay [92]. Serologic assays are of

Table 2-11. EBV diagnostics.

Diagnostic test	Description	Comments
Serology		
Heterophile antibody	Serologic test for antibodies to antigens on erythrocytes of other animal species; rapid Monospot assay uses latex agglutination	Frequently negative in leukemia or HSCT; monospot assay has a sensitivity of 85% in immunocompetent individuals [91]
Viral capsid antigen antibody	Serum assay for IgM or IgG antibodies specific to the EBV viral capsid antigen	IgM levels typically become undetectable after 3 months; may not develop with primary infection in immunocompromised host; IgG levels indicate past infection
Early antigen antibody	Testing of serum IgG for two subsets of early antigens: anti-D and anti-R	Often present in acute infection, but may not develop in immunosuppressed patients
Nuclear antigen antibody	Testing of the serum for IgG toward EBV nuclear antigen	Usually not present during acute infection, but develop after 1–2 months, and may persist throughout life
Culture	Culture of EBV from oropharyngeal washings or blood	Not routinely available; asymptomatic shedding prevents separation of active versus latent infection
PCR	Quantitative amplification of EBV-specific DNA from tissue or body fluid	Does not distinguish latent EBV infection from active invasive disease; PCR of blood can detect active viral replication; optimal cut-off values for each assay unclear
Immunohistochemical staining	In-situ hybridization of tissue samples for EBV-encoded small ribonucleic acid (EBER) using oligonucleotide probes	Highly sensitive and specific for EBV gene expression from tissue samples

HSCT Hematopoietic stem cell transplant; *EBV* Epstein-Barr virus; *PCR* Polymerase chain reaction

little value in diagnosing acute infection in the immunocompromised host as humoral responses may be delayed or absent. There is often a lag in the development of anti-viral capsid and anti-nuclear antigen IgG. Anti-viral capsid antigen IgM and anti-early antigen IgG may fail to appear altogether [93]. Quantitative PCR assays differ between laboratories, but a single assay in an individual should be used for patient management. There is no agreement as to the significance of quantitative values other than within an individual. In studies of HSCT recipients, 1,000 copies/mL has been used to assess risk for the development of PTLD [94]. In situ hybridization of biopsy samples using abundant, small EBV-encoded RNA (EBER) oligonucleotides has become the standard for detecting EBV in lymphoproliferative disorders and malignancies [95].

6.3. Therapy

In the absence of severe complications, there is usually no indication for therapy other than supportive care in primary infection with EBV in the immunocompetent individual. The use of corticosteroids to reduce tonsillar swelling and airway compromise is sometimes necessary [96]. Steroids and antiviral therapy may be employed with other life-threatening complications such as hepatitis and possible liver failure, hematologic crises including aplastic anemia or hemolysis, though there are no prospective studies to support their use. In the immunocompromised individual, therapeutic modalities are diverse and are frequently indicated to either prevent or treat the lymphoproliferative complications and risk for malignancy from EBV. Both acyclovir and ganciclovir have in vitro activity against lytic replication of EBV, with ganciclovir having slightly greater efficacy [97]. However, there are few data to suggest that antivirals have a significant effect on the outcome of infection. EBV-related lymphoproliferative disorders and malignancies in immunocompromised hosts are thought to be dependent on latent infection that relies on cellular enzymes for EBV episomal DNA synthesis, and thus are not inhibited by the routine anti-herpesvirus nucleoside analogues [96]. Both acyclovir and ganciclovir have been used for prophylaxis in patients after solid organ transplantation, with meta-analyses suggesting a benefit to universal prophylaxis against CMV in preventing PTLD [98]. However, no firm conclusions can be drawn because of the small size and heterogeneity of the patient populations and non-randomized nature of these studies. Induction of the EBV thymidine kinase gene through the use of compounds such as arginine butyrate has been attempted in order to induce susceptibility to antiviral therapy with a mixed degree of success [99, 100]. Another antiviral that has been investigated in in vitro assays and in case reports is high-dose zidovudine (AZT) [101]. Maribavir, a newer compound being investigated for the use of treating CMV, also has in vitro activity against EBV through a different mechanism of action than the nucleoside analogues [102]. Yet, there are no trials investigating its use in EBV infection.

Once PTLD is established, therapeutic approaches include reduction of immunosuppression to the degree possible, surgery for isolated lesions, traditional chemotherapy, radiation (especially for CNS lesions), and the use of rituximab, a monoclonal antibody directed toward the CD20 antigen frequently found on B cells, the main site of EBV infection and latency [103]. The use of antiviral therapy in established disease may be used to reduce active viral replication and resultant immunosuppression but does not appear to directly impact tumor progression. In solid organ transplant recipients, CMV is a co-factor for PTLD, and prevention or treatment of CMV may be of benefit. The use of rituximab as a preemptive approach in HSCT to prevent PTLD in patients with otherwise asymptomatic but persistent EBV viremia has not always yielded persistent control in many patients [104]. Investigative approaches include infusion of EBV-primed autologous or allogeneic cytotoxic T-cells and anti-cytokine therapies [103].

7. Human Herpesvirus-8 (Kaposi's Sarcoma Herpesvirus)

HHV-8 is the most recently discovered member of the herpesvirus family, having been isolated in 1994 from a patient with Kaposi's sarcoma and co-infection due to HIV [105]. HHV-8 is a recognized cofactor in Kaposi's sarcoma and in the development of a variety of lymphoproliferative and malignant disorders. The virus is endemic in the Mediterranean region, in central and southern Africa, and much of South America although the route of transmission remains unclear and may vary depending on the population being analyzed [106]. In endemic areas, prevalence increases after 2 years of age, consistent with transmission from family members or close contacts. In low-seroprevalence areas such as the United States, infection is highest among men who have sex with men, suggesting possible sexual transmission [107, 108]. Increased numbers of sexual partners and HIV coinfection also increase risk, though heterosexual transmission and the risk in other HIV-risk groups such as injection drug users appear to be much lower [106]. Among patients with underlying hematologic disorders, there is a suggestion that infection may be higher compared to the general population [109].

7.1. Clinical Syndromes

Primary infection with HHV-8 among immunocompetent children has been associated with a mononucleosis-like syndrome, while in adults, it is a milder illness and frequently asymptomatic. In immunocompromised patients, primary infection has been associated with a wide array of clinical presentations, including mononucleosis in patients with non-Hodgkin's lymphoma after autologous HSCT [110], bone marrow suppression after renal transplantation or autologous HSCT [111], hemophagocytic syndrome in a patient after renal transplantation and others with HIV infection [112, 113], and in one report of an infant with DiGeorge syndrome, disseminated disease with hepatitis, enterocolitis, and pneumonitis [114].

Disease associated with latent or reactivated infection from HHV-8 includes Kaposi's sarcoma, and also primary effusion lymphoma and multi-centric Castleman disease. Kaposi's sarcoma is a mesenchymal neoplasia of the blood and lymphatic vessels with varying presentations and outcomes in different patient populations. Castleman disease, a lymphoproliferative disorder, can lead to HHV-8-positive plasmablastic lymphoma. Other possible associations with HHV-8 that have not been well validated include multiple myeloma and germinotropic lymphoproliferative disorders, as well as non-lymphoid malignancies such as cardiovascular disease, pemphigus vulgaris, and the autoimmune disorder sarcoidosis [115].

7.2. Diagnosis

Current HHV-8 diagnostics may not be available in many clinical centers, and the optimal use of such assays is unclear [115]. The lack of a gold standard test, the inability to assess individual risk for infection among different patient populations, and, in particular, ignorance about the natural history of HHV-8 are barriers to proper management. Among the available assays (Table 2-12), PCR is most commonly used.

HHV-8 antibodies are measured by various techniques, including EIA, immunofluorescence, and Western blot. Sensitivity and specificity vary among these tests, although EIA is technically easier to perform and has been used in large-scale seroprevalence studies [116]. PCR of whole blood has not been well studied and may not offer any value in diagnosing patients with Kaposi's sarcoma or other malignancies with HHV-8 infection. PCR assays vary widely in terms of sensitivity and specificity in diagnosing primary HHV-8 infection. Sensitivity is closer to 100% for detection of HHV-8 in tissue samples such as Kaposi's sarcoma lesions [117].

Table 2-12. HHV-8 diagnostics.

Diagnostic test	Description	Comments
Serology	Presence of HHV-8-specific IgG and IgM antibodies	Presence of past infection; may be negative in acute infection and with hypogammaglobulinemia. Sensitivity and specificity vary by target population
PCR	Quantitative or qualitative amplification of HHV-8-specific DNA from blood, tissue, or body fluid	Sensitivity and specificity vary by tissue studied and clinical syndrome
Immunohistochemical staining of tissue or cells	Staining of fixed cells using antibodies specific to HHV-8 antigens	Detects HHV-8-specific gene expression for diagnosis of Kaposi's sarcoma and other HHV-8-related malignancies

HHV-8 Human herpesvirus-8; *PCR* Polymerase chain reaction

7.3. Therapy

Antiviral therapy with acyclovir, ganciclovir, foscarnet, and cidofovir appears to have activity against HHV-8 viral replication in vitro. Acyclovir may be less active compared to the others [118]. As for EBV, antiviral therapy does not alter latent gene expression, limiting the clinical value of these drugs. There are case reports of antiviral therapy, but no general conclusions are merited [112, 119]. For established Kaposi's sarcoma and lymphoproliferative disorders due to HHV-8, chemotherapy and radiotherapy have been used with some success. Intralesional injections of cidofovir have had little effect in Kaposi's sarcoma compared with the benefit of liposomal doxorubicin, though recurrence and resistant disease have been described with the latter [120]. For primary effusion lymphomas, resistance to traditional chemotherapy is common, and response rates are lower [121]. Therapies targeting latent viral gene expression are under study. Activation of lytic gene expression to make the virus more sensitive to traditional antiviral therapies, similar to EBV, is also under investigation. Hydroxyurea may have activity against latently infected cells in some cases, although resistance has developed frequently [122]. Use of interferon ($-\alpha$ or $-\gamma$) may be able to trigger cell death in infected HHV-8 cells in vitro, but has not undergone clinical evaluation [123]. In HIV infection, immune reconstitution through the use of highly active antiretroviral therapy (HAART) has had a salutatory effect on the treatment and prevention of Kaposi's sarcoma and HHV-8. Immune reconstitution through decreased immunosuppression may also be of benefit in patients with HHV-8-related disease post-transplant.

8. Respiratory Viruses

The viruses primarily affecting the respiratory tract include some closely- and not so closely-related viruses. Adenovirus, influenza, parainfluenza, respiratory syncytial virus (RSV), the other less studied or less clinically significant infections such as rhinovirus, coronavirus, and the relatively newly described metapneumovirus are included in this section. Measles, mumps, and rubella also may cause respiratory syndromes. These viruses spread through the community by air-borne droplet inhalation, physical contact with environmental fomites, or ingestion, and are easily transmitted to patients with hematologic malignancies. Infection control measures, vaccination, and proper hand hygiene for healthcare workers and household contacts is a crucial component in preventing the spread of these infections and their potentially lethal complications in immunocompromised hosts. Reduction in immune suppression and immune reconstitution remains keys to successful outcomes in immunocompromised hosts.

Respiratory viruses cause more severe disease with more frequent complications in immunocompromised individuals. The true incidence of asymptomatic respiratory viral infection is unknown. Atypical presentations often go unrecognized. Although infections limited to the upper respiratory tract are rarely fatal, there is a higher mortality associated with lower respiratory tract infections particularly in allogeneic HSCT recipients.

9. Adenovirus

Adenovirus is a double-stranded, DNA-based, non-enveloped virus associated with diverse clinical findings. Current classification of the virus distinguishes a total of 51 distinct serotypes divided into six subgroups (A–F) based on DNA homology [124]. Infection is usually acquired by inhalation of respiratory droplets, ingestion, or direct contact with the conjunctiva. Infection occurs year-round with no particular peak season, other than that noted in military recruits within the first 4 weeks of fall basic training [125]. Immunocompromised hosts are at high risk for severe disease and dissemination of the virus, leading to significant morbidity and mortality. A case fatality rate has been reported to be as high as 60% among pediatric and young adult HSCT recipients [126].

9.1. Clinical Syndromes

Infection with adenovirus results in upper respiratory tract infection that is usually benign and self-limited. Other clinical syndromes are common, particularly in the immunocompromised host (Table 2-13). Allogeneic HSCT recipients are at the greatest risk for infection and disease due to adenovirus, though complications are reported in patients with other underlying hematologic malignancies.

Risk for infection among HSCT-recipients is reported to be as high as 29%, with the respiratory tract being the most common location of virus isolation. Risk for complicated disease includes GVHD, young age, and presence of other opportunistic infections [130]. Not surprisingly, patients who are more heavily immunosuppressed and who are suffering from other immunologic and infectious complications of transplant are at higher risk for infection and disease due to adenovirus. Mortality is most strongly associated with pneumonia, with or without evidence of dissemination [131].

9.2. Diagnosis

Standard culture-based and serologic methods for detection of adenovirus infection are commonly available but may have limited clinical utility. The availability of newer molecular techniques for diagnosis of active infections may offer opportunities for earlier intervention (Table 2-14) [132].

Table 2-13. Adenovirus Clinical Syndromes.

Anatomic location/syndrome	Symptoms/presentation
Upper respiratory tract infection	Pharyngitis and coryza, laryngitis or otitis media with fever and malaise
Conjunctivitis	Usually with pharyngitis; epidemic form associated with subgroup D and painful bilateral conjunctivitis and blurring of vision
Pneumonitis	Dyspnea, cough and fever, with or without upper respiratory tract signs and symptoms accompanied by often diffuse bilateral pulmonary infiltrates; significant mortality in immunocompromised, especially with bacterial or fungal superinfection
Gastroenteritis	Acute diarrheal illness with fever or other systemic signs and symptoms
Hepatitis	Fever, elevated hepatic transaminases, hepatic necrosis, and fulminant hepatic failure in patients after HSCT [127]
Nephritis	Renal failure with possible prodrome of fever, hematuria, and flank pain after HSCT [128]
Hemorrhagic cystitis	Fever, gross hematuria, anemia, pain
Meningoencephalitis	Fever, headache, and confusion reported in children during an adenovirus outbreak [129]

HSCT Hematopoietic stem cell transplant

Table 2-14. Adenovirus diagnostics.

Diagnostic test	Comments	Limitations
Serology	Adenovirus-specific IgM and IgG antibodies	High prevalence of antibodies in the population limits diagnostic utility for acute infection
Culture	Epithelial cell culture assays with characteristic adenovirus cytopathic effect	Excretion of virus may persist in the stool or urine for months after acute infection; culture can be positive after only 2 days, but may take up to 28 days depending on serotype
Antigen assay	Rapid detection of adenoviral antigens through either direct immunofluorescence or enzyme-linked immunosorbent assays	Not serotype-specific; lacks sensitivity depending on source of specimen
PCR	Molecular amplification and detection of adenovirus-specific DNA	Highly sensitive and specific; not universally available
Pathology with or without immunohistochemical staining	On tissue biopsy, intranuclear inclusions and occasional obscuring of the nuclear membrane, resulting in "smudge cells"	Findings can be nonspecific and not always appreciated; changes confused with other viral processes, particularly CMV; immunohistochemical staining to increase sensitivity and specificity

PCR Polymerase chain reaction; *CMV* Cytomegalovirus

EIA assays for serologic testing are replacing older tests and are likely more sensitive. To diagnose a recent infection with antibodies, however, acute and convalescent sera for testing are required in order to document a ≥ 4-fold increase over time. Serotype-specific neutralizing antibody assays may be useful in therapeutic decision-making. Cultures can be performed on samples from the respiratory tract, conjunctiva, stool, urine, CSF, or other sites. Samples from the stool and urine, in particular, need to be interpreted with caution. Ongoing shedding in asymptomatic immunocompromised individuals limits the utility of culture-based diagnostics. Antigen detection assays can be much more rapid, but lag in sensitivity. Tests for use in conjunctival samples suggest an overall sensitivity of 38%, though this rate was higher when taken earlier in the illness [133]. Among respiratory specimens, the sensitivity of antigen testing may also be relatively low compared to testing for other respiratory viral pathogens. The specificity and predictive values remain close to 100%, however, and ultimately the value of the test is most likely dependent on the adequacy of the sample taken [134]. PCR is emerging as the method of choice for detecting active adenoviral disease from any infected site. Although further studies are needed, there is an association of viremia with end-organ disease and mortality [132]. Asymptomatic viremia appears to be more common than is generally appreciated.

9.3. Therapy

There are no controlled clinical trials regarding the treatment of adenovirus infection to date. There are only limited in vitro susceptibility assays and uncontrolled clinical reports (Table 2-15).

The exact role of antiviral therapy in adenovirus disease remains unclear. Reduction in immune suppression and immune reconstitution is important when feasible. The two most commonly used agents, cidofovir and ribavirin, have significant toxicities. Cidofovir has significant nephrotoxicity, while ribavirin has bone marrow toxicity, risk for anemia, and is a teratogen. Cidofovir appears to be the most active agent against adenovirus in vitro, and clinical experience suggests the capacity to reduce viremia and viruria with subsequent clinical improvement in some patients. Various serotypes differ in response to cidofovir. Dosing and length of therapy remain unclear.

Table 2-15. Adenovirus Therapeutics.

Agent	Comments
Cidofovir	Cidofovir has in vitro activity against all serogroups of adenovirus; case reports and uncontrolled case series suggest clinical effect [135–140]
DLI	Donor lymphocyte infusions have been associated with clearance of adenovirus in a case report of gastroenteritis after HSCT [141] and in a case report of life-threatening hemorrhagic cystitis after HSCT [142]
Ganciclovir	Ganciclovir may have in vitro activity against adenovirus at high levels (which may not be clinically achievable); studies in HSCT patients receiving ganciclovir for CMV prophylaxis may have shown a protective effect [143]
IVIG	Combined use of IVIG with ribavirin or other agents has been reported in at least two cases [144, 145]
Ribavirin	In vitro, ribavirin has mixed activity against adenovirus [146]; case reports are mixed in clinical effect; the largest case series showed no association of ribavirin with survival in HSCT recipients with adenovirus infection [131]
Vidarabine	In vitro activity appears marginal; used in case reports for the treatment of hemorrhagic cystitis [147, 148]
Zalcitabine (ddC)	ddC with some in vitro activity [149]; animal model of adenovirus infection with some efficacy in preventing pneumonia [150]

DLI Donor lymphocyte infusions; *HSCT* Hematopoietic stem cell transplant; *CMV* Cytomegalovirus; *IVIG* Intravenous immunoglobulin

Doses of 5 mg/kg given IV once weekly for two to three doses, followed by infusions every other week, has been most often cited [138]. Cidofovir is usually given concomitantly with probenecid to help prevent some of the renal toxicity of the drug. Hemorrhagic cystitis may be relapsing with immune function, and hydration with urine flow is an essential component of care in these individuals. Despite some case reports, topical administration of antiviral agents has not proven very helpful in therapy of this common syndrome.

10. Influenza, Parainfluenza, and Respiratory Syncytial Virus

The spread of influenza and RSV occurs in outbreaks and epidemics throughout the winter. Parainfluenza infection occurs throughout the year, with epidemics arising occasionally in the fall and spring. For all three, spread within families and household contacts, as well as in the nosocomial setting, is common. Although much emphasis is placed on influenza, RSV is the single most common cause of lower respiratory tract infection in children, and both RSV and parainfluenza infections are likely under-recognized in the elderly and immunocompromised patient populations [151].

Influenza virus A and B are capable of invasive infection in patients with hematologic malignancies. Influenza A is most closely associated with changes in the two major glycoproteins:hemagglutinin (H) and neuraminidase (N). Antigenic shifts in these glycoproteins are associated with epidemics and worldwide pandemics of influenza A, while the role of minor changes, so called antigenic drifts, is more closely associated with localized outbreaks. Influenza B has a lesser propensity for antigenic changes. Parainfluenza is in the paramyxoviridae family and is divided into four major serotypes: Parainfluenza 1–4. Parainfluenza-3 is the most prevalent serotype and is also associated most strongly with the development of pneumonia and bronchiolitis. RSV is also a member of the paramyxoviridae family. There are two subtypes described: A and B. Both can be present simultaneously in community outbreaks, though subtype A typically causes more severe disease [152]. Influenza, parainfluenza, and RSV are all associated with a more prolonged clinical course, risk of pneumonia, co-infection with other pathogens, and death in patients with hematologic malignancies [153].

10.1. Clinical Syndromes

Among immunocompetent non-elderly adults, influenza, parainfluenza, and RSV tend to be self-limited upper respiratory tract illnesses or febrile syndromes. In the setting of hematologic malignancies, the frequency of lower respiratory tract involvement increases dramatically with a risk of dissemination and systemic complications (Table 2-16).

Cardiac and CNS involvement have been reported in parainfluenza, complicating the diagnosis of pulmonary infiltrates with infection and heart failure. Involvement of the lower respiratory tract increases the risk for bacterial or fungal superinfection including *Streptococcus pneumoniae* and *Staphylococcus aureus*.

Table 2-16. Influenza, parainfluenza, and RSV syndromes.

Virus	Syndrome	Symptoms
Influenza	Uncomplicated	Fever, myalgias, malaise, cough, sore throat
	Complicated	
	Pneumonia	Fever, dyspnea, and hypoxia with symptoms of uncomplicated influenza; Superinfection, bacterial and fungal, is common and increases risk for sepsis and death [154]
	Myocarditis	Scattered reports of involvement of influenza with the myocardium during acute illness, leading to congestive heart failure
	Meningoencephalitis	Fever, encephalopathy and seizure with abnormal CSF findings, and a positive PCR for influenza in some children [155]
	Myositis	Myalgia with tenderness of the affected muscles (most commonly the legs), with elevation of serum creatinine phosphokinase, myoglobinuria, and renal failure
Parainfluenza	Upper respiratory tract infection	Fever, cough, sore throat, rhinorrhea, otitis media
	Lower respiratory tract infection	Fever, cough, dyspnea, and hypoxia, with bronchiolitis or pneumonia
RSV	Upper respiratory tract infection	Fever, cough, conjunctivitis, rhinorrhea, sinusitis, otitis media
	Lower respiratory tract infection	Fever, cough, dyspnea, with concomitant bronchospasm and respiratory failure

CSF Cerebrospinal fluid; *PCR* Polymerase chain reaction; *RSV* Respiratory syncytial virus

10.2. Diagnosis

The availability of molecular assays and viral antigen detection testing has altered the clinical approach to respiratory viral infection. Viral culture remains necessary for susceptibility testing, viral typing, and identification of new pathogens. However, laboratories are increasingly utilizing rapid testing methods for identification of respiratory viruses. None of the rapid antigen tests have been well studied in immunocompromised hosts, though in immunocompetent patients, they likely have a sensitivity and specificity in the 80–99% range. Adequacy of the respiratory specimen provided for testing can be a limiting factor [134]. The sensitivity of these assays may also be limited when compared with newer molecular assays (Table 2-17). Rapid diagnostics have significant implications for successful therapy, however.

10.3. Therapy

Therapy for these viruses varies in terms of both efficacy and clinical data. Early diagnosis, and the early initiation of antiviral therapy for influenza, and likely RSV, is of importance. Delaying chemotherapy or HSCT in patients with hematologic malignancy with respiratory viral infections may improve outcomes [160], emphasizing the importance of appropriate and rapid diagnosis (Table 2-18).

Table 2-17. Influenza, parainfluenza, and RSV diagnostics.

Virus	Diagnostic test	Comments	Limitations
Influenza	Serology	Testing of serum for influenza-specific antibodies	Can only diagnose disease retrospectively; requires fourfold increase in titers from both acute and convalescent sera
	Culture	Respiratory samples (sputum, nasal swabs or washings, bronchoalveolar lavage fluid or throat swabs) used on epithelial cell culture assays	48–72 h positive result with rapid shell vial technique, otherwise 5–10 days; remains the "gold standard" of diagnosis
	Antigen assays	Immunofluorescent antigen–antibody staining of respiratory samples (DFA); more rapid, diverse commercially prepared kits for testing of respiratory samples for influenza antigens using enzymc immunoassays	Rapid antigen assays may not test for both influenza A and B, or distinguish between the two (as for DFA and some rapid tests); sensitivity and specificity of rapid tests range from 72–95% and 76–84%, respectively [156]
	PCR	Influenza A- or B-specific molecular amplification of viral RNA from body fluid, nasopharyngeal aspirates, bronchoalveolar lavage fluid, or throat swabs	Highly sensitive and specific, but not available routinely; expensive to perform
Parainfluenza	Serology	Testing of serum for parainfluenza-specific antibodies	Not routinely available, lacks specificity due to some cross-reactivity, and can only diagnose retrospectively (need both acute and convalescent serum to demonstrate at least a fourfold rise)
	Culture	Growth of parainfluenza from respiratory specimens on cell culture lines	Specific assay, though possibly limited sensitivity depending on source and timing of collection [157]
	Rapid antigen assays	Immunofluorescent assays using parainfluenza-specific antibodies for antigen detection in cell samples or tissue	Most readily available sensitive and specific assay
	PCR	Parainfluenza-3-specific molecular amplification of viral RNA has been developed	No clinical experience to clarify its potential role in diagnosing active parainfluenza-3 infection [158]
RSV	Culture	Growth of RSV on cell culture lines using respiratory secretion samples	Culture can take anywhere from 4 to 14 days, limiting clinical utility
	Rapid antigen assays	Detection of RSV-specific antigens on cell surfaces taken from respiratory samples using immunofluorescent antibody techniques	Rapid and widely available, sensitivity may vary depending on patient and quality of sample
	PCR	RSV-specific molecular amplification using respiratory specimens	Sensitive and specific; may be superior to antigen detection in patients with hematologic malignancy [159]

RSV Respiratory syncytial virus; *PCR* Polymerase chain reaction

Table 2-18. Influenza, parainfluenza, and RSV therapeutics.

Virus	Drug	Dosing
Influenza	Oseltamivir	75 mg po bid75 mg po qd (for CrCl<30 mL/min)
	Zanamivir	Two inhalations (5 mg) bid
	Amantidine	100 mg po bid or 200 mg po qd200 mg po x 1, then 100 mg po qd (for CrCl of 30–50 mL/min) 200 mg po x 1, then 100 mg po qod (for CrCl of 15–29 mL/min) 200 mg po every 7 days (for CrCl<15 mL/min)
	Rimantidine	100 mg po bid100 mg po qd (for CrCl < 10 mL/min and for severe liver disease)
	Ribavirin	Dosing unclear, inhalation anecdotally effective in immunocompetent individuals, while oral therapy likely not [161]
Parainfluenza	Ribavirin	Dosing unclear, but reports of using 15–20 mg/kg/day in three divided doses with or without another 6 g/day inhaled therapy has been reported in HSCT recipients [162, 163]
RSV	Ribavirin	Dosing unclear, but reports of using 2 g aerosolized three times daily has been reported in patients with hematologic malignancies and HSCT [164]
	Palivizumab	15 mg/kg IM q monthly during winter season (November through April) for prophylaxis only; no benefit seen in therapy

RSV Respiratory syncytial virus; *CrCl* Creatinine clearance; *HSCT* Hematopoietic stem cell transplant; *IM* Intramuscularly

Oseltamivir has emerged as the most commonly used antiviral therapy for influenza because of its ease of administration and tolerance. Being a neuraminidase inhibitor like zanamivir, it has efficacy against both influenza A and B. Usual treatment in the immunocompetent individual is for 5 days, but in the immunocompromised patient, particularly in HSCT recipients or patients with complicated disease, more prolonged therapy may be warranted [63]. Data specifically in HSCT recipients suggest that early therapy using oseltamivir can possibly reduce viral shedding and risk for pneumonia [165]. The adamantanes, amantidine, and rimantidine, are classified as M2 inhibitors and are efficacious against influenza A only. Although they are less expensive than the neuraminidase inhibitors, they are limited by increasing rates of resistance. In January of 2006, the Centers for Disease Control (CDC) issued an alert to avoid the use of M2 inhibitors during the 2005–2006 influenza season in the United States due to unacceptably high rates of resistance seen in the H3N2 strain circulating at the time. The same precaution has been recommended for the 2006–2007 season as well, until further more definitive susceptibility testing can be established. All of the above agents have also been used for prophylaxis during outbreaks, though dosing, length of therapy, and susceptibilities of circulating strains may vary.

Immunization is a central component of influenza control. Use of the annual trivalent inactivated influenza vaccine among HSCT recipients, healthcare workers, and household contacts may decrease the attack rate both in the community and in the nosocomial setting [165]. Vaccine responses are generally reduced among patients with hematologic malignancies or HSCT, but the potential benefits of prevention far outweigh any risks incurred by administering the vaccine. Accordingly, annual vaccination is recommended in this patient population. The newer live-attenuated influenza vaccine that is administered intranasally has been approved for use in the United States for individuals aged 5–49 years [166] but has not been recommended in immunocompromised individuals or in their household contacts because of risk of transmission [167].

For parainfluenza, the efficacy of therapy is less clear, and there are no established or proven agents. Ribavirin (orally, IV and aerosolized) with and without intravenous immunoglobulin has only anecdotal efficacy. The largest study that evaluated the use of ribavirin in HSCT did not note any difference in mortality or virus shedding, particularly with parainfluenza-3 [163].

Treatment for RSV appears moderately effective in some studies. The use of inhaled ribavirin has not been proven effective in immunocompetent children, while there are data to suggest efficacy in the adult HSCT population [164, 168]. Early diagnosis and intervention may be the key to improving outcomes in this particular group [168]. Repletion of antibodies in hypogammaglobulinemic hosts may be useful. Currently, palivizumab, a monoclonal antibody directed toward RSV, has only been studied as a prophylactic agent in children at risk of respiratory complications from RSV infection. Trials investigating its use as a therapeutic agent in combination with ribavirin are reportedly ongoing [168]. It is well-tolerated in the HSCT population [169] and was successful at treating RSV pneumonitis in combination with corticosteroids in a case report of a women with relapsed Hodgkin's disease after autologous HSCT [170].

11. Human Metapneumovirus

Human metapneumovirus (hMPV) is a recently described respiratory virus in the paramyxovirus family [171]. hMPV is a ubiquitous pathogen, accounting for a substantial portion of respiratory tract illnesses in normal children [172]. Recent studies suggest that hMPV was an unrecognized pathogen for as long as serologic samples have been available. hMPV is not as common as RSV but more common than parainfluenza [173], with a propensity for the winter months [172]. Many questions remain regarding the role of this agent in immunocompromised individuals, the mechanism of spread in the community and prevention and therapy.

hMPV is a likely cause of upper respiratory tract infection as well as bronchiolitis and pneumonia in infants, the elderly and immunocompromised individuals, particularly HSCT recipients. Upper respiratory tract prodromal symptoms are common prior to the onset of lower respiratory tract disease [174]. Death as a result of lower respiratory tract disease has been described in the setting of HSCT, and it may be a relatively common outcome of hMPV pneumonia [174].

PCR for viral RNA is the only established assay for diagnosis. Testing of respiratory secretions or tissue biopsy samples via PCR is sensitive, although the true incidence of asymptomatic viral shedding remains unclear [175]. Biopsies of lung tissue in patients with pneumonia presumably caused by hMPV show changes consistent with viral pneumonitis, but are otherwise non-specific. These changes may include diffuse alveolar damage and mononuclear cell infiltration, but there are no definite viral inclusions [174].

Although there are no clinical data to guide therapy, ribavirin appears to have in vitro activity against hMPV equivalent to that of RSV [176]. A mouse model of hMPV infection suggests that ribavirin may be efficacious in vivo [177]. Prospective clinical studies are needed.

12. Other Respiratory Viruses

Other respiratory pathogens include the rhinoviruses, coronaviruses, measles, mumps, and rubella. Rhinoviruses and coronaviruses are associated with the common cold. Symptoms are generally self-limited and consist of upper respiratory tract-related complaints: rhinorrhea, sinus congestion, pharyngitis and cough. Although these viruses are thought to be limited to the upper respiratory tract for replication, reports isolating them from the lower respiratory tract do exist [178–180]. The outcome of infection due to rhinoviruses or coronaviruses in patients with hematologic malignancies is not well characterized. The incidence of severe infection due to rhinoviruses is unknown. Fatal pneumonia has been attributed to infection from rhinoviruses in patients who have undergone HSCT [181]. Use of reverse-transcriptase PCR (RT-PCR) for rhinoviruses and coronaviruses in bronchoalveolar lavage samples from patients who have undergone HSCT suggests that isolation of rhinoviruses from lower respiratory tract samples is associated with co-infection from other pathogens (e.g., bacteria, fungi and other viruses) [180]. The validity of RT-PCR in respiratory samples remains unclear. Most laboratories do not have the culture techniques or PCR available for the detection of these viruses in clinical samples. There is no established antiviral therapy for these infections.

Measles, mumps, and rubella are uncommon pathogens in the US due to an effective vaccine program. The vaccine is a live attenuated virus vaccine involving all three pathogens. Because it is a live virus vaccine, it is generally avoided in immunocompromised individuals, though it is considered safe and effective in children who had acute lymphoblastic leukemia after they have been effectively treated with chemotherapy [182]. Sporadic cases of all three viruses occur. Measles, or rubeola, is typically associated with cough, coryza, fever, and a maculopapular rash. There are limited data on measles in immunocompromised patients. Cumulative case reports suggest that the case-fatality rate among oncology patients is as high as 70% [183]. Complications from the infection, including pneumonitis and encephalitis, may be more common. The typical rash of measles may be absent in immunocompromised patients, complicating the diagnosis. Serology, culture and RT-PCR can be used to diagnose measles. Serology is commonly available. Acute and convalescent sera are required to demonstrate the requisite fourfold increase over time to confirm the diagnosis. There is no known effective treatment for measles once infection is established. High-dose vitamin A when used in children has been reported to decrease the severity of the disease [184]. Ribavirin remains of unproven benefit [185].

Mumps, a member of the paramyxovirus family, is most commonly associated with parotitis, though its clinical manifestations can be diverse and include meningitis, encephalitis, hearing loss, orchitis, oophoritis, myocarditis, arthritis, and others. Like measles, mumps is usually a rare illness, though a large outbreak in the United States was recently characterized [186]. From January through October of 2006, a total of 5,783 cases of confirmed or probable mumps were reported, involving a total of 45 states. Most cases came from Iowa, Kansas, Wisconsin, and Illinois, and clustered around college campuses. The natural history of this illness in immunocompromised individuals remains unclear. Diagnosis is usually through standard serologic methods. EIA is most often used due to ease of performance and reliability. Therapy is entirely supportive.

Rubella, or German measles, is a member of the Togaviridae family. Although most often associated with only mild, innocuous infections in adults and children, congenital acquisition can have devastating effects on unborn fetuses. Thanks to broad use of the live-attenuated vaccine; rubella is no longer endemic in the United States, with less than 25 cases reported annually among foreign-born persons [187].

12.1. Enteroviruses

Enteroviruses are a heterogeneous group of viruses that along with the rhinoviruses, aphthoviruses, cardioviruses, and Hepatitis A virus, make up the picornaviridae family. The enteroviruses are further subclassified into different groups and 67 total serotypes (Table 2-19). There tends to be a peak season of infection in temperate climates during the summer and autumn months. Spread is generally via the fecal-oral route, though respiratory transmission may be possible. Although cell-mediated immunity generally plays an important role in viral immunology, humoral immunity is thought to be of particular importance in controlling enteroviral infections, and some of the most severe outcomes have been noted in patients with agammaglobulinemia [188, 189].

12.2. Clinical Syndromes

In the immunocompetent host, the vast majority of enteroviral infections produce a completely asymptomatic infection. Occasionally, a mild febrile illness with or without upper respiratory tract symptoms may be present. Other symptoms are rarer, but have been well-characterized (Table 2-20). In patients who have undergone HSCT, fatal complications have been documented [189–196]. Occasionally, these viruses appear to precipitate gastrointestinal GVHD.

Most cases of protracted and fatal enteroviral infections have been among patients with severe B-cell dysfunction, such as hereditary forms of agammaglobulinemia. In these particular clinical scenarios, enterovirus RNA can sometimes be persistently recovered over months to years from multiple anatomic sites such as the CSF, lung, myocardium or bone marrow [188]. In HSCT, the combination of underlying T-cell dysfunction combined

Table 2-19. The enteroviruses.

Virus subgroup	Serotypes
Polio	1–3
Coxsackie A	1–22, 24
Coxsackie B	1–6
Echovirus	1–9, 11–27, 29–33[a]
Enterovirus	68–71[b]

[a]Echovirus 34 is the same virus as a genetic variant of coxsackie
[b]Hepatitis A is often classified as enterovirus 72

Table 2-20. Enteroviral syndromes.

Syndrome	Symptoms
Upper respiratory tract infection	Fever, rhinorrhea, pharyngitis
Pneumonitis	Fever, cough, possibly dyspnea
Rash	Fever, erythematous macular or maculopapular exanthems, with or without other syndromes; occasionally purpuric resembling meningococcemia
Hand-foot-and-mouth syndrome	Fever, oral vesicular lesions and cutaneous maculopapular lesions on the hands, feet, and buttocks
Herpangina	Vesicular lesions on the tonsils and soft palate similar to herpes labialis, sore throat, fever
Conjunctivitis/keratitis	Ocular pain, injection, blurring of vision
Gastroenteritis	Fever, diarrhea
Pericarditis/myopericarditis	Chest pain, congestive heart failure
Aseptic meningitis	Fever, headache, photophobia, nausea/vomiting, meningismus
Pleurodynia	Fever and chest pains with spasms of chest and abdominal muscles that mimic pulmonary emboli
Paralytic poliomyelitis	Weakness or paralysis of one or more extremities following aseptic meningitis

with suppressed humoral responses may contribute to more profound infection as well. However, the true incidence of enteroviral infections in this population remains unclear. Some estimate the incidence of enteroviral infections among HSCT recipients at 10%, though mortality is thought to be low overall and associated with coinfection of other pathogens. No clear independent risk factors for infection among HSCT recipients have been identified [196].

Diagnosis

Diagnosis of enteroviral infections involves the use of serology, culture, or PCR (Table 2-21). Because of many limitations in the other two methods, PCR is becoming a more favored approach.

Microneutralization serologic assays offer the benefit of being serotype-specific. Other methods such as immunofluorescent assays and EIA may show some cross-reactivity between the serotypes. The specificity of measuring serotypes also hampers the clinical utility of these tests. With 67 different serotypes known, routine diagnosis of enteroviruses with serology is not always realistic. Serologies are most useful when looking for evidence of polio infection. Culture can be labor-intensive and can require multiple cell lines to be effective [197]. Because excretion of enteroviruses from the gastrointestinal tract can persist after infection for as long as 8 weeks, [198, 199] isolation of the virus from stool, rectal swabs or possibly the oropharynx may result in a falsely positive assay. The same holds true for PCR when used in samples taken from these anatomic locations. Most experiences with PCR comes from CSF samples in cases of suspected aseptic meningitis where the sensitivity may be higher than culture and much more clinically useful [200].

Table 2-21. Enterovirus diagnostics.

Diagnostic test	Comments	Limitations
Serology	Measurement of IgG and IgM antibodies specific to enteroviruses	Both acute and convalescent sera are required to make a diagnosis; may not be able to determine acute infection in a clinically relevant time period; can be limited in patients with agammaglobulinemia; are serotype specific; cross-reactivity can exist
Culture	Growth of the virus in cell culture, looking for a characteristic cytopathic effect	May take up to 1 week for identification; sometimes may detect carriage of virus rather than true infection
PCR	Reverse transcriptase molecular amplification of RNA specific to enteroviruses	Highly sensitive and specific; not available in all labs; does not identify specific serotypes; sometimes may detect carriage of virus rather than true infection

PCR Polymerase chain reaction

12.3. Therapy

There is no established treatment for enteroviruses [196]. Intravenous immunoglobulin (IVIG) has been used with mixed success in various case reports of patients with persistent meningitis and in children with myocarditis when compared to historical controls [188, 189, 201]. Antibody responses to enterovirus are serotype-specific, and because of this, IVIG may not be clinically useful in all cases [202]. There are no data regarding dosing and duration of use with IVIG. Previous investigations of specific antiviral therapy against enteroviruses resulted in the development of a compound known as pleconaril. Pleconaril acted by binding to the viral capsid antigen, impairing viral binding and uncoating [203]. Clinical trials and various case reports of pleconaril use in aseptic meningitis have shown only modest to no clinical benefit, and its further development was put on hold [189, 204].

Control of polio via vaccination has virtually eliminated wild polio viral infections in the Western hemisphere. Loss of immunity to poliovirus is well-documented in patients after allogeneic HSCT [205, 206], and has led to recommendations for revaccination with inactivated poliovirus vaccine after transplantation [207]. Live virus, vaccines should be avoided in immunosuppressed patients, and the live attenuated oral poliovirus vaccine is no longer available in the United States due to the rare but severe complication of vaccine-associated paralytic polio. Since the implementation of the inactivated vaccine, vaccine-associated paralytic polio has been eliminated in the United States [208].

13. Viral Hepatitides

Viral hepatitis A, B and C are unrelated viruses capable of inducing acute or both acute and chronic liver disease. Hepatitis B virus (HBV) and hepatitis C virus (HCV) are of particular importance because of their abilities to establish chronic infection and reactivate with immunosuppression.

14. Hepatitis A

Hepatitis A is a member of the picornaviridae family that is transmitted via the fecal-oral route from one individual to another. Though most infections are mild, fulminant hepatitis with significant mortality has been reported. However, there are currently no reports of hepatitis A disease in HSCT patients, making the true risk and incidence of infection in this population unknown [209]. Transmission can result from person-to-person contact, sexual contact or ingestion of contaminated food or water. There are also rare reports of transmission via blood products [210]. Once ingested, the virus replicates in the gastrointestinal epithelium and then produces transient viremia, leading to infection of and further replication in the hepatocytes. The average incubation period is close to 4 weeks [211].

Symptoms of infection usually include fever, malaise, and hepatitis with or without jaundice. The differential diagnosis includes numerous infectious and non-infectious etiologies, including other viruses such as CMV, EBV, HSV, VZV, and the other hepatitides. The diagnosis is usually made via the measurement of serum anti-hepatitis A IgM antibodies, in the right clinical setting. These antibodies can usually be detected by 1 week into the illness and persist in immunocompetent individuals for several months. Detection of viral RNA via PCR is only available only in the research setting. Treatment is supportive with no available antiviral therapy. Immune globulin specific for hepatitis A can be administered intramuscularly to provide short-term protection, though long-term prevention is ideally through the use of vaccination. Some groups have recommended that post-HSCT seronegative patients who live in or are traveling to endemic areas receive the inactivated hepatitis A vaccine [212].

15. Hepatitis B

HBV, along with HCV, has the ability to establish chronic infection and occasionally cause a fatal post-transplant hepatitis in HSCT recipients [213]. Despite the availability of an effective vaccine, HBV continues to be an important cause of morbidity and mortality in the United States. Patients from higher-prevalence areas such as Southeast Asia, China and sub-Saharan Africa are at greater risk of exposure to the virus in the perinatal period, and are at greater risk of chronic infection and subsequent complications. The incidence of acute HBV in the United States seems to be declining among pediatric patients, reflecting most likely, the efficacy and implementation of universal vaccination. Among adults, acute infection continues to increase [214]. Among HSCT recipients, the prevalence of HBV infection in the United States is estimated to be about 1% [215]. The most common risk factors for infection include having a history of multiple sex partners, men who have sex with other men and injection drug use. Aside from the usual inoculation by intimate mucocutaneous contact and perinatal infection, transfusion of infected blood products and transplantation of infected organs are well-described modes of transmission.

15.1. Clinical Syndromes

The majority of patients with acute HBV infection are asymptomatic despite active viral replication and elevated hepatic chemistries. The incubation period can last up to 4 months during which time patients may experience constitutional symptoms. About one-third develop icteric hepatitis. Fulminant hepatitis with hepatic failure is unusual with HBV (~1%) [216], and is likely due to immune-mediated complications rather than virally-mediated hepatic necrosis. The risk for developing chronic infection is inversely related to a patient's age, with perinatal infection carrying the highest risk. Chronic infection is diagnosed by persistent (>6 months) elevation of hepatic chemistries, particularly the alanine aminotransferase (ALT) level. Most patients with chronic disease are asymptomatic unless they develop cirrhosis and complications thereof. Immune complex-mediated complications outside the liver can include membranous and membranoproliferative glomerulonephritis as well as polyarteritis nodosa.

15.2. Diagnosis

The diagnosis of HBV is usually with serologies and antigen-detection, with nucleic acid amplification which is now being commonly used. Immunohistochemical staining of liver biopsies are of use to assess hepatic injury and viral replication (Table 2-22).

Hepatitis B surface antigen testing has been the primary marker for identifying acute and chronic infection, and can be detected as early as 9 days into infection with modern automated EIA tests [217]. Occasionally, patients with active infection are found to have a negative hepatitis B surface antigen assay. These patients will usually have serologic evidence of hepatitis B core antibodies and low-level HBV DNA levels. This phenomenon is more common in patients with HBV and HIV coinfection [218]. The development of real-time PCR assays has created the most sensitive assays available for detecting HBV. HBV DNA levels as measured by PCR can be directly correlated to the risk of liver disease, death, and drug resistance in patients on therapy. Though baseline values may vary from individual to individual, monitoring on a regular basis may be useful, particularly in those patients on therapy. Although different algorithms exist, checking a patient's HBV viral load by PCR two to four times yearly while on therapy may provide an assessment of their response. Failure of an antiviral agent to achieve a 1 log or more decrease in viral load over 3 months, or a rebound of viral replication of 1 log or greater after an initial response is often considered evidence of failure [219]. Standardization of quantification in international units (IU)/mL will enhance comparison of different molecular assays [220].

15.3. Therapy

For lamivudine, loading doses of 35–100 mg in the setting of decreased renal function are often given during the first day before starting a lower daily dose. Entacavir doses at the higher end of the range are generally reserved for lamivudine-refractory disease. Other agents being evaluated for treatment of HBV, but less-studied at this time, include emtricitibine (FTC), tenofovir (TDF), telbivudine, valtorcitabine and clevudine [221]. Tenofovir and emtricitibine are currently used in the treatment of HIV infection and have shown particular promise in the setting of HIV and HBV coinfection [222]. Although not studied in detail in the HSCT recipient population, numerous case reports exist regarding the efficacy of these antivirals as both prophylactic agents and as primary therapeutics in chronic carriers and in recipients of HBV positive

Table 2-22. Hepatitis B Diagnostics.

Diagnostic test	Comments	Acute/chronic infection	Limitations
Serology assays			
Hepatitis B surface antibody	IgG antibody	Recovery phase of acute infection and in chronic disease	Immunity due to vaccine or from past exposure; found in acute and chronic infection
Hepatitis B core IgM antibody	IgM antibody	Early acute infection and occasionally during flares of chronic infection	Usually indicates acute infection, but can persist in serum for up to 2 years; increase with flares may be misleading
Hepatitis B core IgG antibody	IgG antibody	Latter part of acute infection (recovery phase), and persist during chronic infection	In combination with hepatitis B surface IgG usually indicates past exposure, but not yet chronic infection
Hepatitis B early antibody	IgG antibody	Latter part of acute infection (recovery phase), and persist in low-level non-replicating chronic infection	Delayed seroconversion can occur in patients who develop chronic infection
Antigen assays			
Hepatitis B surface antigen	Protein found in the viral envelope	Appears early in acute infection; persistence beyond 6 months implies chronic infection	May be absent in brief window period of anti-hepatitis B surface IgG seroconversion in acute infection
Hepatitis B early antigen	Secretory protein from the HBV precore protein	Early acute infection and associated with high levels of HBV DNA replication; occasionally persists into chronic infection when seroconversion (HBV early IgG) does not occur	Perinatally acquired infection may be hepatitis B early antigen positive with normal serum ALT; seroconversion does not always indicate resolution of acute infection
DNA assays			
Hepatitis B viral DNA PCR	Molecular amplification and detection of HBV-specific DNA	Usually detectable in immediate acute infection and throughout chronic infection	Heterogeneity of PCR techniques and absence of standardization
Hepatitis B hybrid capture	Capture oligonucleotide amplification of HBV-specific DNA	Usually detectable very early in acute infection, and can be persistently positive in chronic disease	Less sensitive than PCR, and generally fails to detect <5,000 copies/mL

HBV Hepatitis B virus; *ALT* Alanine aminotransferase; *PCR* Polymerase chain reaction

donor stem cells. Optimal length of therapy is yet to be well-established with many of the agents listed in Table 2-23, and the development of resistance may vary with any of the individual agents.

Implementation of the routine universal immunization protocol is the most effective means of preventing spread of HBV. In patients undergoing allogeneic HSCT, HBV immunization can result in an effective antibody response, though systemic re-immunization of recipients may be necessary to maintain long-term immunity [223].

Table 2-23. Hepatitis B therapeutics.

Drug	Class	Dosing	Limitations
Interferon-α	Immunomodulator	5 million units sq qd, or 10 million units sq tiw	Major side effects
Lamivudine (3TC)	Nucleoside analogue	100 mg po qd for normal CrCl 50 mg po qd for CrCl 30–49 mL/min 15 mg po qd for CrCl 5–14 mL/min 10 mg po qd for CrCl <5 mL/min	Bone marrow suppression
Adefovir	Nucleotide analogue	10 mg po qd for normal CrCl 10 mg po qod for CrCl 20–49 mL/min 10 mg po q 72 h for CrCl 10–19 mL/min 10 mg q week for patients on hemodialysis	Renal insufficiency
Entecavir	Nucleoside analogue	0.5–1 mg po qd for normal CrCl 0.25–0.5 mg po qd for CrCl 30–50 mL/min 0.15–0.3 mg po qd for CrCl 10–29 mL/min 0.05–0.1 mg po qd for CrCl <10 mL/min	Development of resistance poorly understood
Pegylated interferon-α-2a	Immunomodulator	180 μg sq q week	Major side effects; may be better tolerated than interferon-α

16. Hepatitis C

Acquisition of HCV during HSCT has virtually disappeared due to effective testing of donors. HCV, like HBV, causes both acute and chronic infection, and acute infections are frequently asymptomatic. HCV leads to chronic infection in most patients. After HSCT, individuals acquiring HCV have an increased incidence of chronic infection and rapid progression to cirrhosis compared to otherwise healthy controls [224]. Symptoms of acute infection may include malaise and nausea, with or without jaundice. Chronic HCV infection is often asymptomatic with fluctuating transaminase levels. Patients undergoing HSCT who acquire HCV infection rarely develop signs or symptoms of decompensated liver disease during the first 10 years after transplant [225]. Beyond the 10-year mark, a significant portion of HSCT recipients develop cirrhosis and often hepatocellular carcinoma [224].

16.1. Diagnosis

HCV diagnostic testing is based on quantitative molecular assays, though serologic assays are most often used for screening. The second-generation EIA test is widely used with greater sensitivity than the first-generation assay [226]. A third-generation EIA can detect an additional HCV antigen, providing an advantage in high-prevalence settings and in detecting acute infections before seroconversion [227, 228]. Previously, confirmation of HCV infection in the setting of a positive serology was done through the use of a recombinant immunoblot assay (RIBA-2). This immunoblot technique uses the same antigens detected by the second-generation EIA. The RIBA-2 increases the specificity of a positive EIA and reduces false positive results in low-prevalence settings or in patients with normal hepatic chemistries. More commonly now, detection of HCV RNA through the use of molecular amplification is used for confirmation and in patient management. Since patients with acute leukemia after HSCT may be less likely to develop antibody responses to HCV, PCR has significant advantages as a diagnostic tool [229]. Various molecular methods are not directly comparable, but single quantitative assays should be used in individuals. Commercially available assays include both RT-PCR and branched chain PCR methods. Branched chain PCR for HCV is technically easier, but less sensitive than standard RT-PCR techniques. A small percentage of patients with chronic infection have low-grade viremia that may not be detected [230]. PCR assays also have clinical utility in monitoring patients on therapy. Successful virologic response is generally defined as at least a 2 log decline from baseline levels 12 weeks into therapy, whereas those patients who do not experience the same decline are defined as nonresponders. Eradication of infection, or sustained virologic response, is also measured by use of the PCR assay and is defined by undetectable viral levels after completion of therapy and again 6 months later [231].

16.2. Therapy

Patients with chronic HCV infection after HSCT should be considered for therapy. Options are limited, and the current combination of interferon-α plus ribavirin is poorly tolerated. Pegylated interferon may be better tolerated, though the prolonged half-life may be of concern in patients with hematopoietic toxicity [232]. Interferon may be an instigator of reactivation of GVHD as well. Dosing regimens depend on variables such as type of interferon used and patient tolerance. For HCV genotypes 1 and 4, ribavirin is typically dosed at 1,000 mg a day in two divided doses for individuals ≤ 75 kg and 1,200 mg a day in two divided doses for those > 75 kg. With genotypes 2 and 3, 800 mg in two divided doses is likely to be sufficient.

17. Retroviruses

Retroviruses are a group of RNA viruses with a common genetic profile and reproductive machinery using the viral-specific enzyme reverse transcriptase to convert the RNA genome into an integrated DNA sequence within the host genome. The clinically significant retroviruses in human infection include human immunodeficiency virus1- and -2 (HIV-1 and -2), and human T-cell lymphotropic virus-I and -II (HTLV-I and -II).

18. Human Immunodeficiency Virus

HIV infection increases the risk of non-Hodgkin's lymphoma of which diffuse large B-cell lymphoma and Burkitt's lymphoma are the two most common forms [233]. Primary effusion lymphomas and EBV-related polymorphic lymphoproliferative disorders are also well described [234, 235].

18.1. Diagnosis

Testing for HIV infection is via EIA serologic assay from blood with confirmation by Western blot and quantitative molecular assay. The standard third-generation EIA used in clinical practice utilizes recombinant DNA proteins from immunodominant regions of HIV-1 and HIV-2. Some detect both IgM and IgG with a sensitivity in the 96–99% range and a specificity of up to 99% [236]. False negative EIA tests may occur between the time of viral transmission and seroconversion and in hypogammaglobulinemia, replacement transfusions, infection with HIV-1 subtype O [237] or infection with HIV-2 (if an HIV-2 specific-assay is not used) [238].

A positive EIA is confirmed through Western blot using proteins derived from the three major genetic domains of retroviruses (*gag, pol* and *env*). Possible explanations for false positive EIA assays include hematologic malignancies, autoimmune disorders, positive rapid plasma reagin (RPR) tests or infection with syphilis, HIV-2 infection (if an HIV-2 specific western blot is not used) and vaccination. If bands from at least two of the three major proteins are identified, the test is scored as positive. If only a single band is identified, then the test is frequently interpreted as indeterminate. The patients from the latter group usually are not true positives, and represent cross-reactivity due to other retroviruses, autoantibodies, heterophile antibodies, vaccination (most common) or lab error. Rarely, it is reflective of early primary HIV-1 infection prior to full seroconversion. In the presence of primary infection, antibodies to HIV are usually detectable an average of 3–7 weeks after infection. This is occasionally delayed, though 95% have detectable circulating IgG by 6 months [239].

Quantifying cell-free HIV RNA in plasma is now a critical part of assessing and monitoring disease progression and response to therapy. Current RT-PCR techniques can detect viral loads as low as 50 copies/mL and are thought to shorten the window period of HIV detection to within 2–14 days [240]. New rapid serologic tests have been developed in order to increase routine testing [241]. The CDC has recommended that positive tests with these assays be confirmed (usually via western blot) [242].

19. Human T-Cell Lymphotropic Virus

HTLV-I is a member of the retrovirus family known to infect as many as 20 million people worldwide. HTLV-I is a cause of adult T cell leukemia and lymphoma, as well as HTLV-I-associated myelopathy or tropical spastic paresis [243]. HTLV-II has not been consistently linked to any significant disease process. Similar to HIV in that there is a tropism for CD4-positive T cells, HTLV does not lead to cell death, but rather promotes proliferation and transformation. It is endemic in Japan, Indonesia, the Middle East, and parts of the Caribbean, South America and Africa. Prevalence rates are less than 1% in nonendemic areas such as the United States. Transmission is thought to be primarily through breastfeeding, although spread via blood transfusion, transplantation, and sexual contact are factors in endemic areas.

Diagnostic assays for HTLV are similar to those for HIV. Screening is primarily carried out via EIA assays to detect circulating HTLV-specific antibodies. Confirmation can be done with western blot analysis. Western blot confirmation can also distinguish between HTLV-I and HTLV-II [244]. PCR testing is available to detect proviral DNA in whole blood. Treatment for HTLV infection is usually not indicated for asymptomatic patients. In the setting of adult T cell leukemia, the combination of zidovudine, a nucleoside reverse transcriptase inhibitor, and interferon-α have been used with some possible benefit [245]. Once lymphoma is established, use of non-Hodgkin's lymphoma chemotherapy regimens are moderately successful. Allogeneic HSCT has also been reported [246].

20. Polyomaviruses

The two polyomaviruses known to cause infection in humans include JC virus and BK virus. These are both small, non-enveloped, double-stranded DNA viruses closely related to the papillomaviruses. Both groups of viruses are in the Papovaviridae family. JC and BK virus were each first isolated and described in 1971 [247, 248]. JC virus is the cause of progressive multifocal leucoencephalopathy (PML), a demyelinating disease of the central nervous system. PML is best described in patients with acquired immunodeficiency syndrome (AIDS), though it is rarely seen in solid organ and HSCT recipients, and in other immunosuppressed individuals, including patients with hematologic malignancies and in individuals receiving some forms of immunosuppressive antibody therapies. BK virus is associated with nephropathy and ureteric stenosis in renal transplant recipients and with hemorrhagic cystitis in HSCT recipients.

21. JC Virus

JC virus infection is usually acquired during childhood and is not associated with any known illness during the acute phase. Most adults are seropositive, and PML is related to reactivation of the latent virus during significant periods of immunosuppression [249]. Although it has the strongest association with AIDS, PML was originally described in the setting of lymphoproliferative disorders and is thought to have a low prevalence of 0.07% overall among patients with hematologic malignancies [250]. PML presents as a subacute neurologic disease, affecting multiple systems depending on the location of the CNS lesions. Changes in a patient's mental status, ataxia, and motor deficits involving one or more extremities have been described. Infection of the oligodendrocytes by JC virus leads to demyelination of the white matter and the subsequent neurologic consequences. The disease itself is progressive with a median survival of roughly 6 months in patients with AIDS, and probably less than that in non-HIV infected patients with hematologic malignancies [251].

21.1. Diagnosis

The diagnosis is frequently made based on clinical findings. In patients with HIV infection and AIDS, a compatible magnetic resonance imaging (MRI) scan of the head demonstrating one or more white matter lesions without obvious contrast enhancement or mass effect suggests the diagnosis. Computed tomography (CT) scans tend to be less sensitive than MRI scanning [252]. Confirmation of PML and active JC virus infection is made through use of brain biopsy or JC virus molecular testing in CSF. Demyelination with intranuclear inclusions seen in the oligodendrocytes is typical, with or without necrosis and inflammation. In situ hybridization using JC virus DNA probes can increase the sensitivity and specificity of the biopsy findings [253]. Testing for circulating IgG antibodies is of little diagnostic value due to the ubiquity of infection. Likewise, routine CSF analysis is often unhelpful and may or may not reveal any changes consistent with active inflammation such as elevation of cell counts and protein levels. PCR analysis of CSF for JC virus DNA in immunocompromised patients with a consistent clinical history and radiographic findings is most often used to make the diagnosis. CSF PCR for JC virus has a sensitivity close to 90% and a high specificity [254]. Brian biopsy may be needed in the face of a negative CSF PCR to confirm a diagnosis.

21.2. Therapy

There are no therapies with significant value in treating PML. Reversal of immune deficiency is the main modality of therapy. Cidofovir, which has limited in vitro activity against JC virus, has not shown any benefit in clinical trials of patients with HIV infection and PML [255]. Another agent, cytarabine, with some in vitro activity against JC virus [256], has also not been shown to be of benefit in comparative trials in patients with HIV infection and PML. However, a non-comparative, open-label study evaluating non-HIV infected individuals with PML found that cytarabine dosed at 2 mg/kg IV for 5 days had an association with stabilization of neurological function in 36% of individuals [257]. In AIDS the use of highly active antiretroviral therapy (HAART) has been of benefit in some series.

22. BK Virus

BK virus infection in adults has an estimated prevalence of over 80%. Infection is usually acquired during childhood, and tends to be asymptomatic. The route of transmission remains unclear, though respiratory acquisition is postulated. After primary infection, the virus remains latent in the urogenital epithelium, as well as in some lymphoid tissue and circulating leukocytes. Viral reactivation can occur during periods of immunosuppression.

22.1. Clinical Syndromes

BK virus induces in vitro transformation of rodent cells but does not do so as often in human cells. Definitive evidence of a relationship with oncogenesis in humans has not been proven [258]. BK virus has been implicated as a cause of pneumonia in a patient with AIDS and in at least two patients with underlying hematologic malignancies [259–261]. BK virus has a central role in the development of BK nephropathy (polyomavirus nephropathy or PVAN) and ureteral stenosis in renal transplant recipients [262] and in post-engraftment hemorrhagic cystitis of HSCT recipients [263]. The latter syndrome is increasingly being recognized (often in patients previously thought to have adenovirus infection). Symptoms range from microscopic hematuria to painful and severe hemorrhage, with or without bladder obstruction [263]. These symptoms can be persistent in the neutropenic or immunocompromised individual.

22.2. Diagnosis

Though numerous methods may be available to diagnose BK viral infection (Table 2-24), urine cytology and molecular assays are often used as diagnostic tools for hemorrhagic cystitis after HSCT.

Detection of BK viruria with PCR can correlate with active disease, but is limited somewhat by a lack of specificity. Asymptomatic BK viruria can be documented in other non-renal solid organ transplant recipients, elderly patients not on immunosuppression, HIV-infected patients, pregnant women and otherwise healthy individuals [266–270]. BK viruria is uncommon in general and tends to be lower in quantity than in HSCT recipients with hemorrhagic cystitis [271, 272]. HSCT patients with hemorrhagic cystitis have high level viruria (100,000,000–10,000,000,000 copies/mL), and levels of 10,000,000 copies/mL correlate with risk for hemorrhagic cystitis in this patient population [271]. The pattern of BK viruria is also thought to be of potential significance. In one prospective cohort, some patients who went on to develop hemorrhagic cystitis invariably experienced a peaking of their BK viruria as measured by PCR in the 2–3 week period after HSCT, and before clinical hemorrhagic cystitis [273]. Measurement of plasma with PCR for the presence of BK virus may also show a correlation with the development of hemorrhagic cystitis. Levels greater than 10,000 copies/mL strongly correlated with post-engraftment hemorrhagic cystitis in a case-control study among HSCT recipients [274].

22.3. Therapy

Most clinical strategies for hemorrhagic cystitis in HSCT recipients have not been successful. Reduced immunosuppression through the use of related donors or reduced-intensity conditioning regimens may reduce the risk post-HSCT

Table 2-24. BK virus diagnostics.

Diagnostic test	Description	Comments
Serology	BK virus-specific IgG antibodies in serum	Test not commonly available, evidence of prior exposure
Culture	In vitro	Not commonly available and requires weeks to months [264]
Urine cytology	Detection of "decoy cells," uroepithelial cells shed in the urine with changes consistent with active BK virus infection (enlarged nucleus with a large intranuclear inclusion)	Nonspecific, and these changes can possibly be seen with other viral infections (e.g., adenovirus) or malignancy; highly sensitive for screening.
PCR	Quantitative real-time amplification of polyomavirus-specific DNA sequence from either plasma or urine	Highly sensitive assay limited in specificity (see text); real-time assays distinguish JC and BK virus by analysis of the melting curves [265]
Biopsy with in situ hybridization	Viral changes of uroepithelium with in situ hybridization or immunofluorescence increases sensitivity and specificity	Hemorrhagic cystitis often prevents biopsy; often with thrombocytopenia
Electron microscopy	Electron microscopy of viral particles in urine sediment or biopsy specimens	Not widely available

PCR Polymerase chain reaction

[275]. Other factors may contribute to risk including chemotherapy and irradiation injury to bladder mucosa, thrombocytopenia, neutropenia and co-infection with adenovirus or CMV. Reduction of BK viruria or viremia has not been well correlated with reduced incidence or severity of hemorrhagic cystitis.

In vitro suppression of BK viral replication is possible with some fluoroquinolone antibiotics or related compounds that inhibit DNA gyrase [276, 277]. Other in vitro data have suggested that the selectivity index for fluoroquinolones and the inhibition of BK virus replication is too low to be of any clinically significant value [278]. Well-designed clinical trials are needed to validate these data.

Cidofovir has in vitro inhibitory effects on BK virus [279–281]. It has been used in case reports both systemically and through bladder instillation to treat BK virus-related hemorrhagic cystitis [282, 283]. Use of bladder instillation has not been very effective in patients and systemic therapy has been limited by renal toxicity [283].

Leflunomide is an immunosuppressive agent that inhibits CMV, HSV and BK replication in vitro [284]. It has been used to treat PVAN in small numbers of renal transplant recipients in combination with a reduction in immunosuppression [284, 285]. No studies have described its use in HSCT recipients with hemorrhagic cystitis.

References

1. Schillinger JA, Xu F, Sternberg MR et al (2004) National seroprevalence and trends in herpes simplex virus type 1 in the United States, 1976–1994. Sex Transm Dis 31(12):753–60
2. Xu F, Sternberg MR, Kottiri BJ et al (2006) Trends in herpes simplex virus type 1 and type 2 seroprevalence in the United States. JAMA 296(8):964–73
3. Herget GW, Riede UN, Schmitt-Graff A, Lubbert M, Neumann-Haefelin D, Kohler G (2005) Generalized herpes simplex virus infection in an immunocompromised patient – report of a case and review of the literature. Pathol Res Pract 201(2):123–9
4. Roubalova K, Suchankova A, Vitek A, Sajdova J (2000) Presence of herpes simplex virus (HSV) in peripheral leukocytes of patient who developed active HSV infection after bone marrow transplantation. J Clin Virol 17(1):37–42
5. Kaufman B, Gandhi SA, Louie E, Rizzi R, Illei P (1997) Herpes simplex virus hepatitis: case report and review. Clin Infect Dis 24(3):334–8
6. Taplitz RA, Jordan MC (2002) Pneumonia caused by herpesviruses in recipients of hematopoietic cell transplants. Semin Respir Infect 17(2):121–9
7. Jacome DE, Yanez GF (1980) Herpes genitalis and neurogenic bladder and bowel. J Urol 124(5):752
8. Shturman-Ellstein R, Borkowsky W, Fish I, Gershon AA (1976) Myelitis associated with genital herpes in a child. J Pediatr 88(3):523
9. Gonen C, Uner A, Cetinkaya Y, Hascelik G, Haznedaroglu I (2006) Tonsillar abscess formation due to herpes simplex type-1 in a severely immunocompromised stem cell transplant patient with chronic myeloid leukemia. Transpl Infect Dis 8(3):166–70
10. Higgins JP, Warnke RA (1999) Herpes lymphadenitis in association with chronic lymphocytic leukemia. Cancer 86(7):1210–5
11. Mercadal S, Martinez A, Nomdedeu B et al (2006) Herpes simplex and Epstein-Barr virus lymphadenitis in a patient with chronic lymphocytic leukemia treated with fludarabine. Eur J Haematol 77(5):442–4

12. Iwamasa T, Utsumi Y, Sakuda H et al (1989) Two cases of necrotizing myelopathy associated with malignancy caused by herpes simplex virus type 2. Acta Neuropathol (Berl) 78(3):252–7
13. Lakeman FD, Whitley RJ (1995) Diagnosis of herpes simplex encephalitis: application of polymerase chain reaction to cerebrospinal fluid from brain-biopsied patients and correlation with disease. National Institute of Allergy and Infectious Diseases Collaborative Antiviral Study Group. J Infect Dis 171(4):857–63
14. Kennedy PG (2005) Viral encephalitis. J Neurol 252(3):268–72
15. Gargiulo F, De Francesco MA, Nascimbeni G et al (2003) Polymerase chain reaction as a rapid diagnostic tool for therapy of acute retinal necrosis syndrome. J Med Virol 69(3):397–400
16. Skoldenberg B, Forsgren M, Alestig K et al (1984) Acyclovir versus vidarabine in herpes simplex encephalitis. Randomised multicentre study in consecutive Swedish patients. Lancet 2(8405):707–11
17. Whitley RJ, Alford CA, Hirsch MS et al (1986) Vidarabine versus acyclovir therapy in herpes simplex encephalitis. N Engl J Med 314(3):144–9
18. VanLandingham KE, Marsteller HB, Ross GW, Hayden FG (1988) Relapse of herpes simplex encephalitis after conventional acyclovir therapy. JAMA 259(7):1051–3
19. Valencia I, Miles DK, Melvin J et al (2004) Relapse of herpes encephalitis after acyclovir therapy: report of two new cases and review of the literature. Neuropediatrics 35(6):371–6
20. (2005) Drugs for non-HIV viral infections. Treat Guidel Med Lett 3(32):23–32
21. Eisen D, Essell J, Broun ER, Sigmund D, DeVoe M (2003) Clinical utility of oral valacyclovir compared with oral acyclovir for the prevention of herpes simplex virus mucositis following autologous bone marrow transplantation or stem cell rescue therapy. Bone Marrow Transplant 31(1):51–5
22. Liesveld JL, Abboud CN, Ifthikharuddin JJ et al (2002) Oral valacyclovir versus intravenous acyclovir in preventing herpes simplex virus infections in autologous stem cell transplant recipients. Biol Blood Marrow Transplant 8(12):662–5
23. Meyer PA, Seward JF, Jumaan AO, Wharton M (2000) Varicella mortality: trends before vaccine licensure in the United States, 1970–1994. J Infect Dis 182(2):383–90
24. Feldman S, Hughes WT, Daniel CB (1975) Varicella in children with cancer: seventy-seven cases. Pediatrics 56(3):388–97
25. Kilgore PE, Kruszon-Moran D, Seward JF et al (2003) Varicella in Americans from NHANES III: implications for control through routine immunization. J Med Virol 70(Suppl 1):S111–8
26. Heininger U, Seward JF (2006) Varicella. Lancet 368(9544):1365–76
27. Bonhoeffer J, Baer G, Muehleisen B et al (2005) Prospective surveillance of hospitalisations associated with varicella-zoster virus infections in children and adolescents. Eur J Pediatr 164(6):366–70
28. Krah DL (1996) Assays for antibodies to varicella-zoster virus. Infect Dis Clin North Am 10(3):507–27
29. Josephson A, Gombert ME (1988) Airborne transmission of nosocomial varicella from localized zoster. J Infect Dis 158(1):238–41
30. Gregoire SM, van Pesch V, Goffette S, Peeters A, Sindic CJ (2006) Polymerase chain reaction analysis and oligoclonal antibody in the cerebrospinal fluid from 34 patients with varicella-zoster virus infection of the nervous system. J Neurol Neurosurg Psychiatry 77(8):938–42
31. Nagel MA, Forghani B, Mahalingam R et al (2007) The value of detecting anti-VZV IgG antibody in CSF to diagnose VZV vasculopathy. Neurology 68(13):1069–73
32. Quinlivan M, Gershon AA, Steinberg SP, Breuer J (2005) An evaluation of single nucleotide polymorphisms used to differentiate vaccine and wild type strains of varicella-zoster virus. J Med Virol 75(1):174–80
33. (1999) Control CfD. Prevention of Varicella. MMWR Morb Mortal Wkly Rep 48:1–6

34. Garner JS (1996) Guideline for isolation precautions in hospitals. The Hospital Infection Control Practices Advisory Committee. Infect Control Hosp Epidemiol 17(1):53–80
35. Boeckh M, Kim HW, Flowers ME, Meyers JD, Bowden RA (2006) Long-term acyclovir for prevention of varicella zoster virus disease after allogeneic hematopoietic cell transplantation – a randomized double-blind placebo-controlled study. Blood 107(5):1800–5
36. Staras SA, Dollard SC, Radford KW, Flanders WD, Pass RF, Cannon MJ (2006) Seroprevalence of cytomegalovirus infection in the United States, 1988–1994. Clin Infect Dis 43(9):1143–51
37. Spector SA, Hirata KK, Newman TR (1984) Identification of multiple cytomegalovirus strains in homosexual men with acquired immunodeficiency syndrome. J Infect Dis 150(6):953–6
38. Nguyen Q, Estey E, Raad I et al (2001) Cytomegalovirus pneumonia in adults with leukemia: an emerging problem. Clin Infect Dis 32(4):539–45
39. Bigio EH, Haque AK (1989) Disseminated cytomegalovirus infection presenting with acalculous cholecystitis and acute pancreatitis. Arch Pathol Lab Med 113(11):1287–9
40. Zeiser R, Grullich C, Bertz H et al (2004) Late cytomegalovirus polyradiculopathy following haploidentical CD34+-selected hematopoietic stem cell transplantation. Bone Marrow Transplant 33(2):243–5
41. Hernandez-Boluda JC, Lis MJ, Goterris R et al (2005) Guillain-Barre syndrome associated with cytomegalovirus infection after allogeneic hematopoietic stem cell transplantation. Transpl Infect Dis 7(2):93–6
42. Spach DH, Bauwens JE, Myerson D, Mustafa MM, Bowden RA (1993) Cytomegalovirus-induced hemorrhagic cystitis following bone marrow transplantation. Clin Infect Dis 16(1):142–4
43. Tutuncuoglu SO, Yanovich S, Ozdemirli M (2005) CMV-induced hemorrhagic cystitis as a complication of peripheral blood stem cell transplantation: case report. Bone Marrow Transplant 36(3):265–6
44. Nguyen DD, Cao TM, Dugan K, Starcher SA, Fechter RL, Coutre SE (2002) Cytomegalovirus viremia during Campath-1H therapy for relapsed and refractory chronic lymphocytic leukemia and prolymphocytic leukemia. Clin Lymphoma 3(2):105–10
45. Faderl S, Thomas DA, O'Brien S et al (2003) Experience with alemtuzumab plus rituximab in patients with relapsed and refractory lymphoid malignancies. Blood 101(9):3413–5
46. Martin SI, Marty FM, Fiumara K, Treon SP, Gribben JG, Baden LR (2006) Infectious complications associated with alemtuzumab use for lymphoproliferative disorders. Clin Infect Dis 43(1):16–24
47. Zurlo JJ, O'Neill D, Polis MA et al (1993) Lack of clinical utility of cytomegalovirus blood and urine cultures in patients with HIV infection. Ann Intern Med 118(1):12–7
48. Bek B, Boeckh M, Lepenies J et al (1996) High-level sensitivity of quantitative pp 65 cytomegalovirus (CMV) antigenemia assay for diagnosis of CMV disease in AIDS patients and follow-up. J Clin Microbiol 34(2):457–9
49. Brytting M, Xu W, Wahren B, Sundqvist VA (1992) Cytomegalovirus DNA detection in sera from patients with active cytomegalovirus infections. J Clin Microbiol 30(8):1937–41
50. Witt DJ, Kemper M, Stead A et al (2000) Analytical performance and clinical utility of a nucleic acid sequence-based amplification assay for detection of cytomegalovirus infection. J Clin Microbiol 38(11):3994–9
51. Boeckh M, Gallez-Hawkins GM, Myerson D, Zaia JA, Bowden RA (1997) Plasma polymerase chain reaction for cytomegalovirus DNA after allogeneic marrow transplantation: comparison with polymerase chain reaction using peripheral blood leukocytes, pp 65 antigenemia, and viral culture. Transplantation 64(1):108–13

52. Caliendo AM, St George K, Allega J, Bullotta AC, Gilbane L, Rinaldo CR (2002) Distinguishing cytomegalovirus (CMV) infection and disease with CMV nucleic acid assays. J Clin Microbiol 40(5):1581–6
53. Caliendo AM, St George K, Kao SY et al (2000) Comparison of quantitative cytomegalovirus (CMV) PCR in plasma and CMV antigenemia assay: clinical utility of the prototype AMPLICOR CMV MONITOR test in transplant recipients. J Clin Microbiol 38(6):2122–7
54. Biron KK (2006) Antiviral drugs for cytomegalovirus diseases. Antiviral Res 71(2–3):154–63
55. (2000) Guidelines for preventing opportunistic infections among hematopoietic stem cell transplant recipients. Biol Blood Marrow Transplant 6(6a):659–713; 5; 7–27; quiz 29–33
56. Avery RK, Bolwell BJ, Yen-Lieberman B et al (2004) Use of leflunomide in an allogeneic bone marrow transplant recipient with refractory cytomegalovirus infection. Bone Marrow Transplant 34(12):1071–5
57. Cvetkovic RS, Wellington K (2005) Valganciclovir: a review of its use in the management of CMV infection and disease in immunocompromised patients. Drugs 65(6):859–78
58. Foulongne V, Turriere C, Diafouka F, Abraham B, Lastere S, Segondy M (2004) Ganciclovir resistance mutations in UL97 and UL54 genes of Human cytomegalovirus isolates resistant to ganciclovir. Acta Virol 48(1):51–5
59. Boeckh M, Leisenring W, Riddell SR et al (2003) Late cytomegalovirus disease and mortality in recipients of allogeneic hematopoietic stem cell transplants: importance of viral load and T-cell immunity. Blood 101(2):407–14
60. Goodrich JM, Bowden RA, Fisher L, Keller C, Schoch G, Meyers JD (1993) Ganciclovir prophylaxis to prevent cytomegalovirus disease after allogeneic marrow transplant. Ann Intern Med 118(3):173–8
61. Prentice HG, Gluckman E, Powles RL et al (1997) Long-term survival in allogeneic bone marrow transplant recipients following acyclovir prophylaxis for CMV infection. The European Acyclovir for CMV Prophylaxis Study Group. Bone Marrow Transplant 19(2):129–33
62. Ljungman P, de La Camara R, Milpied N et al (2002) Randomized study of valacyclovir as prophylaxis against cytomegalovirus reactivation in recipients of allogeneic bone marrow transplants. Blood 99(8):3050–6
63. Wade JC (2006) Viral infections in patients with hematological malignancies. Hematology Am Soc Hematol Educ Program 368–74
64. Akashi K, Eizuru Y, Sumiyoshi Y et al (1993) Brief report: severe infectious mononucleosis-like syndrome and primary human herpesvirus 6 infection in an adult. N Engl J Med 329(3):168–71
65. Maric I, Bryant R, Abu-Asab M et al (2004) Human herpesvirus-6-associated acute lymphadenitis in immunocompetent adults. Mod Pathol 17(11):1427–33
66. Cone RW, Huang ML, Hackman RC (1994) Human herpesvirus 6 and pneumonia. Leuk Lymphoma 15(3–4):235–41
67. Kuribayashi K, Matsunaga T, Iyama S et al (2006) Human herpesvirus-6 hepatitis associated with cyclosporine-A encephalitis after bone marrow transplantation for chronic myeloid leukemia. Intern Med 45(7):475–8
68. Drobyski WR, Knox KK, Majewski D, Carrigan DR (1994) Brief report: fatal encephalitis due to variant B human herpesvirus-6 infection in a bone marrow-transplant recipient. N Engl J Med 330(19):1356–60
69. Tiacci E, Luppi M, Barozzi P et al (2000) Fatal herpesvirus-6 encephalitis in a recipient of a T-cell-depleted peripheral blood stem cell transplant from a 3-loci mismatched related donor. Haematologica 85(1):94–7
70. Bethge W, Beck R, Jahn G, Mundinger P, Kanz L, Einsele H (1999) Successful treatment of human herpesvirus-6 encephalitis after bone marrow transplantation. Bone Marrow Transplant 24(11):1245–8

71. Drobyski WR, Dunne WM, Burd EM et al (1993) Human herpesvirus-6 (HHV-6) infection in allogeneic bone marrow transplant recipients: evidence of a marrow-suppressive role for HHV-6 in vivo. J Infect Dis 167(3):735–9
72. Hentrich M, Oruzio D, Jager G et al (2005) Impact of human herpesvirus-6 after haematopoietic stem cell transplantation. Br J Haematol 128(1):66–72
73. Ogata M, Kikuchi H, Satou T et al (2006) Human herpesvirus 6 DNA in plasma after allogeneic stem cell transplantation: incidence and clinical significance. J Infect Dis 193(1):68–79
74. Chan PK, Chik KW, To KF et al (2002) Case report: human herpesvirus 7 associated fatal encephalitis in a peripheral blood stem cell transplant recipient. J Med Virol 66(4):493–6
75. Ward KN, White RP, Mackinnon S, Hanna M (2002) Human herpesvirus-7 infection of the CNS with acute myelitis in an adult bone marrow recipient. Bone Marrow Transplant 30(12):983–5
76. Yoshikawa T, Yoshida J, Hamaguchi M et al (2003) Human herpesvirus 7-associated meningitis and optic neuritis in a patient after allogeneic stem cell transplantation. J Med Virol 70(3):440–3
77. Maeda Y, Teshima T, Yamada M et al (1999) Monitoring of human herpesviruses after allogeneic peripheral blood stem cell transplantation and bone marrow transplantation. Br J Haematol 105(1):295–302
78. Suga S, Yoshikawa T, Asano Y et al (1992) IgM neutralizing antibody responses to human herpesvirus-6 in patients with exanthem subitum or organ transplantation. Microbiol Immunol 36(5):495–506
79. Ward KN, Couto Parada X, Passas J, Thiruchelvam AD (2002) Evaluation of the specificity and sensitivity of indirect immunofluorescence tests for IgG to human herpesviruses-6 and -7. J Virol Methods 106(1):107–13
80. Birnbaum T, Padovan CS, Sporer B et al (2005) Severe meningoencephalitis caused by human herpesvirus 6 type B in an immunocompetent woman treated with ganciclovir. Clin Infect Dis 40(6):887–9
81. De Bolle L, Manichanh C, Agut H, De Clercq E, Naesens L (2004) Human herpesvirus 6 DNA polymerase: enzymatic parameters, sensitivity to ganciclovir and determination of the role of the A961V mutation in HHV-6 ganciclovir resistance. Antiviral Res 64(1):17–25
82. Black JB, Burns DA, Goldsmith CS et al (1997) Biologic properties of human herpesvirus 7 strain SB. Virus Res 52(1):25–41
83. Zhang Y, Schols D, De Clercq E (1999) Selective activity of various antiviral compounds against HHV-7 infection. Antiviral Res 43(1):23–35
84. Epstein MA, Achong BG, Barr YM (1964) Virus particles in cultured lymphoblasts from Burkitt's lymphoma. Lancet 15:702–3
85. Volpi A (2004) Epstein-Barr virus and human herpesvirus type 8 infections of the central nervous system. Herpes 11(Suppl 2):120A–7A
86. Gruhn B, Meerbach A, Egerer R et al (1999) Successful treatment of Epstein Barr virus-induced transverse myelitis with ganciclovir and cytomegalovirus hyperimmune globulin following unrelated bone marrow transplantation. Bone Marrow Transplant 24(12):1355–8
87. Corssmit EP, Leverstein-van Hall MA, Portegies P, Bakker P (1997) Severe neurological complications in association with Epstein-Barr virus infection. J Neurovirol 3(6):460–4
88. Mueller GA, Pickoff AS (2003) Pediatric lymphocytic interstitial pneumonitis in an HIV-negative child with pulmonary Epstein-Barr virus infection. Pediatr Pulmonol 36(5):447–9
89. Fujiwara M, Shimozono H, Ono H et al (2003) Polyclonal proliferation of lymphocytes containing the epstein-barr virus genome in a patient dying of myocarditis in chronic active Epstein-Barr virus infection. J Pediatr Hematol Oncol 25(1):85–8

90. Epstein JB, Sherlock CH, Greenspan JS (1991) Hairy leukoplakia-like lesions following bone-marrow transplantation. AIDS 5(1):101–2
91. Linderholm M, Boman J, Juto P, Linde A (1994) Comparative evaluation of nine kits for rapid diagnosis of infectious mononucleosis and Epstein-Barr virus-specific serology. J Clin Microbiol 32(1):259–61
92. Klutts JS, Liao RS, Dunne WM Jr, Gronowski AM (2004) Evaluation of a multiplexed bead assay for assessment of Epstein-Barr virus immunologic status. J Clin Microbiol 42(11):4996–5000
93. Carpentier L, Tapiero B, Alvarez F, Viau C, Alfieri C (2003) Epstein-Barr virus (EBV) early-antigen serologic testing in conjunction with peripheral blood EBV DNA load as a marker for risk of posttransplantation lymphoproliferative disease. J Infect Dis 188(12):1853–64
94. van Esser JW, Niesters HG, van der Holt B et al (2002) Prevention of Epstein-Barr virus-lymphoproliferative disease by molecular monitoring and preemptive rituximab in high-risk patients after allogeneic stem cell transplantation. Blood 99(12):4364–9
95. Niedobitek G, Herbst H (2006) In situ detection of Epstein-Barr virus and phenotype determination of EBV-infected cells. Methods Mol Biol 326:115–37
96. Gershburg E, Pagano JS (2005) Epstein-Barr virus infections: prospects for treatment. J Antimicrob Chemother 56(2):277–81
97. Paya CV, Fung JJ, Nalesnik MA et al (1999) Epstein-Barr virus-induced posttransplant lymphoproliferative disorders. ASTS/ASTP EBV-PTLD Task Force and The Mayo Clinic Organized International Consensus Development Meeting. Transplantation 68(10):1517–25
98. Kalil AC, Levitsky J, Lyden E, Stoner J, Freifeld AG (2005) Meta-analysis: the efficacy of strategies to prevent organ disease by cytomegalovirus in solid organ transplant recipients. Ann Intern Med 143(12):870–80
99. Mentzer SJ, Perrine SP, Faller DV (2001) Epstein-Barr virus post-transplant lymphoproliferative disease and virus-specific therapy: pharmacological reactivation of viral target genes with arginine butyrate. Transpl Infect Dis 3(3):177–85
100. Faller DV, Mentzer SJ, Perrine SP (2001) Induction of the Epstein-Barr virus thymidine kinase gene with concomitant nucleoside antivirals as a therapeutic strategy for Epstein-Barr virus-associated malignancies. Curr Opin Oncol 13(5):360–7
101. Roychowdhury S, Peng R, Baiocchi RA et al (2003) Experimental treatment of Epstein-Barr virus-associated primary central nervous system lymphoma. Cancer Res 63(5):965–71
102. Gershburg E, Hong K, Pagano JS (2004) Effects of maribavir and selected indolocarbazoles on Epstein-Barr virus protein kinase BGLF4 and on viral lytic replication. Antimicrob Agents Chemother 48(5):1900–3
103. Preiksaitis JK (2004) New developments in the diagnosis and management of posttransplantation lymphoproliferative disorders in solid organ transplant recipients. Clin Infect Dis 39(7):1016–23
104. Weinstock DM, Ambrossi GG, Brennan C, Kiehn TE, Jakubowski A (2006) Preemptive diagnosis and treatment of Epstein-Barr virus-associated post transplant lymphoproliferative disorder after hematopoietic stem cell transplant: an approach in development. Bone Marrow Transplant 37(6):539–46
105. Chang Y, Cesarman E, Pessin MS et al (1994) Identification of herpesvirus-like DNA sequences in AIDS-associated Kaposi's sarcoma. Science 266(5192):1865–9
106. Rimar D, Rimar Y, Keynan Y (2006) Human herpesvirus-8: beyond Kaposi's. Isr Med Assoc J 8(7):489–93
107. Dukers NH, Rezza G (2003) Human herpesvirus 8 epidemiology: what we do and do not know. AIDS 17(12):1717–30

108. Blackbourn DJ, Osmond D, Levy JA, Lennette ET (1999) Increased human herpesvirus 8 seroprevalence in young homosexual men who have multiple sex contacts with different partners. J Infect Dis 179(1):237–9
109. Tsai WH, Lee YM, Ing-Tiau Kuo B et al (2005) Increased seroprevalence of human herpesvirus 8 in patients with hematological disorders. Acta Haematol 114(2):95–8
110. Luppi M, Barozzi P, Schulz TF et al (2000) Nonmalignant disease associated with human herpesvirus 8 reactivation in patients who have undergone autologous peripheral blood stem cell transplantation. Blood 96(7):2355–7
111. Luppi M, Barozzi P, Schulz TF et al (2000) Bone marrow failure associated with human herpesvirus 8 infection after transplantation. N Engl J Med 343(19):1378–85
112. Luppi M, Barozzi P, Rasini V et al (2002) Severe pancytopenia and hemophagocytosis after HHV-8 primary infection in a renal transplant patient successfully treated with foscarnet. Transplantation 74(1):131–2
113. Fardet L, Blum L, Kerob D et al (2003) Human herpesvirus 8-associated hemophagocytic lymphohistiocytosis in human immunodeficiency virus-infected patients. Clin Infect Dis 37(2):285–91
114. Sanchez-Velasco P, Ocejo-Vinyals JG, Flores R, Gomez-Roman JJ, Lozano MJ, Leyva-Cobian F (2001) Simultaneous multiorgan presence of human herpesvirus 8 and restricted lymphotropism of Epstein-Barr virus DNA sequences in a human immunodeficiency virus-negative immunodeficient infant. J Infect Dis 183(2):338–42
115. Edelman DC (2005) Human herpesvirus 8 – a novel human pathogen. Virol J 2:78
116. Simpson GR, Schulz TF, Whitby D et al (1996) Prevalence of Kaposi's sarcoma associated herpesvirus infection measured by antibodies to recombinant capsid protein and latent immunofluorescence antigen. Lancet 348(9035):1133–8
117. LaDuca JR, Love JL, Abbott LZ, Dube S, Freidman-Kien AE, Poiesz BJ (1998) Detection of human herpesvirus 8 DNA sequences in tissues and bodily fluids. J Infect Dis 178(6):1610–5
118. Kedes DH, Ganem D (1997) Sensitivity of Kaposi's sarcoma-associated herpesvirus replication to antiviral drugs. Implications for potential therapy. J Clin Invest 99(9):2082–6
119. Dagna L, Broccolo F, Paties CT et al (2005) A relapsing inflammatory syndrome and active human herpesvirus 8 infection. N Engl J Med 353(2):156–63
120. Simonart T, Noel JC, De Dobbeleer G et al (1998) Treatment of classical Kaposi's sarcoma with intralesional injections of cidofovir: report of a case. J Med Virol 55(3):215–8
121. Boulanger E, Gerard L, Gabarre J et al (2005) Prognostic factors and outcome of human herpesvirus 8-associated primary effusion lymphoma in patients with AIDS. J Clin Oncol 23(19):4372–80
122. Klass CM, Offermann MK (2005) Targeting human herpesvirus-8 for treatment of Kaposi's sarcoma and primary effusion lymphoma. Curr Opin Oncol 17(5):447–55
123. Deichmann M, Thome M, Jackel A et al (1998) Non-human immunodeficiency virus Kaposi's sarcoma can be effectively treated with low-dose interferon-alpha despite the persistence of herpesvirus-8. Br J Dermatol 139(6):1052–4
124. Erdman DD, Xu W, Gerber SI et al (2002) Molecular epidemiology of adenovirus type 7 in the United States, 1966–2000. Emerg Infect Dis 8(3):269–77
125. Echavarria M, Sanchez JL, Kolavic-Gray SA et al (2003) Rapid detection of adenovirus in throat swab specimens by PCR during respiratory disease outbreaks among military recruits. J Clin Microbiol 41(2):810–2
126. Hierholzer JC (1992) Adenoviruses in the immunocompromised host. Clin Microbiol Rev 5(3):262–74
127. Wang WH, Wang HL (2003) Fulminant adenovirus hepatitis following bone marrow transplantation. A case report and brief review of the literature. Arch Pathol Lab Med 127(5):e246–8

128. Bruno B, Zager RA, Boeckh MJ et al (2004) Adenovirus nephritis in hematopoietic stem-cell transplantation. Transplantation 77(7):1049–57
129. Simila S, Jouppila R, Salmi A, Pohjonen R (1970) Encephaloningitis in children associated with an adenovirus type 7 epidemic. Acta Paediatr Scand 59(3):310–6
130. Runde V, Ross S, Trenschel R et al (2001) Adenoviral infection after allogeneic stem cell transplantation (SCT): report on 130 patients from a single SCT unit involved in a prospective multi center surveillance study. Bone Marrow Transplant 28(1):51–7
131. La Rosa AM, Champlin RE, Mirza N et al (2001) Adenovirus infections in adult recipients of blood and marrow transplants. Clin Infect Dis 32(6):871–6
132. Lion T, Baumgartinger R, Watzinger F et al (2003) Molecular monitoring of adenovirus in peripheral blood after allogeneic bone marrow transplantation permits early diagnosis of disseminated disease. Blood 102(3):1114–20
133. Wiley LA, Roba LA, Kowalski RP, Romanowski EG, Gordon YJ (1996) A 5-year evaluation of the adenoclone test for the rapid diagnosis of adenovirus from conjunctival swabs. Cornea 15(4):363–7
134. Shetty AK, Treynor E, Hill DW, Gutierrez KM, Warford A, Baron EJ (2003) Comparison of conventional viral cultures with direct fluorescent antibody stains for diagnosis of community-acquired respiratory virus infections in hospitalized children. Pediatr Infect Dis J 22(9):789–94
135. Bordigoni P, Carret AS, Venard V, Witz F, Le Faou A (2001) Treatment of adenovirus infections in patients undergoing allogeneic hematopoietic stem cell transplantation. Clin Infect Dis 32(9):1290–7
136. Legrand F, Berrebi D, Houhou N et al (2001) Early diagnosis of adenovirus infection and treatment with cidofovir after bone marrow transplantation in children. Bone Marrow Transplant 27(6):621–6
137. Hoffman JA, Shah AJ, Ross LA, Kapoor N (2001) Adenoviral infections and a prospective trial of cidofovir in pediatric hematopoietic stem cell transplantation. Biol Blood Marrow Transplant 7(7):388–94
138. Ljungman P, Ribaud P, Eyrich M et al (2003) Cidofovir for adenovirus infections after allogeneic hematopoietic stem cell transplantation: a survey by the Infectious Diseases Working Party of the European Group for Blood and Marrow Transplantation. Bone Marrow Transplant 31(6):481–6
139. Leruez-Ville M, Minard V, Lacaille F et al (2004) Real-time blood plasma polymerase chain reaction for management of disseminated adenovirus infection. Clin Infect Dis 38(1):45–52
140. Yusuf U, Hale GA, Carr J et al (2006) Cidofovir for the treatment of adenoviral infection in pediatric hematopoietic stem cell transplant patients. Transplantation 81(10):1398–404
141. Chakrabarti S, Mautner V, Osman H et al (2002) Adenovirus infections following allogeneic stem cell transplantation: incidence and outcome in relation to graft manipulation, immunosuppression, and immune recovery. Blood 100(5):1619–27
142. Hromas R, Cornetta K, Srour E, Blanke C, Broun ER (1994) Donor leukocyte infusion as therapy of life-threatening adenoviral infections after T-cell-depleted bone marrow transplantation. Blood 84(5):1689–90
143. Bruno B, Gooley T, Hackman RC, Davis C, Corey L, Boeckh M (2003) Adenovirus infection in hematopoietic stem cell transplantation: effect of ganciclovir and impact on survival. Biol Blood Marrow Transplant 9(5):341–52
144. Emovon OE, Lin A, Howell DN et al (2003) Refractory adenovirus infection after simultaneous kidney-pancreas transplantation: successful treatment with intravenous ribavirin and pooled human intravenous immunoglobulin. Nephrol Dial Transplant 18(11):2436–8
145. Flomenberg P, Babbitt J, Drobyski WR et al (1994) Increasing incidence of adenovirus disease in bone marrow transplant recipients. J Infect Dis 169(4):775–81

146. Potter CW, Phair JP, Vodinelich L, Fenton R, Jennings R (1976) Antiviral, immunosuppressive and antitumour effects of ribavirin. Nature 259(5543):496–7
147. Miyamura K, Hamaguchi M, Taji H et al (2000) Successful ribavirin therapy for severe adenovirus hemorrhagic cystitis after allogeneic marrow transplant from close HLA donors rather than distant donors. Bone Marrow Transplant 25(5):545–8
148. Vianelli N, Renga M, Azzi A et al (2000) Sequential vidarabine infusion in the treatment of polyoma virus-associated acute haemorrhagic cystitis late after allogeneic bone marrow transplantation. Bone Marrow Transplant 25(3):319–20
149. Mentel R, Kinder M, Wegner U, von Janta-Lipinski M, Matthes E (1997) Inhibitory activity of 3′-fluoro-2′ deoxythymidine and related nucleoside analogues against adenoviruses in vitro. Antiviral Res 34(3):113–9
150. Mentel R, Wegner U (2000) Evaluation of the efficacy of 2′, 3′-dideoxycytidine against adenovirus infection in a mouse pneumonia model. Antiviral Res 47(2): 79–87
151. Falsey AR, Walsh EE (2000) Respiratory syncytial virus infection in adults. Clin Microbiol Rev 13(3):371–84
152. Walsh EE, McConnochie KM, Long CE, Hall CB (1997) Severity of respiratory syncytial virus infection is related to virus strain. J Infect Dis 175(4):814–20
153. Champlin RE, Whimbey E (2001) Community respiratory virus infections in bone marrow transplant recipients: the M.D. Anderson Cancer Center experience. Biol Blood Marrow Transplant 7(Suppl):8S–10S
154. Simonsen L (1999) The global impact of influenza on morbidity and mortality. Vaccine 17(Suppl 1):S3–10
155. Fujimoto S, Kobayashi M, Uemura O et al (1998) PCR on cerebrospinal fluid to show influenza-associated acute encephalopathy or encephalitis. Lancet 352(9131):873–5
156. Rodriguez WJ, Schwartz RH, Thorne MM (2002) Evaluation of diagnostic tests for influenza in a pediatric practice. Pediatr Infect Dis J 21(3):193–6
157. Frank AL, Couch RB, Griffis CA, Baxter BD (1979) Comparison of different tissue cultures for isolation and quantitation of influenza and parainfluenza viruses. J Clin Microbiol 10(1):32–6
158. Hu A, Colella M, Zhao P et al (2005) Development of a real-time RT-PCR assay for detection and quantitation of parainfluenza virus 3. J Virol Methods 130(1–2): 145–8
159. van Elden LJ, van Kraaij MG, Nijhuis M et al (2002) Polymerase chain reaction is more sensitive than viral culture and antigen testing for the detection of respiratory viruses in adults with hematological cancer and pneumonia. Clin Infect Dis 34(2):177–83
160. Peck AJ, Corey L, Boeckh M (2004) Pretransplantation respiratory syncytial virus infection: impact of a strategy to delay transplantation. Clin Infect Dis 39(5):673–80
161. Gilbert BE, Wilson SZ, Knight V et al (1985) Ribavirin small-particle aerosol treatment of infections caused by influenza virus strains A/Victoria/7/83 (H1N1) and B/Texas/1/84. Antimicrob Agents Chemother 27(3):309–13
162. Sparrelid E, Ljungman P, Ekelof-Andstrom E et al (1997) Ribavirin therapy in bone marrow transplant recipients with viral respiratory tract infections. Bone Marrow Transplant 19(9):905–8
163. Nichols WG, Corey L, Gooley T, Davis C, Boeckh M (2001) Parainfluenza virus infections after hematopoietic stem cell transplantation: risk factors, response to antiviral therapy, and effect on transplant outcome. Blood 98(3):573–8
164. McColl MD, Corser RB, Bremner J, Chopra R (1998) Respiratory syncytial virus infection in adult BMT recipients: effective therapy with short duration nebulised ribavirin. Bone Marrow Transplant 21(4):423–5
165. Nichols WG, Guthrie KA, Corey L, Boeckh M (2004) Influenza infections after hematopoietic stem cell transplantation: risk factors, mortality, and the effect of antiviral therapy. Clin Infect Dis 39(9):1300–6

166. Belshe RB, Nichol KL, Black SB et al (2004) Safety, efficacy, and effectiveness of live, attenuated, cold-adapted influenza vaccine in an indicated population aged 5-49 years. Clin Infect Dis 39(7):920–7
167. Harper SA, Fukuda K, Uyeki TM, Cox NJ, Bridges CB (2005) Prevention and control of influenza. Recommendations of the Advisory Committee on Immunization Practices (ACIP). MMWR Recomm Rep 54(RR-8):1–40
168. Nichols WG, Gooley T, Boeckh M (2001) Community-acquired respiratory syncytial virus and parainfluenza virus infections after hematopoietic stem cell transplantation: the Fred Hutchinson Cancer Research Center experience. Biol Blood Marrow Transplant 7(Suppl):11S–5S
169. Boeckh M, Berrey MM, Bowden RA, Crawford SW, Balsley J, Corey L (2001) Phase 1 evaluation of the respiratory syncytial virus-specific monoclonal antibody palivizumab in recipients of hematopoietic stem cell transplants. J Infect Dis 184(3):350–4
170. Banna GL, Aversa SM, Cattelan AM, Crivellari G, Monfardini S (2004) Respiratory syncytial virus-related pneumonia after stem cell transplantation successfully treated with palivizumab and steroid therapy. Scand J Infect Dis 36(2):155–7
171. van den Hoogen BG, de Jong JC, Groen J et al (2001) A newly discovered human pneumovirus isolated from young children with respiratory tract disease. Nat Med 7(6):719–24
172. Williams JV, Harris PA, Tollefson SJ et al (2004) Human metapneumovirus and lower respiratory tract disease in otherwise healthy infants and children. N Engl J Med 350(5):443–50
173. McIntosh K, McAdam AJ (2004) Human metapneumovirus – an important new respiratory virus. N Engl J Med 350(5):431–3
174. Englund JA, Boeckh M, Kuypers J et al (2006) Brief communication: fatal human metapneumovirus infection in stem-cell transplant recipients. Ann Intern Med 144(5):344–9
175. Debiaggi M, Canducci F, Sampaolo M et al (2006) Persistent symptomless human metapneumovirus infection in hematopoietic stem cell transplant recipients. J Infect Dis 194(4):474–8
176. Wyde PR, Chetty SN, Jewell AM, Boivin G, Piedra PA (2003) Comparison of the inhibition of human metapneumovirus and respiratory syncytial virus by ribavirin and immune serum globulin in vitro. Antiviral Res 60(1):51–9
177. Hamelin ME, Prince GA, Boivin G (2006) Effect of ribavirin and glucocorticoid treatment in a mouse model of human metapneumovirus infection. Antimicrob Agents Chemother 50(2):774–7
178. Imakita M, Shiraki K, Yutani C, Ishibashi-Ueda H (2000) Pneumonia caused by rhinovirus. Clin Infect Dis 30(3):611–2
179. Papadopoulos NG, Bates PJ, Bardin PG et al (2000) Rhinoviruses infect the lower airways. J Infect Dis 181(6):1875–84
180. Ison MG, Hayden FG, Kaiser L, Corey L, Boeckh M (2003) Rhinovirus infections in hematopoietic stem cell transplant recipients with pneumonia. Clin Infect Dis 36(9):1139–43
181. Ghosh S, Champlin R, Couch R et al (1999) Rhinovirus infections in myelosuppressed adult blood and marrow transplant recipients. Clin Infect Dis 29(3):528–32
182. van Tilburg CM, Sanders EA, Rovers MM, Wolfs TF, Bierings MB (2006) Loss of antibodies and response to (re-)vaccination in children after treatment for acute lymphocytic leukemia: a systematic review. Leukemia 20(10):1717–22
183. Kaplan LJ, Daum RS, Smaron M, McCarthy CA (1992) Severe measles in immunocompromised patients. JAMA 267(9):1237–41
184. Hussey GD, Klein M (1990) A randomized, controlled trial of vitamin A in children with severe measles. N Engl J Med 323(3):160–4

185. Forni AL, Schluger NW, Roberts RB (1994) Severe measles pneumonitis in adults: evaluation of clinical characteristics and therapy with intravenous ribavirin. Clin Infect Dis 19(3):454–62
186. (2006) Brief report: update: mumps activity – United States, January 1-October 7, 2006. MMWR Morb Mortal Wkly Rep 55(42):1152–1153
187. (2005) Elimination of rubella and congenital rubella syndrome – United States, 1969-2004. MMWR Morb Mortal Wkly Rep 54(11):279–282
188. McKinney RE Jr, Katz SL, Wilfert CM (1987) Chronic enteroviral meningoencephalitis in agammaglobulinemic patients. Rev Infect Dis 9(2):334–56
189. Tan PL, Verneris MR, Charnas LR, Reck SJ, van Burik JA, Blazar BR (2005) Outcome of CNS and pulmonary enteroviral infections after hematopoietic cell transplantation. Pediatr Blood Cancer 45(1):74–5
190. Galama JM, de Leeuw N, Wittebol S, Peters H, Melchers WJ (1996) Prolonged enteroviral infection in a patient who developed pericarditis and heart failure after bone marrow transplantation. Clin Infect Dis 22(6):1004–8
191. Yolken RH, Bishop CA, Townsend TR et al (1982) Infectious gastroenteritis in bone-marrow-transplant recipients. N Engl J Med 306(17):1010–2
192. Biggs DD, Toorkey BC, Carrigan DR, Hanson GA, Ash RC (1990) Disseminated echovirus infection complicating bone marrow transplantation. Am J Med 88(4):421–5
193. Troussard X, Bauduer F, Gallet E et al (1993) Virus recovery from stools of patients undergoing bone marrow transplantation. Bone Marrow Transplant 12(6):573–6
194. Gonzalez Y, Martino R, Badell I et al (1999) Pulmonary enterovirus infections in stem cell transplant recipients. Bone Marrow Transplant 23(5):511–3
195. Fischmeister G, Wiesbauer P, Holzmann HM, Peters C, Eibl M, Gadner H (2000) Enteroviral meningoencephalitis in immunocompromised children after matched unrelated donor-bone marrow transplantation. Pediatr Hematol Oncol 17(5):393–9
196. Chakrabarti S, Osman H, Collingham KE, Fegan CD, Milligan DW (2004) Enterovirus infections following T-cell depleted allogeneic transplants in adults. Bone Marrow Transplant 33(4):425–30
197. Dagan R, Powell KR, Hall CB, Menegus MA (1985) Identification of infants unlikely to have serious bacterial infection although hospitalized for suspected sepsis. J Pediatr 107(6):855–60
198. Gelfand HM, Holguin AH, Marchetti GE, Feorino PM (1963) A continuing surveillance of enterovirus infections in healthy children in six United States cities. I. Viruses isolated during 1960 and 1961. Am J Hyg 78:358–75
199. Kogon A, Spigland I, Frothingham TE et al (1969) The virus watch program: a continuing surveillance of viral infections in metropolitan New York families. VII. Observations on viral excretion, seroimmunity, intrafamilial spread and illness association in coxsackie and echovirus infections. Am J Epidemiol 89(1):51–61
200. Sawyer MH, Holland D, Aintablian N, Connor JD, Keyser EF, Waecker NJ Jr (1994) Diagnosis of enteroviral central nervous system infection by polymerase chain reaction during a large community outbreak. Pediatr Infect Dis J 13(3): 177–82
201. Drucker NA, Colan SD, Lewis AB et al (1994) Gamma-globulin treatment of acute myocarditis in the pediatric population. Circulation 89(1):252–7
202. Galama JM, Vogels MT, Jansen GH, Gielen M, Heessen FW (1997) Antibodies against enteroviruses in intravenous Ig preparations: great variation in titres and poor correlation with the incidence of circulating serotypes. J Med Virol 53(3):273–6
203. Romero JR (2001) Pleconaril: a novel antipicornaviral drug. Expert Opin Investig Drugs 10(2):369–79
204. Desmond RA, Accortt NA, Talley L, Villano SA, Soong SJ, Whitley RJ (2006) Enteroviral meningitis: natural history and outcome of pleconaril therapy. Antimicrob Agents Chemother 50(7):2409–14

205. Engelhard D, Handsher R, Naparstek E et al (1991) Immune response to polio vaccination in bone marrow transplant recipients. Bone Marrow Transplant 8(4):295–300
206. Ljungman P, Duraj V, Magnius L (1991) Response to immunization against polio after allogeneic marrow transplantation. Bone Marrow Transplant 7(2):89–93
207. (2000) Guidelines for preventing opportunistic infections among hematopoietic stem cell transplant recipients. MMWR Recomm Rep 49(RR-10):1–125, CE1–CE7
208. Alexander LN, Seward JF, Santibanez TA et al (2004) Vaccine policy changes and epidemiology of poliomyelitis in the United States. JAMA 292(14):1696–701
209. Godoi ER, de Souza VA, Cakmak S, Machado AF, Vilas Boas LS, Machado CM (2006) Loss of hepatitis A virus antibodies after bone marrow transplantation. Bone Marrow Transplant 38(1):37–40
210. Brundage SC, Fitzpatrick AN (2006) Hepatitis A. Am Fam Physician 73(12):2162–8
211. Kemmer NM, Miskovsky EP (2000) Hepatitis A. Infect Dis Clin North Am 14(3):605–15
212. Ljungman P, Engelhard D, de la Camara R et al (2005) Vaccination of stem cell transplant recipients: recommendations of the Infectious Diseases Working Party of the EBMT. Bone Marrow Transplant 35(8):737–46
213. Strasser SI, McDonald GB (1999) Hepatitis viruses and hematopoietic cell transplantation: a guide to patient and donor management. Blood 93(4):1127–36
214. (2004) Incidence of acute hepatitis B – United States, 1990-2002. MMWR Morb Mortal Wkly Rep 52(51–52):1252–1254
215. Lau GK, Liang R, Chiu EK, Lee CK, Lam SK (1997) Hepatic events after bone marrow transplantation in patients with hepatitis B infection: a case controlled study. Bone Marrow Transplant 19(8):795–9
216. Lee WM (1993) Acute liver failure. N Engl J Med 329(25):1862–72
217. Biswas R, Tabor E, Hsia CC et al (2003) Comparative sensitivity of HBV NATs and HBsAg assays for detection of acute HBV infection. Transfusion 43(6):788–98
218. Gandhi RT, Wurcel A, Lee H et al (2003) Isolated antibody to hepatitis B core antigen in human immunodeficiency virus type-1-infected individuals. Clin Infect Dis 36(12):1602–5
219. Gish RG, Locarnini SA (2006) Chronic hepatitis B: current testing strategies. Clin Gastroenterol Hepatol 4(6):666–76
220. Hatzakis A, Magiorkinis E, Haida C (2006) HBV virological assessment. J Hepatol 44(1 Suppl):S71–6
221. Keeffe EB, Marcellin P (2007) New and emerging treatment of chronic hepatitis B. Clin Gastroenterol Hepatol 5(3):285–94
222. Benhamou Y (2006) Treatment algorithm for chronic hepatitis B in HIV-infected patients. J Hepatol 44(1 Suppl):S90–4
223. Idilman R, Ustun C, Karayalcin S et al (2003) Hepatitis B virus vaccination of recipients and donors of allogeneic peripheral blood stem cell transplantation. Clin Transplant 17(5):438–43
224. Peffault de Latour R, Levy V, Asselah T et al (2004) Long-term outcome of hepatitis C infection after bone marrow transplantation. Blood 103(5):1618–24
225. Strasser SI, Myerson D, Spurgeon CL et al (1999) Hepatitis C virus infection and bone marrow transplantation: a cohort study with 10-year follow-up. Hepatology 29(6):1893–9
226. Alter HJ (1992) New kit on the block: evaluation of second-generation assays for detection of antibody to the hepatitis C virus. Hepatology 15(2):350–3
227. Kao JH, Lai MY, Hwang YT et al (1996) Chronic hepatitis C without anti-hepatitis C antibodies by second-generation assay. A clinicopathologic study and demonstration of the usefulness of a third-generation assay. Dig Dis Sci 41(1):161–5
228. Uyttendaele S, Claeys H, Mertens W, Verhaert H, Vermylen C (1994) Evaluation of third-generation screening and confirmatory assays for HCV antibodies. Vox Sang 66(2):122–9

229. Lok AS, Chien D, Choo QL et al (1993) Antibody response to core, envelope and nonstructural hepatitis C virus antigens: comparison of immunocompetent and immunosuppressed patients. Hepatology 18(3):497–502
230. Gretch DR, dela Rosa C, Carithers RL Jr, Willson RA, Williams B, Corey L (1995) Assessment of hepatitis C viremia using molecular amplification technologies: correlations and clinical implications. Ann Intern Med 123(5):321–9
231. Strader DB, Wright T, Thomas DL, Seeff LB (2004) Diagnosis, management, and treatment of hepatitis C. Hepatology 39(4):1147–71
232. McDonald GB (2006) Advances in prevention and treatment of hepatic disorders following hematopoietic cell transplantation. Best Pract Res Clin Haematol 19(2):341–52
233. Stebbing J, Marvin V, Bower M (2004) The evidence-based treatment of AIDS-related non-Hodgkin's lymphoma. Cancer Treat Rev 30(3):249–53
234. Carbone A, Gloghini A (2006) HHV-8-associated lymphoma: state-of-the-art review. Acta Haematol 117(3):129–31
235. Martin SI, Zukerberg L, Robbins GK (2005) Reactive Epstein-Barr virus-related polyclonal lymphoproliferative disorder in a patient with AIDS. Clin Infect Dis 41(8):e76–9
236. Burke DS, Brundage JF, Redfield RR et al (1988) Measurement of the false positive rate in a screening program for human immunodeficiency virus infections. N Engl J Med 319(15):961–4
237. Schable C, Zekeng L, Pau CP et al (1994) Sensitivity of United States HIV antibody tests for detection of HIV-1 group O infections. Lancet 344(8933):1333–4
238. Markovitz DM (1993) Infection with the human immunodeficiency virus type 2. Ann Intern Med 118(3):211–8
239. Horsburgh CR Jr, Ou CY, Jason J et al (1989) Duration of human immunodeficiency virus infection before detection of antibody. Lancet 2(8664):637–40
240. Yang Y, Lamendola MH, Mendoza M et al (2001) Performance characteristics of the COBAS AmpliScreen HIV-1 test, version 1.5, an assay designed for screening plasma mini-pools. Transfusion 41(5):643–51
241. van den Berk GE, Frissen PH, Regez RM, Rietra PJ (2003) Evaluation of the rapid immunoassay determine HIV 1/2 for detection of antibodies to human immunodeficiency virus types 1 and 2. J Clin Microbiol 41(8):3868–9
242. Drociuk D, Gibson J, Hodge J Jr (2004) Health information privacy and syndromic surveillance systems. MMWR Morb Mortal Wkly Rep 53(Suppl):221–5
243. de The G, Bomford R (1993) An HTLV-I vaccine: why, how, for whom? AIDS Res Hum Retroviruses 9(5):381–6
244. Wiktor SZ, Alexander SS, Shaw GM et al (1990) Distinguishing between HTLV-I and HTLV-II by western blot. Lancet 335(8704):1533
245. Gill PS, Harrington W Jr, Kaplan MH et al (1995) Treatment of adult T-cell leukemia-lymphoma with a combination of interferon alfa and zidovudine. N Engl J Med 332(26):1744–8
246. Tholouli E, Liu Yin JA (2006) Successful treatment of HTLV-1-associated acute adult T-cell leukemia lymphoma by allogeneic bone marrow transplantation: a 12 year follow-up. Leuk Lymphoma 47(8):1691–2
247. Padgett BL, Walker DL, ZuRhein GM, Eckroade RJ, Dessel BH (1971) Cultivation of papova-like virus from human brain with progressive multifocal leucoencephalopathy. Lancet 1(7712):1257–60
248. Gardner SD, Field AM, Coleman DV, Hulme B (1971) New human papovavirus (B.K.) isolated from urine after renal transplantation. Lancet 1(7712):1253–7
249. Weber T, Trebst C, Frye S et al (1997) Analysis of the systemic and intrathecal humoral immune response in progressive multifocal leukoencephalopathy. J Infect Dis 176(1):250–4
250. Power C, Gladden JG, Halliday W et al (2000) AIDS- and non-AIDS-related PML association with distinct p53 polymorphism. Neurology 54(3):743–6

251. Berger JR, Pall L, Lanska D, Whiteman M (1998) Progressive multifocal leukoencephalopathy in patients with HIV infection. J Neurovirol 4(1):59–68
252. Whiteman ML, Post MJ, Berger JR, Tate LG, Bell MD, Limonte LP (1993) Progressive multifocal leukoencephalopathy in 47 HIV-seropositive patients: neuroimaging with clinical and pathologic correlation. Radiology 187(1):233–40
253. Hulette CM, Downey BT, Burger PC (1991) Progressive multifocal leukoencephalopathy. Diagnosis by in situ hybridization with a biotinylated JC virus DNA probe using an automated histomatic code-on slide stainer. Am J Surg Pathol 15(8):791–7
254. Cinque P, Scarpellini P, Vago L, Linde A, Lazzarin A (1997) Diagnosis of central nervous system complications in HIV-infected patients: cerebrospinal fluid analysis by the polymerase chain reaction. AIDS 11(1):1–17
255. Marra CM, Rajicic N, Barker DE et al (2002) A pilot study of cidofovir for progressive multifocal leukoencephalopathy in AIDS. AIDS 16(13):1791–7
256. Hou J, Major EO (1998) The efficacy of nucleoside analogs against JC virus multiplication in a persistently infected human fetal brain cell line. J Neurovirol 4(4):451–6
257. Aksamit AJ (2001) Treatment of non-AIDS progressive multifocal leukoencephalopathy with cytosine arabinoside. J Neurovirol 7(4):386–90
258. Tognon M, Corallini A, Martini F, Negrini M, Barbanti-Brodano G (2003) Oncogenic transformation by BK virus and association with human tumors. Oncogene 22(33):5192–200
259. Cubukcu-Dimopulo O, Greco A, Kumar A, Karluk D, Mittal K, Jagirdar J (2000) BK virus infection in AIDS. Am J Surg Pathol 24(1):145–9
260. Sandler ES, Aquino VM, Goss-Shohet E, Hinrichs S, Krisher K (1997) BK papova virus pneumonia following hematopoietic stem cell transplantation. Bone Marrow Transplant 20(2):163–5
261. Galan A, Rauch CA, Otis CN (2005) Fatal BK polyoma viral pneumonia associated with immunosuppression. Hum Pathol 36(9):1031–4
262. Nickeleit V, Klimkait T, Binet IF et al (2000) Testing for polyomavirus type BK DNA in plasma to identify renal-allograft recipients with viral nephropathy. N Engl J Med 342(18):1309–15
263. Leung AY, Yuen KY, Kwong YL (2005) Polyoma BK virus and haemorrhagic cystitis in haematopoietic stem cell transplantation: a changing paradigm. Bone Marrow Transplant 36(11):929–37
264. Arthur RR, Shah KV (1989) Occurrence and significance of papovaviruses BK and JC in the urine. Prog Med Virol 36:42–61
265. Whiley DM, Mackay IM, Sloots TP (2001) Detection and differentiation of human polyomaviruses JC and BK by LightCycler PCR. J Clin Microbiol 39(12):4357–61
266. Behzad-Behbahani A, Klapper PE, Vallely PJ, Cleator GM, Khoo SH (2004) Detection of BK virus and JC virus DNA in urine samples from immunocompromised (HIV-infected) and immunocompetent (HIV-non-infected) patients using polymerase chain reaction and microplate hybridisation. J Clin Virol 29(4):224–9
267. Coleman DV, Wolfendale MR, Daniel RA et al (1980) A prospective study of human polyomavirus infection in pregnancy. J Infect Dis 142(1):1–8
268. Markowitz RB, Thompson HC, Mueller JF, Cohen JA, Dynan WS (1993) Incidence of BK virus and JC virus viruria in human immunodeficiency virus-infected and -uninfected subjects. J Infect Dis 167(1):13–20
269. Kitamura T, Aso Y, Kuniyoshi N, Hara K, Yogo Y (1990) High incidence of urinary JC virus excretion in nonimmunosuppressed older patients. J Infect Dis 161(6):1128–33
270. Munoz P, Fogeda M, Bouza E, Verde E, Palomo J, Banares R (2005) Prevalence of BK virus replication among recipients of solid organ transplants. Clin Infect Dis 41(12):1720–5

271. Leung AY, Suen CK, Lie AK, Liang RH, Yuen KY, Kwong YL (2001) Quantification of polyoma BK viruria in hemorrhagic cystitis complicating bone marrow transplantation. Blood 98(6):1971–8
272. Azzi A, Cesaro S, Laszlo D et al (1999) Human polyomavirus BK (BKV) load and haemorrhagic cystitis in bone marrow transplantation patients. J Clin Virol 14(2):79–86
273. Leung AY, Chan MT, Yuen KY et al (2005) Ciprofloxacin decreased polyoma BK virus load in patients who underwent allogeneic hematopoietic stem cell transplantation. Clin Infect Dis 40(4):528–37
274. Erard V, Kim HW, Corey L et al (2005) BK DNA viral load in plasma: evidence for an association with hemorrhagic cystitis in allogeneic hematopoietic cell transplant recipients. Blood 106(3):1130–2
275. Bogdanovic G, Priftakis P, Giraud G, Dalianis T (2006) A related donor and reduced intensity conditioning reduces the risk of development of BK virus-positive haemorrhagic cystitis in allogeneic haematopoetic stem cell-transplanted patients. Anticancer Res 26(2B):1311–8
276. Ferrazzi E, Peracchi M, Biasolo MA, Faggionato O, Stefanelli S, Palu G (1988) Antiviral activity of gyrase inhibitors norfloxacin, coumermycin A1 and nalidixic acid. Biochem Pharmacol 37(9):1885–6
277. Portolani M, Pietrosemoli P, Cermelli C et al (1988) Suppression of BK virus replication and cytopathic effect by inhibitors of prokaryotic DNA gyrase. Antiviral Res 9(3):205–18
278. Randhawa PS (2005) Anti-BK virus activity of ciprofloxacin and related antibiotics. Clin Infect Dis 41(9):1366–7 author reply 7
279. Andrei G, Snoeck R, Vandeputte M, De Clercq E (1997) Activities of various compounds against murine and primate polyomaviruses. Antimicrob Agents Chemother 41(3):587–93
280. Randhawa P, Farasati NA, Shapiro R, Hostetler KY (2006) Ether lipid ester derivatives of cidofovir inhibit polyomavirus BK replication in vitro. Antimicrob Agents Chemother 50(4):1564–6
281. Farasati NA, Shapiro R, Vats A, Randhawa P (2005) Effect of leflunomide and cidofovir on replication of BK virus in an in vitro culture system. Transplantation 79(1):116–8
282. Held TK, Biel SS, Nitsche A et al (2000) Treatment of BK virus-associated hemorrhagic cystitis and simultaneous CMV reactivation with cidofovir. Bone Marrow Transplant 26(3):347–50
283. Bridges B, Donegan S, Badros A (2006) Cidofovir bladder instillation for the treatment of BK hemorrhagic cystitis after allogeneic stem cell transplantation. Am J Hematol 81(7):535–7
284. Josephson MA, Gillen D, Javaid B et al (2006) Treatment of renal allograft polyoma BK virus infection with leflunomide. Transplantation 81(5):704–10
285. Williams JW, Javaid B, Kadambi PV et al (2005) Leflunomide for polyomavirus type BK nephropathy. N Engl J Med 352(11):1157–8

Chapter 3

Bacteria

Pranatharthi H. Chandrasekar and George Alangaden

Abstract Despite the fact that survival among patients with hematologic malignancies has considerably improved, bacterial infections continue to occur as a result of prolonged, profound immunosuppression. Neutropenia, vascular catheters, and chemotherapy-induced mucositis are key risk factors. Data on blood stream infections show the predominance of aerobic gram-positive cocci; however, gram-negative bacilli continue to play a significant role. Better microbiologic data on tissue site infections are needed. Rapid molecular methods of microbiologic diagnosis are entering clinical practice. In an era of ever fewer new antimicrobial drugs developed by pharmaceutical companies, the rising frequency of drug-resistant pathogens among staphylococci, streptococci, enterococci, and aerobic gram-negative bacteria in cancer patients is alarming. Prudent use of available antimicrobial drugs is ever more critical to stem the tide of antibiotic-resistant bacteria.

Keywords Bacterial infections • Antibacterials • Febrile neutropenia • Gram-negative bacteria • Gram-positive bacteria • *Nocardia* • Tuberculosis • Viridans streptococci

1. Introduction

Bacteria, common and opportunistic, cause most infections in patients with hematologic malignancies. Survival rates in cancer patients have significantly improved over the past few decades, and patients with hematological malignancies experience multiple cycles of prolonged periods of immunosuppression with consequent increased risk for infectious complications due to an expanding list of pathogens (Tables 3-1 and 3-2). Episodes of neutropenia, prolonged use of indwelling vascular catheters, chemotherapy-induced mucositis, frequent use of antimicrobial drugs, immunosuppressive therapy, T-lymphocyte deficiency, and administration of blood products are important risk factors for infections in patients with leukemia, lymphoma, or myeloma. Protocol-driven antimicrobial approaches (e.g., empiric and prophylatic strategies) in most

From: *Managing Infections in Patients With Hematological Malignancies*: Contemporary Hematology, Edited by: M. Kleinberg, DOI 10.1007/978-1-59745-415-5_3,

Table 3-1. Gram-positive bacterial pathogens in cancer patients and antibiotics commonly used to treat systemic infections caused by gram-positive bacteria.

Pathogens	
Gram-positive cocci in clusters	Coagulase-positive • *S. aureus* CoNS • *S. epidermidis* • *S. hemolyticus* • *S. saprophyticus* • *S. hominis* • *Staphylococcus lugdunenesis* • *Staphylococcus warnerii*
Gram-positive cocci in pairs or chains	Streptococci Beta hemolytic • *Staphylococcus pyogenes* (Group A streptococcus) • *Staphylococcus agalactiae* (Group B streptococcus) • Group C, F, G streptococci Alpha-hemolytic • Viridans streptococci • *S. pneumoniae* Gamma hemolytic • Group D streptococci Enterococcus • *E. fecalis* • *E. fecium*
Gram-positive bacilli	Aerobic • *Listeria monocytogenes* • *Corynebacterium* sp. • *Bacillus* sp. • *Lactobacillus* sp. • *Propionibacterium* Anaerobic • *Clostridium* species Branching or filamentous • *Nocardia* sp. • *Actinomyces* sp.

Agent	Adult dose	Spectrum of activity	Comments
Nafcillin	2 g IV q 4 h	Gram-positive bacteria	Best agent for *S. aureus* (methicillin-susceptible)No adjustment for renal function
Vancomycin	15 mg/kg IV q12 h	Gram-positive bacteria including methicillin-resistant organisms. (MRSA)	Dose adjustment for renal function. Monitor drug levels.Inferior to Nafcillin against methicillin-susceptible organisms

(continued)

Table 3-1. (continued)

Pathogens			
Quinupristin/ dalfopristin	7.5 mg/kg IV q8 h	Gram-positive bacteria including methicillin- and vancomycin-resistant organisms. No activity against *E. fecalis*	Dose adjustment for renal function. Phlebitis common, therefore central venous access preferred. Arthralgias and myalgias common; consequently, infrequent use.
Linezolid	600 mg PO/ IV q 12 h	Gram-positive bacteria including methicillin- and vancomycin-resistant organisms.	No dose adjustment for renal function. Reversible thrombocytopenia, anemia and leukopenia usually after 2 weeks of therapy. Interaction with SSRIs.
Daptomycin	4–6 mg/kg IVq d	Gram-positive bacteria including methicillin- and vancomycin-resistant organisms.	Dose adjustment for renal function. Can cause myopathy, monitor CPK levels weekly. Not effective in pneumonia since drug is inactivated by pulmonary surfactant

Table 3-2. Gram-negative and acid-fast bacterial pathogens in cancer patients and antibiotics commonly used to treat systemic infections caused by gram-negative bacteria and anaerobic bacteria.

Pathogens	
Gram-negative bacilli	Lactose fermenter
	Oxidase-positive
	• *Aeromonas*
	• *Pasteurella*
	• *Vibrio*
	Oxidase-negative
	• *E. coli*
	• *Klebsiella sp.*
	• *Enterobacter sp.*
	• *Citrobacter sp.*
	Nonlactose fermenter
	Oxidase-positive
	• *P. aeruginosa*
	• *Achromobacter* sp.
	• *Alcaligenes* sp.
	• *Flavobacterium* sp.
	Oxidase-negative
	• *Acinetobacter* sp.
	• *Stenotrophomonas* sp
	• *Morganella* sp.
	• *Proteus* sp.
	• *Providencia* sp.
	• *Salmonella* sp.
	• *Serratia* sp.
	• *Shigella* sp.
	Anaerobes
	Bacteroides spp.

(continued)

Table 3-2. (continued)

Pathogens	
Gram-negative cocci	Cocci • *Neisseria gonorrhoeae* • *Neisseria meningitidis* • *Veillonella* Coccobacilli • *Haemophilus influenzae* • *Moraxella catarrhalis*
Acid-fast bacteria	Mycobacteria • *M. tuberculosis* • *M. avium-intracellulare* complex • *M. chelonae* sp. • *M. fortuitum* • *M. kansasii*

Agent	Adult dose	Activity vs. gram-negative bacteria	Comments
Ceftazidime	1–2 g IV q 8 h. (In neutropenia use 2 g IV q 8 h)	Gram-negative bacteria including *P. aeruginosa*.	Dose adjustment for renal function. No activity against *Enterococcus* sp. and methicillin-resistant gram-positive bacteria. Poor activity against anaerobes.
Cefepime	1–2 g IV q 12 h. (In neutropenia use 2 g IV q 8 h)	Gram-negative bacteria including *P. aeruginosa*.	Dose adjustment for renal function. Better gram-positive (including MSSA) activity than ceftazidime. No activity against *Enterococcus* sp. and methicillin-resistant gram-positive bacteria. Poor activity against anaerobes.
Imipenem/ cilastatin	0.5 g IV q 6 h. (For *P. aeruginosa* use 1 g IV q 6–8 h)	Gram-negative bacteria including *P. aeruginosa*.	Dose adjustment for renal function. Penetration into central nervous system is not well established. Good activity against anaerobes. No activity against *Enterococcus* sp. and methicillin-resistant gram-positive bacteria.
Meropenem	0.5–1 g IV q8 h. In neutropenia use 1 g IV q 8 h	Similar to imipenem	Dose adjustment for renal function. Useful in infection of central nervous system. Similar to imipenem vs. gram-positive bacteria.
Ertapenem	1 g IV q 24 h	Similar to imipenem except poor activity against *P. aeruginosa*.	Dose adjustment for renal function.
Piperacillin/ tazobactam	3.375 g IV q 6 h. (For *P. aeruginosa* and in neutropenia use 4.5 g IV q 6 h.)	Gram-negative bacteria including *P. aeruginosa*	Dose adjustment for renal function. Effective against gram-positive bacteria (streptococci, enterococci and staphylococci except methicillin-resistant organisms). Effective against anaerobes. May cause false-positive test with *Aspergillus* galactomannan.

(continued)

Table 3-2. (continued)

Pathogens			
Aztreonam	1–2 g IV q 8 h. (In neutropenia use 2 g IV q 8 h)	Gram-negative bacteria including *P. aeruginosa*.	Dose adjustment for renal function. Useful if allergy to penicillins or cephalosporins. No activity against gram-positive bacteria or anaerobes.
Ciprofloxacin	400 mg IV q 12 h, or 500–750 mg PO q 12 h	Gram-negative bacteria particularly *P. aeruginosa*.	Dose adjustment for renal function. Avoid monotherapy if treating *P. aeruginosa*. Reduced activity against gram-positive bacteria. No activity against anaerobes. Effective against "atypical pneumonia" pathogens. No activity against anaerobes.
Levofloxacin	500–750 mg IV/PO q 24 h	Gram-negative bacteria	Dose adjustment for renal function. Better activity against *S. pneumoniae* than ciprofloxacin. No activity against anaerobes. Effective against "atypical pneumonia" pathogens.
Antibiotics active against anaerobic bacteria			
Agent	Adult Dose	Spectrum of Activity	Comments
Metronidazole	500 mg IV/PO q 6 h	Anaerobes including *C. difficile*. Poorly active against gram-positive aerobes and anaerobes (e.g., Peptostreptococci)	Dose adjustment for renal function and severe hepatic dysfunction.
Clindamycin	600–900 mg IV q 8 h, 150–450 mg PO q 6 h	Anaerobes, streptococci and staphylococci (MSSA). Some activity against MRSA. No activity against *Enterococcus* sp.	No adjustment for renal function.

cancer centers with potent, broad spectrum antibacterials have greatly reduced infection-related mortality. However, infectious episodes continue to cause high morbidity and interruption of anticancer therapy.

Our understanding of bacterial infections in patients with hematologic malignancies is based largely on data from blood cultures obtained during evaluations of neutropenic fever. Spectrum of bacterial infections in neutropenic patients has undergone periodic changes, and currently, aerobic gram-positive cocci have replaced aerobic gram-negative bacilli as the most frequent pathogens in blood stream infections [1, 2].

2. Gram-Positive Bacteria

In a large, national surveillance program of cancer patients with bacteremia, gram-positive cocci accounted for 62% episodes in 1995 and 76% episodes in 2000 [1]. A Swedish study of 1,402 bacteremia episodes over a 14-year period in patients with hematologic malignancies noted 45% infections to be due to gram-positive cocci [3]. Most common gram-positive pathogens are coagulase-negative staphylococci, *Staphylococcus aureus*, and enterococci.

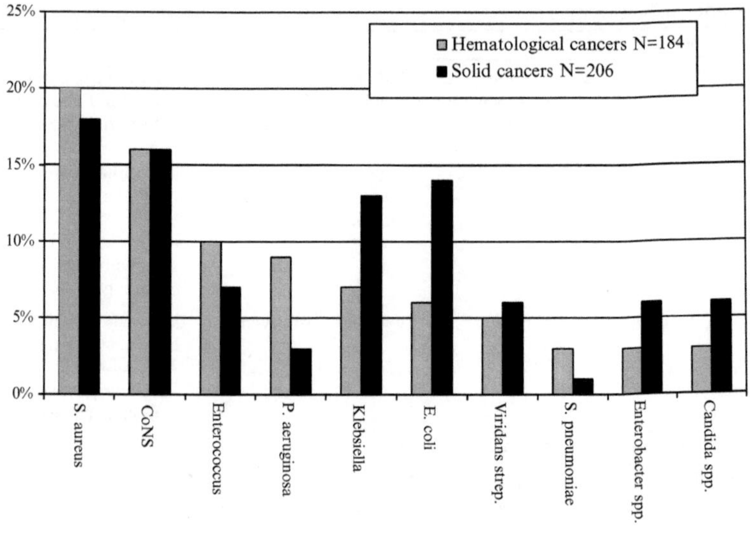

Fig. 3-1. Pathogens causing blood stream infections among patients with hematological malignancies or solid tumor, Karmanos Cancer Institute (2000–2001)

Figure 3.1 shows the frequencies of various species of bacteria and *Candida* recovered from blood stream isolates of patients with hematologic malignancies or solid tumors at the Karmanos Cancer Institute, Detroit, Michigan during 2000–2001. Factors proposed to have caused such a shift towards gram-positive pathogens include widespread use of indwelling catheters, use of quinolone-based prophylactic strategies that effectively eradicate aerobic enteric gram-negative bacilli but not gram-positive cocci, intensive chemotherapeutic regimens causing upper and lower gastrointestinal mucositis, and the use of antacids and H_2 receptor blockers which reduce gastric pH promoting overgrowth with oropharygeal gram-positive microflora [4–8].

2.1. Staphylococci

Coagulase-negative staphylococci (CoNS) are the most common organisms recovered from blood; among these, *Staphylococcus epidermidis* accounts for the majority [9]. Most CoNS bacteremia are believed to be secondary to catheter-related infection, following colonization of the catheter hub during manipulation. A positive blood culture for CoNS may imply true bacteremia or skin contamination during blood collection. Thus, single positive blood cultures for CoNS need to be viewed with suspicion and in those without catheters, such results can be assumed to represent contamination. Many centers initiate therapy only if two or more cultures are positive for CoNS. Simultaneous blood cultures via catheter and peripheral vein may help distinguish true bacteremia from catheter colonization. As these are low-virulence pathogens, antimicrobial therapy alone without catheter removal is adequate in most cases.

Most *S. epidermidis* are penicillin- and methicillin-resistant and only susceptible to vancomycin. Methicillin-resistant staphylococci are resistant to quinolones. Treatment of culture-proven bacteremias due to CoNS and suspected catheter-related infection are the most common reasons for high volume use of vancomycin in most cancer centers. Because of the concern for emergence of resistance in gram-positive bacteria, vancomycin is not used routinely in the initial antibacterial regimen for treatment of neutropenic fever except in some situations– positive blood cultures with smears showing gram-positive bacteria, empirical treatment of critically ill patients pending identification of a pathogen, presence of a skin/soft tissue infection with neutropenic fever, suspicion of a serious catheter-related infection, and known colonization with methicillin resistant *S. aureus*. In vancomycin-intolerant patients, alternate drugs against methicillin-resistant staphylococci include linezolid, daptomycin, and quinupristin-dalfopristin (Tables 3-3 and 3-4). However, these drugs have limitations and are usually reserved for infections caused by vancomycin-resistant enterococci. Already resistance to these newer drugs has been reported among staphylococci. Currently, none of these newer agents have been shown to be superior in efficacy to vancomycin against methicillin-resistant staphylococci.

Less common CoNS include *Staphylococcus hemolyticus, Staphylococcus saprophyticus*, and *Staphylococcus hominis* which like *S. epidermidis,* are methicillin-resistant. Of note, *S. hemolyticus* has reduced susceptibility to glycopeptides like vancomycin and teicoplanin [10–12]. Whether this observation has clinical relevance is unclear [13].

S. aureus, a far more virulent pathogen than CoNS, causes infections which originate mostly from indwelling catheters or skin/soft tissue. *S. aureus* accounts for 20–30% nosocomial blood stream isolates in the general population and 11% blood stream isolates in cancer patients [14–16]. Most skin/soft infections respond promptly to antistaphylococcal therapy but, on occasion, incision and drainage of a large lesion may be required. In bacteremic cases, unlike CoNS, *S. aureus* can cause serious metastatic complications such as deep tissue infection (e.g., splenic abscess), infective endocarditis, septic phlebitis, septic arthritis, and epidural abscess. Predictors of such complications include community-acquired infection, positive blood cultures persisting for more

Table 3-3. Specific features of some "newer" antibiotics.

Agent	Adult dose	Spectrum of activity	Comments
Tigecycline	100 mg IV × 1 then 50 mg IV q 12 h	Gram-positive bacteria including MRSA and VRE. Gram-negative bacteria including *Acinetobacter* spp., *S. maltophilia* and ESBL-producers; Effective against anaerobes. Poor activity against *P. aeruginosa*	No dose adjustment for renal function. Dose adjustment in severe hepatic dysfunction.
Moxifloxacin	400 mg IV/PO q 24 h	Gram-negative bacteria. Better activity against *S. pneumoniae* than ciprofloxacin. Active against "atypical pneumonia" pathogens and anaerobes.	Not appropriate for urinary tract infection.
Colistin	2.5–5 mg/kg IV q 24 h in 2–4 divided doses	Gram-negative bacteria including multidrug resistant *P. aeruginosa* and *Acinetobacter* spp.	Dose adjustment for renal function

Table 3-4. Characteristics of selected antibiotic-resistant gram-positive bacteria.

Bacteria	Resistance profile	Agents with activity	Comments
Methicillin resistant *S. aureus* (MRSA) (nosocomial)	Resistant to penicillins, cephalosporins, quinolones	Vanomycin, linezolid, daptomycin, quinupristin/dalfopristin,	TMP/SMZ, clindamycin may be useful. Quinolones not useful.
Vancomycin-resistant *S. aureus* (VRSA)	Resistant to penicillins, cephalosporins, quinolones	Linezolid, daptomycin, quinupristin-dalfopristin,	TMP/SMZ, rifampin, gentamicin, clindamycin may be useful
Vancomycin-resistant *Enterococcus* spp. (VRE)		Ampicillin, linezolid, daptomycin, tigecycline, quinupristin-dalfopristin,	Gentamicin may be useful for synergy. Quinupristin-dalfopristin not effective against *E. fecalis* Resistance to linezolid or daptomycin may emerge during therapy.
PCN-resistant viridans *Streptococcus*		Advanced generation cephalosporins, vancomycin, quinolones	*S. mitis* more resistant than other viridans strep. May be resistant to macrolides, quinolones

than 48 h, and persistent fever 3 days after the initial positive blood cultures despite therapy [17]. In a retrospective review of 91 patients with cancer and *S. aureus* bacteremia, renal failure significantly increased the likelihood of complications; patients with hematologic malignancies tended to develop more extravascular complications compared to patients with solid tumors [18]. A retrospective review of 85 cancer patients with nosocomial *S. aureus* bacteremia reported a low mortality rate of 3.5% with none developing any complications [19]. Early antimicrobial intervention and prompt catheter removal in hospitalized neutropenic febrile patients may explain such a good outcome.

Against methicillin-susceptible staphylococci, an antistaphylococcal penicillin such as nafcillin is preferred over vancomycin as the former has more rapid bactericidal activity. Antimicrobial resistance in staphylococci, particularly *S. aureus*, in the nosocomial and community settings has justifiably raised major concern. In recent years, specific clones of methicillin-resistant *S. aureus*, distinctly different from nosocomial strains, have emerged in the community [20–22]. Community-associated MRSA (CA-MRSA) tend to cause suppurative skin/soft tissue infections and are transmitted by close physical contact. Unlike nosocomial MRSA, CA-MRSA is susceptible to many non-betalactam drugs (clindamycin, TMP-SMX, quinolones, doxycycline); however, it is anticipated that exposure to multiple antimicrobials will render CA-MRSA in the near future multidrug resistant similar to nosocomial MRSA. As CA-MRSA becomes widespread, empiric therapy with a betalactam drug (e.g., dicloxacillin, cefazolin) for skin/soft tissue infections in cancer patients may no longer be prudent. Dalbavancin and telavancin are two new glycopeptides with promising clinical activity against methicillin-susceptible and –resistant staphylococci [23, 24]. It is unclear if these newer agents offer any advantages over vancomycin.

Explosive vancomycin use has resulted in the appearance of vancomycin resistance among MRSA. These include heteroresistant *S. aureus* (hGISA, hVISA;

MIC 0.5–2 μg/mL), glycopeptide/vancomycin intermediate susceptible *S. aureus* (GISA, VISA; MIC 4–8 μg/mL), and vancomycin resistant *S. aureus* (VRSA; MIC ≥ 16 μg/mL [25]. It is believed that hetero-resistant *S. aureus* (hVISA) is increasing in frequency, and in infections due to hVISA, vancomycin treatment failures have been reported [26–28]. Microbiology laboratories need to be equipped to provide exact MIC data promptly to the clinician. Vancomycin-resistant *S. aureus* may be less susceptible to daptomycin and linezolid as well. As cancer patients receive multiple, frequent courses of IV vancomycin for suspected or proven staphylococcal infection, eventual rapid emergence of VRSA would not be surprising. Most observations regarding vancomycin resistance are in *S. aureus*; little data exist for CoNS.

2.2. Streptococci

At the Karmanos Cancer Institute during 2000–2001, streptococci (mainly viridans streptococci and *Staphylococcus pneumoniae*) accounted for 8% blood stream infection in patients with hematological malignancies. Beta-hemolytic streptococci such as groups A and B streptococci are occasional pathogens. Viridans streptococci are commensals of the oral cavity, upper airway, gastrointestinal and genitourinary tracts, and invade the blood stream during mucositis and neutropenia. While viridans streptococci recovered from blood in noncancer patients may represent contaminants, these are considered true pathogens, even in single blood cultures, in the setting of febrile neutropenia. Bacteremia due to *S. viridans* has increased in recent years in patients with hematologic malignancies with 6–12% mortality rates [8, 29]. Risk factors include profound neutropenia, oral mucositis, quinolone, or trimethoprim-sulfamethoxazole prophylaxis, and exposure to cytotoxic, high dose chemotherapy (particularly cytosine arabinoside) [29–31].

A group of 24 streptococcus species comprise viridans streptococci; the most common species in cancer patients are *S. mitis, S. oralis, S. sanguis* and *S. salivarius*. Most infected patients have fever and mucositis; those with *S. mitis* infection are generally younger with prolonged neutropenia and bacteremias are often associated with development of the adult respiratory distress syndrome (ARDS) and/or septic shock [32]. Bacteremic patients may have persistent fever despite prompt clearance of the organism from the blood stream. Such patients need close follow-up for early diagnosis of respiratory distress.

Though most viridans streptococci are exquisitely susceptible to penicillin, emergence of penicillin-resistant streptococci and macrolide-resistant streptococci has been widespread [33–35]. Prior exposure to quinolones is a common predisposing factor for the emergence of quinolone- and penicillin-resistant streptococci [31]. Resistance rates to penicillin range from 13% to 23% (high grade resistance, MIC ≥4 μg/mL), and 17–43% (intermediate grade resistance, MIC 0.5–2.0 μg/mL). Resistance to penicillin and quinolones is seen more commonly with *S. mitis* than with non-*S. mitis* stains. *S. parasanguis*, a recently described viridans streptococcus, has documented resistance to penicillin as well as azithromycin [32, 36]. Increasing prevalence of antimicrobial-resistant viridans streptococci must serve as a warning against widespread antimicrobial use, particularly in the setting of quinolone prophylaxis.

Unlike viridans streptococci, *S. pneumoniae* causes infection in cancer patients in the community setting, mostly during nonneutropenic periods. *S. pneumoniae* infections in patients with hematological malignancies are characterized by pneumonia and bacteremia [37]. At a tertiary care oncology center, pneumococcal bacteremia occurred in 122 patients over a 5-year period (1998–2002).and 36% of the isolates were penicillin-resistant. Of interest is the fact that factors including initial antibacterial therapy that did not cover *S. pneumoniae*, penicillin-resistant pneumococci, corticosteroid use, and neutropenia were not associated with increased mortality. Investigators from the same institution noted pneumococcal infection to be infrequent but of a serious nature in stem cell transplant (SCT) recipients, particularly those receiving high dose corticosteroid therapy for graft-versus-host disease [38].

2.3. Enterococci

Common infections caused by enterococci in patients with hematologic malignancies include bacteremia, urinary tract infection, biliary tract infection, and vascular-catheter infection. Enterococci *(E. fecalis, E. fecium, E. avium, E. durans)* are normal inhabitants of the gastrointestinal tract and constitute the third most frequent cause of blood stream infection in the U.S [16]. Reported mortality rates in *Enterococcus*-infected patients with hematologic malignancies vary from 19% to 47% [39–42]; however, it remains unclear if death is attributable to the enterococcal bacteremia per se or whether the bacteremia signifies the severity of underlying morbidity and consequent poor outcome. A large, retrospective study of 98 episodes of enterococcal bacteremia during 1984–2001 in the setting of neutropenic patients with hematologic malignancies found that *E. fecalis* (53%) and *E. fecium* (40%) were the most common *Enterococci* species giving rise to mortality rates of 30% [43]. Risk factors for death were age > than 50 years, advanced underlying disease, pneumonia, and shock. Severe neutropenia, enterococcal species, and antibiotic resistance did not affect mortality.

Enterococci, though frequently recovered from the respiratory tract (sputum, bronchoalveolar lavage [BAL] specimen), rarely cause pneumonia. Urinary tract infection or biliary infection caused by enterococci may be seen in the setting of a device (e.g., biliary stent) or after instrumentation (e.g., cystoscopy, ERCP). Clinically useful antibiotics active against enterococci are ampicillin, piperacillin, and vancomycin. Notably, nafcillin, cephalosporins, carbapenems (other than imipenem), macrolides, and quinolones are poorly active. Among the newer antibacterials, quinupristin–dalfopristin (active vs. *E. fecium*, not *E. fecalis*), linezolid, tigecycline, and daptomycin possess good in vitro activity and are clinically useful particularly against vancomycin-resistant organisms. However, resistance to these newer drugs has also been reported. Aminoglycosides, such as gentamicin or streptomycin, are not used in monotherapy but are useful as secondary agents to provide synergistic activity.

Antimicrobial resistance in enterococci is of major clinical importance, particularly in relation to vancomycin and penicillin (or ampicillin). Risk factors for vancomycin-resistant enterococcal (VRE) colonization/infection include prior antimicrobial exposure, severe underlying disease, indwelling foreign devices, and frequent hospitalization or contacts within the health care system [44]. Vancomycin resistance is far more commonly encountered in *E. fecium* than *E. fecalis*; however, the latter is more commonly seen in clinical settings. Vancomycin resistant enterococci (VRE) colonize the gut, frequently as a result of prior antimicrobial (oral vancomycin or other agents that alter gut flora) exposure, and during chemotherapy-induced mucositis, may cause bacteremia. The rates of VRE gut colonization in cancer patients have been studied [45]. VRE colonization, as noted in fecal specimens, was seen in 6% patients with hematologic malignancies. Presence of fecal colonization with VRE had a positive predictive value of 29% for subsequent development of bacteremia, and a high negative predictive value greater than 99% [45]; *E. fecium* was the most common VRE colonizing species. Patients with hematologic malignancies and stem cell recipients were far more likely than solid tumor patients to develop bacteremias and/or other infections because of VRE. Routine surveillance to detect VRE colonization in patients with hematologic malignancies or in any other clinical setting is not currently recommended. However, there are data to show that weekly surveillance programs and isolation of VRE colonized patients have decreased the incidence and density of VRE outbreaks [46–50]. In stem cell recipients, VRE bacteremia has been identified as a marker of critical illness [51, 52].

2.4. Listeria

Listeria monocytogenes, a facultative, gram-positive bacillus believed to gain entry via the gastrointestinal tract, has a tropism for the central nervous system. Common clinical manifestations are bacteremia, meningitis, meningoencephalitis, cerebritis, and rhombencephalitis [53–55]. Listeriosis may be seen in immunocompetent and immunocompromised (primarily those with T-cell immune impairment) hosts. Specific "compromised" populations include neonates, pregnant women, alcoholics, those with diabetes, those receiving corticosteroids, solid organ and stem cell recipients, AIDS patients, and patients with cancer [54, 56–60].

Among cancer patients, listeriosis commonly infects patients with hematologic malignancies, particularly lymphoreticular neoplasms such as chronic lymphocytic leukemia and lymphoma [61, 62] where T-cell impairment is common from both primary disease and therapy. Concurrent steroid use and immunosuppressive drugs such as fludarabine have been associated with listeriosis [56, 63, 64]. In a review of 34 cancer patients with listeriosis encountered over a 11-year period, 59% were at risk because of lymphoma or leukemia (76% had received prior corticosteroids). Bacteremia (74%) and meningoencephalitis (21%) were common clinical presentations. Lymphocytopenia was seen in 62% patients whereas notably, neutropenia was not a risk factor [61].

Diagnosis rests primarily on blood and cerebrospinal fluid cultures. Tiny gram-positive rods in the CSF, almost mimicking pneumococci, provide an early diagnostic clue prior to availability of culture results. Listeriosis is treated with ampicillin in combination with gentamicin in compromised patients [56]. In penicillin-allergic patients, trimethoprim-sulfamethoxazole is the alternative drug. However, patients who are seriously ill (e.g., meningitis) should be treated with ampicillin after penicillin drug desensitization. Vancomycin has also been used successfully for the treatment of listeriosis. Carbapenems, linezolid, and newer fluoroquinolones have good in vitro activity against listeria; whether they play a useful clinical role needs validation [57, 65]. Given the high frequency of CNS involvement in listeriosis, the drug chosen must be able to penetrate the blood brain barrier to achieve adequate concentration in the cerebrospinal fluid. Relapse of listeriosis may occur, thus therapy is recommended for a minimum duration of 3 weeks [53]. Controlled data are lacking for optimal duration of therapy. In general, bacteremic patients have a better prognosis as compared with those with CNS involvement.

Breakthrough cases of listeriosis have been described in allogeneic stem cell recipients receiving daily trimethoprim-sulfamethoxazole for prophylaxis against pneumocystis [66].

2.5. Other Gram-Positive Bacteria

Other emerging gram-positive bacterial pathogens include *Stomatococcus muciclaginosus*, *Bacillus* sp., *Rhodococcus equi*, *Corynebacteria*, *Leuconostoc*, *Pediococcus*, and lactobacilli [9]. Most of these cause blood stream infections in the setting of oral/gastrointestinal mucositis during chemotherapy-related neutropenia or in association with indwelling catheters. These are usually uncomplicated bloodstream infections that respond readily to appropriate antimicrobial therapy. Notably, among these gram-positive bacilli, *Leuconstoc*, *Lactobacillus*, and *Pediococcus* species may be resistant to vancomycin.

3. Gram-Negative Bacteria

Most infections caused by gram-negative bacteria in patients with cancer have been reported in the context of bacteremia. The Surveillance and Control of Pathogens of Epidemiologic Importance (SCOPE) prospectively evaluated 22,631 episodes of bacteremia in 2,340 cancer patients between 1995 and 2001 [1]. Although gram-positive pathogens predominated, gram-negative bacteria accounted for 22% and 15% bacteremic episodes in 1995 and 2000, respectively [1]. Of the gram-negative pathogens, *Escherichia coli* (7.6%),*Klebsiella* species (6.4%), *Pseudomonas aeruginosa* (4.4%), and *Enterobacter* species (3%) were isolated with similar frequency in neutropenic and nonneutropenic patients [1]. Some recent reports show gram-negative bacteria accounting for 53–56% of all bloodstream infections [67, 68], with the predominant pathogens being *E. coli*, *Klebsiella* species, *Enterobacter* species, *P. aeruginosa*, and *Acinetobacter baumannii* (Table 3-5)

Table 3-5. Characteristics of selected antibiotic-resistant gram-negative bacteria.

Bacteria	Resistance profile	Agents with activity	Comments
ESBL producing *E. coli* and *K. pneumoniae*	Generally resistant to all penicillins, cephalosporins. Often resistant to fluoroquinolones	Carbapenems: imipenem, meropenem. Tigecycline active against most strains.	Select drugs based on susceptibility testing. Clinical experience with imipenem
Multidrug resistant *P. aeruginosa*	Resistant to penicillins, cephalosporins, fluoroquinolones carbapenems and aminoglycosides	Colistin (polymixin-E), polymixin B	Select drugs based on susceptibility testing. Limited clinical experience with colistin
Acinetobacter spp.	Resistant to most penicillins, cephalosporins, fluoroquinolones and most aminoglycosides	Some strains susceptible to ampicillin/sulbactam, imipenem, amikacin, colistin and tigecycline	Select drugs based on susceptibility testing
S. maltophilia	Resistant to most penicillins, cephalosporins, fluoroquinolones and most aminoglycosides	Trimethoprim/sulfamethoxazole, chloramphenicol, tigecycline	Select drugs based on susceptibility testing.

Patients with cancer who have infections caused by gram-negative pathogens present with fever and sometimes, hemodynamic instability. Occasionally, symptoms specific to the site of infection, for example, pneumonia or urinary tract infection, may be present. Bacteremia related to central venous catheters (CVCs) are not uncommon. Initial therapy in neutropenic patients generally includes broad-spectrum antibacterials with antipseudomonal activity [69]. Multidrug resistance in many gram-negative bacteria is of major clinical concern [70]. CVC-related bacteremias have better outcomes compared to secondary bacteremias resulting from infections at other sites, for example, pneumonia.

Specific pathogens including their current epidemiology, clinical features, and therapy are discussed below.

3.1. Escherichia coli

E. coli is the commonest cause of gram-negative bacteremia in cancer patients. In the US SCOPE study, *E. coli* accounted for 7.3% and 7.7% of bacteremia in neutropenic and nonneutropenic patients, respectively [1]. *E. coli* was the causative pathogen in 13–27% of bacteremia in patients with leukemia, lymphoma, or myeloma reported from cancer centers in non-US countries [1, 3, 67, 68, 71]. A greater incidence of gram-negative bacteremia was noted in neutropenic patients compared to nonneutropenic cancer patients [67].

Resistance to ampicillin in *E. coli* is common [71]; however, 10% were noted to be resistant to cefotaxime [68] and 5% to gentamicin [1]. Resistance to fluoroquinolones in *E. coli* among cancer patients has been reported from several cancer centers, especially with the widespread use of fluoroquinolone prophylaxis during neutropenia [72–77]. Data from a single center noted an increase in the incidence of bacteremia with fluoroquinolone resistant *E. coli* rising from <0.8% to 4.5%, following routine prophylaxis with ofloxacin in patients with leukemia [72]. With subsequent discontinuation of quinolone prophylaxis, an increase in gram-negative bacteremia occurred but with a decline in the frequency of antibacterial resistance. These trends reversed with resumption of prophylaxis [77, 78]. IDSA guidelines discourage the use of routine antibiotic prophylaxis in cancer patients with hematological malignancies during neutropenia [69]. However, some recent large comparative studies demonstrated the efficacy of fluoroquinolones in decreasing rates of gram-negative bacteremias and fevers and improved infection-related outcomes but not mortality in patients with cancer and neutropenia [79, 80]. Plasmid mediated, extended-spectrum betalactamase (ESBL) producing strains of *E. coli* (resistant to ceftazidime and other third generation cephalosporins) have been reported in cancer patients. The CANCER network reported 3.9% of *E. coli* were ESBL producers [81, 82]. Risk factors associated with ESBL-producing gram-negative bacilli include exposure to fluoroquinolones and other broad-spectrum antibiotics, severity of illness, invasive procedures, CVC, urinary catheters, mechanical ventilation, and tube feeding [83]. ESBL producing gram-negative bacteria are often multidrug resistant and a carbapenem such as imipenem or meropenem is the preferred drug therapy [84]. Tigecycline, a new glycylcycline, has in vitro activity against many ESBL strains and may be a useful agent except in the setting of urinary tract infection since the drug is not excreted in the urine [85]. Mortality due to *E. coli* bacteremia is 17–35%, with increased mortality when associated with polymicrobial bacteremia [86, 87].

3.2. Klebsiella species

In the SCOPE study, *Klebsiella* species were the second most common gram-negative bacteria isolated (6.4%) [1]. Outbreaks of *Klebsiella oxytoca/ Enterobacter cloacae* resulting from contamination of saline flushes in cancer patients have been noted [88]. Frequency of ESBL resistance in Klebsiella has increased up to 20% in ICU isolates in the United States [84]. However, rates of ESBL-producing *Klebsiella* species are less common in cancer patients (2.4%) in the CANCER database [81, 82]. ESBL-producing *Klebsiella pneumoniae* can be multidrug resistant due to the acquisition of plasmid-mediated resistance determinants. Colistin has been used successfully for treatment of carbapenemase-producing *K. pneumoniae* [89]. However, strains resistant to all agents including colistin have been described recently [90].

3.3. Pseudomonas aeruginosa

In the National Nosocomial Survey in 2003 *P. aeruginosa* caused 18.1% of the pneumonias, 3.4% of the bloodstream infections, and 16.3% of the urinary tract infections, twice as many compared to 1975 [91]. In the SCOPE study *P. aeruginosa* accounted for 3.6% and 4.7% of bacteremias in neutropenic and nonneutropenic cancer patients, respectively [1]. Sites of infections in patients with hematological malignancies include bacteremias (35%), pneumonias (38%), and urinary tract infections (11%) [2]. A review of *P. aeruginosa* infections in cancer patients from the 1990s noted an incidence of 5–12% with no decline in the proportion of *P. aeruginosa* among gram-negative bacteria over the last two decades [92]. Significant local and regional differences in the incidence of *P. aeruginosa* bacteremia were seen. Similar rates of infection were noted in patients with hematological and solid malignancies and in neutropenic or nonneutropenic patients. In contrast, data from our institution shows that *P.aeruginosa* is an important and more frequent cause of bacteremia in patients with hematological malignancies as compared to patients with solid tumors (Fig. 3-1). Similar trends were noted from another cancer center where *P. aeruginosa* bacteremia rates of 19/1,000 in hematological cancer patients were less than the 2/1,000 rate seen in solid tumor patients [93].

The clinical presentation of infection with *P. aeruginosa* is nonspecific and is related to the site of infection. Occasionally, *P. aeruginosa* infection during neutropenia may manifest as painful discrete maculopapular skin lesions that rapidly develop central necrosis (ecthyma gangrenosum) [94]. Histopathology of these lesions demonstrates vascular invasion of the skin with *P.aeruginosa* resulting in skin infarction. Ecthyma lesions have also been seen in infections with other gram-negative bacteria, *S. aureus, Aspergillus,* and *Candida.*

In the 1980s, 71–94% of pseudomonal bacteremias in neutropenic patients were treated successfully with an antipseudomonal betalactam such as ceftazidime [95, 96]. Subsequent studies using monotherapy with antipseudomonal agents such as piperacillin, imipenem, meropenem, and cefepime showed comparable outcomes to the combination therapy of a betalactam antibiotic with an aminoglycoside [97]. Monotherapy with any of these potent antipseudomonal antibiotics is currently favored over combination therapy in the empiric treatment of febrile neutropenia [69, 98]. Addition of an aminoglycoside to an antipseudomonal betalactam may be useful in selected patients who are critically ill, especially those at risk for infection with multidrug resistant gram-negative bacteria. Aztreonam is useful in cases of penicillin allergy.

The duration of therapy is a minimum of 14 days for bacteremia or longer until resolution of neutropenia. Factors associated with poor outcome include the presence of shock, associated pneumonia, and lack of neutrophil recovery [93, 95, 99–101].

Increases in resistance of 20%, 15% and 9% to cephalosporins, imipenem and fluoroquinolones, respectively, was noted in *Pseudomonas* strains isolated from ICU patients in 2003 when compared to 1998 [91]. Similar increases in resistant strains has been reported in cancer patients with antibiotic exposure [102, 103]. The increase in multidrug resistant pseudomonal strains has led to the use of polymyxin B or colistin (polymyxin E) with some success [90, 104, 105]. Not surprisingly, reports of colistin resistance have emerged [106, 107]. Removal of indwelling CVC is usually warranted.

3.4. Stenotrophomonas maltophilia

Bacteremia with *S. maltophilia* is increasingly reported in patients with hematological malignancies [108–114]. Risk factors in cancer patients include neutropenia, mucositis, prior antibiotic use, prolonged hospitalization, mechanical ventilation, indwelling central venous and urinary catheters, and corticosteroid use [108, 109, 111, 113, 115, 116]. Common infections include bacteremias, pneumonias, and urinary tract infections. A review of 217 episodes of *S. maltophilia* bacteremia in cancer patients noted that 73% of infected patients had CVC [114]. *S. maltophilia* secondary bacteremias were often associated with pneumonia and were seen mostly in those with hematological malignancy. Breakthrough bacteremia with *S. maltophilia* may occur in patients receiving antibiotics including imipenem [108, 117]. Most isolates are multidrug-resistant and may only be susceptible to trimethoprim/sulfamethoxazole, ticaricillin/clavulanate, chloramphenicol, and ceftazidime [114–116]. Tigecycline is active in vitro against strains of *S. maltophilia* and may be a useful agent [118]. Response to therapy in patients with CVC-related bacteremias was 95% with attributable mortality of 11% as compared to successful responses of 56% and attributable mortality of 57% in patients with secondary bacteremias [114].

3.5. *Enterobacter* species

Enterobacter species are often associated with nosocomial infections including pneumonias, UTI, wound infections, and venous catheter-related infections and account for about 3% of bacteremias in cancer patients [1]. Risk factors include prior exposure to antibiotics and ICU stays [119]. A report of *Enterobacter* bacteremias in 281 cancer patients noted that 74% were acquired nosocomially and 25% of patients presented with septic shock [120]. *Enterobacter* species can develop resistance during therapy to third generation cephalosporins via selection for stable derepressed mutants that overproduce inducible chromosomal AmpC extended spectrum beta-lactamases [84, 121]. Data from the CANCER network noted AmpC mediated resistance to ceftriaxone, ceftazidime, and piperacillin in 8–12% of *Enterobacter* isolates, but most were susceptible to cefepime, a fourth generation cephalosporin, and to imipenem [81, 82]. Resistance may also emerge by acquisition of plasmids containing resistance-determinants such as non-AmpC ESBL [84]. Therapy with antibacterials such as quinolones, carbapenems, cefepime, or trimethoprim/sulfamethoxazole are acceptable alternatives. Pneumonia is the most feared invasive *Enterobacter* infection with successful responses to therapy in only 53% of cases compared to 86% success rate in nonpulmonary infections [120].

3.6. *Acinetobacter* species

Acinetobacter species are an emerging cause of nosocomial infections in cancer patients. Data from the NNIS reported a significant increase in ventilator-associated pneumonias caused by *Acinetobacter* compared to other gram-negative bacteria [91]. *Acinetobacter* can cause CVC-related bacteremias, pneumonias, UTIs, and wound infections, and is associated with poor outcome [122–124]. The most common species isolated is *A. baumannii* associated with CVC infections in 22% and respiratory tract infection in 18% of cases, respectively [125]. Multidrug resistance to four or more classes of antibiotics is not uncommon (around 30%) with imipenem and amikacin being the most active agents [125]. Other useful drugs include ampicillin-sulbactam, meropenem, and polymixins, Tigecycline has good activity in vitro against *Acinetobacter*. Predictors of mortality include older age, diabetes, recent surgery, pneumonia, septic shock, mechanical ventilation, multiorgan failure, decubitus ulcers, and burns [122, 124, 126, 127].

3.7. *Achromobacter* Species and Other Rare Gram-Negative Bacteria

Achromobacter species causing bacteremia have been reported in cancer patients [128–130]. A series of 52 bloodstream infections in 31 patients was reported from a single cancer center [131]. Most patients (67%) had hematological malignancies, only 33% of cases were acquired nosocomially. Polymicrobial infections, particularly with staphylococci, were common (52%), and a quarter of the cases were related to venous catheters. Mortality was around 15%, the commonest species being *Achromobacter xylosoxidans.* Most isolates were resistant to fluoroquinolones, and aminoglycosides [131]. Antibiotic therapy were based upon susceptibility data for the individual isolate. Predictors of mortality were sepsis, mechanical ventilation, and high APACHE score [131].

Other uncommon gram-negative bacteria reported to cause infection in patients with hematological malignancies include *Aeromonas* sp. [132], *Roseomonas* sp. [133], and *Moraxella osoensis* [134].

3.8. Clostidium difficile

Clostridium difficile, is an anaerobic spore-forming, toxin producing colonic bacteria. The number of cases of *C. difficile* associated disease (CDAD) has doubled from 31/100,000 of the US population in 1996 to 61/100,000 in 2003 [135]. Besides antibiotic exposure, other risk factors include age over 65, hospitalization, residence in long-term care facilities, severity of underlying disease, gastrointestinal procedures, nasogastric tube, ICU stay, and long lengths of hospital stay [136, 137]. Gastric acid suppressive agents including proton-pump inhibitors have been recently associated with an increased risk [138, 139]. All classes of antibiotics have been implicated and a recent meta-analysis identified the broad-spectrum cephalosporins cefotaxime and ceftazidime as being associated with the highest risk and tetracyclines with the lowest risk [136]. Newer fluoroquinolones, gatifloxacin, and moxifloxacin, have been strongly associated with CDAD in the context of outbreaks [140–143].

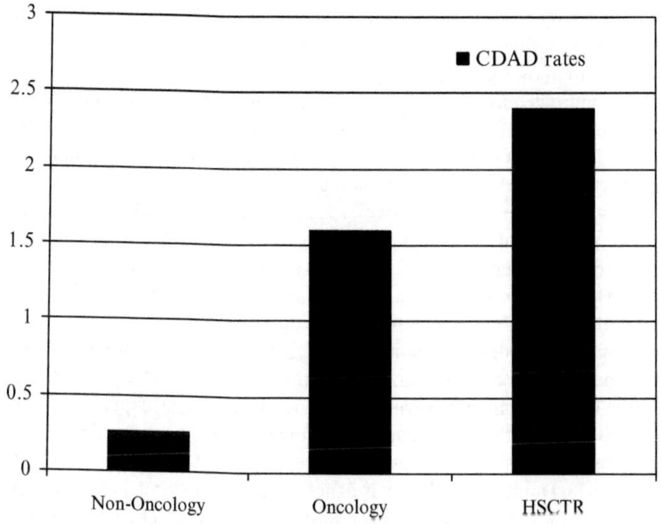

HSCTR=hematopoietic stem cell transplantation recipient

Fig. 3-2. Rates of *Clostridium difficile* Associated Disease per 1,000 Patient Days by Population, Karmanos Cancer Institute/Detroit Medical Center 2006

Several studies have evaluated CDAD in patients with hematological malignancies [144–153]. CDAD occurred in 7% of 875 courses of chemotherapy in patients with hematological malignancies [147]. The reported incidence of CDAD in inpatients with cancer at 2.4/1,000 patient days was no different from other medical and surgical patients [144]. However, surveillance data at our institution during 2006 identified higher rates of CDAD in cancer and SCT patients (Fig. 3-2). Besides traditional risk factors, antineoplastic therapy [154, 155] and graft versus host disease [156] are associated with increased risk for CDAD. The anticancer agents implicated include methotrexate, bleomycin, vinblastine, 5-fluorouracil, cyclophosphamide, doxorubicin, and cytarabine [155]. CDAD has also been associated with paclitaxel [157], cisplatin [158] and interleukin-2 [144].

Recent reports from the USA [159] and Canada [160] noted an increasing incidence of severe CDAD complications such as toxic megacolon, ICU admissions, and need for colectomy [141, 143, 160, 161]. Severe disease often occurred in patients over 65 years of age, leukocyte counts over 20,000/mm^3, renal impairment, and immunosuppression [141, 143, 160–162], and had an attributable mortality of 17% [160]. The outbreak strain designated as North American pulse-field gel electrophoresis strain (NAP-1) produces 16 times and 23 times more toxins A and B, respectively, as compared to traditional strains possibly because of alteration of a toxin repressor gene [159, 163]. An additional binary toxin may contribute to the severity of NAP-1 infections [164].

Diarrhea is the predominant presentation of CDAD which may progress to colitis, pseudomembranous colitis, and fulminant colitis. A grading system for the severity of CDAD based upon the National Cancer Institute Common Terminology Criteria for Adverse Events (CTCAE version 3.0) was recently evaluated in allogeneic SCT recipients [165].

Although detection of *C. difficile* toxin using the slow and labor-intensive tissue culture assay of stool remains the gold standard for the diagnosis of CDAD, it has been largely replaced by the more rapid enzyme immunoassays that detect toxins A and B. Sensitivities of the toxin assays range from 58% to 95% and an overall sensitivity of 75% [166, 167]. A single toxin assay performed on diarrheal stool in patients with suspected CDAD will identify most cases [168]. The sensitivity of toxin assays might be lower in SCT recipients with CDAD and testing two and three stool samples improved detection to 81% and 95% of CDAD infections, respectively [169].

Treatment includes discontinuation of the offending antibiotic, supportive care, and avoidance of antimotility agents [137, 167]. The preferred initial agent is oral metronidazole which is as effective but less expensive than oral vancomycin capsules. Oral vancomycin, the only agent approved by the FDA, is not absorbed systemically and therefore, achieves high levels in the colonic lumen [167]. Duration of therapy is generally for 10 days but may vary depending on the severity of disease and rapidity of response. The response rate to initial therapy with metronidazole was 91% in patients with hematological malignancies and autologous SCT recipients [169]. Oral vancomycin as initial therapy may be considered in severe CDAD [170]. Intracolonic administration of vancomycin has been effective in severe cases [171]. Repeat toxin testing to define cure is not recommended in patients who respond clinically to therapy. In progressive disease or in fulminant cases with bleeding or imminent colon perforation or rupture, colectomy may be necessary [172–174].

Recurrence rates in general are about 15–20% but may be lower (3%) in patients with hematological malignancies [147]. Relapse is managed by avoidance of antibiotics whenever possible and re-treatment with either metronidazole or vancomycin. Other measures may be pulse therapy of vancomycin followed by slow taper [175, 176], serial therapy with vancomycin and rifaximin [177], biotherapy with probiotics using oral *Lactobacillus rhamnosus* or *Saccharomyces boulardii* [178, 179], anion exchange toxin-binding resin cholestyramine [180], fecal implants [181], and intravenous immunoglobulin [182, 183]. Treatment with nitazoxanide and the anionic polymer, tolevamer are promising [184, 185].

4. Nocardia

Nocardia is an aerobic actinomycete that is ubiquitous in nature and most infections are acquired by inhalation. Infections due to this opportunistic pathogen generally occur in patients with chronic lung conditions (e.g., alveolar proteinosis), solid and SCT recipients, corticosteroid recipients, HIV-infected patients, and cancer patients [186]. Over a 13 year period, a single cancer center identified 43 episodes of nocardiosis with an incidence of 60 cases per 100,000 admissions; 64% occurred in patients with hematological malignancies and 31% in bone marrow transplant recipients [187]. The incidence of nocardiosis among SCT recipients is 0.2–1.75% with higher rates among allogeneic recipients with graft versus host disease (GVHD) [188–190]. The lower frequency of nocardiosis in this population might be due to the routine use of trimethoprim/sulfamethoxazole as prophylaxis against *Pneumocystis jiroveci*. In contrast to other bacterial infections in cancer patients, impairment of T cell-mediated immunity rather than neutropenia is the significant risk factor for nocardiosis. Lymphopenia resulting from exposure to corticosteroids, purine analogs, for example, fludarabine, and monoclonal antibodies (e.g., alemtuzumab) is a risk factor [191, 192].

Nocardiosis in cancer patients generally presents as pulmonary infection. Other affected sites include brain, skin, or disseminated disease [187, 193]. Rarely, bacteremia may occur as a consequence of dissemination or catheter-related infection [187, 194–196]. Pulmonary symptoms predominate and are generally subacute with a median duration of 3 weeks before diagnosis [187]. Chest radiograph often demonstrates lobar pneumonia or occasionally lung nodules in SCT recipients [188–190]. The diagnosis is established from cultures and gram stains of respiratory specimens or biopsies of infected tissue. The recovery of *Nocardia* from sputum is about 30–50% compared to 85–90% recovery from specimens obtained from an invasive procedure [186]. It is important for the clinician to notify the laboratory if *Nocardia* is suspected in order to perform the special stains and prolonged incubation of cultures [186]. In cancer patients, the most common species isolated are *Nocardia asteroides* complex. New *Nocardia* species causing invasive disease in hematological cancer patients including *N. otitidiscaviarum, N. transvalensis, N. veterana,* and *N. cyriacigeorgica* have been recently reported [187, 197–199].

Most species of *Nocardia* are susceptible to sulfamethoxazole, third-generation cephalosporins (cefotaxime, ceftriaxone), imipenem, amikacin, and minocycline. Identification of the species and susceptibility testing are recommended as some of the emerging species are resistant to these agents [186, 200]. *Nocardia* species are generally susceptible to linezolid [201]. Recent breakpoints for susceptibility testing for *Nocardia* have been published [202].

Sulfonamides are the drugs of choice with trimethoprim-sulfamethaxozole as the formulation generally used. Combination therapy with amikacin plus imipenem or a third-generation cephalosporin has been recommended for severe disease [200, 203]. Alternatives to oral therapy with TMP/SMX include minocycline or amoxicillin-clavulanate. Linezolid has been used successfully in a few patients including those with brain abscesses [204, 205]. Treatment should be guided by susceptibility testing in case of poor response or relapse on therapy, when a resistant species is isolated, or when initial therapy with sulfonamide is not possible.

The duration of treatment in immunosuppressed patients is guided by the extent of disease, clinical/radiological response to therapy, and underlying immune status and generally lasts at least 6 months in immunosuppressed patients [206]. Surgical resection or drainage of large localized brain abscesses may be considered. TMP-SMX provides effective prophylaxis against *Pneumocystis, Nocardia*, and *Toxoplasma* in the immunosuppressed host but breakthrough nocardiosis has been reported [187, 188]. Mortality in immunosuppressed patients is approximately 50%, with the best response in infections with *N. asteroides* [207].

5. Mycobacteria

Mycobacteria are gram-positive acid-fast bacilli of which *Mycobacterium tuberculosis* complex is the most pathogenic. Nontuberculous mycobacteria (NTM) are less pathogenic, but capable of causing opportunistic infections.

Early reports noted an incidence of mycobacteriosis of 607/100,000 in patients with cancer compared to 95/100,000 in the general hospital population [208]. Most infections occurred in patients with head and neck, lung, or testicular cancers; 50–73% were caused by *M. tuberculosis* with the remainder caused by NTM especially *Mycobacterium kansasii*, *Mycobacterium avium-intracellluare,* and *Mycobacterium fortuitum* [208, 209].

5.1. M. tuberculosis

Even though a third of the world's population is infected with *M. tuberculosis*, it is surprising that tuberculosis is relatively uncommon in patients with cancer and SCT [209–213]. Data from two large cancer centers in the USA from 1950 to 2004 noted a decline in the rates of tuberculosis in cancer patients from 345/100,000 to 55/100,000 [209, 210, 213, 214]. However, the rate of tuberculosis was 50–100 times higher in foreign born patients with hematological malignancies compared to US-born patients [213]. This is consistent with current data from the Centers for Disease Control which reported a steady decline in new cases of tuberculosis in the USA except in foreign-born persons [215]. Similarly, tuberculosis is rare in blood and marrow transplant recipients with an overall frequency of 0.4% [211]. Allogeneic transplant recipients are at greater risk particularly those with GVHD [211, 216]. Recent reports suggest the highest rates of tuberculosis are in patients with hematological malignancies such as non-Hodgkin's lymphoma, Hodgkin's lymphoma, and leukemia [212, 213]. The frequency of tuberculosis was 1.3/1,000 in new leukemia diagnoses compared to 0.2/100 new cancer diagnoses [212]. Tuberculosis and other mycobacterial infections are reported in patients with chronic lymphocytic leukemia treated with fludarabine, an agent that affects T-cell function [217]. The increasing use of monoclonal antibodies, for example, alemtuzumab and TNF-inhibitors in the treatment of GVHD can affect cell mediated immunity, and may further increase the risk of mycobacterial disease [218–220].

The majority of tuberculosis in cancer and bone marrow transplant patients involves the lungs with extrapulmonary disease primarily affecting the lymph nodes and pleura [211, 212, 221]. A high suspicion for tuberculosis should be maintained as the clinical presentation may mimic malignancy, as suggested by several reports of patients with suspected cancers eventually diagnosed correctly as extrapulmonary tuberculosis [221–227]. The delayed diagnosis of tuberculosis in patients with cancer can lead to transmission of infection to other immunocompromised patients and health care workers [228, 229]. Tuberculin skin test (TST) is positive in 60% of patients with tuberculosis and cancer [221]. False positive TST reactions may occur because of infection with NTM or in persons who had received BCG vaccine. New gamma interferon release assays performed on blood samples that improve the specificity of detection of latent tuberculous infection have been recently approved [230].

Most cases of pulmonary tuberculosis have unilateral upper lobe involvement suggesting reactivation of latent tuberculosis [212, 231]. The diagnosis of pulmonary tuberculosis requires microbiological testing of at least three sputum samples for acid-fast staining and mycobacterial cultures. Overall the sputum smear is positive in 50–70% of cases, more so in patients with cavitary disease. Sputum cultures may be negative in about 10–15% of cases [232]. BAL may be appropriate in cases where alternative diagnoses are being considered or if tuberculosis is strongly suspected and the patient is unable to expectorate sputum, or induced sputum testing is inconclusive [233, 234]. In patients with cancer and pulmonary tuberculosis, 35% of the BAL specimens were AFB smear positive and 95% were culture positive [187]. The potential delay in the time to diagnosis of *M. tuberculosis* by conventional AFB smear examination and culturing of clinical specimens has led to the use of molecular methods for the rapid identification of *M. tuberculosis*. FDA approved commercial nucleic acid amplification tests (NAA) have a sensitivity of at least 95% and specificity of 100% when testing respiratory specimens that are AFB smear positive and reduced sensitivity but 99% specificity even in culture positive/smear negative cases [235]. The NAA tests have shown either comparable or slightly lower performance results when tested on nonrespiratory specimens [235]. PCR has been used successfully for the detection of *M. tuberculosis* in smear and culture negative tissue specimens [236, 237]. The time from detection of growth on culture to the identification of mycobacteria has been shortened to a few hours by the use of commercially available species-specific DNA probes which are able to identify *M. tuberculosis* complex, *M. avium* complex, *M. intracellulare, M. kansasii,* and *Mycobacterium gordonae* [236, 238]. Culture remains the only technique for isolating *M. tuberculosis* for testing susceptibility with results available in 6–8 weeks. PCR assays are being evaluated for the rapid detection of specific mutations associated with drug resistance [236, 239, 240]. Routine application of molecular genotyping of *M. tuberculosis* isolated from patients has helped identify transmission of *M. tuberculosis* in epidemiologically unsuspected cases or laboratory contamination, trace genealogy of multidrug resistant-strains, and distinguish relapse from reinfections [236, 240, 241].

Guidelines for the treatment of tuberculosis by the CDC and the American Thoracic Society were updated in 2003 and are available at http://www.cdc.gov/mmwr and http://www.thoracic.org/adobe/statements/treattb.pdf. Close monitoring of patients on treatment is needed as drug interactions are common with rifampin. The mortality attributed to tuberculosis in patients treated appropriately was 12–21%, and occurred mainly in patients receiving high-dose corticosteroids and those with advanced solid-organ cancer [212, 221]. Although baseline tuberculin skin testing (TST) for the detection of latent TB infection (LTBI) in patients with cancer before initiation of immunosuppressive therapy has been recommended by some authors [228], it is not routinely performed in cancer centers in the USA. Recommendations for treatment of LTBI have been published [242, 243].

5.2. Nontuberculous Mycobacteria

NTM infections have been reported in patients with AIDS, transplant recipients, and other immunocompromised hosts, however, they are uncommon in patients with cancer [244]. In general at least three respiratory samples within 1 year positive by culture and/or smears for NTM or isolation of NTM from a tissue sample or sterile extrapulmonary site in appropriate patients is required for diagnosis of infection.

A review of NTM infections in cancer patients from a single center from the 1960s through the 1990s reported colonization with *Mycobacterium chelonei* and *M. fortuitum* in 77 patients and true infection in 14 patients. Most infections occurred in solid tumor patients [245, 246]. Predisposing factors for NTM infection was prior lung disease and chemotherapy. Most infections involved the lungs with nonspecific symptoms, signs, and radiographic findings.

M. avium complex infections and bacteremia were reported in few patients with leukemia [247]. Of 127 cancer patients who had *M. avium* or *M. intracellulare* isolated from a clinical specimen, only 16% had definite or probable infection [248]. Patients with hairy cell leukemia have a predilection for NTM, the commonest are *M. kansasii* and *M. avium-intracellulare* [249–251].

M. kansasii infections were identified in 25 patients with cancer of which 33% occurred in patients with leukemia who had an estimated rate of infection of 115/100,000 compared to only 14/100,000 in patients with solid tumors [252]. Although 92% of the infections involved the lungs, the majority of patients had no fever, cough, or sputum production. Bilateral upper lobe lung infiltrates were common with cavitation noted in 33% of radiographs.

Mycobacterium haemophilum infection has been recently reported in patients with AIDS, SCT recipients, and few patients with hematological malignancies [253, 254]. Patients with hematological malignancies had infections primarily affecting the skin and soft-tissue with a uniformly good treatment outcome. Contamination of chemotherapy with *Mycobacterium bovis* bacilli Calmette-Guerin (BCG) has resulted in nosocomial infections in patients with hematological malignancies [255]. Other unusual NTM reported in patients with hematological malignancies include *Mycobacterium malmoense* [256, 257], *Mycobacterium marinum* [258], and *Mycobacterium vaccae* [259].

Although most NTM infections reported in patients with cancer involve the lungs [245, 246, 260], bacteremia related to CVC have been increasingly reported especially with *M. fortuitum* [261, 262]. CVC has also been reported with *Mycobacterium mucogenicum, Mycobacterium brumae, Mycobacterium senegalense,* and *Mycobacterium szulgai* [263–266].

NTM infections are reported in SCT recipients with incidence of 0.4–4.9%, which is 50–600 times greater than that in the general population [267–269]. The commonly reported species are *M. avium-intracellulare, M. haemophilum, M. fortuitum, Mycobacterium chelonae*, and *Mycobacterium abscessus* [267]. Unlike in cancer patients where pulmonary infections predominate, CVC-associated infections were more common in SCT recipients [267].

The susceptibility of NTM to antibiotics is variable. However, standardization of susceptibility testing of many NTM has facilitated selection of appropriate antimicrobial therapy. The therapy of NTM is summarized in the ATS guidelines [267, 270]. It is important to reduce the degree of immunosuppression whenever possible to improve treatment outcomes. The duration of therapy is often prolonged, and in the absence of large studies, it is guided by the degree of underlying immunosuppression, status of malignancy, and the clinical and radiological response to therapy. Surgical excision of localized cutaneous infections may improve response to therapy. CVC-related NTM infections require removal of the infected catheter [262]. The outcome is generally good and mortality is often related to progression or complication resulting from the underlying malignancy [245, 246, 252, 254].

6. Anaerobic Organisms

Blood stream infections with anaerobic organisms have been perceived to be so uncommon that recent suggestions were made, without success, to discontinue routine use of anaerobic blood culture system. In cancer patients, anaeorbic organisms may be involved as a part of polymicrobial infection in the setting of neutropenic enterocolitis, pneumonia, urinary tract infection, or catheter-related blood stream infection. Cancer patients are at higher risk for an anaerobic infection following disruption of physical barriers (e.g., gastrointestinal tract mucositis, skin breaks, etc.) because of cytotoxic chemotherapy and vascular catheters. Data from the general population in hospitalized patients show 0.5–9% of bacteremia due to anaerobes [271]. Recently, an increase in the incidence of anaerobic blood stream infections has been noted in cancer patients and stem cell recipients [86, 272]. Hematological malignancies, quinolone prophylaxis, surgery, and broad spectrum antibiotic use have been identified as risk factors [272].

A recent French study in nonsurgical cancer patients found 45 patients with anaerobic bacteremia over a 6-year period at a tertiary oncology center (<1% of all positive blood cultures from hospitalized cancer patients) [273]. Abdominal and hematological malignancies were the most common. Most pathogens were suspected to be of oral or gastrointestinal origin; *Bacteroides* spp. (60%) (mainly *B. fragilis*) and *Clostridium* spp.(22%) (mainly *C. perfringens*) were the most frequent. In 20 of 45 patients, *E. coli* was concomitantly recovered. Occasional pathogens producing serious disease included *Bifidobacterium* and *Lactobacillus*. Mortality is high in patients with anaerobic infection [274]. Commonly used antianaerobic drugs include clindamycin, metronidazole, tigecycline, carbapenem, and betalactam – betalactamase inhibitor combinations (e.g., piperacillin-tazobactam, ampicillin-sulbactam). Among the newer fluoroquinolones, moxifloxacin has reliable antianaerobic activity. Aminoglycosides are inactive. In all cases, in addition to antianaerobic drugs, removal of the source of infection must be attempted. Removal of infected indwelling device (e.g., vascular catheter, biliary stent etc.) and open or CT-guided drainage of abscesses are critical for improved outcomes.

Among the specific anaerobic pathogens, *Capnocytophaga* causes bacteremia in patients with neutropenia and cancer [275]. These are facultatively anaerobic fusiform gram-negative bacilli that are part of the normal oral flora. Severe oropharyngeal mucositis after chemotherapy or periodontal disease are frequently associated with *Capnocytophaga* bacteremia. It is often seen in neutropenic patients with hematologic malignancies; uncomplicated bacteremia without organ involvement is the most common clinical presentation. The organism is susceptible to betalactam drugs, however, rising resistance to such drugs, presumably induced by previous exposure, is reported [276, 277]. Emergence of fluoroquinolone-resistant *Capnocytophaga* is also reported [275], and this phenomenon is an important consideration during quinolone prophylaxis.

7. Polymicrobial Infection

Most reports/surveys on infections in cancer patients have paid exclusive attention to monomicrobial blood stream infection. Consequently, polymicrobial infections are inadequately documented. There are scant reports available addressing the involvement of multiple organisms causing bacteremia, pneumonia, perirectal infection, typhlitis/neutropenic enterocolitis, urinary tract infection, and hepatobiliary infection [278–280].

In a large study of 507 polymicrobial bacteremic episodes during 1972–1981 at the MD Anderson Cancer Center in Texas, 76% involved at least 1 gram-negative bacillus and 33% infections involved only gram-negative bacilli [279]. Gram-positive bacteria, anaerobes or fungi were infrequent pathogens. Most frequent gram-negative bacteria were *E. coli, Klebsiella, Pseudomonas* and *Enterobacter*; gram-positive bacteria were streptococci, enterococci and staphylococci. Another large study conducted by the SCOPE project identified 14% polymicrobial infections in 2,340 cancer patients with nosocomial blood stream infection (only 11% with neutropenia) with nosocomial blood stream infection [1]. Several large antibiotic trials involving febrile neutropenic patients have demonstrated 8–32% polymicrobial bacteremia [15, 281–285]. Most polymicrobial blood stream infections are believed to be of oropharyngeal/gastrointestinal origin; the clinical response in polymicrobial infections is lower (≈50%) than that seen with monomicrobial infections.

Typhlitis (neutropenic enterocolitis) is a polymicrobial infection resulting from invasion of enteric microflora following chemotherapy-induced gut mucosal damage and is usually seen in patients with acute leukemia [286, 287]. This entity, best characterized in children, carries a high mortality (around 50%) [288]. Fever, abdominal pain and tenderness, usually starting in the right lower quadrant of the abdomen, and diarrhea are the common clinical features. Microbiologic diagnosis is generally made from blood cultures; common pathogens include aerobic gram-negative bacilli and among anaerobes, *Clostridium septicum*. Antimicrobial therapy consists of drugs targeted against anaerobic and aerobic gut microflora. Whether antifungal coverage must be empirically included is unclear.

Perirectal infections are of polymicrobial origin in patients with cancer. Also infections occurring at the hepatobiliary site or in the urinary tract can be polymicrobial.; these are seen mostly in patients with solid tumors who have undergone invasive procedures (e.g., biliary stents, ureteral stents, percutaneous nephrostomies, previous surgeries) [280, 289].

8. Diagnosis

The traditional, slow culture-based diagnostic method has been used for over 100 years to detect and identify organisms in the blood stream. Results generally take 1–2 days; consequently, inappropriate therapy or a delay in therapy leading to adverse clinical outcomes is commonplace. Recently, a rapid molecular testing method has been introduced – peptide nucleic acid (PNA) fluorescence in situ hybridization (FISH). The peptide probes can specifically target the 16S ribosomal (r) RNA within living bacteria and yeasts. These 16S (r) RNA regions contain highly conserved species-specific sequences as targets [290, 291]. These probes are currently available to identify *S. aureus*, *E. fecalis*, and *Candida albicans*. The tests can identify organisms within 150 min, but has a limit of detection of 10^4 organisms/mL; thus, it can only be performed in specimens with a positive gram stain. Faster identification of organisms using this method has been shown to decrease inappropriate drug use, shorten hospital stay, and even improve survival [292–295]. Real-time PCR testing is another method undergoing evaluation for rapid diagnosis of pathogens in clinical specimens [296]. These tests need validation in cancer patients.

Fever with negative blood cultures necessitating empiric antimicrobial use in cancer wards contributes to enormous antibiotic consumption in most hospitals. Vancomycin and antipseudomonal betalactams (e.g., cefepime, ceftazidine, piperacillin-tazobactam, imipenem, and meropenem) are the most commonly used drugs. Currently, no test can reliably distinguish fevers of infectious and noninfectious origins. A wide variety of inflammatory markers has been examined in febrile cancer patients with or without neutropenia. Such markers include serum C-reactive protein, procalcitonin, neopterin, endotoxin, tumor necrosis factor, and interleukins 6 and 8 [297–299]. Present data suggest that none of these markers provide early and accurate results to reduce inappropriate and empiric antibiotic use in cancer wards.

9. Vascular-Catheter Related Infection

Vascular catheters are indispensable in the care of cancer patients. All catheters, regardless of type and location, constitute a major target of infection, contributing to a large number of cases of coagulase-negative staphylococcal bacteremia in cancer patients. Tunnelled catheters (e.g., Hickman, Broviac catheters), infusaports, and peripherally inserted central catheters (PICC) are the most commonly used catheters. Types of infections are many including asymptomatic bacteremia, exit site infection, superficial cellulitis, and more serious ones such as tunnel infection and symptomatic bacteremia/septic shock. Most catheter related infections present as unexplained fevers and are not accompanied by signs of infection at the exit site or along the tunnel. Absence of inflammation at the catheter exit site does not exclude infection. Malfunction of the catheter, abrupt onset of rigors and fever immediately after starting an infusion via the catheter, or rapid clinical improvement after catheter removal are clues highly suggestive of catheter-related infection. Blood cultures are the mainstay of diagnosis for catheter-related bacteremia. Confirming the catheter to be the source of bacteremia is difficult. More than 15 colonies growing from a catheter tip rolled on solid agar medium suggests that a bacteria is associated with contamination of a CVC [300]. Unfortunately, this method of detection requires sacrificing catheters even when bacteremias are found to be unlikely associated with a catheter source. "Differential time to positivity," where paired blood cultures drawn through the catheter and through a peripheral blood draw, is highly predictive of catheter-related bacteremia when the specimen blood culture drawn from the catheter reveals growth 2 or more hours earlier than from the specimen drawn from a peripheral vein [301–303]. Importantly, this diagnostic method does not warrant catheter removal for diagnosis.

It is estimated that more than 70% of catheters removed as a result of suspected catheter-related infection are removed unnecessarily [304]. Management of catheter-related bacteremia usually requires prompt catheter removal except in cases of coagulase-negative staphylococcal bacteremia in stable patients. This is especially true for organisms such as *S. aureus*, *P. aeruginosa,* or *Candida* where removal of the catheter is mandatory. In cases of *S. aureus* bacteremia, prolonged therapy (4–6 weeks) is indicated if blood cultures are positive over 2–3 days in view of the potential for endovascular or metastatic infection. Duration of therapy may be short in cases of coagulase-negative staphylococcal bacteremia. For catheter-associated gram-negative bacteremia, total duration of 7–10 days of appropriate therapy combined with catheter removal is usually adequate. If blood cultures remain persistently positive for CoNS, despite appropriate antimicrobial therapy, then the catheter needs removal. In catheters with multiple ports, the different ports may be used alternately for antibiotic infusion. On the other hand, if organisms such as *S. aureus*, *P. aeruginosa*, or *Candida* are suspected as the cause of catheter-related bacteremia, prompt removal of the catheter is optimal. If bacteremia persists despite catheter removal, then a thorough search is warranted to look for sites of metastatic infection (e.g., endocarditis, or infected thrombosed vein). Transesophageal echocardiography to detect cardiac vegetations, or an ultrasound examination over the tunnel site to diagnose vascular thrombosis may be required.

References

1. Wisplinghoff H, Seifert H, Wenzel RP, Edmond MB (2003) Current trends in the epidemiology of nosocomial bloodstream infections in patients with hematological malignancies and solid neoplasms in hospitals in the United States. Clin Infect Dis 36:1103–1110
2. Yadegarynia D, Tarrand J, Raad I, Rolston K (2003) Current spectrum of bacterial infections in patients with cancer. Clin Infect Dis 37(8):1144–1145
3. Cherif H, Kronvall G, Bjorkholm M, Kalin M (2003) Bacteraemia in hospitalised patients with malignant blood disorders: a retrospective study of causative agents and their resistance profiles during a 14-year period without antibacterial prophylaxis. Hematol J 4:420–426
4. Lowder JN, Lazarus HM, Herzig RH (1982) Bacteremias and fungemias in oncologic patients with central venous catheters: changing spectrum of infection. Arch Intern Med 142:1456–1459
5. Viscoli C, Bruzzi P, Castagnola E et al (1994) Factors associated with bacteraemia in febrile, granulocytopenic cancer patients. The International Antimicrobial Therapy Cooperative Group (IATCG) of the European Organization for Research and Treatment of Cancer (EORTC). Eur J Cancer 30A:430–437
6. Rotstein C, Mandell L, Goldberg N (1997) Fluoroquinolone prophylaxis for profoundly neutropenic cancer patients: a meta-analysis. Curr Oncol 4:S2–S7
7. Engels EA, Lau J, Barza M (1998) Efficacy of quinolone prophylaxis in neutropenic cancer patients: a meta-analysis. J Clin Oncol 16:1179–1187
8. Elting LS, Bodey GP, Keefe BH (1992) Septicemia and shock syndrome due to viridans streptococci: a case-control study of predisposing factors. Clin Infect Dis 14:1201–1207
9. Rolston KV, Yadegarynia D, Kontoyiannis DP, Raad II, Ho DH (2006) The spectrum of gram-positive bloodstream infections in patients with hematologic malignancies, and the in vitro activity of various quinolones against Gram-positive bacteria isolated from cancer patients. Int J Infect Dis 10:223–230
10. Schwalbe RS, Stapleton JT, Gilligan PH (1987) Emergence of vancomycin resistance in coagulase-negative staphylococci. N Engl J Med 316:927–931
11. Biavasco F, Vignaroli C, Varaldo PE (2000) Glycopeptide resistance in coagulase-negative staphylococci. Eur J Clin Microbiol Infect Dis 19:403–417
12. Sieradzki K, Villari P, Tomasz A (1998) Decreased susceptibilities to teicoplanin and vancomycin among coagulase-negative methicillin-resistant clinical isolates of staphylococci. Antimicrob Agents Chemother 42:100–107
13. Falcone M, Micozzi A, Pompeo ME et al (2004) Methicillin-resistant staphylococcal bacteremia in patients with hematologic malignancies: clinical and microbiological retrospective comparative analysis of *S. haemolyticus*, *S. epidermidis* and *S. aureus*. J Chemother 16:540–548

14. Diekema DJ, Pfaller MA, Jones RN (2002) Age-related trends in pathogen frequency and antimicrobial susceptibility of bloodstream isolates in North America: SENTRY Antimicrobial Surveillance Program, 1997–2000. Int J Antimicrob Agents 20:412–418
15. Wisplinghoff H, Cornely OA, Moser S et al (2003) Outcomes of nosocomial bloodstream infections in adult neutropenic patients: a prospective cohort and matched case-control study. Infect Control Hosp Epidemiol 24:905–911
16. Wisplinghoff H, Bischoff T, Tallent SM, Seifert H, Wenzel RP, Edmond MB (2004) Nosocomial bloodstream infections in US hospitals: analysis of 24, 179 cases from a prospective nationwide surveillance study. Clin Infect Dis 39:309–317
17. Fowler VG Jr, Olsen MK, Corey GR et al (2003) Clinical identifiers of complicated *Staphylococcus aureus* bacteremia. Arch Intern Med 163:2066–2072
18. Ghanem GA, Boktour M, Warneke C et al (2007) Catheter-related Staphylococcus aureus bacteremia in cancer patients: high rate of complications with therapeutic implications. Medicine (Baltimore) 86:54–60
19. Venditti M, Falcone M, Micozzi A et al (2003) Staphylococcus aureus bacteremia in patients with hematologic malignancies: a retrospective case-control study. Haematologica 88:923–930
20. Chambers HF (2005) Community-associated MRSA – resistance and virulence converge. N Engl J Med 352:1485–1487
21. Fridkin SK, Hageman JC, Morrison M et al (2005) Methicillin-resistant *Staphylococcus aureus* disease in three communities. N Engl J Med 352:1436–1444
22. Weber JT (2005) Community-associated methicillin-resistant *Staphylococcus aureus*. Clin Infect Dis 41(Suppl 4):S269–S272
23. Jauregui LE, Babazadeh S, Seltzer E et al (2005) Randomized, double-blind comparison of once-weekly dalbavancin versus twice-daily linezolid therapy for the treatment of complicated skin and skin structure infections. Clin Infect Dis 41:1407–1415
24. Stryjewski ME, Chu VH, O'Riordan WD et al (2006) Telavancin versus standard therapy for treatment of complicated skin and skin structure infections caused by gram-positive bacteria: FAST 2 study. Antimicrob Agents Chemother 50: 862–867
25. Tenover FC, Lancaster MV, Hill BC et al (1998) Characterization of staphylococci with reduced susceptibilities to vancomycin and other glycopeptides. J Clin Microbiol 36:1020–1027
26. Moore MR, Perdreau-Remington F, Chambers HF (2003) Vancomycin treatment failure associated with heterogeneous vancomycin-intermediate Staphylococcus aureus in a patient with endocarditis and in the rabbit model of endocarditis. Antimicrob Agents Chemother 47:1262–1266
27. Howden BP, Ward PB, Charles PG et al (2004) Treatment outcomes for serious infections caused by methicillin-resistant Staphylococcus aureus with reduced vancomycin susceptibility. Clin Infect Dis 38:521–528
28. Charles PG, Ward PB, Johnson PD, Howden BP, Grayson ML (2004) Clinical features associated with bacteremia due to heterogeneous vancomycin-intermediate Staphylococcus aureus. Clin Infect Dis 38:448–451
29. Richard P, Amador Del Valle G, Moreau P et al (1995) Viridans streptococcal bacteraemia in patients with neutropenia. Lancet 345:1607–1609
30. Tunkel AR, Sepkowitz KA (2002) Infections caused by viridans streptococci in patients with neutropenia. Clin Infect Dis 34:1524–1529
31. Razonable RR, Litzow MR, Khaliq Y, Piper KE, Rouse MS, Patel R (2002) Bacteremia due to viridans group Streptococci with diminished susceptibility to Levofloxacin among neutropenic patients receiving levofloxacin prophylaxis. Clin Infect Dis 34:1469–1474
32. Han XY, Kamana M, Rolston KV (2006) Viridans streptococci isolated by culture from blood of cancer patients: clinical and microbiologic analysis of 50 cases. J Clin Microbiol 44:160–165

33. Alcaide F, Benitez MA, Carratala J, Gudiol F, Linares J, Martin R (2001) In vitro activities of the new ketolide HMR 3647 (telithromycin) in comparison with those of eight other antibiotics against viridans group Streptococci isolated from blood of neutropenic patients with cancer. Antimicrob Agents Chemother 45:624–626
34. Doern GV, Ferraro MJ, Brueggemann AB, Ruoff KL (1996) Emergence of high rates of antimicrobial resistance among viridans group streptococci in the United States. Antimicrob Agents Chemother 40:891–894
35. Marron A, Carratala J, Gonzalez-Barca E, Fernandez-Sevilla A, Alcaide F, Gudiol F (2000) Serious complications of bacteremia caused by Viridans streptococci in neutropenic patients with cancer. Clin Infect Dis 31:1126–1130
36. Whiley RA, Fraser HY, Douglas CW, Hardie JM, Williams AM, Collins MD (1990) *Streptococcus parasanguis* sp. nov., an atypical viridans Streptococcus from human clinical specimens. FEMS Microbiol Lett 56:115–121
37. Kumashi P, Girgawy E, Tarrand JJ, Rolston KV, Raad II, Safdar A (2005) *Streptococcus pneumoniae* bacteremia in patients with cancer: disease characteristics and outcomes in the era of escalating drug resistance (1998-2002). Medicine (Baltimore) 84:303–312
38. Youssef S, Rodriguez G, Rolston KV, Champlin RE, Raad II, Safdar A (2007) *Streptococcus pneumoniae* infections in 47 hematopoietic stem cell transplantation recipients: clinical characteristics of infections and vaccine-breakthrough infections, 1989–2005. Medicine (Baltimore) 86:69–77
39. DiazGranados CA, Jernigan JA (2005) Impact of vancomycin resistance on mortality among patients with neutropenia and enterococcal bloodstream infection. J Infect Dis 191:588–595
40. Vergis EN, Hayden MK, Chow JW et al (2001) Determinants of vancomycin resistance and mortality rates in enterococcal bacteremia. a prospective multicenter study. Ann Intern Med 135:484–492
41. Garbutt JM, Ventrapragada M, Littenberg B, Mundy LM (2000) Association between resistance to vancomycin and death in cases of Enterococcus faecium bacteremia. Clin Infect Dis 30:466–472
42. Venditti M, Tarasi A, Visco Comandini U et al (1993) Enterococcal septicemia in patients with hematological malignancies. Eur J Clin Microbiol Infect Dis 12: 241–247
43. Todeschini G, Tecchio C, Borghero C et al (2006) Association between Enterococcus bacteraemia and death in neutropenic patients with haematological malignancies. J Infect 53:266–273
44. Morris JG Jr, Shay DK, Hebden JN et al (1995) Enterococci resistant to multiple antimicrobial agents, including vancomycin. Establishment of endemicity in a university medical center. Ann Intern Med 123:250–259
45. Matar MJ, Tarrand J, Raad I, Rolston KV (2006) Colonization and infection with vancomycin-resistant Enterococcus among patients with cancer. Am J Infect Control 34:534–536
46. Hachem R, Graviss L, Hanna H et al (2004) Impact of surveillance for vancomycin-resistant enterococci on controlling a bloodstream outbreak among patients with hematologic malignancy. Infect Control Hosp Epidemiol 25:391–394
47. Fridkin SK, Steward CD, Edwards JR, Pryor ER, McGowan JE Jr, Archibald LK, Gaynes RP, Tenover FC (1999) Surveillance of antimicrobial use and antimicrobial resistance in United States hospitals: project ICARE phase 2. Project Intensive Care Antimicrobial Resistance Epidemiology (ICARE) hospitals. Clin Infect Dis 29(2):245–252
48. Ostrowsky BE, Trick WE, Sohn AH, Quirk SB, Holt S, Carson LA, Hill BC, Arduino MJ, Kuehnert MJ, Jarvis WR (2001) Control of vancomycin-resistant enterococcus in health care facilities in a region. N Engl J Med 344(19):1427–1433
49. Price CS, Paule S, Noskin GA, Peterson LR (2003) Active surveillance reduces the incidence of vancomycin-resistant enterococcal bacteremia. Clin Infect Dis 37:921–928

50. Montecalvo MA, Jarvis WR, Uman J et al (1999) Infection-control measures reduce transmission of vancomycin-resistant enterococci in an endemic setting. Ann Intern Med 131:269–272
51. Dubberke ER, Hollands JM, Georgantopoulos P et al (2006) Vancomycin-resistant enterococcal bloodstream infections on a hematopoietic stem cell transplant unit: are the sick getting sicker? Bone Marrow Transplant 38:813–819
52. Avery R, Kalaycio M, Pohlman B et al (2005) Early vancomycin-resistant enterococcus (VRE) bacteremia after allogeneic bone marrow transplantation is associated with a rapidly deteriorating clinical course. Bone Marrow Transplant 35:497–499
53. Mylonakis E, Hohmann EL, Calderwood SB (1998) Central nervous system infection with Listeria monocytogenes. 33 years' experience at a general hospital and review of 776 episodes from the literature. Medicine (Baltimore) 77:313–336
54. Mylonakis E, Paliou M, Hohmann EL, Calderwood SB, Wing EJ (2002) Listeriosis during pregnancy: a case series and review of 222 cases. Medicine (Baltimore) 81:260–269
55. Armstrong RW, Fung PC (1993) Brainstem encephalitis (rhombencephalitis) due to Listeria monocytogenes: case report and review. Clin Infect Dis 16:689–702
56. Lorber B (1997) Listeriosis. Clin Infect Dis 24:1–9 quiz 10-1
57. Safdar A, Papadopoulous EB, Armstrong D (2002) Listeriosis in recipients of allogeneic blood and marrow transplantation: thirteen year review of disease characteristics, treatment outcomes and a new association with human cytomegalovirus infection. Bone Marrow Transplant 29:913–916
58. Decker CF, Simon GL, DiGioia RA, Tuazon CU (1991) Listeria monocytogenes infections in patients with AIDS: report of five cases and review. Rev Infect Dis 13:413–417
59. Hantel A, Dick JD, Karp JE (1989) Listeriosis in the setting of malignant disease. Changing issues in an unusual infection. Cancer 64:516–520
60. Jensen A, Frederiksen W, Gerner-Smidt P (1994) Risk factors for listeriosis in Denmark, 1989–1990. Scand J Infect Dis 26:171–178
61. Rivero GA, Torres HA, Rolston KV, Kontoyiannis DP (2003) Listeria monocytogenes infection in patients with cancer. Diagn Microbiol Infect Dis 47: 393–398
62. Vazquez-Boland JA, Kuhn M, Berche P et al (2001) Listeria pathogenesis and molecular virulence determinants. Clin Microbiol Rev 14:584–640
63. Anaissie E, Kontoyiannis DP, Kantarjian H, Elting L, Robertson LE, Keating M (1992) Listeriosis in patients with chronic lymphocytic leukemia who were treated with fludarabine and prednisone. Ann Intern Med 117:466–469
64. Anaissie EJ, Kontoyiannis DP, O'Brien S et al (1998) Infections in patients with chronic lymphocytic leukemia treated with fludarabine. Ann Intern Med 129:559–566
65. Safdar A, Armstrong D (2003) Antimicrobial activities against 84 Listeria monocytogenes isolates from patients with systemic listeriosis at a comprehensive cancer center (1955–1997). J Clin Microbiol 41:483–485
66. Girmenia C, Iori AP, Bernasconi S, Testi AM, Moleti ML, Arcese W, Martino P (2000) Listeriosis in recipients of allogeneic bone marrow transplants from unrelated donors. Eur J Clin Microbiol Infect Dis 19(9):711–714
67. Velasco E, Byington R, Martins CA, Schirmer M, Dias LM, Goncalves VM (2006) Comparative study of clinical characteristics of neutropenic and non-neutropenic adult cancer patients with bloodstream infections. Eur J Clin Microbiol Infect Dis 25:1–7
68. Chen CY, Tang JL, Hsueh PR et al (2004) Trends and antimicrobial resistance of pathogens causing bloodstream infections among febrile neutropenic adults with hematological malignancy. J Formos Med Assoc 103:526–532
69. Hughes WT, Armstrong D, Bodey GP et al (2002) 2002 guidelines for the use of antimicrobial agents in neutropenic patients with cancer. Clin Infect Dis 34:730–751

70. McGowan JE Jr (2006) Resistance in nonfermenting gram-negative bacteria: multidrug resistance to the maximum. Am J Infect Control 34:S29–S37 discussion S64–73
71. Gunther G, Bjorkholm M, Bjorklind A, Engervall P, Stiernstedt G (1991) Septicemia in patients with hematological disorders and neutropenia. A retrospective study of causative agents and their resistance profile. Scand J Infect Dis 23: 589–598
72. Kern WV, Andriof E, Oethinger M, Kern P, Hacker J, Marre R (1994) Emergence of fluoroquinolone-resistant Escherichia coli at a cancer center. Antimicrob Agents Chemother 38:681–687
73. Cometta A, Calandra T, Bille J, Glauser MP (1994) Escherichia coli resistant to fluoroquinolones in patients with cancer and neutropenia. N Engl J Med 330: 1240–1241
74. Carratala J, Fernandez-Sevilla A, Tubau F, Callis M, Gudiol F (1995) Emergence of quinolone-resistant Escherichia coli bacteremia in neutropenic patients with cancer who have received prophylactic norfloxacin. Clin Infect Dis 20:557–560 discussion 61–3
75. Cruciani M, Rampazzo R, Malena M et al (1996) Prophylaxis with fluoroquinolones for bacterial infections in neutropenic patients: a meta-analysis. Clin Infect Dis 23:795–805
76. Murphy M, Brown AE, Sepkowitz KA, Bernard EM, Kiehn TE, Armstrong D (1997) Fluoroquinolone prophylaxis for the prevention of bacterial infections in patients with cancer – is it justified? Clin Infect Dis 25:346–348
77. Kern WV, Klose K, Jellen-Ritter AS et al (2005) Fluoroquinolone resistance of Escherichia coli at a cancer center: epidemiologic evolution and effects of discontinuing prophylactic fluoroquinolone use in neutropenic patients with leukemia. Eur J Clin Microbiol Infect Dis 24:111–118
78. Reuter S, Kern WV, Sigge A et al (2005) Impact of fluoroquinolone prophylaxis on reduced infection-related mortality among patients with neutropenia and hematologic malignancies. Clin Infect Dis 40:1087–1093
79. Cullen M, Steven N, Billingham L et al (2005) Antibacterial prophylaxis after chemotherapy for solid tumors and lymphomas. N Engl J Med 353:988–998
80. Bucaneve G, Micozzi A, Menichetti F et al (2005) Levofloxacin to prevent bacterial infection in patients with cancer and neutropenia. N Engl J Med 353: 977–987
81. Kirby JT, Fritsche TR, Jones RN (2006) Influence of patient age on the frequency of occurrence and antimicrobial resistance patterns of isolates from hematology/ oncology patients: report from the Chemotherapy Alliance for Neutropenics and the Control of Emerging Resistance Program (North America). Diagn Microbiol Infect Dis 56:75–82
82. Mutnick AH, Kirby JT, Jones RN (2003) CANCER resistance surveillance program: initial results from hematology-oncology centers in North America. Chemotherapy Alliance for Neutropenics and the Control of Emerging Resistance. Ann Pharmacother 37:47–56
83. Safdar N, Maki DG (2002) The commonality of risk factors for nosocomial colonization and infection with antimicrobial-resistant Staphylococcus aureus, enterococcus, gram-negative bacilli, *Clostridium difficile*, and Candida. Ann Intern Med 136:834–844
84. Paterson DL (2006) Resistance in gram-negative bacteria: Enterobacteriaceae. Am J Infect Control 34:S20–S28 discussion S64–73
85. Zhanel GG, Karlowsky JA, Rubinstein E, Hoban DJ (2006) Tigecycline: a novel glycylcycline antibiotic. Expert Rev Anti Infect Ther 4:9–25
86. Spanik S, Trupl J, Kunova A et al (1996) Bloodstream infections due to anaerobic bacteria in cancer patients: epidemiology, etiology, risk factors, clinical presentation and outcome of anaerobic bacteremia. Neoplasma 43:235–238

87. Krcmery V, Spanik S, Mrazova M et al (2002) Bacteremias caused by Escherichia coli in cancer patients – analysis of 65 episodes. Int J Infect Dis 6:69–73
88. Watson JT, Jones RC, Siston AM et al (2005) Outbreak of catheter-associated Klebsiella oxytoca and Enterobacter cloacae bloodstream infections in an oncology chemotherapy center. Arch Intern Med 165:2639–2643
89. Falagas ME, Kasiakou SK (2005) Colistin: the revival of polymyxins for the management of multidrug-resistant gram-negative bacterial infections. Clin Infect Dis 40:1333–1341
90. Antoniadou A, Kontopidou F, Poulakou G et al (2007) Colistin-resistant isolates of *Klebsiella pneumoniae* emerging in intensive care unit patients: first report of a multiclonal cluster. J Antimicrob Chemother 59:786–790
91. Gaynes R, Edwards JR (2005) Overview of nosocomial infections caused by gram-negative bacilli. Clin Infect Dis 41:848–854
92. Maschmeyer G, Braveny I (2000) Review of the incidence and prognosis of *Pseudomonas aeruginosa* infections in cancer patients in the 1990s. Eur J Clin Microbiol Infect Dis 19:915–925
93. Chatzinikolaou I, Abi-Said D, Bodey GP, Rolston KV, Tarrand JJ, Samonis G (2000) Recent experience with *Pseudomonas aeruginosa* bacteremia in patients with cancer: retrospective analysis of 245 episodes. Arch Intern Med 160:501–509
94. Pier G, Ramphal R (2005) *Pseudomonas aeruginosa*. In: Mandell GL, Bennett JE, Dolin R (eds) Mandell, Douglas and Bennett's Principles and practice of infectious diseases, 6th edn. Elsevier Churchill Livingston, Philadelphia, PA, pp 2567–2615
95. Bodey GP, Jadeja L, Elting L (1985) Pseudomonas bacteremia. Retrospective analysis of 410 episodes. Arch Intern Med 145:1621–1629
96. Verhagen C, de Pauw BE, Donnelly JP, Williams KJ, de Witte T, Janssen TH (1986) Ceftazidime alone for treating *Pseudomonas aeruginosa* septicaemia in neutropenic patients. J Infect 13:125–131
97. Chamot E, Boffi El Amari E, Rohner P, Van Delden C (2003) Effectiveness of combination antimicrobial therapy for *Pseudomonas aeruginosa* bacteremia. Antimicrob Agents Chemother 47:2756–64
98. (2007) Prevention and treatment of cancer-related infections. http://www.nccn.org. Accessed V.I.2007
99. Carratalà J, Rosón B, Fernández-Sevilla A, Alcaide F, Gudiol F (1998) Bacteremic pneumonia in neutropenic patients with cancer: causes, empirical antibiotic therapy, and outcome. Arch Intern Med 158(8):868–872
100. Todeschini G, Franchini M, Tecchio C et al (1998) Improved prognosis of *Pseudomonas aeruginosa* bacteremia in 127 consecutive neutropenic patients with hematologic malignancies. Int J Infect Dis 3:99–104
101. Maschmeyer G, Noskin GA, Ribaud P, Sepkowitz KA (2000) Changing patterns of infections and antimicrobial susceptibilities. Oncology 14:9–16
102. Jacobson K, Rolston K, Elting L, LeBlanc B, Whimbey E, Ho DH (1999) Susceptibility surveillance among gram-negative bacilli at a cancer center. Chemotherapy 45:325–334
103. Ohmagari N, Hanna H, Graviss L et al (2005) Risk factors for infections with multidrug-resistant *Pseudomonas aeruginosa* in patients with cancer. Cancer 104:205–212
104. Tascini C, Menichetti F, Stefanelli A, Loni C, Lambelet P (2006) Clinical efficacy of intravenous colistin therapy in combination with ceftazidime in severe MDR *P. aeruginosa* systemic infections in two haematological patients. Infez Med 14:41–44
105. Micol JB, de Botton S, Guieze R et al (2006) An 18-case outbreak of drug-resistant *Pseudomonas aeruginosa* bacteriemia in hematology patients. Haematologica 91:1134–1138

106. Landman D, Bratu S, Alam M, Quale J (2005) Citywide emergence of *Pseudomonas aeruginosa* strains with reduced susceptibility to polymyxin B. J Antimicrob Chemother 55:954–957
107. Beno P, Krcmery V, Demitrovicova A (2006) Bacteraemia in cancer patients caused by colistin-resistant Gram-negative bacilli after previous exposure to ciprofloxacin and/or colistin. Clin Microbiol Infect 12:497–498
108. Micozzi A, Venditti M, Monaco M et al (2000) Bacteremia due to *Stenotrophomonas maltophilia* in patients with hematologic malignancies. Clin Infect Dis 31:705–711
109. Victor MA, Arpi M, Bruun B, Jonsson V, Hansen MM (1994) *Xanthomonas maltophilia* bacteremia in immunocompromised hematological patients. Scand J Infect Dis 26:163–170
110. Krcmery V Jr, Pichna P, Oravcova E et al (1996) *Stenotrophomonas maltophilia* bacteraemia in cancer patients: report on 31 cases. J Hosp Infect 34;75–77
111. Elting LS, Bodey GP (1990) Septicemia due to Xanthomonas species and non-aeruginosa Pseudomonas species: increasing incidence of catheter-related infections. Medicine (Baltimore) 69:296–306
112. Khardori N, Elting L, Wong E, Schable B, Bodey GP (1990) Nosocomial infections due to *Xanthomonas maltophilia* (*Pseudomonas maltophilia*) in patients with cancer. Rev Infect Dis 12:997–1003
113. Apisarnthanarak A, Mayfield JL, Garison T et al (2003) Risk factors for *Stenotrophomonas maltophilia* bacteremia in oncology patients: a case-control study. Infect Control Hosp Epidemiol 24:269–274
114. Boktour M, Hanna H, Ansari S et al (2006) Central venous catheter and *Stenotrophomonas maltophilia* bacteremia in cancer patients. Cancer 106: 1967–1973
115. Friedman ND, Korman TM, Fairley CK, Franklin JC, Spelman DW (2002) Bacteraemia due to *Stenotrophomonas maltophilia*: an analysis of 45 episodes. J Infect 45:47–53
116. Muder RR, Harris AP, Muller S et al (1996) Bacteremia due to *Stenotrophomonas* (*Xanthomonas*) *maltophilia*: a prospective, multicenter study of 91 episodes. Clin Infect Dis 22:508–512
117. Elting LS, Khardori N, Bodey GP, Fainstein V (1990) Nosocomial infection caused by *Xanthomonas maltophilia*: a case-control study of predisposing factors. Infect Control Hosp Epidemiol 11:134–138
118. Hoban DJ, Bouchillon SK, Johnson BM, Johnson JL, Dowzicky MJ (2005) In vitro activity of tigecycline against 6792 gram-negative and gram-positive clinical isolates from the global Tigecycline Evaluation and Surveillance Trial (TEST Program, 2004). Diagn Microbiol Infect Dis 52:215–227
119. Sanders WE Jr, Sanders CC (1997) *Enterobacter* spp.: pathogens poised to flourish at the turn of the century. Clin Microbiol Rev 10:220–241
120. Bodey GP, Elting LS, Rodriguez S (1991) Bacteremia caused by Enterobacter: 15 years of experience in a cancer hospital. Rev Infect Dis 13:550–558
121. Chow JW, Fine MJ, Shlaes DM et al (1991) Enterobacter bacteremia: clinical features and emergence of antibiotic resistance during therapy. Ann Intern Med 115:585–590
122. Seifert H, Strate A, Pulverer G (1995) Nosocomial bacteremia due to *Acinetobacter baumannii*. Clinical features, epidemiology, and predictors of mortality. Medicine (Baltimore) 74:340–349
123. Bergogne-Berezin E, Towner KJ (1996) *Acinetobacter* spp. as nosocomial pathogens: microbiological, clinical, and epidemiological features. Clin Microbiol Rev 9:148–165
124. Cisneros JM, Reyes MJ, Pachon J et al (1996) Bacteremia due to *Acinetobacter baumannii*: epidemiology, clinical findings, and prognostic features. Clin Infect Dis 22:1026–1032

125. Wisplinghoff H, Edmond MB, Pfaller MA, Jones RN, Wenzel RP, Seifert H (2000) Nosocomial bloodstream infections caused by Acinetobacter species in United States hospitals: clinical features, molecular epidemiology, and antimicrobial susceptibility. Clin Infect Dis 31:690–697
126. Koprnova J, Svetlansky I, Babel'a R et al (2001) Prospective study of antibacterial susceptibility, risk factors and outcome of 157 episodes of *Acinetobacter baumannii* bacteremia in 1999 in Slovakia. Scand J Infect Dis 33:891–895
127. Chen HP, Chen TL, Lai CH et al (2005) Predictors of mortality in *Acinetobacter baumannii* bacteremia. J Microbiol Immunol Infect 38:127–136
128. Hernandez JA, Martino R, Pericas R, Sureda A, Brunet S, Domingo-Albos A (1998) *Achromobacter xylosoxidans* bacteremia in patients with hematologic malignancies. Haematologica 83:284–285
129. Legrand C, Anaissie E (1992) Bacteremia due to *Achromobacter xylosoxidans* in patients with cancer. Clin Infect Dis 14:479–484
130. Duggan JM, Goldstein SJ, Chenoweth CE, Kauffman CA, Bradley SF (1996) *Achromobacter xylosoxidans* bacteremia: report of four cases and review of the literature. Clin Infect Dis 23:569–576
131. Aisenberg G, Rolston KV, Safdar A (2004) Bacteremia caused by Achromobacter and Alcaligenes species in 46 patients with cancer (1989–2003). Cancer 101: 2134–2140
132. Tsai MS, Kuo CY, Wang MC, Wu HC, Chien CC, Liu JW (2006) Clinical features and risk factors for mortality in Aeromonas bacteremic adults with hematologic malignancies. J Microbiol Immunol Infect 39:150–154
133. De I, Rolston KV, Han XY (2004) Clinical significance of Roseomonas species isolated from catheter and blood samples: analysis of 36 cases in patients with cancer. Clin Infect Dis 38:1579–1584
134. Han XY, Tarrand JJ (2004) Moraxella osloensis blood and catheter infections during anticancer chemotherapy: clinical and microbiologic studies of 10 cases. Am J Clin Pathol 121:581–587
135. McDonald LC, Owings M, Jernigan DB (2006) *Clostridium difficile* infection in patients discharged from US short-stay hospitals, 1996–2003. Emerg Infect Dis 12:409–415
136. Bignardi GE (1998) Risk factors for *Clostridium difficile* infection. J Hosp Infect 40:1–15
137. Barbut F, Richard A, Hamadi K, Chomette V, Burghoffer B, Petit JC (2000) Epidemiology of recurrences or reinfections of *Clostridium difficile*-associated diarrhea. J Clin Microbiol 38:2386–2388
138. Dial S, Alrasadi K, Manoukian C, Huang A, Menzies D (2004) Risk of *Clostridium difficile* diarrhea among hospital inpatients prescribed proton pump inhibitors: cohort and case-control studies. CMAJ 171:33–38
139. Dial S, Delaney JA, Barkun AN, Suissa S (2005) Use of gastric acid-suppressive agents and the risk of community-acquired *Clostridium difficile*-associated disease. JAMA 294:2989–2995
140. Gaynes R, Rimland D, Killum E et al (2004) Outbreak of *Clostridium difficile* infection in a long-term care facility: association with gatifloxacin use. Clin Infect Dis 38:640–645
141. Muto CA, Pokrywka M, Shutt K et al (2005) A large outbreak of *Clostridium difficile*-associated disease with an unexpected proportion of deaths and colectomies at a teaching hospital following increased fluoroquinolone use. Infect Control Hosp Epidemiol 26:273–280
142. Pepin J, Saheb N, Coulombe MA et al (2005) Emergence of fluoroquinolones as the predominant risk factor for *Clostridium difficile*-associated diarrhea: a cohort study during an epidemic in Quebec. Clin Infect Dis 41:1254–1260

143. Loo VG, Poirier L, Miller MA et al (2005) A predominantly clonal multi-institutional outbreak of *Clostridium difficile*-associated diarrhea with high morbidity and mortality. N Engl J Med 353:2442–2449
144. Gifford AH, Kirkland KB (2006) Risk factors for *Clostridium difficile*-associated diarrhea on an adult hematology-oncology ward. Eur J Clin Microbiol Infect Dis 25:751–755
145. Palmore TN, Sohn S, Malak SF, Eagan J, Sepkowitz KA (2005) Risk factors for acquisition of *Clostridium difficile*-associated diarrhea among outpatients at a cancer hospital. Infect Control Hosp Epidemiol 26:680–684
146. Blot E, Escande MC, Besson D et al (2003) Outbreak of *Clostridium difficile*-related diarrhoea in an adult oncology unit: risk factors and microbiological characteristics. J Hosp Infect 53:187–192
147. Gorschluter M, Glasmacher A, Hahn C et al (2001) *Clostridium difficile* infection in patients with neutropenia. Clin Infect Dis 33:786–791
148. Hornbuckle K, Chak A, Lazarus HM et al (1998) Determination and validation of a predictive model for *Clostridium difficile* diarrhea in hospitalized oncology patients. Ann Oncol 9:307–311
149. Gerard M, Defresne N, Daneau D et al (1988) Incidence and significance of *Clostridium difficile* in hospitalized cancer patients. Eur J Clin Microbiol Infect Dis 7:274–278
150. Heard SR, Wren B, Barnett MJ, Thomas JM, Tabaqchali S (1988) *Clostridium difficile* infection in patients with haematological malignant disease. Risk factors, faecal toxins and pathogenic strains. Epidemiol Infect 100:63–72
151. Panichi G, Pantosti A, Gentile G et al (1985) *Clostridium difficile* colitis in leukemia patients. Eur J Cancer Clin Oncol 21:1159–1163
152. Rampling A, Warren RE, Bevan PC, Hoggarth CE, Swirsky D, Hayhoe FG (1985) *Clostridium difficile* in haematological malignancy. J Clin Pathol 38:445–451
153. Morris JG Jr, Jarvis WR, Nunez-Montiel OL et al (1984) *Clostridium difficile*. Colonization and toxin production in a cohort of patients with malignant hematologic disorders. Arch Intern Med 144:967–969
154. Cudmore MA, Silva J Jr, Fekety R, Liepman MK, Kim KH (1982) *Clostridium difficile* colitis associated with cancer chemotherapy. Arch Intern Med 142: 333–335
155. Anand A, Glatt AE (1993) *Clostridium difficile* infection associated with antineoplastic chemotherapy: a review. Clin Infect Dis 17:109–113
156. Chakrabarti S, Lees A, Jones SG, Milligan DW (2000) *Clostridium difficile* infection in allogeneic stem cell transplant recipients is associated with severe graft-versus-host disease and non-relapse mortality. Bone Marrow Transplant 26:871–876
157. Husain A, Aptaker L, Spriggs DR, Barakat RR (1998) Gastrointestinal toxicity and *Clostridium difficile* diarrhea in patients treated with paclitaxel-containing chemotherapy regimens. Gynecol Oncol 71:104–107
158. Emoto M, Kawarabayashi T, Hachisuga MD, Eguchi F, Shirakawa K (1996) *Clostridium difficile* colitis associated with cisplatin-based chemotherapy in ovarian cancer patients. Gynecol Oncol 61:369–372
159. McDonald LC, Killgore GE, Thompson A et al (2005) An epidemic, toxin gene-variant strain of *Clostridium difficile*. N Engl J Med 353:2433–2441
160. Pepin J, Valiquette L, Alary ME et al (2004) *Clostridium difficile*-associated diarrhea in a region of Quebec from 1991 to 2003: a changing pattern of disease severity. CMAJ 171:466–472
161. Dallal RM, Harbrecht BG, Boujoukas AJ et al (2002) Fulminant *Clostridium difficile*: an underappreciated and increasing cause of death and complications. Ann Surg 235:363–372
162. Bartlett JG, Perl TM (2005) The new *Clostridium difficile* – what does it mean? N Engl J Med 353:2503–2505

163. Warny M, Pepin J, Fang A et al (2005) Toxin production by an emerging strain of *Clostridium difficile* associated with outbreaks of severe disease in North America and Europe. Lancet 366:1079–1084
164. Spigaglia P, Mastrantonio P (2002) Molecular analysis of the pathogenicity locus and polymorphism in the putative negative regulator of toxin production (TcdC) among *Clostridium difficile* clinical isolates. J Clin Microbiol 40:3470–3475
165. Dubberke ER, Sadhu J, Gatti R et al (2007) Severity of *Clostridium difficile*-associated disease (CDAD) in allogeneic stem cell transplant recipients: evaluation of a CDAD severity grading system. Infect Control Hosp Epidemiol 28:208–211
166. Sunenshine RH, McDonald LC (2006) *Clostridium difficile*-associated disease: new challenges from an established pathogen. Cleve Clin J Med 73:187–197
167. Bartlett JG (2006) Narrative review: the new epidemic of *Clostridium difficile*-associated enteric disease. Ann Intern Med 145:758–764
168. Mohan SS, McDermott BP, Parchuri S, Cunha BA (2006) Lack of value of repeat stool testing for *Clostridium difficile* toxin. Am J Med 119:356.e7–356.e8
169. Arango JI, Restrepo A, Schneider DL et al (2006) Incidence of *Clostridium difficile*-associated diarrhea before and after autologous peripheral blood stem cell transplantation for lymphoma and multiple myeloma. Bone Marrow Transplant 37:517–521
170. Gerding DN (2005) Metronidazole for *Clostridium difficile*-associated disease: is it okay for Mom? Clin Infect Dis 40:1598–1600
171. Apisarnthanarak A, Razavi B, Mundy LM (2002) Adjunctive intracolonic vancomycin for severe *Clostridium difficile* colitis: case series and review of the literature. Clin Infect Dis 35:690–696
172. Lipsett PA, Samantaray DK, Tam ML, Bartlett JG, Lillemoe KD (1994) Pseudomembranous colitis: a surgical disease? Surgery 116:491–496
173. Koss K, Clark MA, Sanders DS, Morton D, Keighley MR, Goh J (2006) The outcome of surgery in fulminant *Clostridium difficile* colitis. Colorectal Dis 8:149–154
174. Longo WE, Mazuski JE, Virgo KS, Lee P, Bahadursingh AN, Johnson FE (2004) Outcome after colectomy for *Clostridium difficile* colitis. Dis Colon Rectum 47:1620–1626
175. Fekety R, McFarland LV, Surawicz CM, Greenberg RN, Elmer GW, Mulligan ME (1997) Recurrent *Clostridium difficile* diarrhea: characteristics of and risk factors for patients enrolled in a prospective, randomized, double-blinded trial. Clin Infect Dis 24:324–333
176. McFarland LV, Elmer GW, Surawicz CM (2002) Breaking the cycle: treatment strategies for 163 cases of recurrent *Clostridium difficile* disease. Am J Gastroenterol 97:1769–1775
177. Johnson S, Schriever C, Galang M, Kelly CP, Gerding DN (2007) Interruption of recurrent *Clostridium difficile*-associated diarrhea episodes by serial therapy with vancomycin and rifaximin. Clin Infect Dis 44:846–848
178. Dendukuri N, Costa V, McGregor M, Brophy JM (2005) Probiotic therapy for the prevention and treatment of *Clostridium difficile*-associated diarrhea: a systematic review. CMAJ 173:167–170
179. McFarland LV (2006) Meta-analysis of probiotics for the prevention of antibiotic associated diarrhea and the treatment of *Clostridium difficile* disease. Am J Gastroenterol 101:812–822
180. Mogg GA, George RH, Youngs D et al (1982) Randomized controlled trial of colestipol in antibiotic-associated colitis. Br J Surg 69:137–139
181. Aas J, Gessert CE, Bakken JS (2003) Recurrent *Clostridium difficile* colitis: case series involving 18 patients treated with donor stool administered via a nasogastric tube. Clin Infect Dis 36:580–585
182. Aboudola S, Kotloff KL, Kyne L et al (2003) *Clostridium difficile* vaccine and serum immunoglobulin G antibody response to toxin A. Infect Immun 71: 1608–1610

183. McPherson S, Rees CJ, Ellis R, Soo S, Panter SJ (2006) Intravenous immunoglobulin for the treatment of severe, refractory, and recurrent *Clostridium difficile* diarrhea. Dis Colon Rectum 49:640–645
184. Musher DM, Logan N, Hamill RJ et al (2006) Nitazoxanide for the treatment of *Clostridium difficile* colitis. Clin Infect Dis 43:421–427
185. Louie TJ, Peppe J, Watt CK, Johnson D, Mohammed R, Dow G, Weiss K, Simon S, John JF Jr, Garber G, Chasan-Taber S, Davidson DM, Tolevamer Study Investigator Group (2006) Tolevamer, a novel nonantibiotic polymer, compared with vancomycin in the treatment of mild to moderately severe *Clostridium difficile*-associated diarrhea. Clin Infect Dis 43(4):411–420
186. McNeil MM, Brown JM (1994) The medically important aerobic actinomycetes: epidemiology and microbiology. Clin Microbiol Rev 7:357–417
187. Torres HA, Reddy BT, Raad II et al (2002) Nocardiosis in cancer patients. Medicine (Baltimore) 81:388–397
188. van Burik JA, Hackman RC, Nadeem SQ et al (1997) Nocardiosis after bone marrow transplantation: a retrospective study. Clin Infect Dis 24:1154–1160
189. Choucino C, Goodman SA, Greer JP, Stein RS, Wolff SN, Dummer JS (1996) Nocardial infections in bone marrow transplant recipients. Clin Infect Dis 23: 1012–1019
190. Daly AS, McGeer A, Lipton JH (2003) Systemic nocardiosis following allogeneic bone marrow transplantation. Transpl Infect Dis 5:16–20
191. Samonis G, Kontoyiannis DP (2001) Infectious complications of purine analog therapy. Curr Opin Infect Dis 14:409–413
192. Wadhwa PD, Morrison VA (2006) Infectious complications of chronic lymphocytic leukemia. Semin Oncol 33:240–249
193. Berkey P, Bodey GP (1989) Nocardial infection in patients with neoplastic disease. Rev Infect Dis 11:407–412
194. Kontoyiannis DP, Ruoff K, Hooper DC (1998) Nocardia bacteremia. Report of 4 cases and review of the literature. Medicine (Baltimore) 77:255–267
195. Kontoyiannis DP, Jacobson KL, Whimbey EE, Rolston KV, Raad II (2000) Central venous catheter-associated Nocardia bacteremia: an unusual manifestation of nocardiosis. Clin Infect Dis 31(2):617–618
196. Christidou A, Maraki S, Scoulica E, Mantadakis E, Agelaki S, Samonis G (2004) Fatal Nocardia farcinica bacteremia in a patient with lung cancer. Diagn Microbiol Infect Dis 50:135–139
197. McNeil MM, Brown JM, Georghiou PR, Allworth AM, Blacklock ZM (1992) Infections due to *Nocardia transvalensis*: clinical spectrum and antimicrobial therapy. Clin Infect Dis 15:453–463
198. Elsayed S, Kealey A, Coffin CS, Read R, Megran D, Zhang K (2006) *Nocardia cyriacigeorgica* septicemia. J Clin Microbiol 44:280–282
199. Ansari SR, Safdar A, Han XY, O'Brien S (2006) *Nocardia veterana* bloodstream infection in a patient with cancer and a summary of reported cases. Int J Infect Dis 10:483–486
200. Sorrell TC, Mitchell DH, Iredell JR (2005) Nocardia. In: Mandell GL, Bennett JE, Dolin R (eds) Mandell, Douglas and Bennett's Principles and Practice of Infectious Diseases, 6th edn. Elsevier Churchill Livingston, Philadelphia, PA, pp 2916–2924
201. Brown-Elliott BA, Ward SC, Crist CJ, Mann LB, Wilson RW, Wallace RJ Jr (2001) In vitro activities of linezolid against multiple Nocardia species. Antimicrob Agents Chemother 45:1295–1297
202. Clinical and Laboratory Standards Institute. M-24 – Susceptibility testing of mycobacteria, nocardia and other aerobic actinomycetes. Catalog 2-2007.
203. Gombert ME, Aulicino TM (1983) Synergism of imipenem and amikacin in combination with other antibiotics against *Nocardia asteroides*. Antimicrob Agents Chemother 24:810–811

204. Moylett EH, Pacheco SE, Brown-Elliott BA et al (2003) Clinical experience with linezolid for the treatment of nocardia infection. Clin Infect Dis 36:313–318
205. Rupprecht TA, Pfister HW (2005) Clinical experience with linezolid for the treatment of central nervous system infections. Eur J Neurol 12:536–542
206. Lerner PI (1996) Nocardiosis. Clin Infect Dis 22:891–903 quiz 4-5
207. Boiron P, Provost F, Chevrier G, Dupont B (1992) Review of nocardial infections in France 1987 to 1990. Eur J Clin Microbiol Infect Dis 11:709–714
208. Ortbals DW, Marr JJ (1978) A comparative study of tuberculous and other mycobacterial infections and their associations with malignancy. Am Rev Respir Dis 117:39–45
209. Feld R, Bodey GP, Groschel D (1976) Mycobacteriosis in patients with malignant disease. Arch Intern Med 136:67–70
210. Kaplan MH, Armstrong D, Rosen P (1974) Tuberculosis complicating neoplastic disease. A review of 201 cases. Cancer 33:850–858
211. Yuen KY, Woo PC (2002) Tuberculosis in blood and marrow transplant recipients. Hematol Oncol 20:51–62
212. De La Rosa GR, Jacobson KL, Rolston KV, Raad II, Kontoyiannis DP, Safdar A (2004) *Mycobacterium tuberculosis* at a comprehensive cancer centre: active disease in patients with underlying malignancy during 1990–2000. Clin Microbiol Infect 10:749–752
213. Kamboj M, Sepkowitz KA (2006) The risk of tuberculosis in patients with cancer. Clin Infect Dis 42:1592–1595
214. Libshitz HI, Pannu HK, Elting LS, Cooksley CD (1997) Tuberculosis in cancer patients: an update. J Thorac Imaging 12:41–46
215. Centers for Disease Control and Prevention (2006) Reported Tuberculosis in the United States, 2005. U.S. Department of Health and Human Services, CDC, Atlanta, GA. http://www.cdc.gov/tb/. Accessed Sept 2006
216. de la Camara R, Martino R, Granados E et al (2000) Tuberculosis after hematopoietic stem cell transplantation: incidence, clinical characteristics and outcome. Spanish Group on Infectious Complications in Hematopoietic Transplantation. Bone Marrow Transplant 26:291–298
217. Leung WH, Tsang SF, Chim CS (2005) Extrapulmonary tuberculous abscess in chronic lymphocytic leukaemia (CLL) treated with fludarabine: case report and review of literature. Am J Hematol 79:246–247
218. Abad S, Gyan E, Moachon L et al (2003) Tuberculosis due to *Mycobacterium bovis* after alemtuzumab administration. Clin Infect Dis 37:e27–e28
219. Wendtner CM, Ritgen M, Schweighofer CD et al (2004) Consolidation with alemtuzumab in patients with chronic lymphocytic leukemia (CLL) in first remission–experience on safety and efficacy within a randomized multicenter phase III trial of the German CLL Study Group (GCLLSG). Leukemia 18:1093–1101
220. Crum NF, Lederman ER, Wallace MR (2005) Infections associated with tumor necrosis factor-alpha antagonists. Medicine (Baltimore) 84:291–302
221. Aisenberg GM, Jacobson K, Chemaly RF, Rolston KV, Raad II, Safdar A (2005) Extrapulmonary tuberculosis active infection misdiagnosed as cancer: *Mycobacterium tuberculosis* disease in patients at a Comprehensive Cancer Center (2001–2005). Cancer 104:2882–2887
222. Choksey MS, Powell M, Gibb WR, Casey AT, Geddes JF (1989) A conus tuberculoma mimicking an intramedullary tumour: a case report and review of the literature. Br J Neurosurg 3:117–121
223. Wu CS, Wang SH, Kuo TT (1994) Pancreatic tuberculosis mimicking pancreatic head carcinoma: a case report and review of the literature. Infection 22:287–289
224. Rezeig MA, Fashir BM, Al-Suhaibani H, Al-Fadda M, Amin T, Eisa H (1998) Pancreatic tuberculosis mimicking pancreatic carcinoma: four case reports and review of the literature. Dig Dis Sci 43:329–331

225. Piura B, Rabinovich A, Leron E, Yanai-Inbar I, Mazor M (2002) Peritoneal tuberculosis mimicking ovarian carcinoma with ascites and elevated serum CA-125: case report and review of literature. Eur J Gynaecol Oncol 23:120–122
226. Comert FB, Comert M, Kulah C, Tascilar O, Numanoglu G, Aydemir S (2006) Colonic tuberculosis mimicking tumor perforation: a case report and review of the literature. Dig Dis Sci 51:1039–1042
227. Koc S, Beydilli G, Tulunay G et al (2006) Peritoneal tuberculosis mimicking advanced ovarian cancer: a retrospective review of 22 cases. Gynecol Oncol 103:565–569
228. Malone JL, Ijaz K, Lambert L et al (2004) Investigation of healthcare-associated transmission of *Mycobacterium tuberculosis* among patients with malignancies at three hospitals and at a residential facility. Cancer 101:2713–2721
229. Anon (2005) Management of a tuberculosis exposure in an oncology hospital. Can Commun Dis Rep 31:149–156
230. Menzies D, Pai M, Comstock G (2007) Meta-analysis: new tests for the diagnosis of latent tuberculosis infection: areas of uncertainty and recommendations for research. Ann Intern Med 146:340–354
231. Kim DK, Lee SW, Yoo CG et al (2005) Clinical characteristics and treatment responses of tuberculosis in patients with malignancy receiving anticancer chemotherapy. Chest 128:2218–2222
232. Iseman MD (2000) A clinician's guide to tuberculosis. Lippincott Williams and Wilkins, Philadelphia, PA, p 134
233. Fujii H, Ishihara J, Fukaura A et al (1992) Early diagnosis of tuberculosis by fiberoptic bronchoscopy. Tuber Lung Dis 73:167–169
234. Baughman RP, Dohn MN, Loudon RG, Frame PT (1991) Bronchoscopy with bronchoalveolar lavage in tuberculosis and fungal infections. Chest 99:92–97
235. Woods GL (2001) Molecular techniques in myobacterial detection. Arch Pathol Lab Med 125:122–126
236. Palomino JC (2005) Nonconventional and new methods in the diagnosis of tuberculosis: feasibility and applicability in the field. Eur Respir J 26:339–350
237. Kang EY, Choi JA, Seo BK, Oh YW, Lee CK, Shim JJ (2002) Utility of polymerase chain reaction for detecting *Mycobacterium tuberculosis* in specimens from percutaneous transthoracic needle aspiration. Radiology 225:205–209
238. Centers for Disease Control and Prevention (2005) National plan for reliable tuberculosis laboratory services using a systems approach: recommendations from CDC and the Association of Public Health Laboratories Task Force on Tuberculosis. Laboratory Services. MMWR 54:RR-6
239. Rattan A, Kalia A, Ahmad N (1998) Multidrug-resistant *Mycobacterium tuberculosis*: molecular perspectives. Emerg Infect Dis 4:195–209
240. Tenover FC (2007) Rapid detection and identification of bacterial pathogens using novel molecular technologies: infection control and beyond. Clin Infect Dis 44:418–423
241. Li X, Zhang Y, Shen X et al (2007) Transmission of drug-resistant tuberculosis among treated patients in Shanghai, China. J Infect Dis 195:864–869
242. Centers for Disease Control and Prevention (2000) Targeted Tuberculin Testing and Treatment of Latent Tuberculosis Infection. MMWR 49:RR06
243. Centers for Disease Control and Prevention (2003) Update: adverse event data revised American Thoracic Society/CDC recommendations against the use of rifampin and pyrazinamide for treatment of latent tuberculosis infection – United States, 2003. MMWR 52(31):735–738
244. Wallace RJ Jr, Swenson JM, Silcox VA, Good RC, Tschen JA, Stone MS (1983) Spectrum of disease due to rapidly growing mycobacteria. Rev Infect Dis 5:657–679
245. Rolston KV, Jones PG, Fainstein V, Bodey GP (1985) Pulmonary disease caused by rapidly growing mycobacteria in patients with cancer. Chest 87:503–506

246. Jacobson K, Garcia R, Libshitz H et al (1998) Clinical and radiological features of pulmonary disease caused by rapidly growing mycobacteria in cancer patients. Eur J Clin Microbiol Infect Dis 17:615–621
247. Kiehn TE, Edwards FF, Brannon P et al (1985) Infections caused by *Mycobacterium avium* complex in immunocompromised patients: diagnosis by blood culture and fecal examination, antimicrobial susceptibility tests, and morphological and sero-agglutination characteristics. J Clin Microbiol 21:168–173
248. Han XY, Tarrand JJ, Infante R, Jacobson KL, Truong M (2005) Clinical significance and epidemiologic analyses of *Mycobacterium avium* and *Mycobacterium intracellulare* among patients without AIDS. J Clin Microbiol 43:4407–4412
249. Golomb HM, Hadad LJ (1984) Infectious complications in 127 patients with hairy cell leukemia. Am J Hematol 16:393–401
250. Bennett C, Vardiman J, Golomb H (1986) Disseminated atypical mycobacterial infection in patients with hairy cell leukemia. Am J Med 80:891–896
251. Thaker H, Neilly IJ, Saunders PG, Magee JG, Snow MH, Ong EL (2001) Remember mycobacterial disease in hairy cell leukaemia (HCL). J Infect 42:213–214
252. Jacobson KL, Teira R, Libshitz HI et al (2000) *Mycobacterium kansasii* infections in patients with cancer. Clin Infect Dis 31:628–631
253. Shah MK, Sebti A, Kiehn TE, Massarella SA, Sepkowitz KA (2001) *Mycobacterium haemophilum* in immunocompromised patients. Clin Infect Dis 33:330–337
254. Saubolle MA, Kiehn TE, White MH, Rudinsky MF, Armstrong D (1996) *Mycobacterium haemophilum*: microbiology and expanding clinical and geographic spectra of disease in humans. Clin Microbiol Rev 9:435–447
255. Vos MC, de Haas PE, Verbrugh HA et al (2003) Nosocomial *Mycobacterium bovis*-bacille Calmette-Guerin infections due to contamination of chemotherapeutics: case finding and route of transmission. J Infect Dis 188:1332–1335
256. Engervall P, Bjorkholm M, Petrini B, Heurlin N, Henriques B, Kallenius G (1993) Disseminated *Mycobacterium malmoense* infection in a patient with chronic granulocytic leukaemia. J Intern Med 234:231–233
257. Castor B, Juhlin I, Henriques B (1994) Septic cutaneous lesions caused by *Mycobacterium malmoense* in a patient with hairy cell leukemia. Eur J Clin Microbiol Infect Dis 13:145–148
258. Enzensberger R, Hunfeld KP, Elshorst-Schmidt T, Boer A, Brade V (2002) Disseminated cutaneous *Mycobacterium marinum* infection in a patient with non-Hodgkin's lymphoma. Infection 30:393–395
259. Hachem R, Raad I, Rolston KV et al (1996) Cutaneous and pulmonary infections caused by *Mycobacterium vaccae*. Clin Infect Dis 23:173–175
260. Akiyama H, Maruyama T, Uetake T, Kawaguchi K, Sakamaki H, Onozawa Y (1991) Systemic infection due to atypical mycobacteria in patients with chronic myelogenous leukemia. Rev Infect Dis 13:815–818
261. Hoy JF, Rolston KV, Hopfer RL, Bodey GP (1987) Mycobacterium fortuitum bacteremia in patients with cancer and long-term venous catheters. Am J Med 83:213–217
262. Raad II, Vartivarian S, Khan A, Bodey GP (1991) Catheter-related infections caused by the Mycobacterium fortuitum complex: 15 cases and review. Rev Infect Dis 13:1120–1125
263. Kline S, Cameron S, Streifel A et al (2004) An outbreak of bacteremias associated with *Mycobacterium mucogenicum* in a hospital water supply. Infect Control Hosp Epidemiol 25:1042–1049
264. Lee SA, Raad II, Adachi JA, Han XY (2004) Catheter-related bloodstream infection caused by *Mycobacterium brumae*. J Clin Microbiol 42:5429–5431
265. Oh WS, Ko KS, Song JH et al (2005) Catheter-associated bacteremia by *Mycobacterium senegalense* in Korea. BMC Infect Dis 5:107
266. Perandin F, Pinsi G, Signorini L, Soavi L, Signorini C, Manca N (2006) *Mycobacterium szulgai* identification by hsp65 gene sequencing in an HIV-positive patient with non-Hodgkin's lymphoma. New Microbiol 29:215–218

267. Doucette K, Fishman JA (2004) Nontuberculous mycobacterial infection in hematopoietic stem cell and solid organ transplant recipients. Clin Infect Dis 38:1428–1439
268. Gaviria JM, Garcia PJ, Garrido SM, Corey L, Boeckh M (2000) Nontuberculous mycobacterial infections in hematopoietic stem cell transplant recipients: characteristics of respiratory and catheter-related infections. Biol Blood Marrow Transplant 6:361–369
269. Weinstock DM, Feinstein MB, Sepkowitz KA, Jakubowski A (2003) High rates of infection and colonization by nontuberculous mycobacteria after allogeneic hematopoietic stem cell transplantation. Bone Marrow Transplant 31:1015–1021
270. (1997) Diagnosis and treatment of disease caused by nontuberculous mycobacteria. This official statement of the American Thoracic Society was approved by the Board of Directors, March 1997. Medical Section of the American Lung Association. Am J Respir Crit Care Med 156:S1–S25
271. Goldstein EJ (1996) Anaerobic bacteremia. Clin Infect Dis 23(Suppl 1):S97–S101
272. Lark RL, McNeil SA, VanderHyde K, Noorani Z, Uberti J, Chenoweth C (2001) Risk factors for anaerobic bloodstream infections in bone marrow transplant recipients. Clin Infect Dis 33:338–343
273. Zahar JR, Farhat H, Chachaty E, Meshaka P, Antoun S, Nitenberg G (2005) Incidence and clinical significance of anaerobic bacteraemia in cancer patients: a 6-year retrospective study. Clin Microbiol Infect 11:724–729
274. Noriega LM, Van der Auwera P, Phan M et al (1993) Anaerobic bacteremia in a cancer center. Support Care Cancer 1:250–255
275. Martino R, Ramila E, Capdevila JA et al (2001) Bacteremia caused by Capnocytophaga species in patients with neutropenia and cancer: results of a multicenter study. Clin Infect Dis 33:E20–E22
276. Maury S, Leblanc T, Rousselot P, Legrand P, Arlet G, Cordonnier C (1999) Bacteremia due to Capnocytophaga species in patients with neutropenia: high frequency of beta-lactamase-producing strains. Clin Infect Dis 28: 1172–1174
277. Roscoe DL, Zemcov SJ, Thornber D, Wise R, Clarke AM (1992) Antimicrobial susceptibilities and beta-lactamase characterization of Capnocytophaga species. Antimicrob Agents Chemother 36:2197–2200
278. Yadegarynia D, Tarrand J, Raad I, Rolston K (2003) Good interpretation of the results of a diagnostic test. Reply to correspondence. Clin Infect Dis 37:1144–1145
279. Elting LS, Bodey GP, Fainstein V (1986) Polymicrobial septicemia in the cancer patient. Medicine (Baltimore) 65:218–225
280. Rolston KV (2005) Challenges in the treatment of infections caused by gram-positive and gram-negative bacteria in patients with cancer and neutropenia. Clin Infect Dis 40(Suppl 4):S246–S252
281. Giamarellou H, Bassaris HP, Petrikkos G, Busch W, Voulgarelis M, Antoniadou A, Grouzi E, Zoumbos N (2000) Monotherapy with intravenous followed by oral high-dose ciprofloxacin versus combination therapy with ceftazidime plus amikacin as initial empiric therapy for granulocytopenic patients with fever. Antimicrob Agents Chemother 44(12):3264–3271
282. Harter C, Schulze B, Goldschmidt H, Benner A, Geiss HK, Hoppe-Tichy T, Ho AD, Egerer G (2006) Piperacillin/tazobactam vs ceftazidime in the treatment of neutropenic fever in patients with acute leukemia or following autologous peripheral blood stem cell transplantation: a prospective randomized trial. Bone Marrow Transplant 37(4):373–379
283. Del Favero A, Menichetti F, Martino P, Bucaneve G, Micozzi A, Gentile G, Furno P, Russo D, D'Antonio D, Ricci P, Martino B, Mandelli F, Gruppo Italiano Malattie Ematologiche dell'Adulto (GIMEMA) Infection Program (2001) A multicenter, double-blind, placebo-controlled trial comparing piperacillin-tazobactam

with and without amikacin as empiric therapy for febrile neutropenia. Clin Infect Dis 33(8):1295–1301

284. Gonzalez-Barca E, Fernandez-Sevilla A, Carratala J, Granena A, Gudiol F (1996) Prospective study of 288 episodes of bacteremia in neutropenic cancer patients in a single institution. Eur J Clin Microbiol Infect Dis 15:291–296
285. Cometta A, Calandra T, Gaya H, Zinner SH, de Bock R, Del Favero A, Bucaneve G, Crokaert F, Kern WV, Klastersky J, Langenaeken I, Micozzi A, Padmos A, Paesmans M, Viscoli C, Glauser MP (1996) Monotherapy with meropenem versus combination therapy with ceftazidime plus amikacin as empiric therapy for fever in granulocytopenic patients with cancer. The International Antimicrobial Therapy Cooperative Group of the European Organization for Research and Treatment of Cancer and the Gruppo Italiano Malattie Ematologiche Maligne dell'Adulto Infection Program. Antimicrob Agents Chemother 40(5):1108–1115
286. Gorschlüter M, Mey U, Strehl J, Ziske C, Schepke M, Schmidt-Wolf IG, Sauerbruch T, Glasmacher A (2005) Neutropenic enterocolitis in adults: systematic analysis of evidence quality. Eur J Haematol 75(1):1–13
287. Gomez L, Martino R, Rolston KV (1998) Neutropenic enterocolitis: spectrum of the disease and comparison of definite and possible cases. Clin Infect Dis 27(4):695–699
288. Jones GT, Abramson N (1983) Gastrointestinal necrosis in acute leukemia: a complication of induction therapy. Cancer Invest 1(4):315–320
289. Khardori N, Wong E, Carrasco CH, Wallace S, Patt Y, Bodey GP (1991) Infections associated with biliary drainage procedures in patients with cancer. Rev Infect Dis 13(4):587–591
290. Stender H (2003) PNA FISH: an intelligent stain for rapid diagnosis of infectious diseases. Expert Rev Mol Diagn 3:649–655
291. Hartmann H, Stender H, Schafer A, Autenrieth IB, Kempf VA (2005) Rapid identification of Staphylococcus aureus in blood cultures by a combination of fluorescence in situ hybridization using peptide nucleic acid probes and flow cytometry. J Clin Microbiol 43:4855–4857
292. Forrest GN, Mehta S, Weekes E, Lincalis DP, Johnson JK, Venezia RA (2006) Impact of rapid in situ hybridization testing on coagulase-negative staphylococci positive blood cultures. J Antimicrob Chemother 58:154–158
293. Forrest GN (2007) PNA FISH: present and future impact on patient management. Expert Rev Mol Diagn 7:231–236
294. Alexander BD, Ashley ED, Reller LB, Reed SD (2006) Cost savings with implementation of PNA FISH testing for identification of *Candida albicans* in blood cultures. Diagn Microbiol Infect Dis 54:277–282
295. Toombs LS, Forrest GN, Weekes E, Lincalis DP, Johnson JK, Venezia RA (2006) Impact of peptide nucleic acid (PNA) fluorescence in situ hybridization (FISH) for enterococcal blood stream infections. In: Infectious Diseases Society of America Meeting, Toronto, Canada, 12–15 October 2006
296. Xu J, Moore JE, Millar BC et al (2004) Improved laboratory diagnosis of bacterial and fungal infections in patients with hematological malignancies using PCR and ribosomal RNA sequence analysis. Leuk Lymphoma 45:1637–1641
297. Ruokonen E, Nousiainen T, Pulkki K, Takala J (1999) Procalcitonin concentrations in patients with neutropenic fever. Eur J Clin Microbiol Infect Dis 18: 283–285
298. von Lilienfeld-Toal M, Dietrich MP, Glasmacher A et al (2004) Markers of bacteremia in febrile neutropenic patients with hematological malignancies: procalcitonin and IL-6 are more reliable than C-reactive protein. Eur J Clin Microbiol Infect Dis 23:539–544

299. Yonemori K, Kanda Y, Yamamoto R et al (2001) Clinical value of serial measurement of serum C-reactive protein level in neutropenic patients. Leuk Lymphoma 41:607–614
300. Maki DG, Weise CE, Sarafin HW (1977) A semiquantitative culture method for identifying intravenous-catheter-related infection. N Engl J Med 296(23): 1305–1309
301. Raad I, Hanna HA, Alakech B, Chatzinikolaou I, Johnson MM, Tarrand J (2004) Differential time to positivity: a useful method for diagnosing catheter-related bloodstream infections. Ann Intern Med 140:18–25
302. Blot F, Nitenberg G, Chachaty E et al (1999) Diagnosis of catheter-related bacteraemia: a prospective comparison of the time to positivity of hub-blood versus peripheral-blood cultures. Lancet 354:1071–1077
303. Malgrange VB, Escande MC, Theobald S (2001) Validity of earlier positivity of central venous blood cultures in comparison with peripheral blood cultures for diagnosing catheter-related bacteremia in cancer patients. J Clin Microbiol 39:274–278
304. Mermel LA, Farr BM, Sherertz RJ et al (2001) Guidelines for the management of intravascular catheter-related infections. Clin Infect Dis 32:1249–1272

Chapter 4

Fungal and Parasitic Infections

G. Mattiuzzi and L. Ostrosky-Zeichner

Abstract Fungal infections have emerged as major causes of morbidity and mortality among patients with hematological malignancies (Int J Antimicrob Agents 31:193–197, 2008). Although several new antifungal agents have become available for clinical use in the past few years, mortality from fungal infections remains above 20%. Advances in the management of hematological malignancies, including use of more aggressive regimens and expansion of the range of potential recipients to include patients who had previously not been considered for such treatments (e.g., elderly patients or patients with particular types of comorbid conditions), have led to increases in the number of patients at risk for invasive fungal infections (IFIs), as well as potentially more severe suppression of immune function (Int J Antimicrob Agents 31:193–197, 2008).

Remarkable advances in systemic antifungal therapy have occurred in the last decade, offering more options for the treatment of IFI. This chapter will focus on the management of these infections, as well as parasitic diseases that are occasionally seen in this immunocompromised population.

Keywords Fungal infections • Antifungals • Aspergillosis • Candidiasis • Zygomycosis • Pneumocystis • Toxoplasmosis • Parasitic diseases • Fusarium • Scedosporium

1. Fungal Infections

1.1. General Concepts

The management of invasive fungal infections (IFIs) in patients with hematological malignancies is difficult because of the life-threatening nature of these infections, the lack of reliable diagnostic tests, and the need for long-term treatment with agents that are expensive and often associated with toxicity.

Since research has shown that early treatment has a definite impact on patient outcomes [2, 3], contemporary management strategies go well beyond treatment of full-blown disease. These strategies include prophylaxis, pre-emptive

From: *Managing Infections in Patients With Hematological Malignancies*: Contemporary Hematology, Edited by: M. Kleinberg, DOI 10.1007/978-1-59745-415-5_4,

therapy, and empirical therapy, in addition to traditional pathogen-specific curative treatment [4, 5]. Characteristics and examples of these strategies are shown in Table 4-1. It is very important to consider that the bulk of antifungal therapy given to immunocompromised hosts will be as empirical or pre-emptive therapy, as outcomes of delayed therapy are poor.

Candida and *Aspergillus* species are the most common organisms documented in most cases of IFI; however, significant numbers of other fungi, many that had not been considered pathogenic in the past, are now emerging as potential pathogens [6–9]. Table 4-2 shows the most frequent fungal pathogens seen in the hematological malignancy setting. A trend has been noted towards the appearance of infections with non-*albicans Candida* species (*C. glabrata* and *C. krusei*) and non-*fumigatus Aspergillus* species [10–12]. The clinical significance of this shift in the type of infectious organisms is that these species may be more virulent and more difficult to treat.

Table 4-1. Contemporary management strategies for fungal infections in hematological patients.

Strategy	Concept	Examples
Prophylaxis	Prevention of the infection by administering antifungals to high risk hosts	Fluconazole prophylaxis for stem cell transplant recipients or during induction chemotherapy in AML
Pre-emptive therapy	Early initiation of antifungals on asymptomatic patients who have positive results as part of a monitoring strategy	Antifungals on patients with positive galactomannan or with CT findings of fungal pneumonia
Empirical therapy	Early initiation of antifungals in high risk symptomatic patients who have negative diagnostic test	Antifungals on day 3–5 for persistently febrile neutropenic patients
Traditional treatment	Treatment of confirmed disease	Antifungals on a patient with a positive culture or biopsy showing fungal elements

Table 4-2. Fungal pathogens in the hematological malignancy setting.

Yeasts	**Molds**
Common – *Candida* spp.	Common – *Aspergillus* spp.
Rare – *Trichosporon* spp.	Uncommon – *Fusarium* spp.
Cryptococcus neoformans	Zygomycetes
Malasezzia furfur	Rare – *Pseudoallescheria boydii*
	Penicillium spp.
Endemic and dimorphic fungi	**Others**
Common – *Histoplasma capsulatum*	Common – *Pneumocystis jirovecii*
Rare – *Blastomyces dermatitides*	
Coccidiodes immitis	
Sporotrix schenckii	

1.2. Yeast

1.1.1. Candida

Candida species are the fourth most common causes of nosocomial bloodstream infections in the United States [13]. High rates of infections have been reported in infants less than 1 year old, adults over the ages of 65, cancer patients, adults with diabetes, and patients with central venous catheter [11, 14]. *Candida* spp. reside predominantly in the gastrointestinal tract but can be also found as commensal colonizers of the skin, vagina, and urethra. In hospitalized patients, oral carriages rates of *Candida* spp. are higher than in healthy subjects (25–50% and 50–70%, respectively) with *C. albicans* being the most frequent species found. *Candida* spp. can cause a broad variety of infections, from superficial cellulitis to blood stream infections, major organ involvement, and disseminated disease. In most cases, especially in patients with hematological malignancies, invasive candidiasis is of endogenous origin, but person-to-person transmission is possible. Translocation of *Candida* spp. from the gastrointestinal tract to the blood entails overgrowth of the yeast in their commensal habitat in patients treated with broad spectrum antibacterials followed by concomitant loss of integrity of the gastrointestinal mucosa because of graft-versus-host disease (GVHD) or chemotherapy-induced damage.

The most frequent species of invasive *Candida* infection are *C. albicans, C. glabrata, C. tropicalis, C. krusei,* and *C. parapsilosis*. Less frequent species reported are *C. guillermondii, C kefyr*, and *C. rugosa*. Although *C. albicans* remains the most common causative agent of invasive candidiasis (66% of all *Candida* spp.), there has been a shift towards an increase in the isolation of non-*albicans* species such as *C. tropicalis* (from 4.6% to 7.5%) and *C parapsilosis* (from 4.2% to 7.3%) [15]. Factors responsible for this change include the use of fluconazole for prophylaxis and treatment, and changes in demographics of patient whose underlying diseases put them at risk for invasive candidal infections. [16, 17] The use of broad spectrum antibiotics and central venous catheters also may be responsible for an increased risk for developing *C. glabrata*.

C. parapsilosis is an exogenous pathogen that can be found on the skin and can spread by hand carriage. It has a notorious ability to form biofilms on catheters and other implanted devices, and it has been also linked to infections in patients receiving parenteral nutrition. *C. tropicalis* and *C. krusei* are important, though uncommon, pathogens in patients with neutropenia, especially those with hematologic malignancies and bone marrow transplantation (BMT) [11, 18]. While the use of fluconazole prophylaxis has significantly decreased the incidence of *C. tropicalis [*18], infections caused by *C. krusei* have been associated with the use of vancomycin, piperacillin–tazobactam, and fluconazole [16, 18].

Candidemia and acute disseminated candidiasis are the most common forms of infection. Severe immunosuppression, caused by either underlying hematological disease or treatment or both, changes in the integrity of the gastrointestinal mucosa, indwelling central venous catheters, and overgrowth by *Candida* spp. in patients treated with broad spectrum antibacterial agents are the most significant factors related to the development of invasive candidiasis. Candidemia is characterized by the presence of persistent fever that does not respond to broad-spectrum antibacterials and, in the absence of timely therapy, it leads to general deterioration with signs and symptoms of shock. Because many patients who develop candidiasis may already be receiving antifungal medications as prophylaxis or empirical treatment, blood cultures may be negative for *Candida* spp., and treating physicians should be aware of the possibility of such "false-negative" blood cultures even in the face of disseminated *Candida* infections. The organs most commonly involved in acute disseminated candidiasis are the gastrointestinal tract, kidney, heart, liver, skin, and spleen. Skin lesions on the extremities may take the form of nonspecific, hard, nontender nodules or rashes. Endophthalmitis rarely occurs in patients with neutropenia.

Before the routine use of antifungal prophylaxis, candidiasis in patients with hematological malignancies undergoing chemotherapy or BMT often presented as chronic disseminated candidiasis (hepatosplenic candidiasis). Diagnosis of hepatosplenic candidiasis requires a high index of clinical suspicion in febrile patients with treated acute leukemia, who are recovering from chemotherapy-induced neutropenia. Symptoms of chronic disseminated candidiasis typically present as persistent fever, progressive debilitation, abdominal pain, and elevated alkaline phosphatase levels as well as, usually simultaneous or shortly after, increases in neutrophil counts. Other indicators of liver function usually are only moderately elevated. Blood cultures are negative frequently, and the diagnosis is usually made by identification of multiple hypo-echoic lesions in the liver, spleen, and kidneys on abdominal ultrasonography. Computed tomography (CT) or magnetic resonance imaging (MRI) of the abdomen can also be useful for diagnosis. The diagnosis is confirmed by identifying yeast with specific histopathological stains or with a positive culture from the biopsy. However, cultures and histopathology of biopsy specimens may be negative and patients may require empiric treatment if clinical suspicion remains high.

Prompt recognition and treatment of candidemia, as well as other forms of candidal infection, are important because delays in treatment are associated with higher mortality rates and longer hospital stays [2, 3, 19]. The Infectious Diseases Society of America (IDSA) recommends treating candidemia in neutropenic patients with an echinocandin (caspofungin, loading dose of 70 mg, then 50 mg daily; micafungin, 100 mg daily; anidulafungin, loading dose of 200 mg, then 100 mg daily or a lipid formulation of amphotericin B (3-5 mg/kg daily). For patients who are less critically ill and who have no recent azole exposure, fluconazole (loading dose of 800 mg [12 mg/kg], then 400 mg [6 mg/kg] daily. The IDSA candidemia guidelines also recommend prompt removal, when feasible, of indwelling central venous catheters though the benefit in neutropenic patients, in whom the gut may be the source for the *Candida,* is controversial.

Several issues must be considered in choosing the proper antifungal agent, to treat invasive candidiasis in patients with hematological malignancies. First, many patients may already have received antifungal prophylaxis or empirical antifungal therapy before the *Candida* infection is documented; hence infection with potentially azole-resistant *Candida* spp. should be considered. Second, although *Candida albicans* is still the most common species isolated, risk of infection with non-*albicans Candida* species, even in the absence of azole prophylaxis or empirical therapy, may be high in some institutions. Therefore, identification of the species must be accompanied by information on its susceptibility to fluconazole so as to guide the choice of therapy. In

Table 4-3. Antifungals commonly used to treat yeast pathogens.

Agent	Adult dose	Spectrum of activity	Comments
Fluconazole	400–800 mg IV or oral q24h	*Candida* spp. (except *C. krusei, C. glabrata* in areas with high background resistance), *Trichosporon* spp., *Cryptococcus neoformans*	Adjustment for renal function Excellent CNS penetration Excellent oral bioavailability
Caspofungin	70 mg IV load dose q24h once followed by 50 mg IV q24h	*Candida* spp. (*C. parapsilosis* has higher MICs) Not active against *Trichosporon* spp. or *Cryptococcus neoformans*	Dose adjustment for liver function
Micafungin	100 mg IV q24h	*Candida* spp. (*C. parapsilosis* has higher MICs) Not active against *Trichosporon* spp. or *Cryptococcus neoformans*	
Anidulafungin	200 mg IV load dose q24h once followed by 100 mg IV q24h	*Candida* spp. (*C. parapsilosis* has higher MICs) Not active against *Trichosporon* spp. or *Cryptococcus neoformans*	Ethanol diluent
Amphotericin B deoxycholate (AmB-d) and lipid formulations of AmB-d	0.7–1.0 mg/kg IV q24h Lipids: 3–5 mg/kg IV q24h	*Candida* spp., *Cryptococcus neoformans* Poorly active against *Trichosporon* spp.	Frequent renal toxicity may be ameliorated with saline loading before infusion Potassium and magnesium wasting (sometimes profound) High incidence of infusional toxicities including fever and chills but rarely acute pulmonary toxicity, acutely elevated blood pressure, and hypotension. Toxicities less frequent with lipid formulations

many cases, clinicians should be aware that the best approach may involve individualizing initial antifungal choice on the basis of previous antifungal prophylaxis/empirical therapy, history of colonization with non-*albicans* species, epidemiology of non-*albicans* Candida in the institution, etc. Many patients may be treated most effectively by switching from a broad spectrum nonazole class of antifungal agents to fluconazole after species identification and determination of fluconazole susceptibility.

Antifungal prophylaxis with fluconazole or an extended spectrum azole like posaconazole is given in many centers to patients undergoing chemotherapy and likely to produce prolonged neutropenia and to recipients of allogeneic stem cell transplants. The most likely breakthrough infecting *Candida* species in patients with hematological malignancies on fluconazole prophylaxis are fluconazole-resistant *Candida albicans*, *C. glabrata,* and *C. krusei* (the last one being inherently resistant to fluconazole). Although the overall percentage of *C. albicans* susceptible to fluconazole has changed little from 99.2% in 1997 to 99% in 2001 [20], incidences vary widely between institutions and breakthrough candidemia due to *C. albicans* resistant to azoles has been reported in patients with leukemia and taking azoles for prophylaxis [21]. If the isolate is determined to be fluconazole-resistant *C. albicans*, amphotericin B deoxycholate [23], a lipid formulation of amphotericin B [24], or caspofungin [25] can be an appropriate option (Table 4-3).

Two other echinocandins, micafungin [22, 26] and anidulafungin [28, 29] have been approved for use in the United States during the past 2 years for treatment of candidemia. A randomized and blinded clinical trial compared micafungin 100 mg IV daily vs. micafungin 150 mg IV daily vs. caspofungin 70 mg IV loading dose and 50 mg IV daily maintenance dose. This trial showed that neither micafungin dose was inferior to caspofungin and that there was no difference between the two dosing regimens [26]. Anidulafungin was compared to fluconazole for patients with candidemia and other forms of *Candida* infections [29]. Success rates among patients randomly assigned to receive anidulafungin were substantially higher (75.6%) than among those given fluconazole (60.2%). An analysis of response according to *Candida* species also demonstrated that overall success rates were better for recipients of anidulafungin (88.1%) than for those given fluconazole (76.2%, $P=0.02$). Better success rates were seen even in infections with fluconazole-sensitive *C. albicans*. Experience with these two newly-approved echinocandins is limited in neutropenic patients and stem cell transplant recipient populations.

Voriconazole, a broad spectrum azole approved for treatment of candidemia, is an alternative to be considered for patients with hematological malignancies and *C. albicans* infections because of its low minimal inhibitory concentration $(MIC)_{50}$ for this species (less than 0.1 μg/ml) [20]. This agent is also available in an oral dosage form, allowing treatment to be given on an outpatient basis in some cases or shifted from intravenous to oral dosing for completion of therapy.

If the infecting isolate is *C. glabrata*, either an echinocandin or amphotericin B (deoxycholate or lipid formulations) is an appropriate option with similar efficacy [25]. It is unknown if there are significant clinical differences between the different echinocandins against this organism [32]. In many cancer centers, fluconazole resistant rates of *C. glabrata* are high, thereby limiting first-line fluconazole use only to those infections where there is some assurance that *C. glabrata* is sensitive to azoles. Some concerns have been raised about possible cross-resistance of fluconazole-resistant *C. glabrata* species to voriconazole. When the isolated organism is *C. glabrata* that is resistant to fluconazole and to itraconazole, the likelihood that this species is cross-resistant to the new triazoles voriconazole and posaconazole is high because of overexpression of *CDR* genes [33]. Therefore, use of new triazoles in these circumstances should be considered carefully.

C. krusei is resistant to fluconazole and itraconazole. Because some strains of *C. krusei* may be also resistant to amphotericin B [33], the echinocandins are a safe alternative. Voriconazole can also be considered because of its good activity against *C. krusei* in vitro [33–35], which was confirmed in a clinical trial in which voriconazole was used as salvage therapy for patients with candidemia [34]. In that trial of 52 patients, 10 had invasive candidiasis due to *C. krusei*, and 7 of those patients (70%) responded to voriconazole treatment.

C. tropicalis is also common in patients with cancer, particularly in those with hematological malignancies, and is characteristically associated with high mortality rates [36–39]. This species is usually susceptible to amphotericin B and the azoles, but some clinical isolates have been reported that are resistant to azoles, predominantly fluconazole [40–43]. Therefore, amphotericin B, voriconazole, or an echinocandin is an appropriate option for initial therapy, but the final decision about treatment should be made only after the susceptibility of the isolate to fluconazole has been determined.

C. parapsilosis is most commonly isolated in neonates and in patients receiving parenteral nutrition; however, it has also been noted recently in patients with hematological malignancies [37] and in patients receiving caspofungin [44]. Even though the MICs of all echinocandins against *C. parapsilosis* are high, the response rates in several clinical trials have been the same as that of the comparators. In a comparison of caspofungin and amphotericin B for invasive candidiasis, the response rate for *C. parapsilosis* was similar for both drugs (70% and 65%) [25]. Comparable response rates were reported when micafungin was used alone or in combination with caspofungin for newly diagnosed or refractory *C. parapsilosis* candidiasis [22]. However, response failures with echinocandins have been seen. Although these findings indicate that echinocandins may be useful for treating *C. parapsilosis* candidiasis, it seems reasonable in these cases to use a class of antifungal agents other than echinocandins. For clinically stable patients who have not been on antifungal prophylaxis, fluconazole (400 mg/day) should be considered as initial therapy. If the patient cannot tolerate oral medication, intravenous fluconazole should be considered as an alternative.

Azoles interact with cytochrome P450 3A4 which metabolizes many antineoplastic agents used in various chemotherapy strategies for hematological diseases. When possible drug interactions may occur, echinocandins may be preferred over voriconazole, itraconazole, and posaconazole in selected cases. Among patients receiving echinocandins for prophylaxis, *C. parapsilosis* may be the causative organism and therapy with another class of antifungal medication should be started. Both amphotericin B (and its lipid formulations) and the azoles are excellent choices to consider in these situations.

Treatment for patients with candidiasis and acute disseminated candidiasis should be given for at least 14 days after the last positive blood culture and resolution of signs and symptoms of infection and recovery from neutropenia. For patients with chronic disseminated candidiasis, treatment should be given until the resolution of radiologic and clinical signs of infections, usually taking 8–12 weeks. Combination therapy with agents having different mechanisms of action has been recommended for patients with candidiasis refractory to monotherapy who are relatively stable clinically [45]. However, no data are available as yet to demonstrate the superiority of one form of therapy over another in this setting. Only one trial has compared monotherapy versus combination therapy for candidemia in nonneutropenic patients [46]. In that randomized, blinded multicenter study, amphotericin B plus fluconazole was compared with fluconazole plus placebo. The results showed a nonstatistically significant trend toward improved success and more rapid resolution of candidemia in the group given amphotericin B plus fluconazole than in the monotherapy group, but no difference was found in overall mortality (mortality rate at 90 days was 40% for the combination group and 39% for the monotherapy group). Importantly, these findings demonstrated a lack of antagonism between these two drugs.

1.1.2. Trichosporon

Although the incidence of *Trichosporon* infection in immunocompromised patients is relatively low, trichosporonosis is becoming more common in patients with hematological malignancies, particularly those with acute myelogenous leukemia. Breakthrough infections due to *Trichosporon* have been reported during the administration of itraconazole [58], amphotericin B [59], and echinocandins [9, 60]. Clinically, trichosporonosis presents similarly to invasive candidiasis with persistent fever that does not respond to broad-spectrum antibiotics (in neutropenic patients) and often with maculopapular lesions or necrotizing ulcers in the skin. If disseminated, *Trichosporon* can be found in the lungs and kidneys. The diagnosis can be made through blood cultures, which are positive in about 70% of cases, or through microbiologic or histological documentation of the organism in the involved organs. Involvement of the kidneys is associated with flank pain and hematuria and *Trichosporon* can be isolated from the urine.

Although amphotericin B and azoles show in vitro activity against *Trichosporon* species, disease resistance and clinical failure have been reported primarily with amphotericin B, but also with fluconazole, and itraconazole [61–64]. Two new triazoles, posaconazole and voriconazole, seem to be more active than amphotericin B, fluconazole, or itraconazole, and may be fungicidal against *Trichosporon* species [65]. Optimal therapy for trichosporonosis has yet to be determined, particularly in light of the high mortality rates (up to 78%) for patients treated with amphotericin B or azoles (such as fluconazole, itraconazole or micanozole). In addition to in vitro evidence that voriconazole is active against *Trichosporon*, in vivo data also support the superiority of voriconazole over amphotericin B for the treatment of trichosporonosis [66], and several reports have shown successful treatment of disseminated trichosporonosis with voriconazole [9, 64, 67]. Thus, even though few patients have been treated to date and no comparative studies have been done to confirm the superiority of voriconazole over amphotericin B, voriconazole seems to be a good alternative to high dose fluconazole for patients with *Trichosporon* infections.

1.1.3. Cryptococcosis

Cryptococcal infection is now rare among patients with hematologic malignancies. The routine use of fluconazole as a prophylactic agent could be responsible for this low occurrence. It has been thought that patients with Hodgkin's disease or lymphoma are at higher risk for cryptococcosis than are those with other kinds of hematologic malignancies. Yet in a recent series of 17 patients with hematologic malignancies and cryptococcosis, 47% had acute leukemia and only one had Hodgkin's disease [73]. Use of steroids and diabetes mellitus are other additional risk factors.

The most common sign of infection, and the only sign in some patients, is fever. Pneumonia and fungemia are the most common clinical manifestations of disseminated disease. Invasive diagnostic tests such as biopsies cannot be performed in many patients with hematologic malignancies because of associated thrombocytopenia and neutropenia, and therefore, clinical suspicion of infection, with microbiological isolation of the organism (from bronchoalveolar lavage fluid or blood) or a positive serum cryptococcal antigen test, is necessary for the diagnosis.

In general, cryptococcosis in patients with hematologic malignancies is associated with a good prognosis and very low mortality rates if antifungal treatment is started promptly [73, 74]. Nevertheless, in one review, the 3-month survival rate for HIV-negative patients with hematologic malignancies and cryptococcosis was significantly lower than that for HIV-negative patients without hematologic malignancies [75].

Fluconazole or amphotericin B (in either the conventional or liposomal formulation) seems to be effective in cryptococcosis. Combinations of both drugs have been used in some cases, especially meningitis; however no studies have shown that the combination of amphotericin B (conventional or lipid formulation) and fluconazole is better than monotherapy with either one. Because flucytosine can cause bone marrow suppression, this drug should not be used for patients with hematologic malignancies. Patients at high risk for cryptococcosis or those who come from endemic areas may benefit from prophylaxis with fluconazole.

1.3. Molds

1.1.4. Approach to the Patient with a Suspected Mold Infection

The morbidity and mortality of mold infections in the hematological malignancy population are extremely high. This is most likely related to delays in starting antifungal therapy because of poor diagnostics and to the overall state of immunosuppression of infected patients. While the work up of patients with suspected mold infections should be aggressive and expedited, antifungal therapy should never be delayed pending results. Most authors recommend starting antifungals either in the setting of febrile neutropenia despite 3–5 days on broad spectrum antibiotics or for presumed "fungal pneumonia" when the patient has pulmonary infiltrates or nodules detected with chest imaging that are refractory to broad spectrum antibiotics. Recent developments in high resolution CT scanning and serum testing, such as that for galactomannan and (1,3)-β-d-glucan, represent rapid, noninvasive, diagnostic adjuncts that have allowed movement beyond empirical therapy and into a pre-emptive approach (Table 4-1).

1.1.5. Aspergillus

Aspergillus is a filamentous fungus ubiquitous in the environment. The species that most often cause human disease include: *A. fumigatus, A. niger*, and *A. flavus*. Recent reports have mentioned an increase in disease by previously "rare" species, such as *A. terreus* and *A. ustus*. The incidence of invasive aspergillosis among patients with hematological malignancies can be as high as 40%, and the mortality rates in such cases range between 40% and >90%, depending on the sites involved. The lungs are the most common site of infection, but *Aspergillus* can disseminate to any organ. Sino-pulmonary disease and central nervous system infection are relatively common in patients with leukemia. The most important risk factors for invasive aspergillosis are profound and prolonged periods of neutropenia and use of corticosteroids and other antigraft-versus-host disease treatments are involved in allogeneic stem cell transplant recipients. The route of infection is usually inhalation of airborne *Aspergillus* conidia, but some have proposed that molds, including Aspergillosis, can originate from water, especially through aerosolization [47, 48].

Immunocompromised patients with invasive pulmonary aspergillosis can be asymptomatic or present with nonspecific symptoms such as persistent fever, cough, mild hemoptysis, pleuritic chest pain, and dyspnea. Occasionally, patients can present with massive, life-threatening pulmonary hemorrhage.

Radiographically, invasive pulmonary aspergillosis can present in different forms, with one or multiple infiltrates (bronchopneumonia) or as lobar pneumonia similar to a bacterial infection. Chest computed tomography provides more valuable information than conventional chest x-ray, and in addition, detects lesions in earliest stage of the disease; therefore, characteristic chest CT findings have been included as one of the criteria for the case-definition of invasive aspergillosis (IA) in clinical studies.

The most characteristic finding on chest CT is the presence of a macro-nodule with a halo sign. The nodule is seen as a dense core surrounded by a halo of ground glass infiltrate. Pathologically, the core consists of necrotic lung destroyed by the infection and the halo is a combination of edema and local hemorrhage caused by advancing aspergillosis. However, the halo is a fleeting finding and many patients will have a chest CT with one or more nodules, often bilateral. Fewer patients present initially with cavitary lesions, consolidations, or wedge-shaped peripheral pulmonary infarcts. The presence of the halo sign has been considered a distinctive sign of early stages of invasive aspergillosis; however, it can also be seen in patients with cytomegalovirus pneumonia, tuberculosis, or zygomycosis.

Once the patient recovers from immunosuppression, pulmonary lesions may develop cavitations which mark the onset of resolution of the infection.

In immunocompromised patients, sinus infections, with or without antecedent sinusitis, are common and are usually associated with concomitant pulmonary disease. Headaches, sinus discharge, facial pain, fever, and cough are the most common clinical manifestations in such cases. Patients can present with necrotic lesions on the hard palate or nasal turbinates that can spread to the brain, orbits, or to other sinuses, causing thrombosis and infarction. Surgical drainage of infected sinuses has an essential role in the treatment of *Aspergillus* sinusitis.

Central nervous system (CNS) aspergillosis in immunocompromised hosts has been associated with mortality as high as 90%. Cerebral aspergillosis occurs most often after hematogenous dissemination of the infection from the lungs or direct extension from the sinuses, but primary cerebral aspergillosis has been also reported.

CNS aspergillosis can present as solitary or multiple brain lesions, meningitis or granulomas. Patients usually present with persistent fever, altered mental status, focal neurologic deficits, and, less often, meningeal symptoms. In severe immunocompromised patients, symptoms may be absent until late in the infection and progression with neurological deterioration occurs rapidly leading to death. Cerebrospinal fluid (CSF) cultures are usually negative for *Aspergillus* spp. MRI or CT is useful for the diagnosis. The development of poorly defined, low-intensity lesions with little or no mass effect and minimal contrast enhancement on CT is suggestive of infarcts. On MRI scans, *Aspergillus* lesions are evident as heterogeneous high-signal intensity areas surrounded by low-density signal at the peripheral rim, resembling hemorrhagic infarcts.

In immunocompromised patients with invasive aspergillosis, the single most important prognostic factor predicting successful response is timely recovery of immune function. Current therapies have reduced mortality significantly, although rates as high as 30–50% are still being reported in treated patients. The practice guideline published in 2008 by the IDSA [51] recommends voriconazole as the new standard of care and reserves lipid formulations of amphotericin B as alternatives to this drug, in contrast to earlier recommendation [9]. The recommended dose of voriconazole for invasive aspergillosis is two loading doses at 6 mg/kg given 12 h apart followed by 4 mg/kg given every 12 h, as maintenance (Table 4-4). In the 2008 IDSA guidelines for

Table 4-4. Antifungals commonly used to treat mold pathogens.

Agent	Adult dose	Spectrum of activity	Comments
Voriconazole	6 mg/kg q12h load ×2 doses followed by 4 mg/kg q12h IV or oral	*Aspergillus* spp., *Fusarium*, *Scedosporium* spp., many dematiaceous molds, *Candida* spp. (except fluconazole-resistant *C. glabrata*), *Trichosporon* spp. Not active against *Zygomycetes*	Adjustment for hepatic and renal function (IV only due to accumulation of excipient in renal failure), frequent visual effects (photopsia, rarely hallucinations), potential for serious interactions with drugs metabolized through CYP 3A4 and CYP 2C9 (tacrolimus, sirolimus, cyclosporine A, many chemotherapy agents) Excellent CNS penetration Excellent oral bioavailability
Itraconazole	200–400 mg oral suspension q24h (IV formulation no longer available)	Second-line for *Aspergillus* spp.	GI toxicity frequent Adjustment for liver function Variable absorption (use suspension, not tablets) Drug interactions (see voriconazole above)
Caspofungin	70 mg IV load dose q24h once followed by 50 mg IV q24h	Second-line for *Aspergillus* spp. for patients who failed or intolerant of first-line agents	Dose adjustment for liver function
Liposomal amphotericin B (L-AmB)	3–5 mg/kg IV q24h	*Aspergillus* spp. except some *A. terreus* (3 mg/kg/day)*Fusarium*, *Zygomycetes* (5 mg/kg/day) *Candida* spp. Poorly active against *Trichosporon* spp. and *Scedosporium* spp.	Threefold less renal toxicity compared to AmB-d Potassium and magnesium wasting (sometimes profound) Lower incidence of infusional toxicities compared to AmB-d
Amphotericin B lipid complex (ABLC)	5 mg/kg IV q24h	*Aspergillus* spp. except some *A. terreus*, *Fusarium*, *Zygomycetes*, *Candida* spp. Poorly active against *Trichosporon* spp. and *Scedosporium* spp.	Threefold less renal toxicity compared to AmB-d Potassium and magnesium wasting (sometimes profound) Similar incidence of infusional toxicities compared to AmB-d
Posaconazole	200 mg oral suspension q6–8h (IV formulation not available)	Prophylaxis in neutropenic patients with hematological malignancies and allogeneic stem cell recipients with GVHD Second-line treatment of *Zygomycetes* (not FDA approved)	Adjustment for hepatic function Variable absorption (take with fatty meals, avoid agents that suppress gastric acid production, monitor levels when used for treatment) Drug interactions (see voriconazole above)

treatment of aspergillosis, it has been recommended that maintenance treatment with oral voriconazole should be 4 mg/kg per dose rather than the 200 mg oral dose used in the voriconazole versus amphotericin B trial (see below) [52]. An advantage of voriconazole is its availability in both intravenous and oral preparation forms with high bioavailabilities, which is important considering that treatment for invasive aspergillosis in some patients can last for several months. Oral voriconazole is provided as 50 mg and 200 mg tablets or as a liquid suspension. The dose for patients treated with oral tablets should be rounded to the nearest 50 mg increment. Voriconazole has excellent activity against invasive aspergillosis. A randomized study of 277 patients comparing voriconazole and amphotericin B deoxycholate for the initial treatment of invasive aspergillosis showed that response rates (53% and 32%) and survival rates (71% and 58%) favored voriconazole [52]. Principal side effects include visual disturbances (usually transient but can manifest as frank hallucinations), hepatotoxicity, skin rash, and interactions with other drugs metabolized by several cytochrome P450 isoenzymes.

Use of conventional amphotericin B at 1–1.25 mg/kg daily or one of the lipid-based preparations ABLC or liposomal amphotericin B should be used for patients who fail voriconazole therapy or in those who may develop toxicities to voriconazole. The use of lipid formulations is particularly useful for patients with renal dysfunction because of the relatively low nephrotoxicities of these formulations. The recommended dose is 3–5 mg/kg/day depending on the lipid formulation. A recent study [50] reported similar success rates in patients with invasive aspergillosis treated with 3 mg/kg/day versus 10 mg/kg/day of the liposomal formulation, with less toxicity at the lower dose. Therefore, treatment with higher doses of lipid formulated amphotericin B is not recommended.

Among the echinocandins, caspofungin has been approved for invasive aspergillosis in cases of refractory disease or patients who cannot tolerate standard therapies. The efficacy of caspofungin as salvage therapy has been shown in 83 patients with invasive aspergillosis who could not tolerate (or showed no response to) amphotericin B, lipid formulations of amphotericin B, or triazoles. The response rate to caspofungin in that study was 45%, with overall good tolerance and few side effects [53]. Caspofungin has been also used as single-agent first-line therapy for patients with hematological malignancies and proven or probable invasive pulmonary aspergillosis [54]. In that study, 32 patients given the recommended dosage of caspofungin (70 mg on day 1 and 50 mg per day thereafter) showed a successful response (50–100% resolution) rate of 56%, with an additional 6% of patients showing stable or limited (<50%) improvement. However, given this limited experience, echinocandins should be used with caution as initial treatment of aspergillosis because their comparative efficacy versus that of voriconazole and lipid formulations of amphotericin B has not been demonstrated.

Optimal duration of therapy has not been determined. It would be prudent to individualize therapy taking into account response judged from clinical improvement, serial chest CT, serial serum galactomannan antigen levels, and recovery from neutropenia and GVHD/immunosuppression. Patients who have recovered fully from an episode of aspergillosis are at risk for recrudescent infection with neutropenia resulting from subsequent chemotherapy or recurrent GVHD. Many experts advocate secondary prophylaxis with antifungals during these periods of immune deficiency to prevent recurrent aspergillosis. Prophylaxis to prevent aspergillosis and other fungal infections is discussed in Chap. 11.

Combination therapy for invasive aspergillosis is very attractive from a theoretical standpoint as a way to gain synergy and reduce toxicities, as the mortality of this disease remains high despite many therapeutic options. However, this approach cannot be recommended routinely at this point as there are no randomized clinical trials to show its safety and efficacy. Retrospective reports of combination therapy for invasive aspergillosis failed to show any advantages for the combination of caspofungin and liposomal amphotericin B in cancer patients [55] or for the combination of voriconazole and caspofungin in transplant patients [56]. However, another retrospective report in stem cell transplant recipients showed improved survival for patients that received the later combination [57]. Until randomized clinical trials are available, clinicians are discouraged from following this approach routinely.

1.4. Other Molds

1.1.6. Zygomycosis

Zygomycosis is a term used for infections caused by organisms in the orders *Mucorales* and *Entomophthorales*. The most common species include *Mucor* spp., *Rhizopus* spp., and *Absidia* spp. Risk factors for these infections include diabetes (with or without ketoacidosis), systemic or local steroid use, immunosuppressive therapy for solid organ or stem cell transplants, neutropenia, primary immunodeficiency, and deferoxamine therapy. Cases have been described in immunocompetent patients, usually in the setting of trauma or contaminated surgical wounds [70]. The classic syndromes and presentations include pulmonary, rhino-cerebral, and cutaneous diseases, with dissemination occurring typically in the most immunosuppressed patients. Mortality has been reported to be as high as 84% for disseminated disease [70].

In recent years, zygomycosis has been considered as an emerging mycosis. The increase in incidence may be related to an expanding immunocompromised population base or, as many reports have suggested, a possible epidemiological shift related to wide-spread use of antifungals, most notably voriconazole, that are inactive against these organisms [68]. Zygomycosis is a key differential diagnosis in leukemia patients with suspected fungal pneumonia, as it is very difficult to distinguish between clinical disease caused by these organisms and that caused by other filamentous fungi, such as *Aspergillus* [69].

Treatment of these infections includes lipid-based amphotericin B products and surgical debridement. The combined approach of antifungal treatment and surgery has been associated with 73% overall response rate with the best outcomes in sinusitis [70]. Posaconazole, a new oral triazole antifungal agent, has shown encouraging response rates in salvage and open-label settings [71]. Posaconazole is available only as an oral formulation with limited bioavailability. Absorption is enhanced by ingesting posaconazole with food that contains some fat and by stopping gastric acid suppressants commonly given to patients with hematological malignancies. In patients where posaconazole is used for treatment rather than prophylaxis, measuring a serum posaconazole level may be helpful to identify patients who fail to absorb posaconazole. Although echinocandins have no activity against these organisms, combination antifungal therapy with polyenes has shown some encouraging in vitro and in vivo synergy [72].

1.1.7. Fusarium

Local and disseminated fusariosis have been reported in patients with hematologic malignancies with or without bone marrow transplant (BMT). In addition to the well known risk factors for mold infections, patients with fusariosis often have a history of trauma with infection and tissue breakdown at the site of skin trauma. Patients often present with persistent fever and painful skin lesions or cellulitis. Pneumonia, rhinocerebral infection, or endophthalmitis has been also reported in patients with fusariosis.

Three types of cutaneous lesions have been observed in patients with *Fusarium* infections: target lesions (ulcer/eschar lesions surrounded by a thin rim of erythema), multiple subcutaneous nodules, and ecthyma gangrenosum-like lesions. In patients with hematological malignancies, the presence of onychomycosis should alert the physician to the possible presence of *Fusarium* infection. Evaluation by a dermatologist to evaluate the etiology of the onychomycosis is recommended. The isolation of the organism from cultures of skin lesions, sinuses, or lungs specimens is necessary for the diagnosis. In contrast to patients with *Aspergillus*, patients with fusariosis can have positive blood cultures. Patients with pulmonary infection may present with cavitary lesions or nonspecific bilateral infiltrates.

Amphotericin B or its lipid formulations have been the first option for the treatment of fusariosis for several years with response rates as high as 50–70%. Voriconazole has been used in the treatment of fusariosis as a single agent, as well as in combination with amphotericin B, with success rates comparable to those of amphotericin B. However, the lack of a large randomized trial comparing monotherapy versus combination therapy mitigates against a firm recommendation of one over combination antifungals. Posaconazole is another option for the treatment of patients with fusariosis. However, experience is limited and the success rate reported in those cases was only 48%. Debridement of infected tissue should be considered an integral part of treatment in addition to systemic antifungals.

1.1.8. Scedosporium

Although *Scedosporium* infections are not very frequent in immunocompromised patients, the mortality associated with this infection is very high (>60%). There are two *Scedosporium* species: *S. prolificans* and *S. apiospermum*.

Immunocompromised patients with *S. prolificans* usually present with persistent fever despite broad spectrum antibiotics and signs and symptoms of respiratory or skin infection. Involvement of the central nervous system is common with *Scedosporium* infections and has been reported in 37% of the cases. Similar to *Fusarium, Scedosporium* can be isolated in blood cultures and manifest predominately with skin lesions. Because of its histological similarity to *Aspergillus*, isolation of the organism in cultures is necessary to make a microbiological diagnosis. Surgical drainage of the lesions and systemic antifungal therapy are the two mainstays for treatment. *Scedosporium* are resistant to amphotericin B and voriconazole is the drug of choice for treatment of *Scedosporium* spp. infections.

1.5. Other Mycoses

1.1.8. Pneumocystosis

Although pneumocystosis is often associated with HIV and other diseases requiring corticosteroid therapy, it has been well known that this opportunistic pathogen has a high incidence in patients with hematological malignancies, in whom it is also associated with high morbidity and mortality rates up to 50% [76].

Pneumocystis jirovecii is the new accepted nomenclature for the organism formerly known as *Pneumocystis carinii*. This fungal organism is characterized by the formation of trophozoites and cysts, and although it presents most frequently as localized or diffuse pulmonary involvement, it can also present rarely as a disseminated infection or with localized involvement of other organs.

The most frequent signs and symptoms related to Pneumocystis carinii pneumonia (PCP) infections in hematologic patients are fever, nonproductive cough, rales, and shortness of breath. Although the majority of the patients have positive findings at chest radiography (alveolar and/or interstitial opacities), some may present with normal chest x-rays, in particular, patients with neutropenia. Progression to respiratory failure may be very rapid in this group of patients, especially with granulocyte recovery. *Pneumocystis* pneumonia should always be considered in immunocompromised patients with diffuse alveolar involvement [77]. The current diagnostic gold standard is detection of the organism by direct immunofluorescence analysis of bronchoalveolar fluid, although recent research has shown that this organism can be detected by measurement of 1-3-β-d-glucan in serum [78]. The cornerstone of prophylaxis and treatment for pneumocystosis is trimethroprim/sulfamethoxazole [79]. Alternative regimens such as primaquine+clindamycin, or agents such as pentamidine and atovaquone are generally reserved for patients with sulfa allergy, intolerance (bone marrow suppression), or other contraindications to trimethroprim/sulfametoxazole [79–81].

2. Parasitic Diseases

2.1.1. General Concepts

Parasitic diseases are relatively uncommon in the hematological malignancy setting, although they can be devastating, particularly in highly immunosuppressed patients who live in or travel to endemic areas. This section will briefly cover toxoplasmosis as the most frequent endemic parasitic disease, as well as strongyloidiasis, which is associated with high morbidity and can be rapidly fatal.

2.1.2. Toxoplasmosis

Toxoplasmosis is rare in patients with hematologic malignancies, occurring most often in patients with Hodgkin's disease or patients undergoing BMT [82, 83]. In a recent review, Pagano et al. reported an incidence of 8 per 1,000 among patients who had had allogeneic BMT, as compared with only 0.9 per 1,000 in patients who had had autologous BMT [84]. As has been described for patients with AIDS, severe immunosuppression is a major risk factor for toxoplasmosis. In patients undergoing BMT, the main risk factors are the presence of graft-versus-host disease, low lymphocyte counts, and seropositivity for *Toxoplasma* before the transplant [84, 85]. Cerebral toxoplasmosis has also been reported in fludarabine-refractory, elderly patients with chronic lymphocytic leukemia treated with 2-chlorodeoxy-adenosine (2-CDA) [86]. Risk of infection in these patients appears to be associated with chemotherapy-induced profound, long-lasting depression of CD4 lymphocytes.

The most common clinical presentations are fever and central nervous system symptoms such as seizures, headache, lethargy, confusion, and vomiting. In disseminated disease, signs of pulmonary infection such as cough, dyspnea, hypoxemia, and tachypnea can also be present concurrently with the neurologic findings.

The diagnosis of toxoplasmosis can be made by demonstration of brain lesions on CT or MRI scans. Typical findings are multiple hypodense lesions with contrast enhancement that are located mainly in the basal ganglia and the cortico-medullary junction of the cerebral and cerebellar hemispheres. Positive results from polymerase chain reaction analysis of cerebrospinal fluid or tissues can help with the diagnosis. Serologic positivity for *Toxoplasma gondii* is of little help in the diagnosis or follow-up of active disease [87, 88], but serologic testing should be done before allogeneic transplant to determine if the patient is at risk for reactivation of a latent infection.

The worst outcomes have been reported for patients with disseminated disease (64% fatality), patients in whom the infection began between 31 and 100 days after allogeneic transplant (80% mortality), and in patients given total body irradiation and cyclophosphamide as a stem cell transplant conditioning regimen (74% mortality) [85]. Therefore, toxoplasmosis should be suspected in patients who were seropositive before transplant, were given total body irradiation and cyclophosphamide as conditioning regimen, and who develop fever and central nervous symptoms. Patients with disseminated toxoplasmosis will often have pneumonia on chest imaging. *Toxoplasma* can be detected sometimes by careful examination of silver stained cytology preparations from bronchoalveolar lavage samples where *Pneumocystis* is usually the suspected pathogen.

Transplant recipients who received pyrimethamine and sulphadiazine reportedly had better outcomes than those given other treatments (survival rates of 88% vs. 12%, respectively, P=0.05) [78]. Although routine prophylaxis against toxoplasmosis is not recommended generally, a reasonable approach would be to give pyrimethamine and sulfadoxime for toxoplasmosis prophylaxis to seropositive patients who live in endemic areas and who are undergoing allogeneic transplant, until CD4 lymphocyte counts rebound. It is unclear whether trimethoprim/sulfamethoxazole provides the same protective benefit to patients with hematological malignancies as is seen in patients with advanced HIV infections.

2.1.3. Strongyloidiasis

Strongyloidiasis is acquired by inoculation from contaminated soil with subsequent trans-epidermal migration of the larvae of the nematode *Strongyloides stercoralis*. Autoinfections can also occur by ingestion of larvae with trans-rectal migration [89]. The disease is characterized by diarrhea, abdominal pain, and rash (as the larvae migrate). Eosinophilia is a common finding during routine laboratory examinations [90].

Immunocompromised patients, however, commonly present with a "hyperinfection syndrome," which consists of a sepsis-like presentation with fever and hypotension, eosinophilia, diffuse and rapidly changing pulmonary infiltrates, as well as Gram-negative sepsis and meningitis that occur as a result of bacterial gut translocation through the migrating larvae [91].

Strongyloidiasis is diagnosed by stool examination or by enzyme-linked immunosorbent assay of serum or stool. Treatment includes ivermectin 200 μg/kg/day or albendazole 400 mg PO daily for 2–10 days [92]. Paradoxical reactions can occur when treatment is started [93].

References

1. Maschmeyer G, Haas A (2008) The epidemiology and treatment of infections in cancer patients. Int J Antimicrob Agents 31:193–197
2. Garey KW, Rege M, Pai MP, Mingo DE, Suda KJ, Turpin RS, Bearden DT (2006) Time to initiation of fluconazole therapy impacts mortality in patients with candidemia: a multi-institutional study. Clin Infect Dis 43(1):25–31
3. Morrell M, Fraser VJ, Kollef MH (2005) Delaying the empiric treatment of candida bloodstream infection until positive blood culture results are obtained: a potential risk factor for hospital mortality. Antimicrob Agents Chemother 49(9):3640–3645
4. Wingard JR (2007) New approaches to invasive fungal infections in acute leukemia and hematopoietic stem cell transplant patients. Best Pract Res Clin Haematol 20(1):99–107
5. Segal BH, Almyroudis NG, Battiwalla M, Herbrecht R, Perfect JR, Walsh TJ, Wingard JR (2007) Prevention and early treatment of invasive fungal infection in patients with cancer and neutropenia and in stem cell transplant recipients in the era of newer broad-spectrum antifungal agents and diagnostic adjuncts. Clin Infect Dis 44(3):402–409
6. Walsh TJ, Groll A, Hiemenz J, Fleming R, Roilides E, Anaissie E (2004) Infections due to emerging and uncommon medically important fungal pathogens. Clin Microbiol Infect 10(Suppl 1):48–66
7. Bouza E, Munoz P (2004) Invasive infections caused by Blastoschizomyces capitatus and Scedosporium spp. Clin Microbiol Infect 10(Suppl 1):76–85
8. Alvarez M, Lopez Ponga B, Rayon C, Garcia Gala J, Roson Porto MC, Gonzalez M, Martinez-Suarez JV, Rodriguez-Tudela JL (1995) Nosocomial outbreak caused by Scedosporium prolificans (inflatum): four fatal cases in leukemic patients. J Clin Microbiol 33(12):3290–3295
9. Matsue K, Uryu H, Koseki M, Asada N, Takeuchi M (2006) Breakthrough trichosporonosis in patients with hematologic malignancies receiving micafungin. Clin Infect Dis 42(6):753–757
10. Marr KA, Carter RA, Crippa F, Wald A, Corey L (2002) Epidemiology and outcome of mould infections in hematopoietic stem cell transplant recipients. Clin Infect Dis 34(7):909–917
11. Marr KA, Seidel K, White TC, Bowden RA (2000) Candidemia in allogeneic blood and marrow transplant recipients: evolution of risk factors after the adoption of prophylactic fluconazole. J Infect Dis 181(1):309–316
12. Wingard JR, Merz WG, Rinaldi MG, Johnson TR, Karp JE, Saral R (1991) Increase in Candida krusei infection among patients with bone marrow transplantation and neutropenia treated prophylactically with fluconazole. N Engl J Med 325(18):1274–1277
13. Wisplinghoff H, Bischoff T, Tallent SM, Seifert H, Wenzel RP, Edmond MB (2004) Nosocomial bloodstream infections in US hospitals: analysis of 24, 179 cases from a prospective nationwide surveillance study. Clin Infect Dis 39(3):309–317
14. Almirante B, Rodriguez D, Park BJ, Cuenca-Estrella M, Planes AM, Almela M, Mensa J, Sanchez F, Ayats J, Gimenez M et al (2005) Epidemiology and predictors of mortality in cases of Candida bloodstream infection: results from population-based surveillance, Barcelona, Spain, from 2002 to 2003. J Clin Microbiol 43(4):1829–1835

15. Pfaller MA, Diekema DJ, Procop GW, Rinaldi MG (2007) Multicenter comparison of the VITEK 2 yeast susceptibility test with the CLSI broth microdilution reference method for testing fluconazole against Candida spp. J Clin Microbiol 45(3):796–802
16. Lin MY, Carmeli Y, Zumsteg J, Flores EL, Tolentino J, Sreeramoju P, Weber SG (2005) Prior antimicrobial therapy and risk for hospital-acquired Candida glabrata and Candida krusei fungemia: a case-case-control study. Antimicrob Agents Chemother 49(11):4555–4560
17. Malani A, Hmoud J, Chiu L, Carver PL, Bielaczyc A, Kauffman CA (2005) Candida glabrata fungemia: experience in a tertiary care center. Clin Infect Dis 41(7):975–981
18. Abi-Said D, Anaissie E, Uzun O, Raad I, Pinzcowski H, Vartivarian S (1997) The epidemiology of hematogenous candidiasis caused by different Candida species. Clin Infect Dis 24(6):1122–1128
19. Pappas PG, Kauffman CA, Andes D, Benjamin DK, Calandra TF, Edwards JE, Filler AG et al (2009) Clinical Practice Guidelines for the Management of Candidiasis:2009 Update by the Infectious Diseases Society of America. Clin Infect Dis 48 (1 March): 503–535
20. Hazen KC, Baron EJ, Colombo AL, Girmenia C, Sanchez-Sousa A, del Palacio A, de Bedout C, Gibbs DL (2003) Comparison of the susceptibilities of Candida spp. to fluconazole and voriconazole in a 4-year global evaluation using disk diffusion. J Clin Microbiol 41(12):5623–5632
21. Myoken Y, Kyo T, Kohara T, Fujihara M, Sugata T, Mikami Y (2003) Breakthrough fungemia caused by azole-resistant Candida albicans in neutropenic patients with acute leukemia. Clin Infect Dis 36(11):1496–1497
22. Ostrosky-Zeichner L, Kontoyiannis D, Raffalli J, Mullane KM, Vazquez J, Anaissie EJ, Lipton J, Jacobs P, van Rensburg JH, Rex JH et al (2005) International, open-label, noncomparative, clinical trial of micafungin alone and in combination for treatment of newly diagnosed and refractory candidemia. Eur J Clin Microbiol Infect Dis 24(10):654–661
23. Rex JH, Bennett JE, Sugar AM, Pappas PG, van der Horst CM, Edwards JE, Washburn RG, Scheld WM, Karchmer AW, Dine AP et al (1994) A randomized trial comparing fluconazole with amphotericin B for the treatment of candidemia in patients without neutropenia. Candidemia Study Group and the National Institute. N Engl J Med 33(20):1325–1330
24. Anaissie EJ, Darouiche RO, Abi-Said D, Uzun O, Mera J, Gentry LO, Williams T, Kontoyiannis DP, Karl CL, Bodey GP (1996) Management of invasive candidal infections: results of a prospective, randomized, multicenter study of fluconazole versus amphotericin B and review of the literature. Clin Infect Dis 23(5): 964–972
25. Mora-Duarte J, Betts R, Rotstein C, Colombo AL, Thompson-Moya L, Smietana J, Lupinacci R, Sable C, Kartsonis N, Perfect J (2002) Comparison of caspofungin and amphotericin B for invasive candidiasis. N Engl J Med 347(25):2020–2029
26. Pappas PG, Rotstein CM, Betts RF, Nucci M, Talwar D, De Waele JJ, Vazquez JA, Dupont BF, Horn DL, Ostrosky-Zeichner L et al (2007) Micafungin versus caspofungin for treatment of candidemia and other forms of invasive candidiasis. Clin Infect Dis 45(7):883–893
27. Aperis G, Myriounis N, Spanakis EK, Mylonakis E (2006) Developments in the treatment of candidiasis: more choices and new challenges. Expert Opin Investig Drugs 15(11):1319–1336
28. Krause DS, Reinhardt J, Vazquez JA, Reboli A, Goldstein BP, Wible M, Henkel T (2004) Phase 2, randomized, dose-ranging study evaluating the safety and efficacy of anidulafungin in invasive candidiasis and candidemia. Antimicrob Agents Chemother 48(6):2021–2024

29. Reboli AC, Rotstein C, Pappas PG, Chapman SW, Kett DH, Kumar D, Betts R, Wible M, Goldstein BP, Schranz J et al (2007) Anidulafungin versus fluconazole for invasive candidiasis. N Engl J Med 356(24):2472–2482
30. Cornely OA, Maertens J, Winston DJ, Perfect J, Ullmann AJ, Walsh TJ, Helfgott D, Holowiecki J, Stockelberg D, Goh YT et al (2007) Posaconazole vs. fluconazole or itraconazole prophylaxis in patients with neutropenia. N Engl J Med 356(4):348–359
31. Ullmann AJ, Lipton JH, Vesole DH, Chandrasekar P, Langston A, Tarantolo SR, Greinix H, Morais de Azevedo W, Reddy V, Boparai N et al (2007) Posaconazole or fluconazole for prophylaxis in severe graft-versus-host disease. N Engl J Med 356(4):335–347
32. Cota J, Carden M, Graybill JR, Najvar LK, Burgess DS, Wiederhold NP (2006) In vitro pharmacodynamics of anidulafungin and caspofungin against Candida glabrata isolates, including strains with decreased caspofungin susceptibility. Antimicrob Agents Chemother 50(11):3926–3928
33. Pfaller MA, Messer SA, Hollis RJ, Jones RN, Diekema DJ (2002) In vitro activities of ravuconazole and voriconazole compared with those of four approved systemic antifungal agents against 6, 970 clinical isolates of Candida spp. Antimicrob Agents Chemother 46(6):1723–1727
34. Ostrosky-Zeichner L, Rex JH, Pappas PG, Hamill RJ, Larsen RA, Horowitz HW, Powderly WG, Hyslop N, Kauffman CA, Cleary J et al (2003) Antifungal susceptibility survey of 2, 000 bloodstream Candida isolates in the United States. Antimicrob Agents Chemother 47(10):3149–3154
35. Pfaller MA, Diekema DJ, Messer SA, Boyken L, Hollis RJ (2003) Activities of fluconazole and voriconazole against 1, 586 recent clinical isolates of Candida species determined by Broth microdilution, disk diffusion, and Etest methods: report from the ARTEMIS Global Antifungal Susceptibility Program, 2001. J Clin Microbiol 41(4):1440–1446
36. Tortorano AM, Peman J, Bernhardt H, Klingspor L, Kibbler CC, Faure O, Biraghi E, Canton E, Zimmermann K, Seaton S et al (2004) Epidemiology of candidaemia in Europe: results of 28-month European Confederation of Medical Mycology (ECMM) hospital-based surveillance study. Eur J Clin Microbiol Infect Dis 23(4):317–322
37. Dimopoulos G, Karabinis A, Samonis G, Falagas ME (2007) Candidemia in immunocompromised and immunocompetent critically ill patients: a prospective comparative study. Eur J Clin Microbiol Infect Dis 26(6):377–384
38. Nucci M, Colombo AL (2007) Candidemia due to Candida tropicalis: clinical, epidemiologic, and microbiologic characteristics of 188 episodes occurring in tertiary care hospitals. Diagn Microbiol Infect Dis 58(1):77–82
39. Vigouroux S, Morin O, Moreau P, Harousseau JL, Milpied N (2006) Candidemia in patients with hematologic malignancies: analysis of 7 years' experience in a single center. Haematologica 91(5):717–718
40. Vandeputte P, Larcher G, Berges T, Renier G, Chabasse D, Bouchara JP (2005) Mechanisms of azole resistance in a clinical isolate of Candida tropicalis. Antimicrob Agents Chemother 49(11):4608–4615
41. Myoken Y, Kyo T, Fujihara M, Sugata T, Mikami Y (2004) Clinical significance of breakthrough fungemia caused by azole-resistant Candida tropicalis in patients with hematologic malignancies. Haematologica 89(3):378–380
42. Tortorano AM, Rigoni AL, Biraghi E, Prigitano A, Viviani MA (2003) The European Confederation of Medical Mycology (ECMM) survey of candidaemia in Italy: antifungal susceptibility patterns of 261 non-albicans Candida isolates from blood. J Antimicrob Chemother 52(4):679–682
43. Yang YL, Ho YA, Cheng HH, Ho M, Lo HJ (2004) Susceptibilities of Candida species to amphotericin B and fluconazole: the emergence of fluconazole resistance in Candida tropicalis. Infect Control Hosp Epidemiol 25(1):60–64

44. Forrest GN, Weekes E, Johnson JK (2008) Increasing incidence of Candida parapsilosis candidemia with caspofungin usage. J Infect 56:126–129
45. Sims CR, Ostrosky-Zeichner L, Rex JH (2005) Invasive candidiasis in immunocompromised hospitalized patients. Arch Med Res 36(6):660–671
46. Rex JH, Pappas PG, Karchmer AW, Sobel J, Edwards JE, Hadley S, Brass C, Vazquez JA, Chapman SW, Horowitz HW et al (2003) A randomized and blinded multicenter trial of high-dose fluconazole plus placebo versus fluconazole plus amphotericinB as therapy for candidemia and its consequences in nonneutropenic subjects. Clin Infect Dis 36(10):1221–1228
47. Anaissie EJ, Stratton SL, Dignani MC, Lee CK, Summerbell RC, Rex JH, Monson TP, Walsh TJ (2003) Pathogenic molds (including Aspergillus species) in hospital water distribution systems: a 3-year prospective study and clinical implications for patients with hematologic malignancies. Blood 101(7):2542–2546
48. Anaissie EJ, Costa SF (2001) Nosocomial aspergillosis is waterborne. Clin Infect Dis 33(9):1546–1548
49. Stevens DA, Kan VL, Judson MA, Morrison VA, Dummer S, Denning DW, Bennett JE, Walsh TJ, Patterson TF, Pankey GA (2000) Practice guidelines for diseases caused by Aspergillus. Infectious Diseases Society of America. Clin Infect Dis 30(4):696–709
50. Cornely OA, Maertens J, Bresnik M, Ebrahimi R, Ullmann AJ, Bouza E, Heussel CP, Lortholary O, Rieger C, Boehme A et al (2007) Liposomal amphotericin B as initial therapy for invasive mold infection: a randomized trial comparing a high-loading dose regimen with standard dosing (AmBiLoad trial). Clin Infect Dis 44(10):1289–1297
51. Walsh TJ, Anaissie EJ, Denning DW, Herbrecht R, Kontoyiannis DP, Marr KA, Morrison VA, Segal BH, Steinbach WJ, Stevens DA et al (2008) Treatment of aspergillosis: clinical practice guidelines of the Infectious Diseases Society of America. Clin Infect Dis 46(3):327–360
52. Herbrecht R, Denning DW, Patterson TF, Bennett JE, Greene RE, Oestmann JW, Kern WV, Marr KA, Ribaud P, Lortholary O et al (2002) Voriconazole versus amphotericin B for primary therapy of invasive aspergillosis. N Engl J Med 347(6):408–415
53. Maertens J, Raad I, Petrikkos G, Boogaerts M, Selleslag D, Petersen FB, Sable CA, Kartsonis NA, Ngai A, Taylor A et al (2004) Efficacy and safety of caspofungin for treatment of invasive aspergillosis in patients refractory to or intolerant of conventional antifungal therapy. Clin Infect Dis 39(11):1563–1571
54. Candoni A, Mestroni R, Damiani D, Tiribelli M, Michelutti A, Silvestri F, Castelli M, Viale P, Fanin R (2005) Caspofungin as first line therapy of pulmonary invasive fungal infections in 32 immunocompromised patients with hematologic malignancies. Eur J Haematol 75(3):227–233
55. Kontoyiannis DP, Hachem R, Lewis RE, Rivero GA, Torres HA, Thornby J, Champlin R, Kantarjian H, Bodey GP, Raad II (2003) Efficacy and toxicity of caspofungin in combination with liposomal amphotericin B as primary or salvage treatment of invasive aspergillosis in patients with hematologic malignancies. Cancer 98(2):292–299
56. Singh N, Limaye AP, Forrest G, Safdar N, Munoz P, Pursell K, Houston S, Rosso F, Montoya JG, Patton P et al (2006) Combination of voriconazole and caspofungin as primary therapy for invasive aspergillosis in solid organ transplant recipients: a prospective, multicenter, observational study. Transplantation 81(3):320–326
57. Marr KA, Boeckh M, Carter RA, Kim HW, Corey L (2004) Combination antifungal therapy for invasive aspergillosis. Clin Infect Dis 39(6):797–802
58. Krcmery V Jr, Mateicka F, Kunova A, Spanik S, Gyarfas J, Sycova Z, Trupl J (1999) Hematogenous trichosporonosis in cancer patients: report of 12 cases including 5 during prophylaxis with itraconazol. Support Care Cancer 7(1):39–43
59. Walsh TJ, Melcher GP, Rinaldi MG, Lecciones J, McGough DA, Kelly P, Lee J, Callender D, Rubin M, Pizzo PA (1990) Trichosporon beigelii, an emerging pathogen resistant to amphotericin B. J Clin Microbiol 28(7):1616–1622

60. Mattiuzzi GN, Alvarado G, Giles FJ, Ostrosky-Zeichner L, Cortes J, O'Brien S, Verstovsek S, Faderl S, Zhou X, Raad II et al (2006) Open-label, randomized comparison of itraconazole versus caspofungin for prophylaxis in patients with hematologic malignancies. Antimicrob Agents Chemother 50(1):143–147
61. Girmenia C, Pagano L, Martino B, D'Antonio D, Fanci R, Specchia G, Melillo L, Buelli M, Pizzarelli G, Venditti M et al (2005) Invasive infections caused by Trichosporon species and Geotrichum capitatum in patients with hematological malignancies: a retrospective multicenter study from Italy and review of the literature. J Clin Microbiol 43(4):1818–1828
62. Anaissie E, Gokaslan A, Hachem R, Rubin R, Griffin G, Robinson R, Sobel J, Bodey G (1992) Azole therapy for trichosporonosis: clinical evaluation of eight patients, experimental therapy for murine infection, and review. Clin Infect Dis 15(5):781–787
63. Walsh TJ, Lee JW, Melcher GP, Navarro E, Bacher J, Callender D, Reed KD, Wu T, Lopez-Berestein G, Pizzo PA (1992) Experimental Trichosporon infection in persistently granulocytopenic rabbits: implications for pathogenesis, diagnosis, and treatment of an emerging opportunistic mycosis. J Infect Dis 166(1):121–133
64. Fournier S, Pavageau W, Feuillhade M, Deplus S, Zagdanski AM, Verola O, Dombret H, Molina JM (2002) Use of voriconazole to successfully treat disseminated Trichosporon asahii infection in a patient with acute myeloid leukaemia. Eur J Clin Microbiol Infect Dis 21(12):892–896
65. Paphitou NI, Ostrosky-Zeichner L, Paetznick VL, Rodriguez JR, Chen E, Rex JH (2002) In vitro antifungal susceptibilities of Trichosporon species. Antimicrob Agents Chemother 46(4):1144–1146
66. Serena C, Gilgado F, Marine M, Pastor FJ, Guarro J (2006) Efficacy of voriconazole in a guinea pig model of invasive trichosporonosis. Antimicrob Agents Chemother 50(6):2240–2243
67. Asada N, Uryu H, Koseki M, Takeuchi M, Komatsu M, Matsue K (2006) Successful treatment of breakthrough Trichosporon asahii fungemia with voriconazole in a patient with acute myeloid leukemia. Clin Infect Dis 43(4):e39–e41
68. Kauffman CA (2004) Zygomycosis: reemergence of an old pathogen. Clin Infect Dis 39(4):588–590
69. Kontoyiannis DP, Lionakis MS, Lewis RE, Chamilos G, Healy M, Perego C, Safdar A, Kantarjian H, Champlin R, Walsh TJ et al (2005) Zygomycosis in a tertiary-care cancer center in the era of Aspergillus-active antifungal therapy: a case-control observational study of 27 recent cases. J Infect Dis 191(8):1350–1360
70. Roden MM, Zaoutis TE, Buchanan WL, Knudsen TA, Sarkisova TA, Schaufele RL, Sein M, Sein T, Chiou CC, Chu JH et al (2005) Epidemiology and outcome of zygomycosis: a review of 929 reported cases. Clin Infect Dis 41(5):634–653
71. van Burik JA, Hare RS, Solomon HF, Corrado ML, Kontoyiannis DP (2006) Posaconazole is effective as salvage therapy in zygomycosis: a retrospective summary of 91 cases. Clin Infect Dis 42(7):e61–e65
72. Spellberg B, Fu Y, Edwards JE Jr, Ibrahim AS (2005) Combination therapy with amphotericin B lipid complex and caspofungin acetate of disseminated zygomycosis in diabetic ketoacidotic mice. Antimicrob Agents Chemother 49(2):830–832
73. Pagano L, Fianchi L, Caramatti C, D'Antonio D, Melillo L, Caira M, Masini L, Todeschini G, Girmenia C, Martino B et al (2004) Cryptococcosis in patients with hematologic malignancies. A report from GIMEMA-infection. Haematologica 89(7):852–856
74. Valero G, Graybill JR (1995) Successful treatment of cryptococcal meningitis with amphotericin B colloidal dispersion: report of four cases. Antimicrob Agents Chemother 39(11):2588–2590
75. Dromer F, Mathoulin-Pelissier S, Launay O, Lortholary O (2007) Determinants of disease presentation and outcome during cryptococcosis: the CryptoA/D study. PLoS Med 4(2):e21
76. Sepkowitz KA (2002) Opportunistic infections in patients with and patients without Acquired Immunodeficiency Syndrome. Clin Infect Dis 34(8):1098–1107

77. Roblot F, Le Moal G, Godet C, Hutin P, Texereau M, Boyer E, Prazuck T, Lacroix C, Souala MF, Raffi F et al (2003) Pneumocystis carinii pneumonia in patients with hematologic malignancies: a descriptive study. J Infect 47(1):19–27
78. Marty FM, Koo S, Bryar J, Baden LR (2007) (1→3)beta-D-glucan assay positivity in patients with Pneumocystis (carinii) jiroveci pneumonia. Ann Intern Med 147(1):70–72
79. Madhi SA, Albrich W (2007) WHO guidelines for treatment of severe pneumonia. Lancet 370(9585):386–387
80. Sepkowitz KA (1992) Pneumocystis carinii pneumonia among patients with neoplastic disease. Semin Respir Infect 7(2):114–121
81. Patel N, Koziel H (2004) Pneumocystis jiroveci pneumonia in adult patients with AIDS: treatment strategies and emerging challenges to antimicrobial therapy. Treat Respir Med 3(6):381–397
82. Israelski DM, Remington JS (1993) Toxoplasmosis in patients with cancer. Clin Infect Dis 17(Suppl 2):S423–S435
83. Chandrasekar PH, Momin F (1997) Disseminated toxoplasmosis in marrow recipients: a report of three cases and a review of the literature. Bone Marrow Transplant Team. Bone Marrow Transplant 19(7):685–689
84. Pagano L, Trape G, Putzulu R, Caramatti C, Picardi M, Nosari A, Cinieri S, Caira M, Del Favero A (2004) Toxoplasma gondii infection in patients with hematological malignancies. Ann Hematol 83(9):592–595
85. Mele A, Paterson PJ, Prentice HG, Leoni P, Kibbler CC (2002) Toxoplasmosis in bone marrow transplantation: a report of two cases and systematic review of the literature. Bone Marrow Transplant 29(8):691–698
86. Byrd JC, Peterson B, Piro L, Saven A, Vardiman JW, Larson RA, Schiffer C (2003) A phase II study of cladribine treatment for fludarabine refractory B cell chronic lymphocytic leukemia: results from CALGB Study 9211. Leukemia 17(2):323–327
87. Mechain B, Garin YJ, Robert-Gangneux F, Dupouy-Camet J, Derouin F (2000) Lack of utility of specific immunoglobulin G antibody avidity for serodiagnosis of reactivated toxoplasmosis in immunocompromised patients. Clin Diagn Lab Immunol 7(4):703–705
88. Derouin F, Devergie A, Auber P, Gluckman E, Beauvais B, Garin YJ, Lariviere M (1992) Toxoplasmosis in bone marrow-transplant recipients: report of seven cases and review. Clin Infect Dis 15(2):267–270
89. Lewthwaite P, Gill GV, Hart CA, Beeching NJ (2005) Gastrointestinal parasites in the immunocompromised. Curr Opin Infect Dis 18(5):427–435
90. Vijayan VK (2007) How to diagnose and manage common parasitic pneumonias. Curr Opin Pulm Med 13(3):218–224
91. Al-Hasan MN, McCormick M, Ribes JA (2007) Invasive enteric infections in hospitalized patients with underlying strongyloidiasis. Am J Clin Pathol 128(4):622–627
92. Keiser PB, Nutman TB (2004) Strongyloides stercoralis in the Immunocompromised Population. Clin Microbiol Rev 17(1):208–217
93. Wehner JH, Kirsch CM (1997) Pulmonary manifestations of strongyloidiasis. Semin Respir Infect 12(2):122–129

Hematological Malignancies

Chapter 5

Acute Myelogenous Leukemia and Febrile Neutropenia

Alexandra Herbers and Ben E. de Pauw

Abstract Aggressive chemotherapy has a deleterious effect on all components of the defense system of the human body. The resulting neutropenia as well as injury to the pulmonary and gastrointestinal mucosa allow pathogenic micro-organisms easy access to the body. The symptoms of an incipient infection are usually subtle and limited to unexplained fever due to the absence of granulocytes. This is the reason why prompt administration of antimicrobial agents while waiting for the results of the blood cultures, the so-called empirical approach, became an undisputed standard of care. Gram-negative pathogens remain the principal concern because their virulence accounts for serious morbidity and a high early mortality rate. Three basic intravenous antibiotic regimens have evolved: initial therapy with a single antipseudomonal β-lactam, the so-called monotherapy; a combination of two drugs: a β-lactam with an aminoglycoside, a second β-lactam or a quinolone; and, thirdly, a glycopeptide in addition to β-lactam monotherapy or combination. As there is no single consistently superior empirical regimen, one should consider the local antibiotic susceptibility of bacterial isolates in the selection of the initial antibiotic regimen. Not all febrile neutropenic patients carry the same risk as those with fever only generally respond rapidly, whereas those with a clinically or microbiologically documented infection show a much slower reaction and less favorable response rate.

Once an empirical antibiotic therapy has been started, the patient must be monitored continuously for nonresponse, emergence of secondary infections, adverse effects, and the development of drug-resistant organisms. The average duration of fever in serious infections in eventually successfully treated neutropenic patients is 4–5 days. Adaptations of an antibiotic regimen in a patient who is clearly not responding is relatively straightforward when a micro-organism has been isolated; the results of the cultures, supplemented by susceptibility testing, will assist in selecting the proper antibiotics. The management of febrile patients with pulmonary infiltrates is complex. Bronchoscopy and a high resolution computer-assisted tomographic scan represent the cornerstones of all diagnostic procedures, supplemented by serological tests for relevant viral pathogens and for aspergillosis. Fungi have been

From: *Managing Infections in Patients With Hematological Malignancies*: Contemporary Hematology, Edited by: M. Kleinberg, DOI 10.1007/978-1-59745-415-5_5,

found to be responsible for two thirds of all superinfections that may surface during broad-spectrum antibiotic treatment of neutropenic patients. Antibiotic treatment is usually continued for a minimum of 7 days or until culture results indicate that the causative organism has been eradicated and the patient is free of major signs and symptoms. If a persistently neutropenic patient has no complaints and displays no evidence of infection, early watchful cessation of antibiotic therapy or a change to the oral regimen should be considered.

Keywords Neutropenic fever • Empirical antibacterial therapy • Unexplained fever • Immunodeficiency • Invasive fungus

1. Introduction

Only 50 years ago, dealing with a patient with a disseminated malignant disease was relatively simple. There were no curative options and information on the inevitable dismal prognosis was not shared with the patient or his family. The mid sixties of the twentieth century witnessed the first successes of chemotherapeutic agents. This encouraged investigators to explore this route further, thereby escalating the dosage of the cytostatic drugs in the expectation of better results. It became rapidly clear that the destructive effects of cytotoxic compounds were not limited to malignant cells. Infection has emerged as a prominent complication of chemotherapy, which was particularly worrisome in the sixties, a decade without powerful broad-spectrum antimicrobial agents. Since a possible cure of the cancer was seen as the primary goal, complications of rigid cytotoxic regimens were taken for granted and when they occurred, treatment was more or less improvised. This situation remained unchanged until Bodey [1] pointed out that patients in remission of their underlying disease could die suddenly of an overwhelming infection during cytotoxic therapy-induced neutropenia. Neutropenia was and remains defined as an absolute neutrophil count of less than 0.5×10^9/l (500/mm^3) or a count less than 1.0×10^9/l (1,000/mm^3) expected to fall below 0.5×10^9/l (500/mm^3) [1]. He even showed a positive correlation between the severity and duration of neutropenia and the risk of acquiring a life-threatening bacterial infection. This risk appeared even more pronounced in individuals who were treated for an acute leukemia or lymphoma as these disorders interfered directly with vital components of the immune system. Next to gram-negative bacilli, *Staphylococcus aureus* earned a notably bad reputation [2]. A few years later, Schimpff and co-workers demonstrated convincingly that early administration of antimicrobial agents covering the above suspected pathogens while waiting for the results of the blood cultures saved lives. His so-called empirical approach became an undisputed standard of care [3]. However, better options to manage infections encouraged hematologists to intensify their antileukemic regimens further in an attempt to improve the remission rates in previously refractory cases. These intensifications, in turn, inspired more thorough clinical research into potentially more effective antimicrobial regimens, which was facilitated by the booming development of new antimicrobial agents such as broad-spectrum synthetic penicillins, third and fourth generation cephalosporins, fluoroquinolones, and carbepenems in conjunction with a keen eagerness of the respective pharmaceutical companies to put their compounds to test in large clinical trials that were usually conducted by cooperative trial groups [4, 5]. A cycle of several subsequent rounds of broader-spectrum antibiotics and further intensification of chemotherapeutic regimens has eventually lessened the mortal risk of neutropenia to only one of many problems in today's clinical practice.

Modern anti-leukemic therapy is inherently associated with ulceration of the pulmonary and gastrointestinal mucosa thereby allowing micro-organisms originating from the damaged mucosal tracts easy access to the body [6, 7]. These pathogens may be part of the original indigenous flora but are commonly acquired during hospitalization [8]. In the 1970s, it was considered logical to prevent invasion of the body by indigenous flora by prophylactic administration of anti-infective agents. Since such prophylactic agents were mainly targeted against the gram-negative enterobacteriaceae, a shift from gram-negative to gram-positive micro-organisms, including coagulase-negative staphylococci, viridans streptococci, and enterococci, as the primary cause of fever in neutropenic patients was seen [9–15]. In the meantime, therapeutic regimens in the treatment of hematological malignancies have become so complex that use of surgically implanted venous access devices became universal in spite of the risk of catheter-associated infections and thrombosis [16, 17]. An epidemiological survey among hospitalized patients treated for hematological malignancies between 1995 and 2001 in the United States showed that approximately 70% (64% in 1995 and 76% in 2001) of all microbiologically confirmed febrile episodes were due to gram-positive bacteria and 18% (22% in 1995 and 14% in 2001) due to gram-negative bacilli [18]. This change in pathogens was facilitated by increased use of central venous catheters and other medical devices.

Introduction of immunomodulatory monoclonal antibodies into the therapeutic arena has extended the treatment-related immunodeficiency to T-cell functions and innate immunity. This, in turn, has brought viral and fungal infections, including *Pneumocystis jeroveci*, into play, particularly when impaired cellular immunity coincided with prolonged, severe neutropenia [19, 20]. The modern chemotherapeutic regimens designed to treat acute lymphoblastic leukemia incorporate high doses of corticosteroids. As a result, patients treated with such regimens are at increased risk of infections typically related to an impaired cellular immunity. In addition, allogeneic bone marrow transplantations have become a fully accepted treatment modality for many hematological malignancies. Nowadays, infections still account for substantial morbidity and mortality among patients who undergo myeloablative therapy for a hematological malignancy. In spite of all changes in the spectrum of infectious agents, gram-negative pathogens remain the principal concern because their virulence accounts for serious morbidity and high early mortality rate [21, 22].

2. Management of New Fever and Infections

2.1. Principles

Administration of potentially curative chemotherapy is the starting point in treating acute leukemias. Giving cytotoxic drugs is relatively straightforward since internationally accepted antitumor protocols have defined the optimal dosages. Once the chemotherapy has been administered, the hematologist must wait patiently for the desired outcome a few weeks later. However, while the scientist in the hematologist has completed this first task, the general clinician in him or her has to step forward to monitor the patient, as the natural host defense system gradually disintegrates. Close surveillance of the patients with attention to the emergence of infectious complications is mandatory. Management of infections during this time of danger must be individualized because fixed protocols and algorithms are of limited usefulness given the complexity of infectious diseases management [23, 24]. It is here that the science and art of medicine meet; listening to the patient's complaints and meticulous physical examinations constitute the crucial factors for timely therapeutic interventions and eventual success. This applies to both patients who are treated with intensive chemotherapeutic regimens and to recipients of a stem cell transplant. During this period of neutropenia, appropriate coordination of information coming from different sources is important, since, next to the patient, family members, nurses, microbiologists, pulmonologists, radiologists, and pathologists can assist in the timely discovery of an emerging complication. Different cancer centers approach these tasks in different ways but it occurs to us that the hematologist who is responsible for treating the underlying hematological disease must also act as the captain of the ship. This coordinating role obliges him or her to have at least some basic knowledge of likely infection problems and, perhaps even more importantly, to have fine communication skills to keep all parties on board as well as incorrect on the same course. Since the symptoms of an incipient infection are usually rather subtle due to the absence of granulocytes, teamwork is crucial to ensure that antibiotics are administered at the first signs or symptoms of infection [25]. In most cases, fever defined as a single oral temperature of more than 38,3°C (101°F) or a temperature of more than 38,0°C (100,5°F) for more than 1 h, will serve as a trigger for action. At the onset of fever, attempts to identify the cause of fever deserve absolute priority (see Table 5-1), immediately followed by institution of appropriate broad-spectrum antibiotic therapy preferably within one hour of fever [22]. Fever in a neutropenic patient is a warning sign that should be taken very seriously because self-limiting infection is virtually

Table 5-1. Diagnostic procedures at the onset of fever.

- Short history of the patient with recent complaints
- Physical examination with special attention to:
  - o Vital signs
  - o Gastrointestinal tract: abdomen, perineum
  - o Respiratory tract: oropharyngeal area and lungs
  - o Skin, including bone marrow aspiration sites, vascular access sites, and tissue around the nails
- Cultures of blood (minimal 15 ml) and any clinical suspicious body site, including urine
- CT scanning of the chest
- Check medication list, results of surveillance cultures, compliance with prophylaxis, course of the leukocyte count
- Consider determination of CRP, galactomannan antigen, and viral serology

nonexistent in neutropenic patients irrespective of whether they have been treated for acute leukemia or lymphoma or received a stem cell transplantation. In anticipation of the results of the diagnostic evaluation, fever denotes infection until proven otherwise. Absence of phagocytic cells in combination with a damaged skin and mucosal surfaces allows micro-organisms residing at a superficial site of infection easy access to the bloodstream. Under these circumstances, a relatively small inoculum, that easily can escape detection when limited volumes of blood are sampled for culturing, can cause a serious septic syndrome [3]. Therefore, withholding antibiotics while waiting for a blood culture to become positive is a bad idea, even though fever can be of noninfectious origin [26]. A sudden onset of fever accompanied by chills, tachycardia with or without a drop in blood pressure, and tachypnea is associated with a higher rate of positive blood cultures. Shock at the onset of fever is an ominous clinical sign but neither clinical manifestations nor the pattern of fever during neutropenia can serve as an indicator of a particular causative agent, not even when the most notorious pathogens such as *Pseudomonas aeruginosa* or *Staphylococcus aureus* are involved [19, 27]. A substantial minority of patients with true infections will have an insidious onset of fever. Although more frequently related to noninfectious causes than acute fever, a slow rise of temperature does not exclude an infectious origin, although gram-negative rods, viridans streptococci, and *Staphylococcus aureus* are less prevalent amongst these patients. Acute fever following transfusion is often related to the presence of irregular blood group antigens or to cytotoxic antibodies acquired during previous transfusions or a pregnancy [28]. Of note, relative bradycardia in patients who did not receive antiarrhythmic medication suggests either a viral or noninfectious origin of the fever. A possible relation between fever and frequently used drugs such as allopurinol, antibiotics, bleomycin, and cytarabine or with the underlying disease process itself should always be kept in mind [29, 30]. A dysfunctional immune system is presumed to be responsible for the high rate of drug allergy in patients with active acute leukemia; the allergy may abate when complete remission is achieved [29]. This phenomenon is well known in patients with infectious mononucleosis or acquired immunodeficiency syndrome.

Until recently, coagulase-negative staphylococcal bacteremia was thought to be entirely related to the use of central venous catheters but recent work points at mucosal sites as important portals of entry [31–33]. The clinical spectrum of catheter-related infections ranges from asymptomatic bacteremia as a manifestation of intraluminal colonization or a process confined to the site of insertion to marked inflammation of the tunnel tract and septicemia with metastatic emboli in the skin and other organs. Suspicion of a tunnel or exit line infection should arise when the catheter tract becomes painful, red, or swollen or when signs of inflammation are visible at the exit site. Malfunction of the catheter, illustrated by problems drawing blood through the line, is a common first warning of a possible lumen infection [16, 17].

2.2. Selection of Antimicrobial Agents for the Empiric Phase

2.2.1. Basic Regimens

In the selection of the initial antibiotic regimen, one should consider the type, frequency of occurrence, and antibiotic susceptibility of bacterial isolates recovered from other patients at the same hospital. In addition, the use of certain antibiotics may be limited by special circumstances, such as drug allergy, liver function disturbances, or renal insufficiency. Despite numerous clinical studies, since the 1970s, no single empirical antibiotic regimen has been shown to be superior for initial treatment of patients who become febrile during a neutropenic episode after therapy with chemotherapy drugs for hematological malignancies (see Table 5-2) [4, 9, 34–44]. However, there is world-wide consensus that any initial antibiotic regimen should include drugs with reliable activity against *Escherichia coli*, *Pseudomonas aeruginosa*, *Klebsiella* species, other enterobacteriaceae, and *Staphylococcus aureus* [22]. Three basic intravenous antibiotic regimens have evolved: initial therapy with a single β-lactam, the so-called monotherapy; a combination of two drugs, a β-lactam with an aminoglycoside, a second β-lactam or a quinolone but without a glycopeptide; and, thirdly, a glycopeptide in addition to β-lactam monotherapy or combination. Numerous extensive studies have shown that traditional combinations, consisting of an antipseudomonal β-lactam and an aminoglycoside, are not more effective than monotherapy in the empiric treatment of uncomplicated episodes of fever in neutropenic patients. A third or fourth generation cephalosporin, a carbapenem, as well as piperacillin–tazobactam, have been found to be effective single agents in the majority of cases [43, 45]. It appears appropriate to reserve two-drug regimens for complicated cases or if antimicrobial resistance is a potential problem. The major disadvantages of an aminoglycoside are nephrotoxicity and ototoxicity, and the necessity to monitor serum levels [46–48]. Combination of drugs such as amphotericin B, cyclosporine, and cisplatinum with an aminoglycoside is best avoided because of their additive renal toxicity, whereas high sodium content may limit the simultaneous use of two β-lactam antibiotics in elderly patients. An extensive study by European Organization for Research and Treatment of Cancer – National Cancer Institute of Canada [11] showed unambiguously that vancomycin can be withheld and not administered empirically for persistent fever despite appropriate initial monotherapy or combination antibiotic treatment until the results of the cultures indicate the need for vancomycin. Vancomycin must be included in an initial empiric regimen for patients known to be colonized with penicillin- and cephalosporin-resistant pneumococci, viridans streptococci, or methicillin-resistant *Staphylococcus aureus* or in situations where β-lactam resistance is likely such as a catheter-associated cellulitis where coagulase-negative staphylococci predominate .

The choice to implement a particular antibiotic regimen is, at least partly, based on the results of clinical trials as reported in the literature. Yet, the results of such trials should be interpreted with great caution. Definitions for response as well as inclusion and exclusion criteria for clinical study protocols are usually very rigid and quite different from common clinical practice [23, 24].

2.2.2. Specifically Tailored Regimens

Conduct of clinical trials in febrile neutropenic patients was a booming business in the mid-seventies and eighties when many new broad-spectrum antibiotics became available. The data derived from these trials expanded our knowledge of the possible infectious complications tremendously. For instance, analyses of these studies revealed that only half of the patients who develop fever during neutropenia will have a clinically or microbiologically

Table 5-2. Efficacy of antibacterial regimens in the treatment of neutropenic patients with fever.

Study	No of evaluable episodes (patients)	Treatment	Favorable responses/documented infections	Favorable responses/ bacteremia
Wade et al. [33]	121 (92)	Piperacillin + Amikacin	22/38 (58%)	5/15 (33%)
		Ticarcillin + Amikacin	19/34 (56%)	6/11 (55%)
Duprez and Michaux [34]	(118)	Piperacillin + Amikacin	26/34 (76%)	9/14 (64%)
		Cefotaxime + Amikacin	27/37 (78%)	15/20 (75%)
Winston et al. [35]	297 (244)	Piperacillin + Amikacin	38/53 (72%)	16/25 (64%)
		Carbenicillin + Amikacin	48/66 (73%)	20/36 (56%)
Winston et al. [36]	272 (219)	Piperacillin + Moxalactam	45/61 (74%)	17/23 (74%)
		Moxalactam + Amikacin	41/50 (82%)	13/18 (72%)
EORTC [9]	(872)	Azlocillin + Amikacin full course	75/138 (54%)	12/47 (26%)
		Ceftazidime + Amikacin short.	69/118 (58%)	12/35 (34%)
		Ceftazidime + Amikacin full course	95/145 (66%)	19/41(46%)
Winston et al. [37]	(187)	Piperacillin + Cefoperozone	39/50 (78%)	22/29 (76%)
		Piperacillin + Moxalactam	31/38 (82%)	16/22 (73%)
Sage et al. [38]	174 (225)	Piperacillin + Netilmicin	12/15 (80%)	1/2 (50%)
		Ticarcillin + Netilmicin	11/14 (79%)	1/2 (50%)
		Mezlocillin +Netilmicin	11/18 (61%)	1/5 (20%)
		Cefoperozone + Netilmicin	4/10 (40%)	0/2 (0%)
Feliu et al. [39]	170 (118)	Piperacillin + Amikacin	24/44 (55%)	9/21 (43%)
		Ceftazidime +Amikacin	30/51 (59%)	14/23 (61%)
De Pauw et al. [4]	784 (696)	Ceftazidime	127/367 (35%)	33/118 (28%)
		Piperacillin + Tobramycin	117/335 (33%)	25/132 (19%)
Cometta et al. [13]	706 (475)	Piperacillin–tazobactam + Amikacin	210/342 (61%)	40/50 (50%)
		Ceftazidim + Amikacin	196/364 (54%)	35/101 (35%)
De Pauw et al. [40]	304 (225)	Meropenem	54/110 (44%)	37/79 (47%)
		Ceftazidime	35/105 (41%)	24/79 (30%)
Cometta et al. [14]	483 (475)	Meropenem	270/483 (56%)	47/113 (42%)
		Ceftazidime + Amikacin	245/475 (52%)	34/114 (30%)
Feld et al. [41]	409 (471)	Meropenem	33/77 (54%)	14/31 (45%)
		Ceftazidime	33/82 (44%)	22/43 (51%)
Del Favero et al. [42]	(733)	Piperacillin–tazobactam	67/186 (36%)	42/140 (30%)
		Piperacillin tazobactam + Amikacin	60/176 (34%)	44/137 (32%)
Bow et al. [43]	(528)	Piperacillin–tazobactam	71/265 (27%)	11/81 (14%)
		Cefepime	54/263 (21%)	7/86 (8%)

documented infection, the majority being pulmonary infiltrates and bacteremias (see Table 5-3) [49, 50]. Furthermore, it was obvious that neutropenic patients without a documented infection generally defervesced within a few days, whereas those with a clinically or microbiologically documented infection showed a much slower and less frequent fever defervescence rate [19, 27, 51]. This very consistent observation suggests that it might be prudent to select different antibiotic regimens for patients with different symptoms. Although there is no statistically valid evidence to support a more individually tailored approach, it appears reasonable to assume that patients might benefit from timely administration of the antibiotics with the highest intrinsic potency against a given micro-organism. A known or suspected focus of infection, if present at the time of initial fever, could help in the selection of additional case-specific anti-infective agents because the location of an infection is, at least to a certain extent, predictive of specific infective pathogens (see Table 5-4)[52]. Likewise, results of surveillance cultures and knowledge of

Table 5-3. Classification of febrile neutropenic episodes.

FUO-fever of unknown origin	**New fever, not accompanied by clinical or microbiological evidence of infection**
Clinically documented infection	Fever accompanied by a clinical infection, but pathogens cannot be identified, e.g., cellulitis, pneumonia
Microbiologically documented infection	Fever accompanied by a localized infection and microbiologically plausible evidence, or fever without a localized infection, but infectious agents can be demonstrated in a (blood) culture

Table 5-4. Sites of infection and prevalent causative micro-organisms.

Site	**Prevalent pathogens**	**Preferred antimicrobial agents**
Upper respiratory tract	Streptococci	Amoxicillin, clindamycin
Lower respiratory tract	Gram-negative bacilli	Combination therapy <<?>>
	Streptococci	Amoxicillin, clindamycin, macrolides
	Moulds	Consider antifungal agents in an early phase
	Diffuse infiltrates	Antiviral agents
	Cytomegalovirus	Trimethoprim–sulfamethoxazole
	Pneumocystis jeroveci	
Skin and soft tissue	Staphylococci	Glycopeptides
	Streptococci, anaerobes	Amoxicillin, clindamycin, macrolides, glycopeptides
Abdominal	Anaerobes	Metronidazole, glycopeptides
Perianal abscess	Gram-negative bacilli	Combination therapy <<?>>

the common complications associated with particular antileukemic regimens may offer valuable input to individualizing appropriate initial treatment of a neutropenic patient with fever.

2.2.2.1. Gastrointestinal Tract

A damaged integument probably plays a major etiologic role in virtually all infections that occur following aggressive cytoreductive therapy for a hematological malignancy but its involvement is most obvious in infections of the skin and gastrointestinal tract. The use of high-dose cytarabine in conjunction with the occurrence of diarrhea were found to be independent risk factors for streptococcal infections among 513 patients evaluated during first episodes of neutropenic fever [53]. It has been recognized that bacteremias due to oral *Streptococcus mitis* and *Streptococcus oralis* may result in serious complications such as sepsis or adult respiratory distress syndrome, which carry high mortality [54–56]. Similarly, bacteremias due to *Staphylococcus aureus, Pseudomonas aeruginosa,* and *Clostridium* species as well as candidemias are more frequently encountered in patients with acute leukemia who suffer from neutropenic enterocolitis or typhlitis, the most serious disturbance of the delicate balance between mucosal damage and microbial flora in the setting of prolonged exposure to antibiotics after intermediate or high-dose cytarabine chemotherapy. The signs and symptoms of chemotherapy-induced enterocolitis or typhlitis vary considerably from patient to patient and include nausea, vomiting, abdominal cramps, and severe abdominal pain with virtually no formed bowel movements but accompanied by profuse, watery diarrhea. Many patients are in such pain that they only gain relief from narcotic analgesics which, in turn, induce constipation by reduction of bowel movements. This may create a very alarming situation as the clinical picture in severe cases resembles that of gut perforation, acute pancreatitis, or even toxic megacolon. Because there is a high mortality rate for surgical interventions in neutropenic and thrombocytopenic patients with acute leukemia, it is essential for physicians to be aware of the existence of neutropenic enterocolitis/typhlitis with the accompanying symptoms. Ultrasonography or CT, showing pathological thickening of the bowel walls, may be useful to establish the diagnosis of typhlitis. Patients treated for acute myeloid leukemia with a bowel wall thickness of more than 10 mm had a significantly higher mortality rate than did those with a bowel thickness of less than 10 mm [57]. Disproportional bacterial overgrowth in the gastrointestinal tracts of neutropenic patients with damaged mucosa can serve as a source of bacteremia for the endogenous gastrointestinal flora as well as for otherwise exclusively enteric pathogens such as *Clostridium septicum* [58, 59] and *Bacteroides fragilis*. In contrast, *Salmonella* species are rarely found in the stool or blood of granulocytopenic patients; these organisms are obviously not major players in this field. This is also true for pathogens like *Campylobacter* and *Shigella* species. Therefore, an adequate antibiotic regimen for patients with abdominal symptoms should cover gram-negative rods but due consideration should be given to the use of compounds with activity against anaerobes. Next to glycopeptides and carbapenems, metronidazole is an attractive adjunct to a standard monotherapy/combination regimen under these circumstances. Pseudomembranous colitis caused by *Clostridium difficile* [60–64] constitutes a related but distinct entity that can be severe and even fatal. The stool should be tested immediately for *Clostridium difficile* toxin if the diagnosis is suspected. Enteric *Clostridia* infections necessitate oral antibiotic therapy with either vancomycin or metronidazole. Relapses are frequent and may follow cancer chemotherapy or courses with antibiotics such as clindamycin. Relapse is harder to document because toxin may persist in the stool of successfully treated patients.

Diagnostic problems account for underestimating enteric viruses as causative agents in gastrointestinal infections. Although a compromised cell-mediated immunity is known to predispose for parasitic and protozoan infections, their incidence is surprisingly low in patients who are treated for a hematological malignancy [65, 66].

2.2.2.2. Skin

Folliculitis and cellulitis are the most common manifestations of infectious processes in the skin. Sometimes it is difficult to differentiate infectious lesions from drug-induced toxic skin eruptions. Infection-associated erythema and swelling are usually mild but, if left untreated, infiltration and abscess formation will involve extensive areas of the skin with necrosis and gangrene. Since the lesions associated with the various organisms are rather alike, a simple needle aspiration or biopsy should be performed to establish an accurate diagnosis as early as possible in the course of the disease. Causative micro-organisms include streptococci, staphylococci, and, less commonly, gram-negative bacilli and fungi [67–70]. Localized infections of the skin, particularly in the face, are usually caused by gram-positive bacteria that arise more frequently in carriers of organisms like *Staphylococcus aureus*. None of the standard empiric regimens is the optimal choice for treating skin infections caused by the prevalent but usually indolent non*S. aureus* gram-positive cocci that are often methicillin-resistant, but the morbidity from these infections should not be underestimated either. *Pseudomonas aeruginosa* acquired in a hot Jacuzzi may cause a folliculitis that occasionally progresses to a destructive ecthyma gangrenosum [71]. This characteristic entity should be distinguished from similar lesions caused by other rare pathogens, such as actinomyces, *Stenotrophomonas maltophilia* [68] and fungi [69, 70] as well as from pyoderma gangrenosum, a noninfectious cutaneous process in patients with a myeloid malignancy [72, 73]. Sweet's syndrome, a dense, tender infiltration by neutrophils of the dermis on the head, neck, and upper extremities is associated with a leukocytosis [74]. Varicella zoster is the leading dermatologic complication in patients with impaired cell-mediated immunity [75–77]. If skin or mucous membrane lesions due to herpes simplex or varicella-zoster viruses are present, even if they are not the cause of fever, treatment with valacyclovir or another suitable antiviral is indicated with the intention to speed healing of lesions that could become potential portals of entry for bacteria and fungi.

The results of several prospective studies do not indicate a general need for a glycopeptide as part of the front-line therapeutic regimen unless one has a particular reason to suspect the presence of methicillin-resistant *Staphylococcus aureus* or penicillin-resistant *viridans* Streptococci on the basis of local patterns of resistance or surveillance cultures. Nevertheless, most physicians intuitively prefer an up-front glycopeptide-containing regimen to cover catheter-related infections as these are frequently due to coagulase-negative staphylococci, although early glycopeptide treatment does not contribute to improved survival from these usually indolent infections. Hence, when coagulase-negative staphylococci are involved, a few days of watchful waiting for a possible clinical response and the results of the cultures will have no detrimental impact.

Most catheter-associated infections will respond to antibiotic therapy without the removal of the catheter. Rotation of antibiotics through each lumen of multilumen catheters to avoid microbial sequestration in one of the lines and the use of antibiotic-containing heparin lock solutions to supplement systemic therapy have been proposed by some investigators but such practices remain controversial. Pulling the catheter is most likely to be required for the cure if a concurrent venous thrombosis is found, the tunnel tract appears involved, or if the infection, regardless of the etiology, is recurrent, or if after several days of therapy an eventual response to antibiotics appears doubtful [78].

2.2.2.3. Upper Respiratory Tract

Gingivostomatitis and periodontal lesions occur frequently in patients with acute leukemia [79]. Oral mucositis is characterized by pain, edema, erythema, superficial lesions, pseudomembranous formation in conjunction with excessive mucous production, reduced saliva secretion, and bleeding. A wide array of pathogens can be found and include *Herpes simplex*, gram-negative bacilli, streptococci, anaerobes, and *Candida* species [80]. With the introduction of aggressive chemotherapeutic regimens, hitherto unusual pathogens such as *Stomatococcus* and *Aerococcus* are increasingly seen in patients with mucositis. Mixed and polymicrobial infections are more or less standard [80, 81]. Given the range of prevalent pathogens, there is little need to deviate from one of the standard regimens, although, on theoretical grounds one might prefer to select a carbapenem, fourth generation cephalosporin, or extended-spectrum penicillin given their superior intrinsic activity against viridans streptococci and pneumococci. The course of *Herpes simplex* stomatitis is usually prolonged in patients treated for leukemia or lymphoma, and relapses are common [82]. *Herpes simplex* lesions are most commonly white painful plaques with or without serpiginous borders on the gums, tongue, buccal mucosa, or oropharynx and may be difficult to discriminate from oropharyngeal candidiasis and, indeed, co-infections do occur. Swallowing can be so painful that saliva is expectorated and intake of food and fluids drastically reduced. It is not uncommon for oropharyngeal *Herpes simplex* and *Candida* infections to extend to the esophagus. Although neither herpes nor candidiasis belong to the category of diseases that requires an empiric approach, it is generally accepted that early treatment with valacyclovir and fluconazole, respectively, is important to prevent extension into the esophagus and further dissemination, particularly among bone marrow transplant recipients. When the paranasal sinuses are involved in the infectious process, moulds have to be considered as possible causes. Direct inspection of the nasal turbinates and a computer-assisted tomographic scan of the sinuses can be helpful to establish or reject the diagnosis.

2.2.2.4. Lower Respiratory Tract

Management of pulmonary infiltrates that are responsible for 70% of all fatal infections in febrile neutropenic patients is complex [83–85]. The importance of classic clinical complaints of cough, pain, and dyspnea should not be neglected but bronchoscopy and radiological examination of the chest by a computer-assisted tomographic scan represent the cornerstones of all diagnostic procedures. Typically, chest radiographs performed early in the evolution of infection in patients with profound granulocytopenia fail to show infiltrates. It may take more than 3 days for the infection to generate enough necrosis with hemorrhage and edema to produce a visible infiltrate. The critical decision faced by the clinician at the bedside of patients with pulmonary infiltrates is whether to undertake invasive procedures such as bronchoscopy with or without bronchoalveolar lavage, transbronchial biopsy, transthoracic aspiration, thoracoscopy-guided biopsy, or open lung biopsy. The exact role of these diagnostic procedures in the optimal management of patients is still controversial because the yield depends on the collaboration and skills of various specialists. Moreover, concurrent thrombocytopenia precludes simple invasive diagnostic procedures such as transbronchial biopsies in many patients.

The radiologic pattern of a possible infiltrate is often suggestive of its cause. A diffuse opacity, usually of both lungs, is seldom of bacterial or fungal origin. Although viruses and *Pneumocystis jeroveci* typically cause diffuse, bilateral pulmonary infiltrations, it should be kept in mind that a similar picture of pneumonitis can be seen secondary to radiation, fluid overload, cytotoxic drugs such as methotrexate, cytarabine and bleomycin, and in pulmonary hemorrhage. *Pneumocystis jeroveci* pneumonia is manifested in patients with deficient cellular immunity as fever, progressive hypoxemia with dry cough, and dyspnea, typically beginning after discontinuation of corticosteroid therapy given for other reasons [85]. High-dose trimethoprim–sulfamethoxazole with adjuvant corticosteroids for hypoxemic patients ($PO_2 < 70$ mmHg) has become the preferred therapy for these infections [86]. Alternatives include intravenous pentamidine, oral dapsone in combination with trimethoprim, or oral atovaquone suspension alone.

Antiviral drugs are indicated only if there is clinical or laboratory evidence of viral disease. With the exception of a cytomegalovirus-related pneumonitis in allogeneic bone marrow transplant recipients with graft-versus-host disease, there appears to be no need for empiric coverage of respiratory viruses, such as respiratory syncytial virus, influenza [87, 88], and adenoviruses. Ganciclovir, valganciclovir, and foscarnet have established activity in the treatment of cytomegalovirus infection and their timely use might be lifesaving. *Mycoplasma pneumoniae* with or without cold agglutinins is remarkably infrequent in patients treated for leukemia. In more acutely ill patients, the possibility of acute lung injury following transfusion of a cellular blood product or respiratory distress syndrome related to streptococcal sepsis should be considered.

Patients with an infection by *Streptococcus mitis,* which has been linked with severe mucositis and high-dose cytarabine are at particular risk [53, 54]. The incidence of acute respiratory distress syndrome in such cases is more than 20% and mortality is substantial. The pathophysiology of adult respiratory distress syndrome following streptococcal bacteremia in a neutropenic patient is poorly understood. Probably several factors are involved, such as deleterious effects of sepsis superimposed on preexisting tissue damage. Even patients who had received appropriate antimicrobials at the onset of fever were reported to experience shock and death [54–56]. Therefore, in addition to antibiotics, corticosteroids should be considered in the management of patients affected by ARDS and streptococcal bacteremia.

Bacterial infections of the lung, accompanied by bacteremia in about 50% of cases, usually create infiltrates on a computer-assisted tomographic scan that are confined to one or more lobes. Pneumonias caused by *Pseudomonas aeruginosa* and *Staphylococcus aureus* do have a bad reputation but enterobacteriaceae [89, 90], *Haemophilus influenzae* and *Streptococcus* species are hardly less dangerous. Given the uniformly poor outcomes of pulmonary infections in clinical trials, the empiric use of a combination of antibiotics is recommended with the addition of vancomycin in centers that face resistance of *S. pneumoniae* to penicillin and macrolides. Outbreaks of *Legionella pneumophila,* an infection characterized by patchy interstitial or nodular pulmonary infiltrates and sometimes accompanied by headache or gastrointestinal symptoms, have been observed among compromised patients in units with contaminated water systems [91]. Therefore, if a case of legionellosis is encountered, other patients with similar symptoms on the same ward should be treated with a macrolide or a fluoroquinolone from the start of antimicrobial therapy.

A nodular pattern of pulmonary infiltrates should lead the physician to consider the possibility of atypical pneumonia or, more commonly, a pulmonary fungal infection. In the latter case, diagnostic procedures rather than immediate institution of antifungal drugs should be given priority. Especially in patients with concomitant impairment of the cell-mediated immunity, pulmonary aspergillosis has to be distinguished from tuberculosis. Infections with *Mycobacterium tuberculosis* in patients with impaired cell-mediated immunity are manifested as either localized pulmonary disease or devastating miliary tuberculosis. Nontuberculous mycobacteria are still rather rare in patients with acute leukemia, but the introduction of purine analogues such as cladribine and fludarabine, which cause severe and prolonged depression of cellular immunity, may change this picture in the near future [92].

2.2.2.5. Other Foci of Infection

Urinary tract infections are astonishingly uncommon in patients who are treated for leukemia or lymphoma and, since gram-negative bacteria are the predominant urinary tract pathogens, the choice for a single broad-spectrum β-lactam is fully justified.

Malignant otitis externa is a very serious infectious complication that can emerge after administration of aggressive chemotherapy for a hematological malignancy. At the outset, the patient will complain of a painful, discharging ear, and physical examination will reveal a reddened edematous ear canal. Local maceration and humid conditions favor the growth of *Pseudomonas aeruginosa* which, indeed, can be isolated frequently from swabs taken from superficial lesions of the external canal. Untreated, the infection will penetrate into underlying soft tissues, threatening the retromandibular and parotid area. Likewise, spread to the middle ear, the mastoid air cells, and adjacent temporal bone is possible. Once osteomyelitis becomes established, extension to the base of the skull with invasion of the cranial nerves and local thrombosis poses a direct danger to the patient's life. A computer-assisted tomographic scan may be helpful to identify tissue damage in the early phase. Prolonged antibiotic therapy with ceftazidime, ciprofloxacin, or other antipseudomonal antibiotics in combination with surgical debridement constitutes the treatment of choice [93]. Occasionally, a similar clinical picture can be the result of an infection by *Staphylococcus aureus* or *Aspergillus fumigatus*. In such cases, surgery should be combined with an antistaphylococcal penicillin or vancomycin, or with voriconazole, respectively.

An insidious onset of fever accompanied by headache and confusion might be indicative of meningitis when causation by leukemia or lymphoma has been excluded by cytologic examination of the cerebrospinal fluid. In cases of infection, the cerebrospinal fluid is usually clear with moderate protein elevation. The prevalent pathogens are *Listeria monocytogenes, Cryptococcus neoformans,* and *Toxoplasma gondii* [65]. Recovery of one of *Listeria monocytogenes* [94] and *Cryptococcus neoformans* from blood cultures should, provided that no intracranial hypertension is detected, always prompt a lumbar puncture even in the absence of neurological symptoms. Considering their low incidence and the relatively reliable diagnostic possibilities, there is no need to cover for these infections with a specific empiric regimen.

2.2.3. Management on an Out-Patient Basis

Outpatient management of infections in patients with hematological malignancies is discussed in more depth in Chap. 6. When potent oral broad-spectrum antibiotics became available in the late eighties, many clinicians felt tempted to use these drugs in the treatment of febrile neutropenic patients. Several groups around the world assessed the options and limitations of this seemingly revolutionary approach [95–97] systematically. These analyses showed that it is possible to define risk factors that can be used to classify patients into low or high-risk categories. In fact, these studies offered nothing more than identification of objective parameters that corroborate the gut's feeling of the experienced clinician. Since the time of Bodey [1], it was already obvious that patients with absolute neutrophil count between 0,1 and 0.5×10^9/l (100–500/ml) carry a minor risk compared to those with a granulocyte count of less than 0.1×10^9/l (100/ml). But now other risk factors have been identified. Patients with concurrent mucosal damage or impaired cellular immunity, as well as those with clinically documented infections or unstable vital signs, are at high risk and deserve increased vigilance. Patients with these additional risks cannot be considered candidates for antibiotic treatment on an out-patient basis. The vast majority of patients with acute leukemia are considered high-risk patients and should continue to receive intravenous broad-spectrum antibiotics in the hospital or similar setting. The remaining low-risk patients, namely those with unexplained fever who are clinically stable, may be safely treated with oral antibiotics provided that they have been seen at a qualified medical center promptly after the onset of fever [95, 96]. The possible use of antibiotic prophylaxis does not pre-empt the need for a thorough check-up but limits the choice of drugs that can be used for treatment. Patients with increasing granulocyte counts are considered to be better candidates for outpatient therapy than are patients without an indication of bone marrow recovery. Among the oral regimens that have been evaluated are ofloxacin, ciprofloxacin, and ciprofloxacin plus amoxicillin–clavulanate. It is crucial to make sure that the patient is informed about the risk of unremitting fever during a neutropenic episode and that he or she fully understands the importance of seeking immediate medical advice in case any unexpected incident occurs. Vigilant observation at home by a relative or professional health care worker and prompt access to appropriate medical care must be available 24 h per day, 7 days a week [98–101]. As an alternative to initial outpatient therapy, early discharge with continued outpatient therapy for selected patients may be considered after a brief admission during which intravenous therapy is initiated, fulminant infection is excluded, and appropriate culture specimens are taken [102, 103].

Two studies have demonstrated that children who lack signs of sepsis and severe mucositis, who are afebrile for >48 h, who have neutrophil counts of >100 cells/mm^3 (>0.5 × 10^9/l), and who are at low risk for complications may have their intravenous antibiotic treatment safely stopped to be substituted by oral cefixime [104, 105].

3. Management of Fever After the Empiric Episode

3.1. Principles

After starting empiric antibacterial treatment, fevers will persist or return in about one third of patients. The average duration of fever in serious infections, in eventually successfully treated neutropenic patients is 4–5 days (Table 5-2, Fig. 5-1) [4, 9, 13, 14, 34–44]. Although fever can be inconvenient for the patient, it is important to realize that it is part of the body's defense system [106]. Indeed, some retrospective studies have suggested that fever is associated with improved survival and shortened disease. Uncontrolled studies have reported an association of increased mortality with the absence of fever in polymicrobial or gram-negative sepsis and in elderly patients with community acquired pneumonia [107, 108]. So, when the body temperature remains above normal during 3 or 4 days on apparently effective broad-spectrum antibiotics, this should not be considered a complete waste of time, particularly not if the time is used for an appropriate diagnostic work-up. It should be kept in mind that empiric administration of antibiotics is only meant as an immediate cover for rapidly fatal bacteria such as gram-negative rods and *Staphylococcus aureus*, thereby, so to say, buying time for consideration of the next therapeutic interventions and for waiting for the results of the diagnostic procedures. When the results of the cultures become available and the infection has had time to blossom clinically, there is a more solid basis for decisions on necessary adjustments of an antibiotic regimen.

Unfortunately, all large, randomized clinical trials on empiric antibiotic therapy in the febrile neutropenic patients during the past 30 years have been pharmaceutical company-driven for purposes of attaining governmental agency approval [23, 24]. As a consequence, the design of these studies focused primarily on the efficacy of a particular drug in comparison with another drug

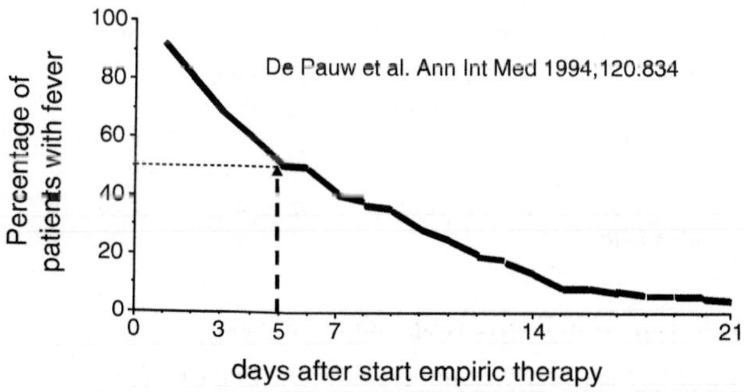

Fig. 5-1. Typical course of fever after institution of empiric antimicrobial therapy in neutropenic patients.

or combination of drugs. According to the protocols for these trials, only patients who survived the febrile episode without a change in the allocated regimen could be labeled as successes, whereas any change in therapy, independent of the trigger, was denoted a failure, even if the patient survived unscathed and the infection was eradicated. Therefore, modification of the test regimens was discouraged, which constitutes a rather artificial situation, as clinicians are inclined to adjust an antibiotic regimen for no other reason than a subjective feeling of unease with the original choice of antibiotics. Changes often reflect impatience, nervousness, and lack of confidence on the part of the clinician concerned over the still febrile neutropenic patient rather than any deficiency in the original antibiotic regimen used. When restrictions surrounding a clinical trial do not apply, juggling antibiotics against an undulating line on a temperature chart is a well-known frequent occurrence on a ward full of patients suffering with hematological malignancies. Indeed, in daily practice, many modifications are not based on objective criteria and are made outside office hours, i.e., by less experienced physicians on call [103, 109]. However, it is generally recognized that exposure to many different antibiotics as a result of haphazard changes of regimens enhances the risk of drug-related adverse events and seldom improves the outcome of the patient under treatment. Moreover, such a policy of endless therapeutic trials of antibiotic changes might wrongly decrease the perceived need for further diagnostic procedures in poorly responding patients. Since there is evidence from clinical trials on what to do after the empiric phase, some experts have been promoting the so-called algorithms of planned progressive antibiotic therapy to treat neutropenic patients with fever. A planned progressive strategy involves adjustment of therapy every 2–3 days, until the patient becomes febrile or until all the potential causes of infection are covered by the best available microbial agents, irrespective of the development of additional symptoms. It is clear that algorithms featuring planned progressive therapy are destined to lead to overtreatment with unnecessary expenses and drug exposures [108]. It appears more intellectually attractive not to rely on fixed algorithms but to weigh several different, patient-specific parameters, including fever and clinical response, as a guide for modification of an empiric regimen. It goes without saying that spending time at the bedside is crucial for those who feel attracted to the role of attending physician because careful observation often provides early clinical clues for a rational adaptation of the original empirical antibiotic regimen. The need for individualization is not only dictated by variations in the signs and symptoms of the patient that accompany persisting fever but also by differences in skills and expertise amongst attending specialists in various centers. For example, centers with excellent and interested departments of medical microbiology and pathology will rely more heavily on their findings than do centers with poorly functioning departments, whereas units with an active radiology service may benefit from the locally available know-how in this particular field.

3.2. Modifications in Poorly Responding Patients

3.2.1. Case-by-Case Modification of an Initial Empiric Regimen

Once an empiric antibiotic therapy has been started, the patient must be monitored continuously for nonresponse, emergence of secondary infections, adverse effects, and the development of drug-resistant organisms. This implies that the start of antibacterial agents cannot be seen as an impetus to stop diagnostic procedures. Daily blood cultures are certainly justified as long as patients remain febrile and when a new temperature peak occurs because breakthrough bacteremia or fungemia may develop. Close monitoring of sites that are prone to infection should start before the onset of fever and has to be continued after empirical antibacterial therapy has commenced. Subtle changes must bring diagnostic tools into play to confirm or exclude the presence of an infectious focus. Regular CT-scans of the chest, preferably in combination with serological monitoring for *Aspergillosis* antigen, have an established value in patients who are at increased risk of fungal infections [92].

As a rule, approximately 65% of patients without a focus of infection, which includes 30% overall with positive blood cultures, will show some clinical improvement after 3 days of broad-spectrum empiric coverage in spite of persisting fever. In most cases, defervescence will follow rapidly. Elements that should be incorporated in clinical decision making include the course of fever and clinical condition with special attention to the vital signs, evolving symptoms of infection in relation to the granulocyte count, C-reactive protein levels, antigen monitoring, and risk for relapses of latent viral infections determined by pretreatment antiviral titers. The results of all cultures taken at the onset of fever have to be assessed and it is recommended to analyze surveillance cultures, if any, to identify possibly colonizing resistant organisms. Without clinical deterioration or proof of an infection caused by a micro-organism resistant to the initial antibiotic regimen, persisting fever after 72–96 h of empiric therapy in and of itself is an unsatisfactory basis for changing the original empirical antibacterial regimen. It is better to alter the regimen only when there are objective reasons to do so: deterioration of vital signs, isolation of a resistant pathogen without clinical improvement, persistence of a pathogen, antibiotic-related adverse events, occurrence of a new focus of infection or progression of an existing focus in the absence of granulocyte recovery, unexplained fever persisting for more than 5 days, new fever, a new pathogen or recognition of a local outbreak with a resistant organism (Tables 5-5 and 5-6). In most patients, antimicrobial therapy can be adjusted objectively on the basis of clinical or microbiologic findings but such an individually tailored approach requires careful daily assessment of all possible parameters collaborating with consulting specialists, including microbiologists, pulmonologists, and radiologists. In contrast to the moment of the onset of fever, there is ample time for deliberation and contemplation in a situation where the patient's fever persists for 3 or more days while on antibiotics because the origin of fever is obviously not a rapidly fatal micro-organism that needs immediate treatment. Fever that persists for more than 3 days suggests that the patient has a nonbacterial infection, a resistant bacterial infection, a second infection, or a drug fever [22, 110].

Despite extensive cultures, only around 30% of all febrile patients will be shown to have microbiologically defined infections. In 30% of patients, organ involvement is already apparent with the initial fever and an additional 10% will show clinically defined infection within the next 72 h (see Fig. 5-2). Others have neither a focus of infection, nor a positive culture and are defined as unexplained fevers. Using clinical well-being as a leading parameter, there are

Table 5-5. Reasons to modify an empirical antibiotic regimen.

- Deteriorations of vital signs
- Development of a new clinical focus
- Progression of an existing focus
- Persistence of a presumed causative pathogen
- Isolation of an in vitro resistant organism in the absence of clinical improvement
- Occurrence of a new fever
- Isolation of a new pathogen
- Adverse event attributable to one of the current antibiotics
- Known local outbreak with an unusual micro-organism such as Legionella

Table 5-6. Possible causes for the lack of response to antibiotics.

- A bacterial infection resistant to the antibiotics
- Cell wall-deficient bacteremia
- Infections at a avascular site (e.g., abscesses or catheters)
- Inadequate serum and tissue levels of the antibiotics
- Slow response to the drugs in use
- The emergence of a second infection
- A nonbacterial infection
  - o Fungal
  - o Viral
  - o Posttransplant lymphoproliferative disease (in allogeneic stem cell transplant recipients)
  - o Parasitic
- Pyrogenic substances
  - o Cytokines
  - o (Auto)immune reactions
  - o Blood product antigens
  - o Toxins
  - o Drugs (antibiotics)
  - o Tissue (tumor) products

roughly three possible situations after 3 days of treatment: the patient's condition is (a) improving (approximately 55% of cases); (b) stable (approximately 35%); or (c) deteriorating (10%; see Fig. 5-3 and Table 5-7). Patients belonging to each of these three categories may have either a microbiologically documented infection, a clinically documented infection, or an explained fever. All these factors that are partly subjective and partly objective can be exploited to steer the modification of an empiric regimen when there is a perceived need to do so. Ultimately, only 15–20% of patients with a persisting unexplained fever should require a continued empirical rather than a clinical or microbiologically directed approach after 72 h of broad-spectrum antibacterial therapy.

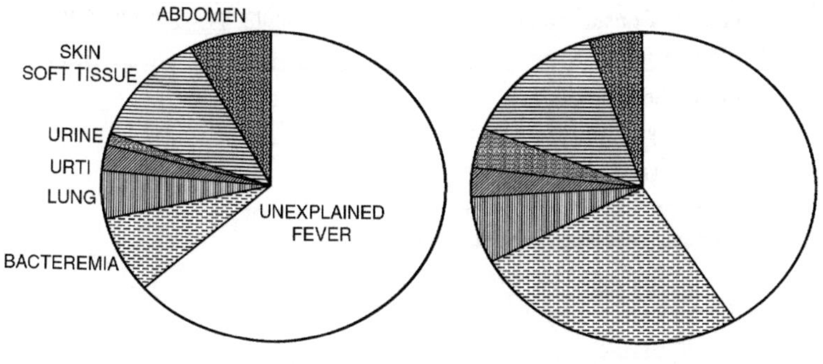

Fig. 5-2. Identified causes of infection at the onset of fever and at the end of the empiric episode.

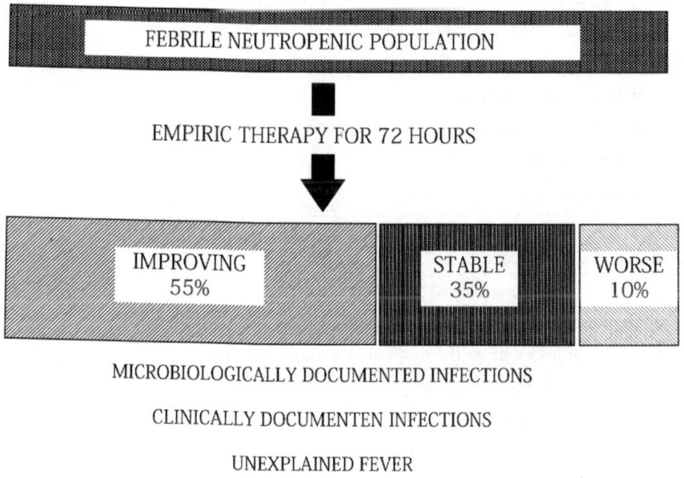

Fig. 5-3. Evolution of clinical condition during the first 72 h of empiric antimicrobial therapy.

Whichever modification is planned, it cannot be overemphasized that maintenance of appropriate antigram-negative cover is mandatory as long as a patient is febrile and neutropenic.

3.2.1.1. Microbiologically Documented Infections

When the patient is improving or stable, there appears to be no imminent need to adjust an antibiotic regimen. Depending on the micro-organism isolated, a change to an oral regimen could be considered with caution. When a gram-negative isolate is identified, broad-spectrum antibiotic coverage should be maintained in full dose. Whereas the clinical relevance of a blood culture

Table 5-7. Considerations for modification of antibiotic regimens in febrile neutropenic patients.

Improving clinical condition
- Microbiologically documented infection
  - o Maintain gram-negative coverage
  - o Consider adjustment on the basis of susceptibility pattern
  - o Consider switching to an oral regimen
- Clinically documented infection
  - o Continue existing regimen
- Unexplained fever
  - o Maintain gram-negative coverage
  - o Consider switching to an oral regimen

Stable clinical condition
- Microbiologically documented infection
  - o Maintain gram-negative coverage
  - o Consider adjustment on the basis of susceptibility pattern
  - o Consider switch to an oral regimen
- Clinically documented infection
  - o Continue existing regimen
  - o Consider change on the basis of organ- or syndrome-specific pathogens
- Unexplained fever
  - o Maintain gram-negative coverage
  - o Consider further diagnostic procedures

Deteriorating clinical condition
- Microbiologically documented infection
  - o Maintain gram-negative coverage at maximally tolerated doses
  - o Consider adjustment on the basis of susceptibility patterns
- Clinically documented infection
  - o Maintain gram-negative coverage at maximally tolerated doses
  - o Broaden coverage of organ- or syndrome-specific pathogens
- Unexplained fever
  - o Cover relevant potential gaps in the spectrum of the existing regimen
  - o Consider further diagnostic procedures
  - o Consider institution of intravenous antifungals

positive for gram-negative bacilli is never a matter of controversy, the implication of recovery of particular gram-positive cocci is less clear. Single blood cultures positive for *S. aureus*, *S. pneumoniae*, or *Enterococcus faecalis* in neutropenic patients should be regarded as significant and indicative of the need for further treatment. Viridans group streptococci, with an average mortality of 15–20%, are perhaps the most feared among the bacteremias today [54–56]. Although viridans streptococci are common blood contaminants in the general population, positive blood cultures in patients with oral mucositis should not be disregarded, certainly not when *S. mitis* or related streptococci are isolated [53, 54]. Isolation of rare micro-organisms should prompt evaluation of the appropriateness of the starting antibiotic regimen, especially when the patient is not responding optimally. On the other hand, isolation of in vitro resistant organisms such as coagulase-negative staphylococci and, more rarely, *Stenotrophomonas maltophilia,* from the blood of a clinically, evidently improving patient, pose an interesting challenge. Many would be inclined to modify the initial regimen but in many cases other bacteria that were not recovered on the culture plate may have been the culprits in the current fever. A blood culture that yields *Candida* species or another fungus should be taken very seriously and dictates immediate institution of antifungal therapy [111–113]. The availability of the candins has extended the therapeutic options [114–116].

Adaptations of an antibiotic regimen in a patient who is clearly not responding is relatively straightforward when a micro-organism has been isolated; the results of the cultures, supplemented by susceptibility testing, will assist in selecting the proper antibiotics.

3.2.1.2. Clinically Documented Infections

All clinical trials so far have demonstrated consistently that patients diagnosed with a clinically documented infection respond much slower and remain febrile for a longer time than those without a focus of infection [19, 27, 51]. Moreover, due to problematic penetration into avascular sites, infections associated with abscesses or prosthetic devices usually respond poorly to antimicrobial therapy. Attending physicians should, therefore, be more hesitant to change antibiotics in patients who are not deteriorating. On the other hand, there are indications that early addition of specific agents might be useful for more rapid control of clinically documented infections. For instance, considering the probable involvement of anaerobes, switching to a carbapenem, if not given initially, or addition of metronidazole to a standard anti-gram-negative regimen, appears a logical choice when fever is accompanied by abdominal symptoms. In cases with a clinically documented site who do not improve or stabilize, coverage of micro-organisms known to prevail at the involved site of infection (see Table 5-4) appears appropriate. Clinically documented infections that emerge later during the course of febrile neutropenia carry a dismal prognosis and are presumed to be related to the occurrence of resistant micro-organisms, including invasive fungi, in combination with persisting immunodeficiency often as a result of a refractory underlying disease.

3.2.1.3. Persistent Unexplained Fever or Fever of Unknown Origin

If the patient with an unexplained fever clinically improves or remains stable after 72 h of empirical treatment and re-evaluation by physical examination and diagnostic tests yields no new information, and no isolate was found, the initial antibiotic regimen can be continued or can be switched to an oral compound. The latter option is more reasonable clinically if neutropenia is expected to resolve within the ensuing days. If vancomycin is a component of the initial antimicrobial regimen, withdrawal of the drug should be considered if the results of the cultures do not support its use.

Deteriorating cases without any microbiological or clinical sign of infection pose a dilemma. Unexplained fever accompanied by deterioration can imply that the patient has a nonbacterial infection or a noninfectious cause of fever, but foremost, a resistant bacterial infection or the emergence of a second infection should be taken into account [19, 110]. An initial response rate of about 35% may be expected in patients with shock, compared with 70% in patients without shock, which suggests the possible presence of an undetected toxin-producing pathogen in the former. Addition to the original empirical antibacterial regimen is mandatory in critically ill patients, independent of the level of fever. Escalation might include filling theoretical gaps in antibiotic spectrum and enhanced monitoring for any changes in the patient's condition. Under these circumstances, the selection of agents should be guided by knowledge of locally prevalent virulent pathogens and actual susceptibility patterns, which implies the necessity of close cooperation with the local microbiology laboratory. Addition of vancomycin appears reasonable in view of the fact that the spectrum of antibacterial drugs in traditional empiric regimens usually does not cover coagulase-negative staphylococci, methicillin-resistant *Staphylococcus aureus*, enterococci, and some strains of penicillin-resistant *S. pneumoniae* and viridans streptococci. On the other hand, liberal use of vancomycin has confronted the medical community with vancomycin-resistant enterococci and staphylococci, which has led to increasing use of new agents like quinupristin-dalfopristin and linezolid in the treatment of febrile neutropenic patients. When the starting regimen consists of a single, broad-spectrum β-lactam, addition of an aminoglycoside is an attractive option to provide a better coverage when infections by resistant gram-negative rods are suspected. However, it has to be emphasized that development of resistance during therapy is extremely rare and that aggressive gram-negative organisms typically cause the infection to deteriorate rapidly to a stage beyond cure within a few days after first fever in most cases. Hence, if the local resistance pattern or a particular concern in an individual patient prompts the use an aminoglycoside for resistant gram-negative bacteria, then aminoglycosides should be prescribed from the start in optimal doses with monitoring of the peak and trough serum levels. Clinical deterioration in a persistently neutropenic patient with unexplained fever is an important but rather rare event in daily practice and applies to only a quarter of the overall 10% of cases that deteriorate while on broad-spectrum antibacterial treatment. Moreover, it is noteworthy that the success rate of empiric modifications is less than 20%, whereas more than 50% of cases will respond to specifically customized modifications [41].

3.3. Specific Considerations

3.3.1. Invasive Fungal Disease

Invasive fungal infections are encountered in up to 40% of autopsies in patients with hematological malignancies. Fungi have been found to be responsible for two thirds of all superinfections, which surface during broad-spectrum antibiotic treatment of neutropenic patients. More than 20 years ago, when diagnostic capabilities were virtually nonexistent and the choice of effective antifungal agents limited, two prospective, randomized trials laid the scientific foundation for the addition of systemically active antifungals even though neither study was adequately powered to reach a statistically valid conclusion [111, 112]. This strategy appeared to reduce the incidence of invasive fungal infections in patients without any further sign of a clinically documented infection. Solid statistical evidence to support the validity of this empiric approach was never obtained subsequently in further placebo-controlled trials because empirical antifungal treatment had become widely accepted as the standard of care. This so-called empiric antifungal therapy has remained popular as it seemed to make life easy for clinicians. The lack of reliable diagnostic tools combined with very poor outcomes of invasive fungal infections that were not timely treated contributed greatly to this popularity [117–119]. However, in most cases in 2007, antifungals prescribed empirically for fever alone are unnecessary because invasive fungal infection is present in a minority of cases. A better understanding of the pathophysiology of invasive fungal disease in combination with use of better diagnostics allows for a more individualized approach [117, 120]. An optimal diagnostic work-up in conjunction with careful clinical observation will likely render routine empiric antifungal therapy superfluous in most cases because appropriate application of presently available diagnostic tools enables timely pre-emptive institution of appropriate antifungal therapy by experienced clinicians [121–123]. The most common initial presentation of invasive aspergillosis is unremitting fever despite broad-spectrum antibacterial treatment, accompanied eventually in most patients by pulmonary infiltrates or sinusitis. Clinicians should suspect the diagnosis in a patient with pleuritic pain, hemoptysis, or a localized pleural rub. The halo sign (a dense central nodule with surrounding less dense infiltrate) on a computer-assisted tomographic scan of the chest, though not pathognomonic, is highly suggestive of an early phase of pulmonary aspergillosis or other mould pneumonia in immunosuppressed patients [124–126]. Even when gram-negative pathogens, including *Pseudomonas aeruginosa* and *Enterobacter cloacae*, are isolated from the sputum or blood of such patients, aspergillosis should be the leading consideration when nodular chest CT findings are present. If no infiltrate is found in a high-risk patient with persisting fever, the investigation should be repeated within a few days, preferably supported by bronchoalveolar lavage if indicated and additional assays such as screening for the presence of galactomannan in the blood [121]. Even in patients with aspergillosis who are responding adequately to antifungals, the computer-assisted tomographic chest scan will usually show some enhancement of the lesion when the neutrophils return with eventual development of cavitation within the infiltrate, the so-called air-crescent sign [124–126]. This finding is suggestive of aspergillosis, although mucormycosis and other moulds may cause an identical picture. Whether the increased incidence of non *Aspergillus* mould is due to more extensive use of the new azoles like voriconazole or to the use of more intensive immunosuppressive treatment schemes remains to be seen [127, 128]. Isolation of an *Aspergillus* species from sputum or bronchoalveolar lavage specimens connotes either invasive infection or bronchial colonization, the latter conferring high risk for invasive aspergillosis. When voriconazole or posaconazole have been used as prophylaxis, it is sensible to select an antifungal compound with a different mode of action when therapy becomes mandatory [129, 130]. Surgery is indicated for patients in whom lesions near the pulmonary hilus pose a direct threat of invasion of a major vessel with the risk of fatal hemorrhage or for debridement of dead tissue after a period of antifungal therapy [126]. Low risk patients who test negative for *Aspergillus* in all diagnostic procedures do not need to be started on intravenous antifungals. Treatment should be stopped for those patients started on antifungals pending diagnostic test results. A more conservative wait-and-see approach can be implemented successfully once clinicians learn to accept that negative diagnostic results constitute sufficient evidence that there is no fungal infection in many persistently febrile neutropenic patients [121, 123].

Fluconazole given as prophylaxis has virtually eliminated infections with *Candida albicans*. However, *Candida* species or other fungi are still occasionally identified as causes of disseminated infections in humans, albeit with a shift from *Candida albicans* to nonalbicans species [131, 132]. A candidemic patient typically presents with an irregular fever sometimes accompanied by polymyalgia and polyathralgia. In about 10% of cases, characteristic pinkish-purple, nontender subcutaneous nodules may arise anywhere on the body. Biopsy specimens should be cultured and histologically screened at multiple levels in an attempt to establish a final diagnosis. *Candida* ophthalmitis is seldom seen in leukemic patients since the distinctive retinal exudates are the result of an inflammatory response that involves granulocytes. Upon the return of the neutrophils or tapering of corticosteroids, complaints of abdominal discomfort and elevation of alkaline phosphatase levels with or without hepatosplenomegaly may emerge. At this stage, an abdominal ultrasound or computer-assisted tomographic scan will display rather distinctive multiple abscesses in the liver and/or spleen, known as "bull's-eyes" [133, 134]. Mortality from an invasive yeast infection may be as high as 40%, particularly when the start of antifungal therapy has been delayed. Trichosporonosis and fusariosis can produce a clinical syndrome identical to candidemia [135–137].

3.3.2. Biological Response Modifiers

Up to now, empirical antimicrobial therapy has been the backbone of improving survival of febrile neutropenia in leukemic patients. Hematopoietic growth factors have been studied as adjunctive therapy for febrile neutropenic patients in several randomized, controlled trials. G-CSF (filgrastim) and granulocyte-macrophage colony-stimulating factor (sargramostim) when used as part of the treatment of febrile neutropenic patients were shown to consistently shorten the duration of neutropenia defined as a neutrophil count below $0.5 \times 10^9/l$ (500/ml). However, the duration of absolute neutropenia, i.e., count of less than $0.1 \times 10^9/l$ (100/ml), was not influenced, which might help to explain why neither a decrease in infection-related mortality rates nor a significant effect on morbidity, including duration of fever and use of anti-infectives, were observed [138, 139]. Therefore, the use of growth factors should be restricted to complicated cases for which there appears to be no rational alternative therapeutic option [140–142]. This concept also applies to the use of granulocyte transfusions. Transfusion of high numbers of granulocytes harvested after administration of G-CSF, with or without dexamethasone, to a donor is done by some clinicians without there being any unequivocal evidence of its efficacy. Patients with prolonged profound neutropenia and an uncontrolled clinically documented infection, such as severe cellulitis or sinusitis, appear to be the primary candidates for treatment with granulocyte transfusions, whereas administration of a colony-stimulating factor (G-CSF) should be preferred when a return of the neutrophils is imminent. Significant toxicities in granulocyte-transfusion recipients include transmission of cytomegalovirus, alloimmunization associated with fever, graft-versus-host reactions if granulocytes are not irradiated, progressive platelet refractoriness, and, possibly, respiratory insufficiency associated with concomitant administration of amphotericin B. New approaches with agents designed to protect the mucosa, like recombinant human interleukin 11 and keratinocyte growth factor palifermin, show promising results in terms of reducing severity of mucositis and occurrence of fever and bacteremia in neutropenic patients [143–145].

4. Cessation of Antimicrobial Therapy

4.1. Antibacterial Therapy

It is widely believed that antibiotic treatment should be continued for a minimum of 7 days or until culture results indicate that the causative organism has been eradicated, infection at all sites has resolved, and the patient is free of major signs and symptoms. Ideally, the neutrophil count should be >500 mm^3 (0.5×10^9/l) before treatment is stopped [146]. When no infection has been identified after 3 days of treatment and the patient has become afebrile for 48 h in association with a neutrophil count that has exceeded 500 cells/mm^3 (0.5×10^9/l), antibiotic therapy may be stopped. In addition, if a persistently neutropenic patient has no complaints and displays no clinical, radiological, or laboratory evidence of infection, cessation of antibiotic therapy or a change to oral antimicrobials should be considered after 4 days without symptoms. If antibiotics are discontinued while the patient is still neutropenic, the patients must be monitored closely and intravenous antibiotics restarted immediately with recurrence of fever or any other evidence of bacterial infection, since the initial infection may have only been suppressed, not eradicated. One should consider continuous administration of antibiotics throughout the neutropenic period in patients who have profound neutropenia, mucous membrane lesions of the gastrointestinal tract, or any other identified risk factor. Some experts suggest, in patients in whom hematological recovery cannot be anticipated, a change from the therapeutic regimen to a prophylactic scheme after 2 weeks of therapy with intravenous antimicrobials. When the suspicion of a noninfectious cause of the fever is high, interruption of antibiotic therapy after ~4 days seems warranted in clinically well patients without any evidence of infection apart from persisting fever. Under these conditions, meticulous monitoring has to be maintained to guarantee the patients timely protection against subsequent infections that are likely to occur.

4.2. Antifungal Therapy

The decision to start antifungals may appear complex but is not as difficult as the decision to discontinue. If a systemic fungal infection has been identified, the course of antifungal therapy will be determined by the causative agent and the extent of the disease. In patients with pulmonary infiltrates or other suspicious lesions, it is essential to see a clinical and, preferably, a radiological response before one ponders cessation of antifungal therapy. However, if no fungal infection is found, it is not clear how long antifungal drugs should be administered [147]. For clinically well patients with prolonged neutropenia, it is suggested that antifungal agents can be stopped after 2 weeks of treatment, provided that no conspicuous lesions can be found by clinical evaluation or by computer-assisted tomographic scanning of the chest and the abdominal organs. In the patient who appears ill or is at high risk, continuation of antifungal therapy throughout the neutropenic episode is recommended. Conversely, when neutropenic fever subsides, the patient is clinically well and computer-assisted tomographic scan of the abdomen and chest reveals no suspicious lesions; antifungals may be discontinued, particularly when the criterion for commencing antifungal therapy had been simply fever unresponsive to antibiotics. This approach also applies when the presumptive diagnosis becomes questionable during the course of granulocytopenia. When a patient diagnosed with and treated for a proven or probable invasive fungal disease requires further chemotherapy or bone marrow transplantation, protection against the offending pathogen has to be provided, even if the patient responded completely to initial antifungal therapy. The risk of relapse of invasive fungal disease is so high that secondary prophylaxis is warranted, requiring that a full dose of the most effective antifungal is administered [148, 149]. After introduction of routine CT scanning it became apparent that solitary lesions caused by invasive fungal disease are rare and this observation reduced the enthusiasm for surgical interventions. However, if the number of lesions is limited or a difficult-to-treat pathogen, such as a zygomycosis, has been found, surgical excision has to be considered, especially when the lesions are located close to a large vessel [150].

5. Concluding Remarks

Modern chemotherapy offers hope of a cure to many cancer patients, but it confronts the medical community with new challenges continuously. Infection remains an inevitable side-effect of the myeloablative therapy for acute leukemia and is the principal cause of morbidity and mortality amongst these patients. Optimal care can be delivered only by those who pay scrupulous attention to the patient's clinical condition and are aware of the evolving therapeutic and diagnostic modalities. It cannot be denied that time remains an important factor in the management of infectious complications but we must try to distinguish more accurately between patients truly in need of immediate therapy and those who are not. Fixed treatment algorithms are only acceptable if they allow individual interpretation and reasonable deviations. Maintaining guidelines that dictate second line treatment of a population in which more than half of the patients do not have true infection is not justifiable in view of potential adverse events and the economical burden. The demand for an alternative strategy, built on clinical skills, modern and more accurate laboratory tests and imaging techniques, has become apparent and a broad application of this principle may change the approach to antimicrobial treatment in neutropenic patients completely. Overuse of antimicrobial agents, both antibacterial and antifungal, has become all too common in the belief that broader coverage will benefit the patient. Unfortunately, prescription of antimicrobials according to a preset scheme may give a false sense of security with reduced or delayed diligence in pursuing a diagnosis. Diagnostic considerations should prevail whenever patients do not respond satisfactorily to an antibacterial regimen. In addition, neutropenia can no longer be seen as the major compass to steer antimicrobial therapy in a febrile patient because neutropenia is not the one and only factor predisposing for infection. A damaged integument and impairment of T cell-mediated immunity have altered the incidences of causative micro-organisms. This change not only has consequences for the selection of antimicrobial agents but may also foster development of totally different future treatment modalities such as biological response modifiers that might reduce the need for antimicrobial agents. Undoubtedly, unwarranted widespread use of antibiotics has contributed to the development of resistance amongst micro-organisms. Resistance of previously susceptible pathogens to drugs like penicillins, cephalosporins, glycopeptides, fluoroquinolones, and azoles has become all too familiar of extended spectrum macrolides, carbapenems, and other agents . The primary purpose of prophylactic or empiric use of antimicrobial agents is not to make the physician's life easier but rather to help patients most at risk survive a difficult and dangerous episode.

References

1. Bodey GP, Buckley M, Sathe YS, Freireich EJ (1966) Quantitative relationships between circulating leukocytes and infection in patients with acute leukemia. Ann Intern Med 64(2):328–340
2. Hersh EM, Bodey GP, Nies BA, Freireich EJ (1965) Causes of death in acute leukemia. A ten-year study of 414 patients from 1954-1963. JAMA 193:105–109
3. Schimpff SC, Young VM, Greene WH, Vermeulen GD, Moody MR, Wiernik PH (1972) Origin of infection in acute nonlymphocytic leukemia: significance of hospital acquisition of potential pathogens. Ann Intern Med 77(5):707–714
4. De Pauw BE, Deresinski SC, Feld R, Lane-Allman EF, Donnelly JP (1994) Ceftazidime compared with piperacillin and tobramycin for the empiric treatment of fever in neutropenic patients with cancer. A multicenter randomized trial. The Intercontinental Antimicrobial Study Group. Ann Intern Med 120(10): 834–844
5. Viscoli C, EORTC International Antimicrobial Therapy Group (2002) Management of infections in cancer patients. Studies of the EORTC International Antimicrobial Therapy Group (IATCG). Eur J Cancer 38(Suppl 4):S82–S87
6. Sonis ST, Oster G, Fuchs H et al (2001) Oral mucositis and the clinical and economic outcomes of hematopoietic stem-cell transplantation. J Clin Oncol 19(8):2201–2205
7. Blijlevens NMA (2005) Implications of treatment-induced mucosal barrier injury. Curr Opin Oncol 17(6):605–610
8. Fainstein V, Rodriguez V, Turck M, Hermann G, Rosenbaum B, Bodey GP (1981) Patterns of oropharyngeal and fecal flora in patients with acute leukemia. J Infect Dis 144(1):10–18
9. The EORTC International Antimicrobial Therapy Cooperative Group (1987) Ceftazidime combined with a short or long course of amikacin for empiric therapy of Gram-negative bacteremia in cancer patients with granulocytopenia. N Engl J Med 317(27):1692–1698
10. Klastersky J, Zinner SH, Calandra T et al (1988) Empiric antimicrobial therapy for febrile granulocytopenic cancer patients: lessons from four EORTC trials. Eur J Cancer Clin Oncol 24(Suppl 1):S35–S45
11. (1991) The EORTC International Antimicrobial Therapy Cooperative Group and National Cancer Institute of Canada. Vancomycin added to empirical combination antibiotic therapy for fever in granulocytopenic cancer patients. J Infect Dis 163(5): 951-958
12. (1993) The International Antimicrobial Therapy Cooperative Group of the European Organisation for Research and Treatment of Cancer. Efficacy and toxicity of single daily doses of amikacin and ceftriaxone versus multiple daily doses of amikacin and ceftazidime for infection in patients with cancer and neutropenia. Ann Intern Med 119:584–593

13. Cometta A, Zinner S, De Bock R et al (1995) Piperacillin-tazobactam plus amikacin versus ceftazidime plus amikacin as empiric therapy for fever in granulocytopenic patients with cancer. Antimicrob Agents Chemother 39(2):445–452
14. Cometta A, Calandra T, Gaya H et al (1996) Monotherapy with meropenem versus combination therapy with ceftazidime plus amikacin as empiric therapy for fever in granulocytopenic patients with cancer. Antimicrob Agents Chemother 40(5):1108–1115
15. Marchetti O, Calandra T (2002) Infections in neutropenic cancer patients. Lancet 359(9308):723–725
16. Press OW, Ramsey PG, Larson EB, Fefer A, Hickman RO (1984) Hickman catheter infections in patients with malignancies. Medicine (Baltimore) 63:189–200
17. Raad II, Bodey GP (1992) Infectious complications of indwelling vascular catheters. Clin Infect Dis 15:197–210
18. Wisplinghoff H, Seifert H, Wenzel RP, Edmond MB (2003) Current trends in the epidemiology of nosocomial bloodstream infections in patients with hematological malignancies and solid neoplasms in hospitals in the United States. Clin Infect Dis 36:1103–1110
19. Nucci M, Spector N, Bueno AP et al (1997) Risk factors and attributable mortality associated with superinfection in neutropenic patients with cancer. Clin Infect Dis 25:572–579
20. Gerson SL, Talbot GH, Hurwitz S, Strom BL, Lusk EJ, Cassileth PA (1984) Prolonged granulocytopenia: the major risk factor for invasive pulmonary aspergillosis in patients with acute leukemia. Ann Intern Med 100:345–351
21. Chang HY, Rodrigues V, Narboni G et al (1976) Causes of death in adults with acute leukemia. Medicine 55:259–268
22. Hughes WT, Armstrong DA, Bodey GP et al (2002) Guidelines for the use of antimicrobial agents in neutropenic patients with cancer. Clin Infect Dis 34:730–751
23. Donelly JP (1991) For debate: assessment and reporting of clinical trials of empirical therapy in neutropenic patients. J Antimicrob Chemother 27:377–378
24. Feld R (1998) Criteria for response in patients in clinical trials of empiric antibiotic regimens for febrile neutropenia. Is there agreement? Support Care Cancer 6:444–448
25. Sickles EA, Greene WH, Wiernik PH (1975) Clinical presentation of infection in granulocytopenic patients. Arch Intern Med 135:715–719
26. Slavin MA, Grigg AP, Schwartzer AP et al (2007) A randomized comparison of empiric or pre-emptive antibiotic therapy after hematopoietic stem cell transplantation. Bone Marrow Transplant 40:157–163
27. Elting LS, Rubenstein EB, Rolston KVI, Bodey GP (1997) Outcomes of bacteremia in patients with cancer and neutropenia: observations from two decades of epidemiological and clinical trials. Clin Infect Dis 25:247–259
28. Anderson KC, Lew MA, Gorgone BC, Martel J, Leamy CB, Sullivan B (1986) Transfusion-related sepsis after prolonged platelet storage. Am J Med 81:405–411
29. Verhagen C, Stalpers LJA, De Pauw BE, Haanen C (1987) Drug induced skin reactions in patients with acute non-lymphocytic leukaemia. Eur J Haematol 38:225–230
30. Klastersky J (1994) Non-infectious causes of fever in cancer patients. In: Glauser MP, Calandra T (eds) Baillière's clinical infectious diseases. Baillière Tindall, London, pp 439–53
31. Wade JC, Schimpff SC, Newman KA, Wiernik PH (1982) Staphylococcus epidermidis: an increasing cause of infection in patients with granulocytopenia. Ann Intern Med 97:503–508
32. Lina B, Forey F, Troncy J, Greenland T, Fleurette J, Etienne J (1994) Oral source of staphylococcus epidermidis septicaemia in a neutropenic patient. Eur J Clin Microbiol Infect Dis 13(9):773–775
33. Costa SF, Barone AA, Miceli MH et al (2006) Colonization and molecular epidemiology of coagulase-negative Staphylococcal bacteremia in cancer patients: a pilot study. Am J Infect Control 34:36–40

34. Wade JC, Schimpff SC, Newman KA, Fortner CL, Standiford HC, Wiernik PH (1981) Piperacillin or ticarcillin plus amikacin: a double-blind prospective comparison of empiric antibiotic therapy for febrile granulocytopenic cancer patients. Am J Med 71:983–990
35. Duprez P, Michaux JL (1981) Piperacillin or cefotaxime plus amikacin: result of empirical antibiotic therapy for febrile episodes in granulocytopenic patients. Proceedings of the 12th International Congress of chemotherapy. Florence, Italy; July 19–24
36. Winston DJ, Ho WG, Young LS et al (1982) Piperacillin plus amikacin therapy v carbenicillin plus amikacin therapy in febrile granulocytopenic patients. Arch Intern Med 142:1663–1667
37. Winston DJ, Barnes RC, Ho WG, Young LS, Champlin RE, Gale RP (1984) Moxalactam plus piperacillin versus moxalactam plus amikacin in febrile granulocytopenic patients. Am J Med 77:442–450
38. Winston DJ, Ho WG, Bruckner D, Gale RP, Champlin RE (1988) Controlled trials of double beta-lactam therapy with cefoperazone plus piperacillin in febrile granulocytopenic patients. Am J Med 85(1a):21–30
39. Sage R, Han I, Prentice HG et al (1988) A randomized trial of empirical antibiotic therapy with one of four beta-lactam antibiotics in combination with netilmicin in febrile neutropenic patients. J Antimicrob Chemother 22:237–247
40. Feliu J, Artal A, Gonzlaez Baron M et al (1992) Comparison of two antibiotic regimens (piperacillin plus amikacin versus ceftazidime plus amikacin) as empiric therapy for febrile neutropenic patients with cancer. Antimicrob Agents Chemother 36:2816–2820
41. De Pauw BE, Boogaerts MA, Demuynck H et al (1995) Equivalent efficacies of meropenem and ceftazidime as empirical monotherapy of febrile neutropenic patients. J Antimicrob Chemother 36:185–200
42. Feld R, de Pauw BE, Berman S, Keating A, Ho W (2000) Meropenem versus ceftazidime in the treatment of cancer patients with febrile neutropenia: a randomized, double-blind trial. J Clin Oncol 18:3690–3698
43. Del Favero A, Menichetti F, Martino P et al (2001) A multicenter, double-blind, placebo-controlled trial comparing piperacillin-tazobactam with and without amikacin as empiric therapy for febrile neutropenia. Clin Infect Dis 33:1295–1301
44. Bow EJ, Rotstein C, Noskin GA et al (2006) Randomized, open-label, multicenter comparative study of the efficacy and safety of piperacillin-tazobactam and cefepime for the empirical treatment of febrile neutropenic episodes in patients with hematologic malignancies. Clin Infect Dis 43:447–459
45. Paul M, Soares-Weiser L, Leibovici L (2003) β lactam monotherapy versus β lactam-aminoglycoside combination therapy for fever with neutropenia: systematic review and meta-analysis. BMJ 326(7399):1111
46. Galloe AM, Graudal N, Christensen HR et al (1995) Aminoglycosides: single or multiple daily dosing? A meta-analysis in efficacy and safety. Eur J Clin Pharmacol 48:39–43
47. Munckhof WJ, Grayson ML, Turnodge JD (1996) A meta-analysis of studies on the safety and efficacy of aminoglycosides given either once daily or as divided doses. J Antimicrob Chemother 37:645–663
48. Ali MZ, Goetz MB (1997) A meta-analysis of the relative efficacy and toxicity of single daily dosing versus multiple daily dosing of aminoglycosides. Clin Infect Dis 24:796–809
49. Donnelly JP, Novakova IRO, Raemakers JMM, De Pauw BE (1993) Empiric treatment of localized infections in the febrile neutropenic patients with monotherapy. Leuk Lymphoma 9:193–203
50. Castagnola E, Fontanma V, Caviglia I et al (2007) A prospective study on the epidemiology of febrile episodes during chemotherapy-induced neutropenia in children with cancer or after hematopoietic stem cell transplantation. Clin Infect Dis 45:1296–1304

51. Viscoli C, Bruzzi P, Castagnola E et al (1994) Factors associated with bacteremia in febrile granulocytopenic cancer patients. Eur J Cancer 30:430–437
52. De Pauw BE, Donnelly JP, Elves A et al (1990) Towards individually tailored empiric antibiotic therapy in febrile granulocytopenic patients. Neth J Med 37: 111–119
53. Cordonnier C, Buzyn A, Leverger G et al (2003) Epidemiology and risk factors for gram-positive coccal infections in neutropenia: toward a more targeted antibiotic strategy. Clin Infect Dis 36:149–158
54. Kern W, Jurrie E, Schmeiser T (1990) Streptococcal bacteremia in adult patients with leukemia undergoing aggressive chemotherapy. A review of 55 cases. Infection 18:138–145
55. Engelhard D, Elishoov H, Or R et al (1995) Cytosine arabinoside as a major risk factor for Streptococcus viridans septicemia following bone marrow transplantation: a 5-year prospective study. Bone Marrow Transplant 16:565–570
56. Bochut P-Y, Calandra T, Francioli P (1994) Bacteremia due to viridans streptococci in neutropenic patients: a review. Am J Med 97:256–264
57. Blijlevens NMA, Donnelly JP, De Pauw BE (2000) Mucosal barrier injury: biology, pathology, clinical counterparts and consequences of intensive treatment for haematological malignancy: an overview. Bone Marrow Transplant 25:2469–2478
58. Pouwels MJM, Donnelly JP, Raemaekers JMM, Verweij PE, De Pauw BE (1997) Clostridium septicum sepsis and neutropenic enterocolitis in a patient treated with intensive chemotherapy for acute myeloid leukemia. Ann Hematol 74:153–157
59. Tikko SK, Distenfield A, Davidson M (1985) Clostridium septicum septicemia with identical metastatic myonecroses in a granulocytopenic patient. Am J Med 79:256–258
60. Gerard M, Defresne N, Daneau D et al (1988) Incidence and significance of Clostridium difficile in hospitalized cancer patients. Eur J Clin Microbiol Infect Dis 7:274–278
61. Rampling A, Warren RE, Bevan PC et al (1985) Clostridium difficile in haematological malignancy. J Clin Pathol 38:445–451
62. Delmé M, Vandercam B, Avesani V et al (1987) Epidemiology and prevention of Clostridium difficile infection in a leukemia unit. Eur J Clin Microbiol 6:623–627
63. Heard SR, O'Farrell S, Holland D et al (1986) The epidemiology of Clostridium difficile with use of a typing scheme: nosocomial acquisition and cross-infection among immunocompromised patients. J Infect Dis 153:159–162
64. Gorschlüter M, Glasmacher A, Hahn C et al (2001) Clostridium difficile infection in patients with neutropenia. Clin Infect Dis 33:786–791
65. Luft BJ, Remington JS (1985) Toxoplasmosis of the central nervous system. Curr Clin Top Infect Dis 6:315–358
66. Longworth DL, Weller PF (1986) Hyperinfection syndrome with strongyloidiasis. Curr Clin Top Infect Dis 7:1–26
67. Sanders CC (1991) New b-lactams: new problems for the internist. Ann Intern Med 115:650–651
68. Muder RR, Harris AP, Muller S et al (1996) Bacteremia due to Stenotrophomonas (Xanthomonas) maltophilia: a prospective multicenter study of 91 episodes. Clin Infect Dis 22:508–512
69. Anaissie E (1992) Opportunistic mycoses in the immunocompromised host: experience at a cancer center and review. Clin Infect Dis 43(Suppl 1):14–53
70. Fine JD, Miller JA, Harrist TJ et al (1981) Cutaneous lesions in disseminated candidiasis mimicking ecthyma gangrenosum. Am J Med 70:1133–1135
71. Bodey GP, Jadeja L, Elting L (1985) Pseudomonas bacteremia: retrospective analysis of 410 episodes. Arch Int Med 145:1621–1629
72. Suster S, Rose LB (1987) Intradermal bullous dermatitis due candidiasis in an immunocompromised patient. JAMA 258:2106–2107

73. Hay CRM, Messenger AG, Cotton DWK et al (1987) Atypical bullous pyoderma gangrenosum associated with myeloid malignancies. J Clin Pathol 40:387–392
74. Cohen PR, Kurzrock R (1987) Sweet's syndrome and malignancy. Am J Med 82:1120–1126
75. Bookman MA, Longo DL (1986) Concomitant illness in patients treated for Hodgkin's disease. Cancer Treat Rev 13:77–111
76. Miliauskas JR, Webber BL (1984) Disseminated varicella at autopsy in children with cancer. Cancer 53:1518–1525
77. Strauss SE (1988) Varicella zoster virus infections: biology, natural history, treatment and prevention. Ann Intern Med 108:221–237
78. Lordick F, Hentrich M, Decker T et al (2003) Ultrasound screening for internal jugular vein thrombosis aids the detection of central venous catheter-related infections in patients with haemato-oncological diseases: a prospective observational study. Br J Haematol 120(6):1073–1078
79. Overholser CD, Peterson DE, William LT et al (1982) Periodontal infections in patients with acute nonlymphocytic leukemia: prevalence of acute exacerbations. Arch Intern Med 142:551–554
80. Bergmann OJ (1989) Oral infections and fever in immunocompromised patients with haematologic malignancies. Eur J Clin Microbiol Infect Dis 8:207–213
81. Noriega LM, van der Auwera P, Phan M et al (1993) Anaerobic bacteremia in a cancer center. Support Care Cancer 1:250–255
82. Corey L, Spear PG (1986) Infections with herpes simplex viruses. N Engl J Med 314:686–691, 749–757
83. Shelhamer JH, Toews GB, Masur H et al (1992) Respiratory disease in the immunosuppressed patient. Am Intern Med 117:415–431
84. Nováková IRO, Donnelly JP, De Pauw B (1993) Potential sites of infection that develop in febrile neutropenic patients. Leuk Lymphoma 10:461–467
85. Varthalitis I, Meunier F (1993) Pneumocystis carinii pneumonia in cancer patients. Cancer Treat Rev 19:387–413
86. Hughes WT, Rivera GK, Schell MJ et al (1987) Successful intermittent chemoprophylaxis for Pneumocystis carinii pneumonitis. N Engl J Med 316:1627–1632
87. Whimbey E, Couch RB, Englund JA et al (1995) Respiratory syncytial virus pneumonia in hospitalized adult patients with leukemia. Clin Infect Dis 21:376–379
88. Whimbey E, Champlin RE, Couch RB et al (1996) Community respiratory virus infections among hospitalized adult bone marrow transplant recipients. Clin Infect Dis 22:778–782
89. Schimpff SC, Greene WH, Young VM et al (1973) Pseudomonas septicemia: incidence, epidemiology, prevention and therapy in patients with advanced cancer. Eur J Cancer 9:449–455
90. Vidal F, Mensa J, Almela M et al (1996) Epidemiology and outcome of Pseudomonas aeruginosa bacteremia, with special emphasis in the influence of antibiotic treatment. Analysis of 189 episodes. Arch Int Med 156:2121–2126
91. Ampel NM, Wing EJ (1988) Legionellosis in the compromised host. In: Rubin RH, Young LS (eds) Clinical approach to infection in the compromised host, 2nd edn. Plenum, New York, pp 305–319
92. Mayaud C, Cadranel J (2000) A persistent challenge: the diagnosis of respiratory disease in the non-AIDS immunocompromised host. Thorax 55:511–517
93. Johnson MP, Ramphal R (1990) Malignant external otitis: report on therapy with ceftazidime and review of therapy and prognosis. Rev Infect Dis 12:173–180
94. Chang J, Powles R, Mehta J, Paton S, Treleaven J, Jameson B (1995) Listeriosis in the bone marrow transplant recipient. Clin Infect Dis 21:1289–1290
95. Talcott JA, Siegel RD, Finberg R, Goldman L (1992) Risk assessment in cancer patients with fever and neutropenia: a prospective, two-center validation of a prediction rule. J Clin Oncol 10:316–322

96. Klastersky J, Paesmans M, Rubenstein EB et al (2000) The multinational Association for supportive Care in Cancer risk index: a multinational scoring system for identifying low-risk febrile neutropenic cancer patients. J Clin Oncol 18:3038–3051
97. Vidal L, Paul M, Ben dor I, Pokroy E, Soares-Weiser K, Leibovici L (2004) Oral versus intravenous antibiotic treatment for febrile neutropenia in cancer patients: a systematic review and meta-analysis of randomized trials. J Antimicrob Chemother 54:29–37
98. Malik IA, Abbas Z, Karim M (1992) Randomised comparison of oral ofloxacin alone with a combination of parenteral antibiotics in neutropenic febrile patients. Lancet 339:1092–1096
99. Rubenstein EB, Rolston K, Benjamin RS (1993) Outpatient treatment of febrile episodes in low-risk neutropenic patients with cancer. Cancer 71:3640–3646
100. Talcott JA, Whalen A, Clark J, Rieker PP, Finberg R (1994) Home antibiotic therapy for low-risk cancer patients with fever and neutropenia: a pilot study of 30 patients based on a validated prediction rule. J Clin Oncol 12:107–114
101. Malik IA, Khan WA, Karim M, Azziz Z, Khan MA (1995) Feasibility of outpatient management of fever in cancer patient with low-risk neutropenia: results of a prospective randomized trial. Am J Med 98:224–231
102. Horowitz DW, Holmgren D, Seiter K (1996) Stepdown single antibiotic therapy for the management of the high risk adult with hematologic malignancies. Leuk Lymphoma 23:159–163
103. Aquino VM, Tkaczewski I, Buchanan GR (1997) Early discharge of low-risk febrile neutropenic children and adolescents with cancer. Clin Infect Dis 25:74–78
104. Jones GR, Konsler GK, Dunaway RP, Gold SH, Cooper HA, Wells RJ (1994) Risk factors for recurrent fever after discontinuation of empiric antibiotic therapy for fever and neutropenia in pediatric patients with a malignancy or hematologic condition. J Pediatr 124:703–708
105. Lucas KG, Brown AE, Armstrong D, Chapman D, Heller G (1996) The identification of febrile, neutropenic children with neoplastic disease at low risk for bacteremia and complications of sepsis. Cancer 77:791–798
106. Su F, Nguyen ND, Wang Z, Cay Y, Rogiers P, Vincent J-L (2005) Fever control in septic shock: beneficial or harmful? Shock 23:516–520
107. Kreger BE, Craven DE, McCabe WR (1980) Gram-negative bacteremia. IV. Re-evaluation of clinical features and treatment in 612 patients. Am J Med 68:344–355
108. O' Hanley P, Easaw J, Rugo H, Easaw S (1989) Infectious disease management of adult leukemic patients undergoing chemotherapy: 1982 to 1986 experience at Stanford University Hospital. Am J Med 87:605–613
109. De Pauw BE, Dompeling EC (1996) Antibiotic strategy after the empiric phase in patients treated for a hematological malignancy. Ann Hematol 72:273–279
110. Akova M, Paesmans M, Calandra T, Viscoli C, International Antimicrobial Therapy Group of the European Organization of Research and Treatment of Cancer (2005) A European Organization for Research and treatment of Cancer-International Antimicrobial Therapy Group Study of secondary infections in febrile, neutropenic patients with cancer. Clin Infect Dis 40:239–245
111. Pizzo PA, Robichaud KJ, Gill FA, Witebsky FG (1984) Empiric antibiotic and antifungal therapy for cancer patients with prolonged fever and granulocytopenia. Am J Med 72:101–107
112. EORTC International Antimicrobial Therapy Cooperative Group (1989) Empiric antifungal therapy in febrile neutropenic patients. Am J Med 86:668–672
113. Edwards JE, Bodey GP, Bowden RA et al (1997) International conference for the development of a consensus on the management and prevention of severe candidal infections. Clin Infect Dis 25:43–59

114. Kuse E-R, Chetchotisakd P, Arns da Cunha C, Micafungin Invasive Candidiasis Working Group et al (2007) Micafungin versus liposomal amphotericin B for candidaemia and invasive candidosis: a phase III randomised double-blind trial. Lancet 369:1519–1527
115. Kullberg BJ, Sobel JD, Ruhnke M et al (2005) Voriconazole versus a regimen of amphotericin B followed by fluconazole for candidaemia in non-neutropenic patients: a randomised non-inferiority trial. Lancet 366:1435–1442
116. Sobel JD, Revankar SG (2007) Echinocandins – first-choice or first-line therapy for invasive candidiasis? N Engl J Med 356:2525–2526
117. Walsh TJ, Hathorn JW, Sobel JD et al (1991) Detection of circulating candida enolase by immunoassay in patients with cancer and invasive candidiasis. N Engl J Med 324:1026–1031
118. Verweij PE, Stynen D, Rijs AJMM, de Pauw BE, Hoogkamp-Korstanje JA, Meis JF (1995) Sandwich enzyme-linked immunosorbent assay compared with Pastorex latex agglutination test for diagnosing invasive aspergillosis in immunocompromised patients. J Clin Microbiol 33:1912–1914
119. Pagano L, Caira M, Nosari A et al (2007) Fungal infections in recipients of hematopoietic stem cell transplants: results of the SEIFEM B-2004 study – Sorveglianza Epidemiologica Infezioni Fungine nelle Empatie Maligne. Clin Infect Dis 45:1161–1170
120. Verweij PE, Rijs AJMM, De Pauw BE, Horrevorts AM, Hoogkamp-Korstanje JAA, Meis JFGM (1995) Clinical evaluation and reproducibility of the Pastorex Aspergillus antigen latex agglutination test for diagnosing invasive aspergillosis. J Clin Pathol 48:474–476
121. Maertens J, Theunissen K, Verhoef G et al (2005) Galactomannan and computed tomography-based preemptive antifungal therapy in neutropenic patients at risk of invasive fungal infection: a prospective feasibility study. Clin Infect Dis 41:1242–1250
122. De Pauw BE (2005) Between over- and undertreatment of invasive fungal disease. Clin Infect Dis 41:1251–1253
123. Oshima K, Kanda Y, Asono-Mori Y et al (2007) Presumptive treatment strategy for aspergillosis in allogeneic haematopoietic stem cell transplant recipients. J Antimicrob Chemother 60:350–355
124. Greene RE, Schlamm HT, Oestmann J-W et al (2007) Imaging findings in acute invasive pulmonary aspergillosis: clinical significance of the halo sign. Clin Infect Dis 44:373–379
125. Kuhlman JE, Fishman EK, Siegelman SS (1985) Invasive pulmonary aspergillosis in acute leukemia: characteristics findings on CT, the CT halo sign, and the role of CT in early diagnosis. Radiology 157:611–614
126. Caillot D, Casasnovas O, Bernard A et al (1997) Improved management of invasive pulmonary Aspergillosis in neutropenic patients using early thoracic computed tomographic scan and surgery. J Clin Oncol 15:139–147
127. Marr KA, Carter RA, Crippa F, Wald A, Corey L (2002) Epidemiology and outcome of mould infections in hematopoietic stem cell transplant recipients. Clin Infect Dis 34:909–917
128. Kontoyiannis DP, Lionakis MS, Lewis RE et al (2005) Zygomycosis in a tertiary-care cancer center in the era of Aspergillus-active antifungal therapy: a case-control observational study of 27 recent cases. J Infect Dis 191:1350–1360
129. Cornely OA, Maertens J, Winston DJ et al (2007) Posaconazole vs. fluconazole or itraconazole prophylaxis in patients with neutropenia. N Engl J Med 356: 348–359
130. Cornely OA, Maertens J, Bresnik M, AmBiLoad Trial Study Group et al (2007) Liposomal amphotericin B as initial therapy for invasive mold infection: a randomized trial comparing a high-loading dose regimen with standard dosing (AmBiLoad Trial). Clin Infect Dis 44:1289–1297

131. Meunier F, Aoun M, Bitar N (1992) Candidemia in immunocompromised patients. Clin Infect Dis 14(Suppl 1):S120–S125
132. Girmenia C, Martino P, De Bernardis F et al (1996) Rising incidence of Candida parapsilosis fungemia in patients with hematologic malignancies: clinical aspects, predisposing factors, and differential pathogenicity of the causative strains. Clin Infect Dis 23:506–514
133. Thaler M, Pastakia B, Shawker TH, O'Leary T, Pizzo PA (1988) Hepatic candidiasis in cancer patients: the evolving picture of the syndrome. Ann Intern Med 108: 88–100
134. Anaissie EJ, Vartivarian SE, Abi-Said D et al (1996) Fluconazole versus amphotericin B in the treatment of hematogenous candidiasis: a matched cohort study. Am J Med 101:170–176
135. Walsh TJ, Pizzo PA (1989) Fungal infections in granulocytopenic patients: current approaches to classification, diagnosis, and treatment. In: Holmberg K, Meyer R (eds) Diagnosis and therapy of systemic fungal infections. Raven, New York, pp 47–70
136. Krcmery V, Jesenska Z, Spanik S et al (1997) Fungemia due to Fusarium spp in cancer patients. J Hosp Infect 36:223–228
137. Boutati EI, Anaissie EJ (1997) Fusarium, a significant emerging pathogen in patients with hematologic malignancy: ten years' experience at a cancer center and implications for management. Blood 90:999–1008
138. Maher DW, Lieschke GJ, Green M et al (1994) Filgrastim in patients with chemotherapy-induced febrile neutropenia. A double-blind, placebo controlled trial. Ann Intern Med 121:492–501
139. Anaissie EJ, Vartivarian S, Bodey GP et al (1996) Randomized comparison between antibiotics alone and antibiotics plus granulocyte-macrophage colony-stimulating factor (Escherichia coli-derived) in cancer patients with fever and neutropenia. Am J Med 100:17–23
140. American Society of Clinical Oncology (1996) Update of recommendations for the use of hematopoietic colony-stimulating factors: evidence-based clinical practice guidelines. J Clin Oncol 14:1957–1960
141. Croockewit AJ, Bronchud MH, Aapro MS et al (1997) A European perspective on haematopoietic growth factors in haemato-oncology: report of an expert meeting of the EORTC. Eur J Cancer 33:1732–1746
142. Levenga TH, Timmer-Bonte JNH (2007) Review of the value of colony stimulating factors for the prophylaxis of febrile neutropenic episodes in adult patients treated for haematological malignancies. Br J Haematol 138: 146–152
143. Ellis M, Zwaan F, Hedstrom U et al (2003) Recombinant human interleukin 11 and bacterial infection in patients with haematological malignant disease undergoing chemotherapy: a double-blind placebo-controlled randomised trial. Lancet 25:275–280
144. Spielberger R, Stiff P, Bensinger W et al (2004) Palifermin for oral mucositis after intensive therapy for hematologic cancer. N Engl J of Med 351:2590–2598
145. Beaven AW, Shea TC (2006) Palifermin: a keratinocyte growth factor that reduces oral mucositis after stem cell transplant for hematological malignancies. Expert Opin Pharmacother 7:2287–2299
146. Joshi JH, Schimpff SC, Tenney JH et al (1984) Can antibacterial therapy be discontinued in persistently febrile granulocytopenic cancer patients? Am J Med 76:450–457
147. Oude Lashof AML, Donnelly JP, Meis JFGM, van der Meer JWM, Kullberg BJ (2003) Duration of antifungal treatment and development of delayed complications in patients with candidaemia. J Haematol 22:43–48
148. Karp JE, Burch PA, Merz WG (1988) An approach to intensive antileukemic therapy in patients with previous invasive aspergillosis. Am J Med 85:203–206

149. Offner F, Cordonnier C, Ljungman P et al (1998) Impact of previous aspergillosis on the outcome of bone marrow transplantation. Clin Infect Dis 26:1098–1103
150. Nosari A, Ravini M, Cairoli R et al (2007) Surgical resection of persistent pulmonary fungus nodules and secondary prophylaxis are effective in preventing fungal relapse in patients receiving chemotherapy or bone marrow transplantation for leukemia. Bone Marrow Transplant 39:631–635

Chapter 6

Lymphomas and Chronic Lymphocytic Leukemia

Kenneth V. I. Rolston

Abstract Many solid tumor cancer patients are considered to be at "low-risk" for developing complications even during episodes of neutropenic fever and are routinely managed without hospitalization. Low-risk subsets are now being recognized in patients with hematologic malignancies (CLL/lymphomas) as well. The spectrum of infection in most of these patients is different from that seen in neutropenic patients, with fungal, viral, and bacterial infections primarily associated with defects in cellular immunity predominating. With improvements in supportive care and infusion technology, and the availability of many anti-infective agents for parenteral and oral administration, outpatient management of low-risk patients with hematologic malignancies is being practiced with increasing frequency. This approach has several advantages and very few disadvantages but does require substantial initial investment in infrastructure by individual institutions. Nevertheless, it is an investment well worth making by institutions that care for cancer patients, as cancer survivorship continues to rise.

Keywords Hematologic malignancies • Low-risk patients • Fungal infections • Viral infections • Outpatient therapy

1. Introduction

Patients with hematologic malignancies are at substantial risk of developing infections as a result of immunologic deficits associated with underlying diseases, and those caused by antineoplastic therapy [1]. For a long time clinicians have been aware that not all patients with hematologic malignancies have the same risk of developing infections or infection-related complications. Nevertheless, until very recently, most patients particularly those with neutropenia, were managed in the hospital when they developed fever or other symptoms and signs of infection [2]. This was considered prudent because (a) there were no reliable risk-assessment strategies which could accurately identify low-risk patients and, (b) most institutions did not have the necessary

From: *Managing Infections in Patients With Hematological Malignancies*: Contemporary Hematology, Edited by: M. Kleinberg, DOI 10.1007/978-1-59745-415-5_6,

infrastructure and multi-disciplinary teams necessary to support an active program of outpatient management. The situation has changed considerably over the past decade, particularly, at Comprehensive Cancer Centers and other institutions caring for patients with hematologic malignancies.

Several risk-assessment strategies have been developed which can identify with acceptable accuracy febrile neutropenic patients who are at low-risk for life-threatening outcomes from infections [3, 4]. Although majority of patients categorized as low-risk have solid tumors such as breast cancer or sarcoma, several subsets of patients with hematologic malignancies have also been identified to be at low-risk. Many of these low-risk neutropenic patients do not need to be hospitalized when they develop an infection. With the ability to identify large numbers of low-risk patients came the commitment from many institutions to invest in the infrastructure required to manage patients in the outpatient setting, because of several advantages associated with this approach.

Newer therapeutic modalities for the treatment of lymphoproliferative disorders including purine nucleoside analogs and monoclonal antibodies have now become commonplace. These modalities have changed the spectrum of infections seen in patients with hematologic malignancies. They have also created a subpopulation of patients that are at intermediate-to-low risk for the development of serious infection-related morbidity/mortality. In the real world, the majority of such patients are being managed without hospitalization. In this chapter, I will discuss various risk-assessment strategies, the changing spectrum of infections encountered in patients with lymphoma/CLL, and the feasibility of outpatient management for intermediate/low-risk patients.

2. Risk Assessment

Several risk prediction rules have recently been developed and validated in neutropenic patients presenting with fever. Some of these are based on statistically derived models whereas others utilize simple clinical characteristics and some laboratory data that are part of initial work-up of such patients [5–7]. The most widely accepted and used model is MASCC Risk Index developed by the Multinational Association of Supportive Care in Cancer. This index is derived by ascribing weighed points to various characteristics including age, clinical stability, severity of underlying disease, concurrent comorbidity, etc. which have been shown factors that predict good/bad responses in febrile neutropenic patients [4]. These points are then added up to achieve a cumulative score with a maximum possible score of 26. A cumulative score of >20 is predictive of low-risk status with <5% chance of developing serious medical complications such as septic shock during an episode of fever and neutropenia (Table 6-1). Several studies have used MASCC risk index to identify low-risk patients for early discharge or outpatient therapy, with acceptable accuracy as mentioned above [8, 9]. This model is particularly useful when conducting multicenter trials or comparing data from different centers. It, however, may not be the most practical model for risk-assessment in a busy emergency center or clinical practice setting due to the need for calculating the index, and the time involved.

Several institutions/organizations (The University of Texas M. D. Anderson Cancer Center – Houston, Texas; The National Cancer Institute – NCI; The European Organization for Research and Treatment of Cancer (EORTC) have also used simple clinical criteria to reliably identify low-risk patients,

Table 6-1. The scoring system for the MASCC risk-index.

Clinical characteristic	Numerical weight assigned
Burden of illness: No symptoms, or mild symptoms	5
No hypotension (systolic BP >90 mmHg)	5
Absence of chronic obstructive pulmonary disease (COPD)	4
Underlying solid tumor/absence of previous fungal infection[a]	4
Absence of dehydration (i.e., parenteral fluids not required)	3
Burden of illness: Moderate symptoms	3
Outpatient status on development of neutropenic infection (fever and neutropenia)	3
Age <60 years	2

Note: Maximum possible score is 26 as points from "burden of illness" are not cumulative. A cumulative score of >20 is considered to be predictive of low-risk (<5%) for the development of serious medical complications and <1% for death, during an episode of neutropenic fever [4]
MASCC Multinational Association for Supportive Care in Cancer
[a]May be marker for underlying hematologic malignancy

without having to calculate a risk index [6, 7, 10]. These criteria include the following:

> Hemodynamic stability; absence of hepatic, renal, respiratory abdominal or central nervous system dysfunction; absence of documented catheter-related infection or pneumonia; expected duration of neutropenia not to exceed 7–10 days. Some clinicians include age >65 years and the presence of hematologic malignancies as markers of increased risk although MASCC risk prediction rules do not confirm this.

There is close correlation (>95%) between the MASCC statistically derived risk-prediction rule and simple clinical criteria [11]. The latter are probably more user-friendly for the identification of low-risk patients in busy clinical practices and emergency room settings. Regardless of which method is used for risk assessment, a small proportion of patients will get misclassified. This is not a major issue in low-risk patients who get misclassified as intermediate or high-risk and get hospitalized for inpatient treatment of an episode of febrile neutropenia. It can be problematic when truly high-risk patients get misclassified as low-risk, and are sent home with outpatient therapy [5]. If there is any doubt, a short period of hospitalization is the prudent thing to do. In fact, many investigators admit all low-risk patients for a 24–48 h observation period to ensure clinical stability before discharging them to receive outpatient therapy.

These risk-assessment strategies apply only to febrile neutropenic patients. However, many patients with lymphoma/CLL develop infections when they are not neutropenic. These infections can be bacterial, mycobacterial, fungal, viral or parasitic. The majority of these patients are stable enough not to require hospital admission either for diagnostic purposes, or for treatment, once a specific infection has been documented. Specific treatment recommendations are discussed below.

3. Infections in Patients with Non-Hodgkin's Lymphomas

Non-Hodgkin's lymphomas (NHL) are a diverse group of disorders. They are relatively common with approximately 63,190 new cases diagnosed in the United States each year [12]. The most common types are diffuse large B cell lymphomas and relatively indolent follicular cell lymphomas. Current treatment modalities for many NHL include purine nucleoside analogs like fludarabine as a single agent or in various combinations, rituximab, a chimeric anti CD20 antibody, radio-immunotherapy, high dose chemotherapy with autologos stem cell rescue, and allogeneic stem-cell transplantation using either nonmyeloablative or high-dose regimens [13]. The immunological defects and infections associated with these modalities are listed in Table 6-2.

Fludarabine is a purine nucleoside analog that inhibits DNA repair. It is used singly and in combination to treat low-grade NHL and is also active in both newly diagnosed and refractory CLL [14, 15]. It causes a marked decrease in CD_{4+} lymphocytes and has been associated with a number of opportunistic infections. The most common pathogens in fludarabine-treated patients include unusual bacteria such as *Listeria monocytogenes* and mycobacteria; fungal organisms such as *Candida* species, *Aspergillus* species and *Cryptococcus neoformans*; viruses including herpes-simplex virus, varicella-zoster viruses, and Epstein–Barr virus, cytomegalovirus; and pneumonia caused by *Pneumocystis jiroveci* (PCP) (previously *Pneumocystis carinii*) considered by many to be a fungus, and *Toxoplasma gondii*, a unicellular parasite that can cause pneumonia, retinitis, and other infections. [16–19]. The use of trimethoprim/sulfamethoxazole for prophylaxis against PCP is strongly

Table 6-2. Infections frequently associated with various defects in host defence mechanisms.

Prominent defect[a]	Predominant infections
Neutropenia	Gram-positive organisms (staphylococci, streptococci, enterococci, *Corynebacterium* spp., *Stomatococcus mucilaginosus*) Gram-negative bacilli (*Enterobacteriaceae*, nonfermentative gram-negative bacilli) *Candida* spp., *Aspergillus* spp., and other molds
Hypogammaglobulinemia	Encapsulated organisms (*streptococcus pneumoniae, Haemophilus influenzae, Neisseria meningitis*)
Impaired T-lymphocyte response	*Listeriosis, Salmonellosis*, mycobacterial infections, *Rhodococcus equi*, Cryptococcosis, Endemic fungi, *Pneumocystis jiroveci* pneumonia, viral reactivation (HSV, VZV, CMV, EBV), adenoviruses; toxoplasmosis
Splenectomy	Encapsulated organisms *(S. pneumoniae, H. influenzae); Capnocytophaga canimorsus*; gram-negative bacilli (*E. coli, P. aeruginosa*) *Plasmodium* spp., *Babesia* spp.

[a]Multiple defects are often present in the same patient, widening the spectrum of infection that needs to be considered as part of the diagnostic work-up and empiric therapy

recommended even after discontinuation of fludarabine therapy. Use of prophylactic antifungal and antiviral agents is recommended by some, but left to the discretion of the treating physician in most cases. Although no definitive data exist, some experts recommend monitoring CD_4 counts in such patients and administering antifungal and antiviral prophylaxis in patients with CD_4 counts below 200/mm^3.

Rituximab is a chimeric monoclonal antibody directed against the pan-B-cell marker CD20. Although initially approved for the treatment of B-cell-NHL, its usage has been expanded to include any CD20 positive NHL [20]. Rituximab targets and depletes both malignant and normal B-lymphocytes resulting in sustained reductions of immunoglobulins (IgM and IgG) levels causing impaired humoral immunity [21]. In the pivotal single agent trial of rituximab conducted at The University of Texas M. D. Anderson Cancer Center, hypogammaglobulinemia occurred in only 14% of cases and was not considered to cause significant morbidity [21]. Rituximab-treated patients developed only minor infectious complications which were predominantly bacterial (37 of 68 episodes of infection). Viral infections including ten episodes caused by HSV and five episodes caused by VZV were also reported. Overall, infection-related morbidity and mortality was low. Rituximab is also used in combination with CHOP-14 regimens with some success [22]. R-CHOP-14 causes Grade 3–4 granulocytopenia in most patients and febrile neutropenic episodes are not uncommon. Pegfilgrastim used as hematopoeitic support enhances neutrophil recovery, reduces the frequency and intensity of neutropenia, and facilitates the timely administration of multiple cycles of the regimen. Many patients with episodes of fever and neutropenia may be stable enough to be treated with outpatient antibiotic therapy for the entire febrile episode or after a short period of hospitalization, .

Sporadic cases of viral infection or reactivation associated with rituximab have been reported including CMV, VZV, HSV, hepatitis B, parvovirus B19, West Nile Virus and progressive multifocal leucoencephalopathy associated with JC virus [23–33]. At least one case of fulminant and fatal adenoviral hepatitis has also been documented in a rituximab treated patient [34]. High incidence of fungal infections and non-neutropenic infections have been reported with rituximab+CHOP and rituximab+fludarabine regimens [35, 36]. Increased vigilance for such infections is recommended when using rituximab based regimens as the recovery period from the immunosuppression is prolong. Adoptive immunotherapy might be a potential therapeutic option with potential benefits seen in adenoviral infections [37].

The main risk factor for infection in patients with NHL is treatment related neutropenia. Most agents used for chemotherapy (cyclophosphamide, etoposide, vincristine) cause myelosuppression with the risk of neutropenia increasing with each cycle. Approximately 30–40% of patients receiving combination chemotherapy for aggressive NHL develop an episode of neutropenic fever. The most common infections in this setting are bacterial, with a clear predominance of gram-positive pathogens, and enteric gram-negative bacilli. An increasing number of infections in this setting are polymicrobial [38]. Broad-spectrum antimicrobial therapy based on local susceptibility/resistant patterns is the standard of care [2, 39, 40]. Parenteral or oral outpatient antibiotic therapy may be an option in some stable, low to intermediate risk patients [39, 40].

4. Infections in Patients with Hodgkin's Disease

The American Cancer Society estimates that approximately 8,190 new cases of Hodgkin's Disease will be diagnosed in the United States in 2007, a number that has not changed much over the past several years [12]. Hodgkin's disease cells – the Reed Sternberg cells – are usually CD15 and CD30 T cells. T cell mediated immunity which is depleted in patients with HD provides protection against a wide variety of viral, fungal, and predominantly intracellular bacterial and mycobacterial pathogens (Table 6.2). Common bacterial infections in this setting include *Listeria monocytogenes*, *Nocardia* spp., *Salmonella* spp., and occasionally *Rhodococcus equi*. *Mycobacterium tuberculosis* and nontuberculosis mycobacteria (*M. avium* complex, *M. abscessus, M. chelonae, M. kansasii*, and *M. fortuitum*) are not uncommon. Viral infections caused by HSV, VZV, CMV, EBV and other virus have been recognized. Pneumonia caused by *Pneumocystis jiroveci* and other fungal infections including those caused by *Candida* spp., *Cryptococcus* spp., and *Aspergillus* spp., have also been described. Additionally, endemic mycosis such as Histoplasmosis and Blastomycosis may also be more common in patients with HD [41]. Patients living in endemic areas also have a higher frequency of developing parasitic/helminth infestations such as Strongyloidiosis, including the hyperinfection syndrome which is associated with high morbidity and mortality [42]. Knowledge of a patient's residence in or travel to such endemic areas may provide important historical information and lead one towards making appropriate diagnostic and therapeutic decisions.

A splenectomy is sometimes performed as part of the diagnostic work up and staging of HD. Asplenic individuals are susceptible to infections caused by encapsulated organisms such as *Haemophilus influenzae* and *Streptococcus pneumoniae* [43]. Other organisms that cause infections in such patients include *Neisseria meningitis, Capnocytophaga canimorsus*, and gram negative bacilli such as *Escherichia coli* and *Pseudomonas aeruginosa*. Since *S. pneumoniae* and *H. influenzae* cause >90% of post splenectomy sepsis, patients undergoing elective splenectomy should receive the pneumococcal and *H. influenzae* type B (HIB) vaccines 2 weeks prior to surgery.

Chemotherapy for HD often results in neutropenia. Bacterial and fungal infections common in this setting need to be considered in addition to the infections related to the immunologic deficits already mentioned, when investigating and treating such patients (Table 6.2). A substantial proportion of HD patients with fever and neutropenia are at intermediate-to-low risk for complications and candidates for early discharge or outpatient management.

5. Infections in Patients with Chronic Lymphocytic Leukemia

CLL is the most frequent hematologic malignancy in the United States and accounts for approximately 30% of all leukemias [12]. The number of new cases of CLL expected to be diagnosed in the US in 2007 is 15,340. As with many other hematologic malignancies, multiple factors predispose patients with CLL to develop infectious complications. These include hypogammaglobulinemia, which is a well-known feature of CLL, and as discussed earlier, is associated with infections caused by encapsulated organisms. Chemotherapy induced neutropenia is not uncommon. Cell-mediated immune function is also altered in patients with CLL, which leads to impaired immune responses to intracellular bacteria and viruses. Splenectomy is infrequently performed in patients with CLL, unless autoimmune hemolytic anemia or immune thrombocytopenia is present. Infections associated with all these risk-factors have already been discussed. So have infections associated with fludarabine use, which is one of the cornerstones of CLL treatment.

Alemtuzumab is a humanized monoclonal IgG1 antibody directed against CD52, a cell surface antigen expressed on B and T lymphocytes, monocytes and NK cells [44, 45]. Alemtuzumab has efficacy in the treatment of various malignancies including NHL, B cell chronic lymphocytic leukemia, and T cell prelymphocytic leukemia. Almost all clinical trials with alemtuzumab have reported an increased risk of infectious complications [46, 47]. This is probably due to the loss of circulating T cells resulting in defective cell mediated immunity. Treatment with alemtuzumab causes a profound and prolonged state of lymphopenia in all patients and can also cause neutropenia in approximately one-third of patients [44].

The most frequently observed opportunistic infection associated with ale mtuzumab therapy is CMV reactivation which occurs in 15–25% of patients [48]. This usually takes place between weeks 4 and 6 of therapy, shortly after the T-cell nadir. Other opportunistic infections include HSV and VZV reactivation, *Pneumocystis jiroveci* pneumonia, candidiasis, cryptococcosis, mold infections (aspergillosis, mucormycosis) and toxoplasmosis [47, 49–52]. Antiviral prophylaxis (acyclovir, famciclovir, valacyclovir) is effective for the prevention of HSV and VZV reactivation and is recommended for all patients receiving alemtuzumab. Although CMV reactivation can also be prevented by valgancyclovir prophylaxis, most clinicians perform weekly monitoring for CMV reactivation during therapy and for 2 months after discontinuation, and administer pre-emptive treatment (ganciclovir or foscarnet) if evidence of CMV viremia is detected [47, 53] .

Nonopportunistic infections are also common and include listeriosis, salmonellosis, and infections caused by *Staphylococcus* spp., *Streptococcus* spp., *Enterococcus* spp., the *Enterobacteriaceae*, and nonfermentative gram-negative bacilli [46, 47, 50, 51, 54].

6. Site of Care

The change in the spectrum of infection in patients with lymphoma/CLL (with a significant proportion of chronic viral and fungal infections), the development of accurate and reliable risk-assessment strategies for patients with neutropenic fever, and improvements in the supportive care of the cancer patient including infusion therapy has shifted the site of care for many of these patients from the hospital to the outpatient center/clinic [2, 5, 55]. In many patients the entire episode including diagnostic work-up, therapy, maintenance and follow-up can all be conducted without hospitalization. There are several advantages and very few disadvantages associated with managing patients outside the hospital inpatient wards, as outlined in Table 6.3. This has led to the development of multidisciplinary teams of health-care providers to meet the varied needs of these patients. Most institutions that take care of large numbers of patients with cancer including lymphoma/CLL have

Table 6-3. The advantages and disadvantages of outpatient management of cancer patients with infections (Adapted from Refs. [5, 10, 11, 40, 55]).

Advantages
• Avoidance of iatrogenic/logistic/and environmental hazards of hospitalization
• Lower frequency of "Healthcare Associated Infections"
• Lower overall cost of care
• Increased convenience (patient, family, or other caregiver)
• Improved quality of life and patient satisfaction
• More efficient utilization of expensive resources (hospital or other healthcare organization)
Potential disadvantages
• Possibility of development of serious events (sepsis, hemorrhage, seizure) in a relatively unsupervised environment (most likely to occur in patients who are misclassified as being low-risk)
• Need to develop and maintain infrastructure, multidisciplinary team, and monitoring capability (e.g., 24 h hotline)
• Potential for noncompliance with therapy

Table 6-4. Requirements for a successful program of outpatient management of cancer patients with infections (Adapted from Refs. [5, 8, 10, 11, 55]).

• Dedicated multidisciplinary team of healthcare providers (e.g., Physicians, Nurses, Pharmacists, Laboratory technicians)
• Institutional support of adequate infrastructure (Emergency Center, Outpatient Pharmacy, Infusion services, Laboratory services, Radiology services) on a 24/7 schedule
• Availability of real time, local epidemiological, and susceptibility/resistance data
• Selection of microbiologically appropriate (not merely convenient) treatment regimens
• Adequate and frequent outpatient monitoring for response/failure or progression of infections, development of medical complications or comorbidity, or toxicity
• Motivated and compliant patients supported by family members or other caretakers
• Adequate transportation and communication (automobile, city transport, telephone) between patient and medical center
• Access 24 h a day to multidisciplinary team (Hotline, Ambulatory or Emergency Center)

invested in the creation of such teams and the infrastructure necessary to maintain a successful program of outpatient treatment. The salient features of such a program are summarized in Table 6.4.

Multidisciplinary teams consist of the primary hematology/oncology services with consultative input from Infectious Diseases, Pulmonary Medicine, and other medical or surgical specialties as needed, along with support from nursing, pharmacy, laboratory medicine, radiology, transfusions and infusion teams, the Emergency Center/outpatient clinics, and, last but not least, from administration/scheduling services. Most of these services need to be available on a 24/7. Of key importance is the monitoring and tracking of patients who are receiving outpatient therapy. Our institution has created a "neutropenic fever clinic" where all patients come for their follow-up visits. There is a mechanism for tracking and contacting patients who have failed to keep their appointments, and ensuring that they "do not fall through the cracks." This is an expensive and time-consuming undertaking. However, benefits associated with such a program generally justify the investment needed to sustain these resources. These benefits include avoidance of some of the potential hazards (iatrogenic, logistic, environmental) associated with hospitalization, reduced frequency of healthcare-associated infections (many of which are caused by resistant pathogens), increased convenience and quality of life for the patient and family or other caregivers, and more efficient utilization of resources leading to lower overall cost of care [5, 55, 56].

Most non-neutropenic patients and many neutropenic patients with documented or suspected bacterial infections can be evaluated and treated as outpatients using parenteral, sequential (IV →PO), or oral treatment regimens. Most patients with a pulmonary infiltrate can be evaluated (microbiology, serology, CT or other imaging, bronchoscopy) as outpatients if their respiratory status is stable. The availability of newer antiviral and antifungal agents, many of which can be administered orally, has made outpatient therapy (both acute and maintenance) of these infections feasible. Infusion services have also gained recognition and popularity and outpatient antimicrobial therapy (OPAT) has now become commonplace [57].

7. Specific Recommendations

7.1. Neutropenic patients

Antibacterial, antifungal, and antiviral prophylaxis is not generally recommended unless severe (ANC < 100) and prolonged neutropenia (>10–14 days) is expected [2, 39]. Low-risk patients with neutropenia can safely be treated with oral regimens if they do not have significant (>grade II) mucositis and are able to tolerate oral intake [2, 39, 40, 58]. Patients who are otherwise stable but are unable or unwilling to take oral therapy can be treated with parenteral outpatient regimens. Intermediate and high-risk patients should be hospitalized and treated at least initially with parenteral antibiotics [2, 39]. Some of these patients can subsequently be discharged on outpatient anti-infective therapy (OPAT) if they stabilize over 24–72 h [8, 58–60].

7.2. Patients with Impaired Cellular Immunity

Patients with impaired cellular immunity are at increased risk for developing *Pneumocystis jiroveci* pneumonia, consequently prophylaxis with trimethoprim/sulfamethoxazole (TMP/SMX) is recommended. TMP/SMX prophylaxis may also protect against bacterial infections including listerosis, and possibly toxoplasmosis. Inpatients unable to tolerate TMP/SMX, alternative agents such as pentamidine, dapsone, or atovaquone will provide protection against *P. jiroveci*. Additional antibacterial prophylaxis with a fluoroquinolone is not recommended unless severe (ANC < 100) and prolonged (>10–14 days) neutropenia is anticipated. Some authors recommend avoidance of food items known to contain *L. monocytogenes* (soft cheeses, unpasteurized milk, raw vegetables, and undercooked poultry or meats) and advocate self-administration of amoxicillin/clavulanate before transit to the hospital, clinic, or emergency department if signs and symptoms of infection such as fever and chills develop [61]. Acyclovir, famciclovir, and valacyclovir are active against Herpes viruses (HSV, VZV) and their use should be considered in patients with positive herpes serology, past history of recurrent HSV or VZV infections, especially if the CD_4 count is ≤50 cells/ml. These agents are not active against CMV. Although valgancyclovir can prevent reactivation of CMV in high-risk patients, most authors recommend pre-emptive therapy with ganciclovir or foscarnet if CMV antigenemia testing is positive, rather than CMV prophylaxis [62]. Routine antifungal prophylaxis is not recommended. However, it should be considered if prolonged neutropenia is anticipated or mucositis and fungal colonization are present [61].

The management of documented infections in patients with lymphoma/CLL who have significant impairment in cellular immunity (e.g., those treated with purine analogs or alemtuzumab) depends upon the recognition of patients at high-risk of life-threatening infections and associated complications (pneumonia, meningitis) and the initiation of prompt antimicrobial therapy along with initiation of appropriate diagnostic workup. Most viral infections can be treated in the outpatient setting (HSV, VZV, CMV pre-emptive therapy). Similarly patients with fungal infections can be treated without hospitalization unless they have meningitis or worsening respiratory function. Patients with mild to moderate PCP can also be treated with a short period of hospitalization for initial workup or, without hospitalization as long as close monitoring is available.

7.3. Impaired Humoral Immunity

The association between hypogammaglobulinemia and infections with encapsulated organisms (*S. pneumoniae, H. influenzae*) is well known. Consequently the use of pneumococcal polysaccharide vaccine, and *Haemophilus influenzae* B (Hib) vaccine is recommended. Unfortunately, antibody responses to the pneumococcal polysaccharide vaccine particularly in patients with CLL are often suboptimal or poor [63]. There is evidence that the conjugate vaccine might be beneficial in patients who have poor antibody response to the polysaccharide vaccine [64, 65].

Staging laparotomy with splenectomy was used until recently for patients with HD. With the availability of sophisticated imaging and sampling techniques, splenectomy for this indication is performed very rarely nowadays. Splenectomy is a therapeutic procedure for some hematologic disorders and is occasionally performed after trauma as well. Vaccination against pneumococcal infections, *H. influenzae* type B and meningococci is recommended 2 weeks prior to elective splenectomy [66–68]. Patients should also be offered annual influenza vaccination. The role of antimicrobial prophylaxis in asplenic patients remains unclear. Intravenous immunoglobulin (IVIG) may lower the incidence of bacterial infection in patients with hypogammaglobulinemia (IgG levels lower than 400 mg/dl). However, the high cost and limited availability of IVIG precludes its use in most patients.

Bacterial infections in patients with hypogammaglobulinemia, particularly in splenectomized patients can be fulminant and associated with significant morbidity and mortality [69–72]. Prompt treatment with effective antimicrobial agents is critical, and most of these patients need to be hospitalized. Additional measures such as the use of recombinant human activated protein C may be of benefit in patients with fulminant infections [69]. Many authorities recommend that such high-risk patients should keep a supply of antibiotics with them and self medicate themselves at the first sign of a febrile illness, before seeking prompt medical attention [64].

As mentioned previously, many patients have a number of immunologic defects present at the same time. The treating physician should take all of these into consideration when ordering diagnostic studies and initiating antimicrobial therapy. Some physicians prefer the more conservative approach of a short period of hospitalization, prior to outpatient therapy, for all low-risk patients.

8. Summary

Lymphomas and chronic lymphocytic leukemias are relatively common disorders with approximately 86,720 new cases expected to be diagnosed each year in the U.S. These disorders are associated with multiple immunological defects that increase the risk of infection. Although some infections (such as those caused by encapsulated organisms, gram-negative bacilli, *L. monocytogenes*, and some fungi) can be fulminant, the majority of bacterial, viral and fungal infections in this setting are indolent or slowly progressive. The use of therapeutic modalities such as the purine nucleoside analogs (fludarabine) and monoclonal antibodies (rituximab, alemtuzumab) have changed the spectrum of infection towards predominance of viral and fungal infections. Specific infection prevention and treatment strategies have been developed for infections associated with the various immunologic defects. Advances in supportive care have shifted the site of patient management from the hospital to various outpatient settings, based on the relative risk of each patient. This has resulted in better utilization of valuable resources, and, more importantly in a substantially enhanced quality of life for patients and their loved ones.

References

1. Rolston KVI, Bodey GP (2006) Infections in patients with cancer. In: Kufe DW, Bast RC Jr, Hait WN, Hong WK, Pollock RE, Weichselbaum RR, Holland JF, Frei E III (eds) Cancer Medicine, e7. BC Decker, Hamilton, Ontario, pp 2222–2245
2. Hughes WT, Armstrong D, Bodey GP et al (2002) 2002 Guidelines for the use of antimicrobial agents in neutropenic patients with cancer. Clin Infect Dis 34:730–751
3. Talcott JA, Siegel RD, Finberg R et al (1992) Risk assessment in cancer patients with fever and neutropenia: A prospective, two-center validation of a prediction rule. J Clin Oncol 10:316–322
4. Klastersky J, Paesmans M, Rubenstein E et al (2000) The MASCC Risk Index: A multinational scoring system to predict low-risk febrile neutropenic cancer patients. J Clin Oncol 18:3038–3051
5. Rolston K (1999) New trends in patient management: Risk-based therapy for febrile patients with neutropenia. Clin Infect Dis 29:515–521
6. Kern WV, Cometta A, De Bock R, Langenaeken J, Paesmans M, Gaya H, for the International Antimicrobial Therapy Cooperative Group of the European

Organization for Research and Treatment of Cancer (1999) Oral versus intravenous empirical antimicrobial therapy for fever in patients with granulocytopenia who are receiving cancer chemotherapy. N Engl J Med 341:312–318
7. Freifeld A, Marchigiani D, Walsh T et al (1999) A double-blind comparison of empirical oral and intravenous antibiotic therapy for low-risk febrile patients with neutropenia during cancer chemotherapy. N Engl J Med 341:305–311
8. Klastersky J, Paesmans M, Georgala A et al (2006) Outpatient oral antibiotics for febrile neutropenic cancer patients using a score predictive for complications. J Clin Oncol 24:4129–4134
9. Uys A, Rapoport BL, Anderson R (2004) Febrile neutropenia: A prospective study to validate the Multinational Association of Supportive Care of Cancer (MASCC) risk-index scores. Support Care Cancer 12:555–560
10. Rubenstein EB, Rolston K, Benjamin RS et al (1993) Outpatient treatment of febrile episodes in low risk neutropenic cancer patients. Cancer 71:3640–3646
11. Rolston KVI, Manzullo EF, Elting LS et al (2006) Once daily, oral, outpatient quinolone monotherapy for low-risk cancer patients with fever and neutropenia. Cancer 106:2489–2494
12. American Cancer Society. Cancer Facts & Figures 2007. Atlanta, Ga. http://www.cancer.org/docroot/stt/stt_0.asp
13. Smith MR (2003) Rituximab (monoclonal anti-CD20 antibody): Mechanisms of action and resistance. Oncogene 22:7359–7368
14. Monserrat E, Moreno C, Esteve J, Urbano-Ispizua A, Gine E, Bosch F (2006) How I treat refractory CLL. Blood 107:1276–1283
15. Gartenhaus NC, RB TMS (2004) Purine nucleoside analogues and combination therapies in B-cell chronic lymphocytic leukemia: Dawn of a new era. Leuk Res 28:429–442
16. Samonis G, Kontoyannis DP (2001) Infectious complications of purine analog therapy. Curr Opin Infect Dis 14:409–413
17. Vilchez RA, Linden P, Lacomis J, Costello P, Fung J, Kusne S (2001) Acute respiratory failure associated with pulmonary cryptococcosis in non-AIDS patients. Chest 119:1865–1869
18. Nishida H, Ogura Y, Yoshimizu N et al (2007) Cryptococcus lung infection complicating fludarabine treatment in a chronic lymphocytic leukemia patient. Leuk Res 31:119–120
19. Mercadal S, Martinez A, Nomdedeu B et al (2006) Case Report. Herpes simplex and Epstein–Barr virus lymphadenitis in a patient with chronic lymphocytic leukemia treated with fludarabine. Eur J Haematol 77:442–444
20. Field T (2004) Non-hodgkin's lymphoma. In: Green JN (ed) Infections in Cancer Patients. Marcel Dekker, Inc., New York, pp 127–143
21. McLaughlin P, Grillo-Lopez AJ, Link BK et al (1998) Rituximab chimeric anti-CD20 monoclonal antibody therapy for replaced indolent lymphoma: Half of patients respond to a four-dose treatment program. J Clin Oncol 16: 2825–2833
22. Mey UJM, Maier A, Schmidt-Wolf IG et al (2007) Pegfilgrastim as hematopoietic support for dose-dense chemoimmunotherapy with R-CHOP-14 as first-line therapy in elderly patients with diffuse large B cell lymphoma. Support Care Cancer 15:877–884
23. Haura EB, Winden PA, Proia AD, Trotter JR (2002) Infections in oncology: Fulminant hepatic failure due to disseminated adenovirus infection in a patient with chronic lymphocytic leukemia. Cancer Control 9:248–253
24. Suzan F, Ammor M, Ribrag V (2001) Fatal reactivation of cytomegalovirus infection after use of rituximab for a posttransplantation lymphoproliferative disorder. N Engl J Med 345:1000
25. Bermudez A, Marco F, Conde E, Mazo E, Recio M, Zubizarreta A (2000) Fatal visceral varicella-zoster infection following rituximab and chemotherapy treatment in a patient with follicular lymphoma. Haematologica 85:894–895

26. Devite I, Hober D, Morel P (2001) Acute hepatitis B in a patient with antibodies to hepatitis B surface antigen who was receiving rituximab. N Engl J Med 344:68–69
27. Westhoff TH, Jochimsen F, Schmittel A et al (2003) Fatal hepatitis B virus reactivation by an escape mutant following rituximab therapy. Blood 102:1930
28. Sharma VR, Fleming DR, Slone SP (2000) Pure red cell aplasia due to parvovirus B19 in a patient treated with rituximab. Blood 96:1184–1186
29. Huang C, Slater B, Rudd R et al (2002) First isolation of West Nile virus from a patient with encephalitis in the United States. Emerg Infect Dis 8:1367–1371
30. Picardi M, Pane F, Quintarelli C et al (2003) Hepatitis B reactivation after fludarabine-based regimens for indolent nonHodgkins lymphomas: High prevalence of acquired viral genomic mutations. Haematologica 88:1296–1303
31. Goldberg SL, Pecora AL, Alter RS et al (2002) Unusual viral infections (progressive multifocal leukoencephalopathy and cytomegalovirus disease) after high dose chemotherapy with autologous stem cell rescue and peritransplantation rituximab. Blood 99:1486–1488
32. Klepfish A, Rachmilevitch E, Schattner A (2006) Parvovirus B19 reactivation presenting as neutropenia after rituximab. Eur J Intern Med 17:505–507
33. Freim Wahl SG, Folvik MR, Torp SH (2007) Progressive multifocal leukoencephalopathy in a lymphoma patient with complete remission after treatment with cytostatics and rituximab: Case report and review of the literature. Clin Neuropathol 26:68–73
34. Iyer A, Mathur R, Deepak BV, Sinard J (2006) Fatal adenoviral hepatitis after rituximab therapy. Arch Pathol Lab Med 130:1557–1560
35. Lin PC, Hsiao LT, Poh SB et al (2007) Higher fungal infection rate in elderly patients (more than 80 years old) suffering from diffuse large B cell lymphoma and treated with rituximab plus CHOP. Ann Hematol 86:95–100
36. Cabanillas F, Liboy I, Pavia O, Rivera E (2006) High incidence of non-neutropenic infections induced by rituximab plus fludarabine and associated with hypogammaglobulinemia: A frequently unrecognized and easily treatable complication. Ann Oncol 17:1424–1427
37. Feuchtinger T, Lang P, Hamprecht K et al (2004) Isolation and expansion of human adenovirus-specific CD4 and CD8 T cells according to IFN-gamma secretion for adjuvant immunotherapy. Exp Hematol 32:282–289
38. Rolston KVI, Bodey GP, Safdar A (2007) Polymicrobial infection in patients with cancer: An underappreciated and underreported entity. Clin Infect Dis 45:228–233
39. Freifeld AG, Baden LR, Brown AE, Guidelines Panel Member (2004) Fever and neutropenia NCCN Clinical Practice Guidelines in Oncology. JNCCN (J Natl Compr Canc Netw) 2:390–432
40. Rolston KVI (2005) Challenges in the treatment of infections caused by gram-positive and gram-negative bacteria in patients with cancer and neutropenia. Clin Infect Dis 40:S246–S252
41. Winwuist EW, Walmsley S, Berinstein NL (1993) Reactivation and dissemination of Balstomycosis complication of Hodgkin's disease: A case report and review of the literature. Am J Hematol 43:129–132
42. Safdar A, Malathum K, Rodriguez SJ, Husni R, Rolston KVI (2004) Strongyloidiasis in patients at a comprehensive cancer center in the United States. Cancer 100: 1531–1536
43. Lynch AM, Kapila R (1996) Overwhelming postsplenectomy infection. Infect Dis Clin North Am 10:693–707
44. James DF, Kipps TH (2007) Alemtuzumab in chronic lymphocytic leukemia. Future Oncol 3:29–42
45. Wierda WG (2006) Current and investigational therapies for patients with CLL. Hematology 2006:285–294
46. Martin SI, Marty FM, Fiumara K, Treon SP, Gribben JG, Baden LR (2006) Infectious complications associated with alemtuzumab use for lymphoproliferative disorders. Clin Infect Dis 43:16–24

47. Alinari L, Lapalombella R, Andritsos L, Baiocchi RA, Lin TS, Byrd JC (2007) Alemtuzumab (Campath-1H) in the treatment of chronic lymphocytic leukemia. Oncogene 26:3644–3653
48. Nguyen DD, Cao TM, Dugan K, Starcher SA, Fechter RL, Coutre SE (2002) Cytomegalovirus viremia during Campath-1H therapy for relapsed and refractory chronic lymphocytic leukemia and prolymphocytic leukemia. Clin Lymphoma 3:105–110
49. Rafailidis PI, Kakisi O, Vardakas K, Falagas M (2007) Infectious complications of monoclonal antibodies used in cancer therapy. A systematic review of the evidence from randomized controlled trials. Cancer 109:2182–2189
50. Lim Z, Baker B, Zuckermann M et al (2007) Toxoplasmosis following alemtuzumab based allogeneic haematopoietic stem cell transplantation. J Infect 54:e83–e86
51. Ferrajoli A, Faderl S, Keating MJ (2006) Monoclonal antibodies in chronic lymphocytic leukemia. Expert Rev Anticancer Ther 6:1231–1238
52. Wendtner C-M, Ritgen M, Schweighofer CD et al (2004) Consolidation with alemtuzumab in patients with chronic lymphocytic leukemia (CLL) in first remission – experience on safety and efficacy within a randomized multicenter phase III trial of the German CLL study group (GCLLSC). Leukemia 18:1093–1101
53. O'Brien S, Ravandi-kashani F, Wierda W et al (2005) A randomized trial of Valacyclovir versus Valganciclovir to prevent CMV reactivation in patients with CLL receiving alemtuzumab. Blood 106:830 (abstract 2960)
54. Silveira FP, Marcos A, Kwak EJ et al (2006) Bloodstream infections in organ transplant recipients receiving alemtuzumab: No evidence of occurrence of organisms typically associated with profound T cell depletion. J Infect 53:241–247
55. Kern WV (2006) Risk assessment and treatment of low-risk patients with febrile neutropenia. Clin Infect Dis 42:533–540
56. Kohn L, Corrigan J, Donaldson M (eds) (2000) To Err is Human: Building a Safer Health System. Committee on Quality of Health Care in America, Institute of Medicine Report, National Academy Press, Washington, DC
57. Chary A, Tice AD, Martinelli LP et al (2006) Experience of infectious diseases consultants with outpatient parenteral antimicrobial therapy: Results of an emerging infections network survey. Clin Infect Dis 43:1290–1295
58. Klastersky J, Paesmans M (2007) Risk-adapted strategy for the management of febrile neutropenia in cancer patients. Support Care Cancer 15:477–482
59. Innes HE, Smith DB, O'Reilly SM et al (2003) Oral antibiotics with early hospital discharge compared with inpatient intravenous antibiotics for low-risk febrile neutropenia in patients with cancer: A prospective randomized controlled single centre study. Br J Cancer 89:43–49
60. Rolston KVI (2003) Oral antibiotic administration and early hospital discharge is a safe and effective alternative for treatment of low-risk neutropenic fever. Cancer Treat Rev 29:551–554
61. Anaissie EJ, Kontoyiannis DP, O'Brien S, Kantarjian H, Robertson L, Lerner S, Keating MJ (1998) Infections in patients with chronic lymphocytic leukemia treated with fludarabine. Ann Intern Med 129:559–566
62. Cheung WW, Tse E, Leung AYH, Yuen KY, Kwong YL (2007) Regular virologic surveillance showed very frequent cytomegalovirus reactivation in patients treated with alemtuzumab. Am J Hematol 82:108–111
63. Cherif H, Landgren O, Konradsen HB, Kalin M, Björkholm M (2006) Poor antibody response to pneumococcal polysaccharide vaccination suggests increased susceptibility to pneumococcal infection in splenectomized patients with hematological diseases. Vaccine 24:75–81
64. O'Brien SN, Blijlevens NMA, Mahfouz TH, Anaissie EJ (2003) Infections in patients with hematological cancer: Recent developments. Hematology 2003:4 38–472

65. Musher DM, Ceasar H, Kojic EM et al (2005) Administration of protein-conjugate pneumococcal vaccine to patients who have invasive disease after splenectomy despite their having received 23-valent pneumococcal polysaccharide vaccine. J Infect Dis 191:1063–1067
66. Davies JM, Barnes R, Milligan D (2002) Update of guidelines for the prevention and treatment of infection in patients with an absent or dysfunctional spleen. Clin Med 2:440–443
67. (1996) Guidelines for the prevention and treatment of infection in patients with an absent or dysfunctional spleen. Working Party of the British Committee for Standards in Haematology Clinical Haematology Task Force. BMJ 312:430–434.
68. Centers for Disease Control and Prevention (1997) Prevention of pneumococcal disease. Recommendations of the Advisory Committee on Immunization Practices (ACIP). MMWR Morb Mortal Wkly Rep 46:1–18
69. Schumann C, Triantafilou K, Kamenz J et al (2006) Septic shock caused by Streptococcus pneumoniae in a post-splenectomy patient successfully treated with recombinant human activated protein C. Scand J Infect Dis 38:139–142
70. Sims KD, Barton TD (2006) Group B streptococcal toxic shock syndrome in an asplenic patient: Case report and literature review. Eur J Clin Microbiol Infect Dis 25:208–210
71. Cerquetti M, Cardines R, Giufrè M et al (2006) Detection of six copies of the capsulation b locus in a *Haemophilus influenzae* type b strain isolated from splenectomized patient with fulminant septic shock. J Clin Microbiol 44:640–642
72. Dudley MH, Czarnecki LA, Wells MA (2006) Fatal capnocytophaga infection associated with splenectomy. J Forensic Sci 51:664–666

Chapter 7

Multiple Myeloma

Marcio Nucci and Elias J. Anaissie

Abstract Infection is the leading cause of death in patients with multiple myeloma (MM). Over the past decade, significant changes have occurred in the spectrum of infections in patients with multiple myeloma, paralleling the changes in the treatment of the disease. Although bacteria (particularly Gram-negative organisms) remain the most frequent etiologic agents, invasive fungal infections caused by moulds (*Aspergillus* sp. and *Fusarium* sp.) have been increasingly reported. While the increase in the intensity of the treatment of multiple myeloma represents a major advance having a positive impact on survival, problems related to new infections have emerged. Therefore, a practical approach to managing infections in MM patients must include recognition of likely pathogens depending on several factors, such as past medical history, status of the underlying disease, and past and current treatment for MM. Specific strategies of diagnosis, prophylaxis, and empiric and specific therapy are driven according to this approach.

Keywords Myeloma • Multiple myeloma • Infection • Complication • Epidemiology • Prophylaxis • Treatment

1. Introduction

Infection has long been considered a significant cause of morbidity and the leading cause of death in patients with MM [1–4]. The increased susceptibility to infection is partly due to disease-related immunodeficiency characterized by a reduction in the production of normal immunoglobulins, defects in the complement cascade [5], and others [6]. Historically, these abnormalities predisposed patients to infections by encapsulated bacteria, such as *Streptococcus pneumoniae* [7] and *Haemophylus influenzae* [8]. More recently, it has been suggested that increased susceptibility for infections is more likely due to the cumulative immunosuppressive effects of an ever expanding number of myeloma-specific therapies. Indeed, myeloma has become, in most patients, a chronic disease with multiple relapses and salvage therapies as a result of more

From: *Managing Infections in Patients With Hematological Malignancies*: Contemporary Hematology, Edited by: M. Kleinberg, DOI 10.1007/978-1-59745-415-5_7,

effective treatments, including high doses of dexamethasone, bortezomib, lenalidomide, and autologous and allogeneic hematopoietic stem cell transplant (HSCT). Sequential, and often continuous, treatment with these therapies leads to cumulative immunosuppression affecting various components of the immune system with the emergence of infections not associated with myeloma a decade ago, such as cytomegalovirus (CMV) [9], *Varicella zoster* virus (VZV) [10], *Aspergillus* spp. [11], and *Fusarium* spp. [12]. In addition to the immunosuppression associated with the underlying disease and its treatment, patients with MM have other risk factors for infection (Table 7-1).

2. Infection in Different Phases of the Treatment of MM (Table 7-2)

2.1. Infections After Induction Therapy

The regimen of oral melphalan and prednisone (MP) is associated with a greater risk of infection during the first 2 months of treatment. In a study of 60 patients evaluating risk factors for infection, the incidence of infectious episodes per year for patients treated with MP-based regimens was 4.68 during the first 2 months, compared to 1.04 thereafter. Pre-existing renal dysfunction (serum creatinine >2 mg/dl) and low serum immunoglobulin levels were identified as risk factors for infection [13]. Pathogens included enterobacteriaceae and *Staphylococcus aureus* [14–17]. Randomized trials comparing MP with melphalan plus dexamethasone (3 trials) or with melphalan, prednisone and thalidomide (1 trial) showed lower rates of infection in the MP arms [18–21].

Infections after VAD (vincristin, doxorubicin and dexamethasone) chemotherapy occurred in a significant proportion of cases despite the absence of significant neutropenia, and they were related to dexamethasone-induced T-cell immunodeficiency. Hyperglycemia and central venous catheters may have been contributing factors [22]. Like in MP, the frequency of infection with VAD chemotherapy was higher in the first 4 months of therapy. Pneumonia accounted for the large majority of major infections, and the risk factors for infection included renal failure and hypogammaglobulinemia [23].

Other induction regimens include dexamethasone alone or in combination with thalidomide, bortezomib alone, in combination with dexamethasone, or with dexamethasone and thalidomide, and lenalidomide plus dexamethasone [24]. Thalidomide is not significantly myelotoxic, and the risk of infection does not necessarily increase with its use. However, thalidomide may indirectly increase the risk for infection because of a higher frequency of other complications associated with its use, such as deep vein thrombosis and peripheral neuropathy. In a randomized study in elderly (≥60 years) patients with MM, 129 patients receiving melphalan, prednisone and thalidomide (MPT) were compared with 126 receiving MP. The frequency of grade III–IV adverse events was much more frequent in the MPT group, especially deep vein thrombosis, peripheral neuropathy and infection. The incidence of infection (mostly pneumonia) was 10% in the MPT group compared to only 2% in the MP group ($p = 0.01$) [20]. However, the addition of thalidomide to standard MP did not increase serious infectious complications in another randomized controlled

Table 7-1. Risk factors for and strategies to prevent infection in patients with multiple myeloma.

Risk factor	Pathogen/infection	Prevention/management
Related to the disease		
Hypogammaglobulinemia	Encapsulated bacteria	IVIG (if serum Ig G < 400 mg/dl), TMP–SMX, fluoroquinolones (if not on TMP–SMX), vaccine against *S. pneumoniae*, *H. influenzae* (vaccination rarely protective)
Renal failure	Various	Prevention of conditions that result in renal failure (hypovolemia, drugs, tumor lysis, obstruction, hypercalcemia, others)
Fractures	Discitis, osteomyelitis	Osteolysis inhibitors (clodronate, pamidronate, zoledronate)
Related to its treatment		
Dexamethasone-induced T-cell immunodeficiency	Virus (CMV, HSV, VZV, Influenza), fungi (oral and esophageal candidiasis, *P jiroveci*), tuberculosis	TMP–SMX (*P. jiroveci*), acyclovir (HSV), CMV antigenemia, isoniazid (*M. tuberculosis*) if PPD positive or prior history of tuberculosis, vaccine against Influenza
Iron overload (red blood cells transfusion)	Various	Erythropoietin instead of transfusions, iron chelation (deferoxamine, deferasirox)
Dexamethasone-induced hyperglycemia	Various	Strict control of glycemia
Renal failure	Various	Prevention of conditions that result in renal failure (hypovolemia, drugs, tumor lysis, obstruction, hypercalcemia, others)
Bisphosphonate-induced osteonecrosis of the jaw	Various	Avoid bisphosphonates 3 months before and 3 months after dental surgeryIntensive oral hygiene Early diagnosis (pain, exposed bone)
Deep vein thrombosis	Various	Low-molecular weight heparin, others
Chemo-radiotherapy-induced mucositis	Viridans streptococci (oral), Gram-negative and Gram-positive bacteria, *Candida* spp. (gut)	Amifostine, keratinocyte growth factor, oral/dental hygiene
Chemotherapy-induced prolonged and severe neutropenia	Gram-negative (enterobacteriaceae, *P. aeruginosa*) and Gram-positive (staphylococci, viridans streptococci)	G-CSF, high cell dose (>5 × 10^6 CD34+ cells/kg) in autologous transplant
Exposure to pathogens		
History of infection	Various (e.g., fungal, *P. jiroveci*, tuberculosis, viruses)	Antimicrobial prophylaxis/pre-emptive therapy (e.g., CMV, others)
Colonization with pathogens	Various	Decolonization (e.g., *S. aureus*); specific prophylaxis (e.g., fungi)
Environmental exposure	Respiratory viruses, water-borne or food-borne pathogens, others	Immunizations; patient education and appropriate infection control measures

IVIG Intravenous immunoglobulin; *TMP–SMX* trimethoprim–sulfamethoxazole; *CMV* cytomegalovirus; *HSV* herpes simplex virus; *VZV* varicella–zoster virus; *G-CSF* granulocyte colony-stimulating factor

Table 7-2. Type and pattern of infections among patients with multiple myeloma according to treatment regimen.

Phase of treatment	Regimen	Type and pattern of infection, agent
Induction	MP	Pneumonia, bacteremia (Encapsulated bacteria, *S. aureus*, enterobacteriaceae); higher incidence in the first 2 months after diagnosis of MM
Induction/Relapse	VAD and other Dexamethasone-based regimens	Pneumonia, bacteremia (Encapsulated bacteria, *S. aureus*, enterobacteriaceae), herpes zoster, oral candidiasis; higher incidence in the first 4 months after diagnosis of MM
Induction	MP + Thalidomide	Higher incidence of infection (mostly pneumonia) in elderly patients
Induction/Relapse	Bortezomib	Herpes zoster
Induction/Relapse	Lenalidomide	Higher incidence of neutropenia and neutropenia-related infections
Early after autologous HSCT	Any	Infections associated with neutropenia and mucositis (enterobacteriaceae, *P. aeruginosa*, staphylococci, viridans streptococci)
Late after autologous HSCT		Herpes zoster, CMV reactivation

MP melphalan + oral prednisone; *MM* multiple myeloma; *VAD* vincristina, doxorubicin, dexamethasone; *HSCT* hematopoietic stem cell transplant; *CMV* cytomegalovirus

trial in elderly patients [25], and in a large trial of MM patients receiving more intensive cytotoxic therapies, including tandem autologous HSCT [26]. In addition to an indirect effect on the risk for infection, thalidomide inhibits tumor necrosis factor alpha but stimulates T-cell proliferation with an increase in interleukin-12 [27]. The potential immunosuppressive effect of thalidomide may be illustrated by a case report of disseminated herpes simplex and VZV infection in a myeloma patient who was taking single agent thalidomide for 5 years after an autologous HSCT [28].

Data on infectious complications associated with the use of bortezomib as first line therapy are scarce. Bortezomib is associated with a low incidence of neutropenia. The frequencies of grade III and grade IV neutropenia in a phase II study were 13 and 3%, respectively [29]. In another study, bortezomib was added to MP as primary treatment for 60 MM patients aged ≥65 years [30]. Seventy-five percent of patients developed at least one episode of infection (16% grade III–IV). Of note was the incidence of herpes zoster: 13% in the first 38 patients, and reduced to 7% after the introduction of acyclovir prophylaxis. A low rate of herpes zoster was also observed when prophylactic acyclovir was given to bortezomib recipients in a randomized trial of MP with or without bortezomib [31].

Preliminary data on lenalidomide suggests that neutropenia is relatively common. In a phase II study, lenalidomide and dexamethasone were given to 34 newly diagnosed patients with MM. Grade III–IV neutropenia occurred in 12% of the patients. Granulocyte colony stimulating factor (G-CSF) was given in subsequent courses of treatment if the patient developed neutropenia, and grade III–IV infection occurred in only 3% of patients [32]. In a randomized clinical trial of 445 newly diagnosed MM patients treated with lenalidomide plus two different doses of dexamethasone, grade III–IV neutropenia occurred in 14% of the patients[33]. No increase in viral infection was observed.

2.2. Infection After HSCT

2.2.1. Autologous HSCT

Autologous HSCT may be divided into two risk periods for infection; the first is associated with chemotherapy-induced neutropenia and mucositis, and the second, which begins with the resolution of neutropenia, is related to the slow recovery of T-cell mediated immunity [34]. In the first phase, the incidence and severity of infection is related to the duration of neutropenia which varies according to the conditioning regimen. In general, conditioning regimens that include total body irradiation (TBI) are associated with higher rates of infectious complications [35, 36]. During the neutropenic period, infectious complications are comparable to those seen with other underlying diseases receiving autologous HSCT [37, 38], and consist mainly of bacteremia, pneumonia, soft tissue infection and mucositis-associated gastrointestinal infection. Typical agents of infection are Gram-negative (enterobacteriaceae and *Pseudomonas aeruginosa*) and Gram-positive (staphylococci and viridans streptococci) bacteria. In addition to neutropenia, some myeloma-specific co-morbidities, such as renal failure and iron overload, may increase the risk for infection. In one study, the rate of pneumonia was higher in patients with renal failure than in patients with normal renal function (17% vs. 1%, respectively) [39], while in another study, rates of infection after autologous HSCT were similar, even though mucositis was more frequent and severe in patients with renal failure [40]. Iron overload, associated with multiple transfusions, was associated with aspergillosis in an autopsy study [41], and was an independent risk factor for infection (together with smoking) in another study [42].

Infections associated with T-cell immunodeficiency predominate during the post-engraftment period. T-cell reconstitution occurs slowly and is influenced by the status of the underlying disease, the stem cell manipulation (CD34 positive selection, CD19 negative selection), the conditioning regimen (TBI), and more importantly, the intensity of subsequent MM therapy [34]. Late infections (mostly dermatomal VZV infection) are more likely to occur in MM patients compared to patients who undergo autologous HSCT for other underlying diseases [43]. Besides VZV infection, patients not receiving appropriate prophylaxis are at increased risk to develop *Pneumocystis jiroveci* pneumonia. CMV reactivation may also occur, and may present as fever without other clinical manifestations. In one study, CMV reactivation occurred in 39% of 41 CMV seropositive patients who presented with non-neutropenic fever after autologous HSCT [9]. The increased risk for late infections in myeloma patients is likely the result of a combination of intensive conditioning regimens and extensive pre-transplant induction therapy with regimens containing high-dose dexamethasone.

2.2.2. *Allogeneic HSCT*

The use of allogeneic HSCT with myeloablative conditioning regimen in MM is associated with a high rate of complications, with transplant-related mortality (TRM) exceeding 40%. The main cause of death is infection (bacteremia, fungal infections and interstitial pneumonia) [44]. By contrast, non-myeloablative HSCT was associated with lower TRM (10%) in a series of 31 patients with MM treated at a single center [45]. More recently, in a randomized trial in patients with newly diagnosed MM, double autologous HSCT followed by allogeneic HSCT showed a slightly higher TRM rate compared with allogeneic HSCT alone (10% vs. 2%), but the difference was not statistically significant [46]. The spectrum of infections after allogeneic HSCT in patients with MM is not different from infections in allogeneic HSCT overall, and a detailed description of these complications is discussed in Chap. 8.

2.3. Infections After Consolidation and Maintenance: Total Therapy and Other Intensive Therapy Approaches

A Total Therapy MM treatment protocol consisting of induction chemotherapy, consolidation with one or two HSCT, and post-transplant maintenance therapy prolonged event-free and overall survival in a non-randomized comparison with historical controls [47]. However, as expected, the frequency of infections was higher. In the Total Therapy I protocol, bacteremia or pneumonia occurred in 17% after VAD; in 28% after high-dose cyclophosphamide; in 11% after EDAP protocol (etoposide, dexamethasone, cytarabine and cisplatin) induction chemotherapies; in 25% after the first autologous HSCT; in 31% after the second autologous HSCT given without TBI; and in 40% after the second HSCT given with TBI [48].

In a randomized study, the use of post-transplant maintenance dexamethasone was associated with higher rates of infection when compared with no maintenance (40% vs. 27%, $p = 0.02$) [21]. Thalidomide maintenance was evaluated in a three-arm randomized trial comparing pamidronate plus thalidomide, to pamidronate alone, or to no therapy. While neutropenia was more frequent among thalidomide recipients (6% vs. 2% and 0%, respectively), the frequencies of overall infections were similar (6%, 7% and 4%, respectively) [49].

2.4. Infections After Salvage Therapy

Different salvage regimens have been given to patients with MM who have had a relapse or disease progression after the completion of induction chemotherapy with or without autologous HSCT. The rates of infectious complications tend to be higher with salvage therapy because of the presence of severe organ dysfunction that is associated with advanced myeloma disease. In addition to the risks of the chemotherapeutic regimen itself (the intensity and duration of neutropenia and mucositis), the risk of infection after salvage therapy depends on other factors as well, such as the extent and intensity of prior therapy (including the dose and duration of corticosteroids), control of MM, and other co-morbidities which tend to worsen with myeloma progression.

Bortezomib has been increasingly used as salvage therapy in MM. In a randomized study comparing bortezomib with dexamethasone for relapsed MM, grade III and IV neutropenia occurred more frequently (12 and 2%, respectively) with bortezomib [10]. An unexpected finding of this study was the 13% incidence of herpes zoster infection in patients receiving bortezomib compared to 2% in patients receiving dexamethasone. A similar rate of herpes zoster infection was observed in 38 elderly MM patients who received bortezomib, melphalan, and prednisone as primary therapy [30] Bortezomib exerts potent immunosuppressive effects on T-cells [50–55], and its use increases the risk for infection due to *Varicella zoster* virus, and possibly other infections associated with T-cell mediated immunodeficiency.

The use of lenalidomide in relapsed or refractory patients is associated with a higher incidence of neutropenia, compared to lenalidomide use in newly diagnosed MM patients. In a randomized study comparing dexamethasone plus lenalidomide or dexamethasone plus placebo, grade III–IV neutropenia occurred in 16.5% of patients in the lenalidomide arm and only 1.2% in the placebo arm. However, grade III–IV infections occurred with similar frequencies in both arms [56]. In another study, 102 relapsed/refractory MM patients were randomized to receive oral lenalidomide at a dose of 30 mg once-daily or 15 mg twice-daily every 28 days. Grade III–IV neutropenia was observed in 69 and 61% of patients in each group (the difference not statistically significant), but the time to first clinically significant Grade III–IV myelosuppression was shorter in the patients receiving the twice-daily dose of 15 mg[57].

3. Changing Spectrum of Infections in Multiple Myeloma

In recent years, a significant change in the spectrum of infections in patients with MM has been reported, with an increase in severe fungal infections, such as aspergillosis and fusariosis [11]. Although speculative, it is possible that this is a reaction to an increase in the intensity of treatment of MM, with sequential chemotherapeutic strategies coupled with double transplants and post-transplant maintenance, rendering these patients functionally neutropenic and immune suppressed for prolonged periods of time.

In a recent study of invasive aspergillosis after HSCT, late onset aspergillosis (occurring after day +30) was increasingly observed. Patients with MM were at higher risk to develop late aspergillosis by multivariate analysis, with a 4.5 greater risk compared to patients with chronic myeloid leukemia in the chronic phase [58]. This finding was unexpected because MM is not a hematological malignancy classically associated with invasive aspergillosis [59]. That the risk for aspergillosis in patients with MM may be increasing is illustrated by the observation that among the 31 cases of invasive aspergillosis occurring in non-HSCT recipients reported from 15 European centers, eight cases were diagnosed between 1984 and 1991, compared to 23 cases between 1992 and 1996. Neutropenia was present in 51% of patients with aspergillosis with a median duration of neutropenia before the diagnosis of 19 days. Forty-five percent of patients had received high doses of corticosteroids within 1 month before diagnosis, and 36% had received high doses of melphalan. All non-neutropenic patients were on corticosteroids at the time of the diagnosis of aspergillosis [60].

In an autopsy study of 69 cases of MM, 38 deaths were attributed to infection. In 21 of these 38 deaths, a mould infection was diagnosed (20/21 aspergillosis), with a 45% incidence in autopsied MM patients after allogeneic HSCT (nine of 20 cases), 21% after autologous HSCT, and 25% after receiving chemotherapy [11]. In another study describing the incidence and characteristics of non-*Aspergillus* mould infections in HSCT, MM was associated with a 6.9 higher risk for the development of fusariosis compared to other underlying hematological malignancies [12].

4. Approach to Infection in MM

4.1. Infections at Diagnosis and During Induction Therapy

4.1.1. Risk Assessment and Prevention (Table 7-1)

Risk assessment for newly diagnosed patients should include past medical history, with emphasis on prior infections that may recur (tuberculosis, herpes simplex (HSV), VZV, CMV, chronic sinusitis, endemic fungi), assessment of co-morbidities (renal function, iron overload), and serology (herpes simplex, VZV, CMV). For patients from areas endemic to tuberculosis, a tuberculin skin test should also be performed before starting induction therapy [61]. Serum levels of immunoglobulins should be obtained both for future comparisons, and for identifying patients with IgG levels <600 mg/dl who may benefit from antibacterial prophylaxis.

Most of the recommendations for prophylaxis in MM patients are inferential, and lack strong scientific support from randomized clinical trials. The decision to offer prophylaxis and the appropriate prophylactic regimens depend on the induction regimen and, importantly, on whether or not the patient will receive dexamethasone or other corticosteroids. All patients with MM, including those recently diagnosed and those receiving induction without dexamethasone, are at increased risk for bacterial infections because of deficiencies in humoral immunity. In addition, the use of high doses of dexamethasone is associated with T-cell mediated immunodeficiency besides rendering patients at increased risk for viral and fungal infections. Patients treated with corticosteroid-containing induction regimens should receive prophylaxis against *P. jiroveci* pneumonia with trimethoprim–sulfamethoxazole (TMP–SMX – 800 mg/160 mg per day). Alternative regimens, such as aerosolized pentamidine (150 mg every 2 weeks or 300 mg/month) or dapsone (100 mg/day) may be used, but they are associated with more breakthrough infections than TMP/SMX [62]. Antiviral prophylaxis against HSV and /or VZV (acyclovir 400 mg TID, valacyclovir 500 mg TID or famciclovir 500 mg TID) may be used if the patient is seropositive for HSV or, importantly, presents a history of recurrent fever blisters, cold sores, or other indications of recurrent HSV infections, especially if the CD4 counts are low (<50/mm^3). However, the benefit of prophylaxis must be weighted against the cost, toxicity, and the potential for resistance [63]. The same is true for mucosal candidiasis, which occurs frequently in patients receiving dexamethasone, especially after a course of broad-spectrum antibiotics. Although primary prophylaxis (fluconazole 100 mg/day) is effective, there is the danger that prolonged exposure to fluconazole will lead to replacement of the sensitive *Candida albicans* colonizing the GI tract and skin with fluconazole resistant *Candida* species. An alternative is to monitor closely and to treat appropriately with fluconazole (200 mg daily for 7–14 days) if oral and/or esophageal candidiasis develops. Patients with a past history of tuberculosis (or a positive tuberculin test) should receive isoniazid (500 mg daily) or alternative regimens [64].

Intravenous immunoglobulin (400 mg/kg) every 4 weeks may be effective for the prevention of bacterial infections, and this recommendation is supported by a randomized controlled study [65]. However, since its use is costly, intravenous immunoglobulin should be reserved for the population of patients with repeated episodes of severe infections. A cheaper alternative to immunoglobulin is quinolone prophylaxis with levofloxacin (500 mg/day), moxifloxacin (400 mg/day), or TMP–SMX [66]. Routine vaccination against *S. pneumoniae*, *H. influenzae* and influenza has been advised, but response rates to vaccination may be very low [67].

4.1.2. Management of Infections (Fig. 7-1)

Fever in MM patients must be considered as caused by infection until proven otherwise. However, in occasional patients, especially those with relapsed or advanced disease, fever may be caused by MM disease itself. These patients usually have obvious signs of active MM, sometimes with extramedullary plasmacytoma or pancytopenia secondary to massive bone marrow infiltration by

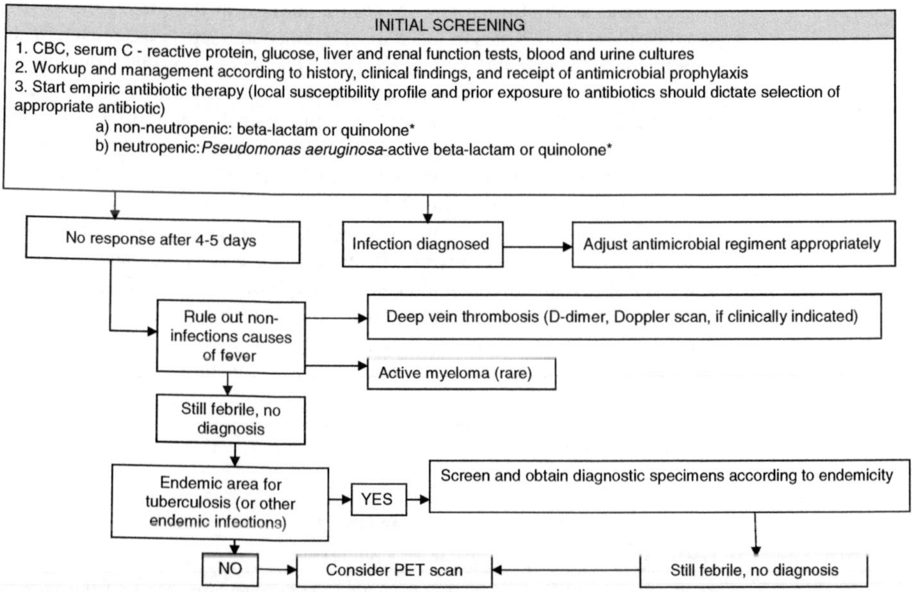

CBC = complete blood counts; CMV = cytomegalovirus; PCR = polymerase chain reaction;*levofloxacin (500 -750 mg/d PO) or moxifloxacin (400 mg/d PO); PET = positron emission tomography

HSV = Herpes simplex virus; VZV = Varicella-zoster virus; *Valaciclovir (500 mg PO TID) or famciclovir (500 mg PO TID); ** Acyclovir (400 mg PO 5x/d) or valaciclovir (1 g PO TID); TMP-SMX = trimethoprim-sulfamethoxazole; ***Moxifloxacin (400 mg/d PO); CMV = cytomegalovirus; PCR = polimerase chain reaction

Fig. 7-1. Initial management of fever in myeloma patients receiving induction therapy.

plasma cells. Nevertheless, every febrile patient must be screened for infection and treated appropriately. This includes an understanding of the most frequent pathogens associated with that particular phase of MM disease and its treatment, as well as the appropriate use of empirical antimicrobial therapy. All these actions must be guided by an assessment of the risks of specific infections, taking into account the medical history (past history of recurrent infections such as aspergillosis, tuberculosis, sinusitis, reactivated latent herpes infections, contact with patients with tuberculosis, geographic origin of the patient), co-morbidities (renal failure, chronic pulmonary disease or sinusitis, fractures, deep vein thrombosis), and past and current treatment for MM.

Infections in newly diagnosed patients and in those receiving induction therapy are usually caused by encapsulated bacteria, *Staphylococcus aureus* and Gram-negative bacilli, and the airways, the urinary tract, and the bloodstream are the most frequent sites of infections. Therefore, the workup of fever must include a search for respiratory tract infections, including a chest X-ray (and computed tomography [CT] scans if the X-ray is non-informative), a sinus CT scan, blood and urine cultures, C-reactive proteins, complete blood counts, and liver enzyme tests. If the initial tests are negative, non-infectious causes of fever, such as deep vein thrombosis (very frequent in MM patients [68, 69]) must be ruled out. In addition, depending on the number of cycles of dexamethasone received and other past medical history, tuberculosis (especially in endemic areas) is another possibility that should be ruled out.

Empirical antibiotic therapy should be initiated at the same time as the diagnostic workup because the risk of rapid, fatal sepsis associated with *Streptococcus pneumoniae* is high [70]. The choice of the appropriate antibacterial agent depends on the local rates of penicillin-resistant pneumococci, as well as on the patient's general clinical condition. Reasonable options for ambulatory patients include cefuroxime, semi-synthetic penicillins with beta-lactamase inhibitors (amoxacillin/clavulanate, amoxacillin/sulbactam or ampicillin/sulbactam), quinolones with good activities against streptococci (levofloxacin or moxifloxacin), and macrolides (erythromycin, azithromycin and clarithromycin). If resistance is a concern, vancomycin or linezolid are good options. Patients requiring hospitalization should receive broad-spectrum betalactam antibiotics. Empirical therapy is also indicated for febrile neutropenic patients. Because induction therapy of MM is seldom associated with severe and prolonged neutropenia, oral empirical therapy with a broad spectrum quinolone such as moxifloxacin or levofloxacin (but not ciprofloxacin which lacks potent anti-streptococcal activity) is an acceptable choice [71].

4.2. Infections During Autologous HSCT

4.2.1. Risk Assessment and Prevention

Risk assessment before autologous HSCT must take into account the factors that increase the risk of infection, as well as those associated with severe complications and death from infection (Table 7-3). Prophylaxis during the neutropenic phase of autologous HSCT for low-risk patients is not different from that for other diseases. In most instances, the transplant is performed in an outpatient setting, and the patient receives prophylaxis against HSV (acyclovir 250 mg/m^2 IV TID or 400 mg PO TID, valacyclovir 500 mg TID or

Table 7-3. Risk assessment of infection in patients with multiple myeloma prior to autologous hematopoietic stem cell transplantation.

Factor	Low risk	High risk
Extent of prior therapy	Minimal	Extensive, including prior transplant
Status of myeloma	Remission	Progressive disease
Conditioning regimen	Melphalan	Melphalan-total-body-irradiation-based-regimens
In vitro manipulation of stem cells	No	CD34 selection
Cell dose	≥5 × 10^6 CD34/kg	<2 × 10^6 CD34/kg
Co-morbidities	None	Smoking, iron overload, poor performance status, organ dysfunction (renal failure, particularly hemodialysis, cardiac disease, liver dis ease), bone fractures

famciclovir 500 mg TID) and G-CSF (5 μg/kg/day SC) to accelerate neutrophil recovery. Prophylaxis for chemotherapy-induced mucositis includes the use of amifostine [72] and keratinocyte growth factor (palifermin) [73]. Antibacterial prophylaxis with quinolones may be also given, especially if the frequency of Gram-negative bacteremia is high. However, close monitoring for the potential of induction of resistance is mandatory. Antifungal prophylaxis with fluconazole 200–400 mg/day PO is not universally recommended, but should be considered in patients who develop severe mucositis. In high-risk patients (HSCT performed after repeated courses of chemotherapy, second HSCT), special attention should be given to the occasional occurrence of a systemic fungal infection, such as aspergillosis, zygomycosis or fusariosis. In this situation, one may consider obtaining *Aspergillus* antigenemia twice weekly and / or PCR, serum beta-glucan, and giving fluconazole prophylaxis or a mould-active prophylactic agent (posaconazole 200 mg PO TID, voriconazole 200 mg BID PO, micafungin 50 mg/day IV, lipid amphotericin B 3 mg/kg/day IV).

4.2.2. Fever During Neutropenia

Immediately after autologous HSCT, the patient becomes neutropenic and usually develops fever. The management of fever in MM patients is similar to that in other autologous transplant recipients. The choice of the antibiotic regimen for febrile neutropenia must be guided by the local epidemiology and the past history of colonization and / or infection due to resistant organisms. With an adequate cell dose (>5 × 10^6 CD34+ cells/kg), bone marrow recovery occurs by the 10–11th day of transplant, with a median duration of neutropenia of 7 days.

4.2.3. Infections After Bone Marrow Recovery of an Autologous HSCT (Fig. 7-2)

4.2.3.1. Fever of Unknown Origin

After bone marrow recovery of autologous HSCT, T-cell immunodeficiency predominates, and its intensity depends largely on the type of additional therapies used for the treatment of MM. This is a distinguishing feature of

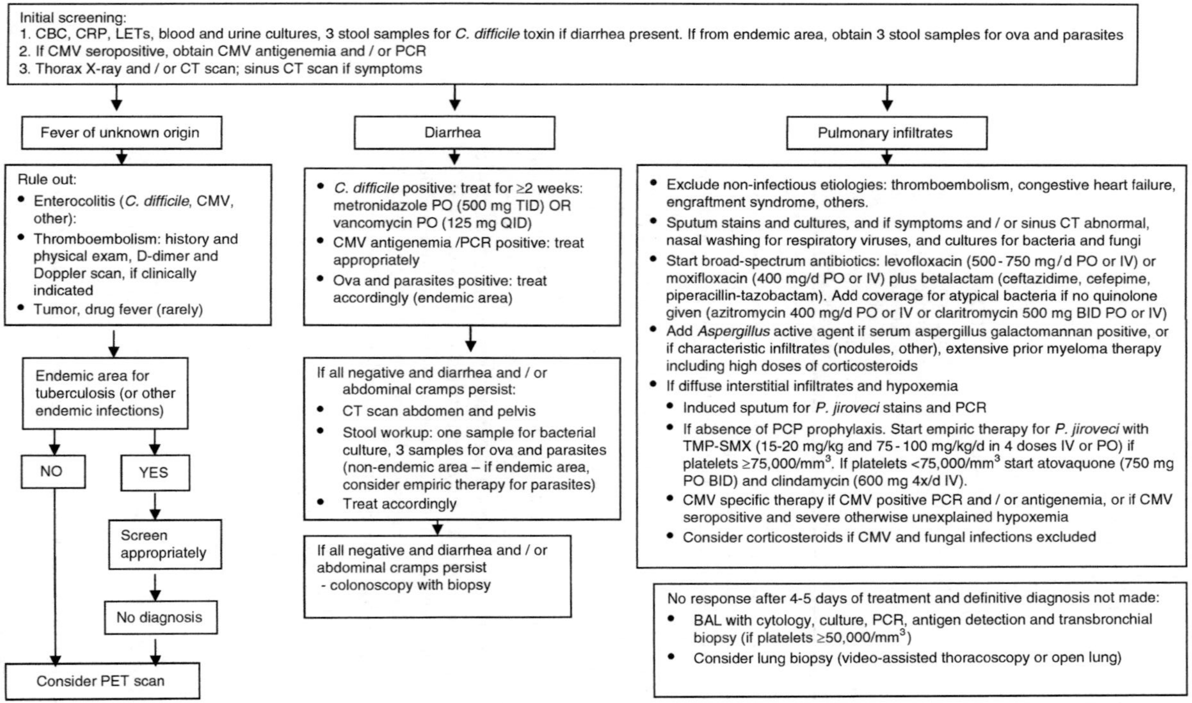

CBC = complete blood counts; CRP = C-reactive protein; LFTs = liver function tests; CMV = cytomegalovirus; PCR = polymerase chain reaction; PET = positron emission tomography

Fig. 7-2. Initial management of myeloma patients with suspected infection after autologous HSCT.

MM when compared with other diseases such as lymphomas or leukemia. Therefore, in addition to the common pathogens (encapsulated bacteria and enterobacteriaceae), the workup of fever must include CMV antigenemia or PCR for those who are seropositive because CMV reactivation may be the cause of fever. In a retrospective study that analyzed fever after bone marrow recovery from autologous HSCT in different underlying diseases (mostly MM and lymphoma), CMV antigenemia was positive in 39% of 41 seropositive patients, and appropriate anti-CMV therapy resulted in the resolution of fever in all but two patients [9]. If CMV antigenemia (and / or PCR) is positive, a course of anti-CMV treatment is recommended (gancyclovir 5 mg/kg BID, or valganciclovir 900 mg daily or foscarnet 60 mg/kg BID for 2 weeks).

Because occasional patients with *Clostridium difficile*-associated diarrhea may present with fever before overt diarrhea is manifested (especially if accompanied by abdominal cramps) [74], stool samples should be screened for the presence of toxin A and B [75]. If positive, metronidazole (500 mg TID PO for 10–14 days) or vancomycin (125 mg PO QID for 10–14 days) should be given.

If all the tests are negative, non-infectious causes of fever, such as deep vein thrombosis and active MM should be investigated (serum D-dimer and Doppler ultrasonography, if clinically indicated). If a cause of fever is still not reveaed, other tests, such as CT scan (head, thorax and abdomen) or a positron emission tomography (PET) may be helpful in selected patients. PET may diagnose occult infection that is not evident from other image exams, particularly in a patient with MM, a disease in which neoplastic lung involvement is exceedingly rare [76–78]. In a study in 1,100 MM patients who had at least one PET performed, infection was present in 20 of 125 patients (16%) with no clinical manifestations of infection, as well as in all 49 patients whose PET was performed as part of the workup for infection, and in 74 patients with the signs and symptoms present at the time of PET but whose PET was performed for the staging of MM. The sites of infection were the respiratory tract (99 episodes), bone, joint and soft tissues (26 episodes), the vascular system (18 episodes), the gastrointestinal tract (12 episodes), and dentition (10 episodes) [79].

4.2.3.2. Diarrhea

Diarrhea is frequent in the neutropenic phase following autologous HSCT, and may have different causes, both infectious and non-infectious. In addition, diarrhea may occur after bone marrow recovery. Infectious causes in this period include *Clostridium difficile*-associated diarrhea, viral diseases (CMV, adenovirus, rotavirus, calicivirus, others) and parasitic diseases (strongyloidiasis [80], cryptosporidiosis [81], and others). The workup for patients with diarrhea in the post-engraftment period must include non-specific tests such as C-reactive proteins, complete blood counts and liver enzyme tests, as well as CMV antigenemia and / or PCR (in CMV seropositive patients), and stool screening for *Clostridium difficile* toxins A and B. In the case of unrevealing and persistent diarrhea, stool examination for ova and parasites, stool cultures for bacteria, and stool and serum tests for viruses (culture, PCR, enzyme immunoassay, others) and *Strongyloides stercoralis* [82] should be performed. If all the tests are negative and diarrhea is still present, colonoscopy with biopsy is indicated.

4.2.3.3. Pulmonary Infiltrates

After bone marrow recovery from autologous HSCT, the spectrum of pathogens causing pneumonia is much broader, and includes bacteria (Gram positive, Gram-negative, *Legionella*, *Nocardia*), viruses (CMV, respiratory syncytial virus [RSV], influenza, and parainfluenza viruses), fungi (especially *Aspergillus*, but also other moulds, such as *Fusarium*, Zygomycetes and *Scedosporium*), mycobacteria, and rarely parasites (*Strongyloides stercoralis*, *Toxoplasma gondii*). These infections are more likely to occur in patients with severe T-cell immunodeficiency, typically after intensive and prolonged periods of treatment, including two or more HSCT. In addition, non-infections causes of pneumonia, such as engraftment syndrome [83], conditioning-induced pneumonitis, and pulmonary embolism, may be present. The patient's medical history must detail his/her exposure (contact with patients with tuberculosis or respiratory viral infection, contact with dust or constructions), travel (to areas endemic to specific pathogens), and a latent infection that may recur (tuberculosis, aspergillosis, toxoplasmosis, CMV). In addition, the timing of the appearance of pulmonary manifestations is important because some conditions occur specifically in certain periods, such as the engraftment syndrome that usually occurs within 10 days from neutrophils engraftment [83].

The initial workup for patients with pulmonary infiltrates and / or hypoxemia in the post-engraftment period may include non-specific tests such as C-reactive proteins, complete blood counts, and liver enzyme tests, as well as pathogen-specific testing such as CMV antigenemia and / or PCR (in CMV seropositive patients), *Aspergillus* antigenemia or PCR, and 1-3 beta-D-glucan. In addition, a thorax X-ray should be obtained, and if the X-ray is normal or shows discrete abnormalities, a CT scan is mandatory.

The pattern of pulmonary infiltrates helps to define the additional tests that are needed. Because non-cardiogenic pulmonary edema is a relatively common cause of diffuse pulmonary infiltrates, the physician should rule out fluid overload (and give diuretics) before ordering additional tests. If this is not the case, additional investigation should include: (a) a nasal wash with culture, PCR and / or antigen detection for viruses; (b) bronchoalveolar lavage with cytology, Gomori methenamine-silver or alternative stains for *P. jiroveci*, Gram stain, cultures for bacteria, viruses, fungi and mycobacteria, immunofluorescence for *Legionella*, and PCR for virus and mycobacteria. The performance of transbronchial biopsy depends on the platelet counts (usually safe if the platelet counts are >50,000/mm^3). If all the tests are negative, a non-infectious cause of diffuse pulmonary infiltrates should be considered (chemo and / or radiotherapy, lung injury, engraftment syndrome, pulmonary embolism). In the case of engraftment syndrome or lung toxicity of cancer treatment, the physician should consider giving a course of intravenous corticosteroids (methylprednisolone 0.5–1.0 g daily for 3 days). The next step, if this extensive evaluation fails to identify a cause, may be a second broncho-alveolar lavage or an open lung biopsy, depending on the patient's clinical condition.

Empiric antibiotic therapy is usually indicated, especially if the patient is hypoxemic. If the pneumonia is likely community-acquired, and the patient is not hypoxemic, the coverage for respiratory pathogens common in outpatients (*Streptococcus pneumoniae* and *Haemophylus influenzae*) is enough (cefuroxime, a semi-synthetic penicillin associated with betalactamase inhibitors, newer quinolones or macrolides). In hospital-acquired pneumonia, empiric therapy should include broad-spectrum antibiotics for bacteria potentially resistant to usual first-line outpatient antibiotics. In addition, if the patient is hypoxemic, empiric treatment-dose TMP–SMX (especially if the prophylactic regimen for *P. jiroveci* was pentamidine or dapsone), or ganciclovir (if the patient is seropositive for CMV) may be considered in selected patients pending further diagnostic evaluation.

Workup for patients with localized pulmonary infiltrates includes sputum analysis (cytology, culture), but interpretation may be difficult because positive cultures may represent colonization of the oropharynx. Empiric antibiotic therapy targeting encapsulated bacteria is indicated, but if the patient is hospitalized, broad-spectrum coverage is needed to cover hospital-acquired pathogens. If the patient does not respond to treatment, bronchoalveolar lavage is indicated (cytology, Gram stain, cultures for bacteria, viruses, fungi and mycobacteria, immunofluorescence for *Legionella*, PCR for virus and mycobacteria). Some additional tests may be necessary, depending on the other characteristics of the preliminary exams. Patients with nodular lesions (especially with a halo sign) should have serum galactomannan or 1-3 beta-D-glucan tests, because invasive aspergillosis (or other mould infection) may be the cause. This diagnosis must be specially considered if the patient has received more than one transplant, has been on prolonged use of corticosteroids, or has received a transplant with stem cell manipulation (positive or negative selection). If all the tests are negative, a pulmonary biopsy should be undertaken.

4.3. Prophylactic Measures to Reduce the Impact of Co–morbidities on the Risk of Infection

Every effort should be made to avoid conditions that may worsen or cause renal failure, such as dehydration and hypercalcemia. Patients should be encouraged to quit smoking [42]. Likewise, iron overload should be minimized by avoiding unnecessary red blood cell transfusions, giving erythropoietin to control anemia, and giving chelating agents (subcutaneous deferoxamine or oral deferiprone or deferasirox), if significant iron overload is present [84]. Other measures include the use of bisphosphonates (clodronate, pamidronate or zoledronate) to reduce the risk of bone fractures, strict control of glucose metabolism during treatment with corticosteroids, and low-molecular weight heparin for patients at high risk for deep vein thrombosis.

5. Special Considerations

Infection in patients with MM represents a great challenge to physicians. A broad list of pathogens may cause infection, including Gram-negative and Gram-positive bacteria, fungi, viruses and parasites. In addition, the signs and symptoms of infection may be masked by manifestations of the underlying disease or its complications. On the other hand, the pathogens causing infection may vary over time, because severe immunodeficiency tends to develop as the disease progresses, and the patient receives different courses of treatment. In this context, the physician must be alert to the possibility of infection due to uncommon pathogens, as well as to the recurrence of infection.

Patients with MM may require prolonged courses of treatment for specific infections because of organ damage caused by the disease, such as bone fractures, bed restriction and renal failure. This is the case for bacteremia due to *Staphylococcus aureus* and other microorganisms with high potential to complicate with septic emboli. In these situations, the duration of treatment may be prolonged to 4–6 weeks. Likewise, in the choice of particular antimicrobial agents, the physician should consider the potential for additional toxicity to the kidneys, as well as drug–drug interactions (P450 competitors or inducers which may interfere with metabolism of corticosteroids, thalidomide, bortezomib, and drugs that prolong the QT interval). Finally, the physician should be familiar with new diagnostic tools (such as PET scan) that may help to discriminate between infectious and non-infectious complications.

6. Conclusions

Infections represent a major problem in patients with MM. Changes in the spectrum of infections parallel changes in the way MM is treated. A practical approach to infections in MM patients must include the recognition of the likely pathogens, depending on several factors, such as past medical history, status of the underlying disease, and past and current treatment for MM. Specific strategies of diagnosis, prophylaxis, and empiric and specific therapy are driven according to this approach

References

1. Augustson BM, Begum G, Dunn JA et al (2005) Early mortality after diagnosis of multiple myeloma: analysis of patients entered into the United kingdom Medical Research Council trials between 1980 and 2002 – Medical Research Council Adult Leukaemia Working Party. J Clin Oncol 23(36):9219–9226
2. Kapadia SB (1980) Multiple myeloma: a clinicopathologic study of 62 consecutively autopsied cases. Medicine (Baltimore) 59(5):380–392
3. Kyle RA (1975) Multiple myeloma: review of 869 cases. Mayo Clin Proc 50(1): 29–40
4. Oshima K, Kanda Y, Nannya Y et al (2001) Clinical and pathologic findings in 52 consecutively autopsied cases with multiple myeloma. Am J Hematol 67(1): 1–5
5. Kraut EH, Sagone AL Jr (1981) Alternative pathway of complement in multiple myeloma. Am J Hematol 11(4):335–345
6. Prabhala RH, Neri P, Bae JE et al (2006) Dysfunctional T regulatory cells in multiple myeloma. Blood 107(1):301–304
7. King K (1980) Septicaemia in patients with haematological malignant disease. Med J Aust 1(12):603–606
8. Saba HI, Hartmann RC, Herion JC (1979) Hemophilus influenzae septicemia and polyarthritis in multiple myeloma. South Med J 72(6):743–746
9. Fassas AB, Bolanos-Meade J, Buddharaju LN et al (2001) Cytomegalovirus infection and non-neutropenic fever after autologous stem cell transplantation: high rates of reactivation in patients with multiple myeloma and lymphoma. Br J Haematol 112(1):237–241
10. Richardson PG, Sonneveld P, Schuster MW et al (2005) Bortezomib or high-dose dexamethasone for relapsed multiple myeloma. N Engl J Med 352(24): 2487–2498

11. Koneru B, Hough A, Fassas A et al (1007) Autopsy review in multiple myeloma reveals aspergillosis as a significant cause of death after high dose therapy especially with allo-transplants. Blood 90(Suppl 1):353a. doi:353a abstract 1573
12. Marr KA, Carter RA, Crippa F, Wald A, Corey L (2002) Epidemiology and outcome of mould infections in hematopoietic stem cell transplant recipients. Clin Infect Dis 34(7):909–917
13. Perri RT, Hebbel RP, Oken MM (1981) Influence of treatment and response status on infection risk in multiple myeloma. Am J Med 71(6):935–940
14. Espersen F, Birgens HS, Hertz JB, Drivsholm A (1984) Current patterns of bacterial infection in myelomatosis. Scand J Infect Dis 16(2):169–173
15. Rayner HC, Haynes AP, Thompson JR, Russell N, Fletcher J (1991) Perspectives in multiple myeloma: survival, prognostic factors and disease complications in a single centre between 1975 and 1988. Q J Med 79(290):517–525
16. Savage DG, Lindenbaum J, Garrett TJ (1982) Biphasic pattern of bacterial infection in multiple myeloma. Ann Intern Med 96(1):47–50
17. Shaikh BS, Lombard RM, Appelbaum PC, Bentz MS (1982) Changing patterns of infections in patients with multiple myeloma. Oncology 39(2):78–82
18. Facon T, Mary JY, Pegourie B et al (2005) Dexamethasone-based regimens versus melphalan-prednisone for elderly multiple myeloma patients ineligible for high-dose therapy. Blood 107(4):1292–1298
19. Hernandez JM, Garcia-Sanz R, Golvano E et al (2004) Randomized comparison of dexamethasone combined with melphalan versus melphalan with prednisone in the treatment of elderly patients with multiple myeloma. Br J Haematol 127(2):159–164
20. Palumbo A, Bringhen S, Caravita T et al (2006) Oral melphalan and prednisone chemotherapy plus thalidomide compared with melphalan and prednisone alone in elderly patients with multiple myeloma: randomised controlled trial. Lancet 367(9513):825–831
21. Shustik C, Belch A, Robinson S et al (2007) A randomised comparison of melphalan with prednisone or dexamethasone as induction therapy and dexamethasone or observation as maintenance therapy in multiple myeloma: NCIC CTG MY.7. Br J Haematol 136(2):203–211
22. Anderson H, Scarffe JH, Lambert M et al (1987) VAD chemotherapy – toxicity and efficacy – in patients with multiple myeloma and other lymphoid malignancies. Hematol Oncol 5(3):213–222
23. Cesana C, Nosari AM, Klersy C et al (2003) Risk factors for the development of bacterial infections in multiple myeloma treated with two different vincristine-adriamycin-dexamethasone schedules. Haematologica 88(9):1022–1028
24. Rajkumar SV, Kyle RA (2005) Multiple myeloma: diagnosis and treatment. Mayo Clin Proc 80(10):1371–1382
25. Facon T, Mary JY, Hulin C et al (2007) Melphalan and prednisone plus thalidomide versus melphalan and prednisone alone or reduced-intensity autologous stem cell transplantation in elderly patients with multiple myeloma (IFM 99–06): a randomised trial. Lancet 370(9594):1209–1218
26. Barlogie B, Tricot G, Anaissie E et al (2006) Thalidomide and hematopoietic-cell transplantation for multiple myeloma1230. N Engl J Med 354(10):1021–1030
27. Corral LG, Kaplan G (1999) Immunomodulation by thalidomide and thalidomide analogues. Ann Rheum Dis 58(Suppl 1):I107–I113
28. Curley MJ, Hussein SA, Hassoun PM (2002) Disseminated herpes simplex virus and varicella zoster virus coinfection in a patient taking thalidomide for relapsed multiple myeloma. J Clin Microbiol 40(6):2302–2304
29. Jagannath S, Barlogie B, Berenson J et al (2004) A phase 2 study of two doses of bortezomib in relapsed or refractory myeloma. Br J Haematol 127(2):165–172
30. Mateos MV, Hernandez JM, Hernandez MT et al (2006) Bortezomib plus melphalan and prednisone in elderly untreated patients with multiple myeloma: results of a multicenter phase I/II study. Blood 108(7):2165–2172

31. San Miguel J, Schlag R, Khuageva N et al (2007) A phase 3 study comparing bortezomib-melphalan-prednisone (VMP) with melphalan-prednisone (MP) in newly diagnosed multiple myeloma. Blood 110(11):31a
32. Rajkumar SV, Hayman SR, Lacy MQ et al (2005) Combination therapy with lenalidomide plus dexamethasone (REV/DEX) for newly diagnosed myeloma. Blood 106(13):4050–4053
33. Rajkumar SV, Jacobus S, Callander N et al (2007) A randomized trial of lenalidomide plus high-dose dexamethasone (RD) versus lenalidomide plus low-dose dexamethasone (Rd) in newly diagnosed multiple myeloma. Blood 110(11):30a
34. Anaissie E, Nucci M (2003) Risks and epidemiology of infections after autologous stem cell transplantation. In: Bowden RA, Ljungman P, Paya CV (eds) Transplant infections. Lippincott Williams & Wilkins, Philadelphia, pp 39–50
35. Moreau P, Facon T, Attal M et al (2002) Comparison of 200 mg/m(2) melphalan and 8 Gy total body irradiation plus 140 mg/m(2) melphalan as conditioning regimens for peripheral blood stem cell transplantation in patients with newly diagnosed multiple myeloma: final analysis of the Intergroupe Francophone du Myelome 9502 randomized trial. Blood 99(3):731–735
36. Abraham R, Chen C, Tsang R et al (1999) Intensification of the stem cell transplant induction regimen results in increased treatment-related mortality without improved outcome in multiple myeloma. Bone Marrow Transplant 24(12): 1291–1297
37. Auner HW, Sill H, Mulabecirovic A, Linkesch W, Krause R (2002) Infectious complications after autologous hematopoietic stem cell transplantation: comparison of patients with acute myeloid leukemia, malignant lymphoma, and multiple myeloma. Ann Hematol 81(7):374–377
38. Reich G, Mapara MY, Reichardt P, Dorken B, Maschmeyer G (2001) Infectious complications after high-dose chemotherapy and autologous stem cell transplantation: comparison between patients with lymphoma or multiple myeloma and patients with solid tumors. Bone Marrow Transplant 27(5):525–529
39. Knudsen LM, Nielsen B, Gimsing P, Geisler C (2005) Autologous stem cell transplantation in multiple myeloma: outcome in patients with renal failure. Eur J Haematol 75(1):27–33
40. Carlson K (2005) Melphalan 200 mg/m2 with blood stem cell support as first-line myeloma therapy: impact of glomerular filtration rate on engraftment, transplantation-related toxicity and survival. Bone Marrow Transplant 35(10):985–990
41. Altes A, Remacha AF, Sarda P et al (2004) Frequent severe liver iron overload after stem cell transplantation and its possible association with invasive aspergillosis. Bone Marrow Transplant 34(6):505–509
42. Miceli MH, Dong L, Grazziutti ML et al (2006) Iron overload is a major risk factor for severe infection after autologous stem cell transplantation: a study of 367 myeloma patients. Bone Marrow Transplant 37(9):857–864
43. Ketterer N, Espinouse D, Chomarat M et al (1999) Infections following peripheral blood progenitor cell transplantation for lymphoproliferative malignancies: etiology and potential risk factors. Am J Med 106(2):191–197
44. San Miguel JF, Blade CJ, Garcia-Sanz R (1999) Treatment of multiple myeloma. Haematologica 84(1):36–58
45. Badros A, Barlogie B, Siegel E et al (2002) Improved outcome of allogeneic transplantation in high-risk multiple myeloma patients after nonmyeloablative conditioning. J Clin Oncol 20(5):1295–1303
46. Bruno B, Rotta M, Patriarca F et al (2007) A comparison of allografting with autografting for newly diagnosed myeloma. N Engl J Med 356(11):1110–1120
47. Barlogie B, Shaughnessy J, Tricot G et al (2004) Treatment of multiple myeloma. Blood 103(1):20–32
48. Barlogie B, Jagannath S, Desikan KR et al (1999) Total therapy with tandem transplants for newly diagnosed multiple myeloma. Blood 93(1):55–65

49. Attal M, Harousseau JL, Leyvraz S et al (2006) Maintenance therapy with thalidomide improves survival in patients with multiple myeloma. Blood 108(10): 3289–3294
50. Uy GL, Peles S, Fisher NM, Tomasson MH, DiPersio JF, Vij R (2006) Bortezomib prior to autologous transplant in multiple myeloma: effects in mobilization, engraftment, and markers of immune function. Biol Blood Marrow Transplant 12(Suppl 1):116
51. Blanco B, Perez-Simon JA, Sanchez-Abarca LI et al (2006) Bortezomib induces selective depletion of alloreactive T lymphocytes and decreases the production of Th1 cytokines. Blood 107(9):3575–3583
52. Nencioni A, Schwarzenberg K, Brauer KM et al (2006) Proteasome inhibitor bortezomib modulates TLR4-induced dendritic cell activation. Blood 108(2): 551–558
53. Nencioni A, Garuti A, Schwarzenberg K et al (2006) Proteasome inhibitor-induced apoptosis in human monocyte-derived dendritic cells. Eur J Immunol 36(3): 681–689
54. Sun K, Welniak LA, Panoskaltsis-Mortari A et al (2004) Inhibition of acute graft-versus-host disease with retention of graft-versus-tumor effects by the proteasome inhibitor bortezomib. Proc Natl Acad Sci USA 101(21):8120–8125
55. Hideshima T, Richardson P, Chauhan D et al (2001) The proteasome inhibitor PS-341 inhibits growth, induces apoptosis, and overcomes drug resistance in human multiple myeloma cells. Cancer Res 61(7):3071–3076
56. Dimopoulos MA, Spencer A, Attal M et al (2005) Study of lenalidomide plus dexamethasone versus dexamethasone alone in relapsed or refractory multiple myeloma (MM): results of a phase 3 study (MM-010). ASH Annu Meet Abstr 106(11):6
57. Richardson PG, Blood E, Mitsiades CS et al (2006) A randomized phase 2 study of lenalidomide therapy for patients with relapsed or relapsed and refractory multiple myeloma. Blood 108(10):3458–3464
58. Marr KA, Carter RA, Boeckh M, Martin P, Corey L (2002) Invasive aspergillosis in allogeneic stem cell transplant recipients: changes in epidemiology and risk factors. Blood 100(13):4358–4366
59. Cornet M, Fleury L, Maslo C, Bernard JF, Brucker G (2002) Epidemiology of invasive aspergillosis in France: a six-year multicentric survey in the Greater Paris area. J Hosp Infect 51(4):288–296
60. Lortholary O, Ascioglu S, Moreau P et al (2000) Invasive aspergillosis as an opportunistic infection in nonallografted patients with multiple myeloma: a European Organization for Research and Treatment of Cancer/ Invasive Fungal Infections Cooperative Group and the Intergroupe Francais du Myelome. Clin Infect Dis 30(1):41–46
61. Taylor Z, Nolan CM, Blumberg HM (2005) Controlling tuberculosis in the United States. Recommendations from the American Thoracic Society, CDC, and the Infectious Diseases Society of America. MMWR Recomm Rep 54(RR-12): 1–81 54
62. Vasconcelles MJ, Bernardo MV, King C, Weller EA, Antin JH (2000) Aerosolized pentamidine as pneumocystis prophylaxis after bone marrow transplantation is inferior to other regimens and is associated with decreased survival and an increased risk of other infections. Biol Blood Marrow Transplant 6(1):35–43
63. Stranska R, Schuurman R, Nienhuis E et al (2005) Survey of acyclovir-resistant herpes simplex virus in the Netherlands: prevalence and characterization. J Clin Virol 32(1):7–18
64. Chaisson RE (2000) New developments in the treatment of latent tuberculosis. Int J Tuberc Lung Dis 4(Suppl 2):S176–S181
65. Chapel HM, Lee M, Hargreaves R, Pamphilon DH, Prentice AG (1994) Randomised trial of intravenous immunoglobulin as prophylaxis against infection in plateau-phase

multiple myeloma. The UK Group for Immunoglobulin Replacement Therapy in Multiple Myeloma. Lancet 343(8905):1059–1063
66. Oken MM, Pomeroy C, Weisdorf D, Bennett JM (1996) Prophylactic antibiotics for the prevention of early infection in multiple myeloma. Am J Med 100(6):624–628
67. Robertson JD, Nagesh K, Jowitt SN et al (2000) Immunogenicity of vaccination against influenza, Streptococcus pneumoniae and Haemophilus influenzae type B in patients with multiple myeloma. Br J Cancer 82(7):1261–1265
68. Zangari M, Barlogie B, Thertulien R et al (2003) Thalidomide and deep vein thrombosis in multiple myeloma: risk factors and effect on survival. Clin Lymphoma 4(1):32–35
69. Zangari M, Anaissie E, Barlogie B et al (2001) Increased risk of deep-vein thrombosis in patients with multiple myeloma receiving thalidomide and chemotherapy. Blood 98(5):1614–1615
70. Chou MY, Brown AE, Blevins A, Armstrong D (1983) Severe pneumococcal infection in patients with neoplastic disease. Cancer 51(8):1546–1550
71. Hughes WT, Armstrong D, Bodey GP et al (2002) 2002 guidelines for the use of antimicrobial agents in neutropenic patients with cancer. Clin Infect Dis 34(6): 730–751
72. Spencer A, Horvath N, Gibson J et al (2005) Prospective randomised trial of amifostine cytoprotection in myeloma patients undergoing high-dose melphalan conditioned autologous stem cell transplantation. Bone Marrow Transplant 35(10):971–977
73. Freytes CO, Ratanatharathorn V, Taylor C et al (2004) Phase I/II randomized trial evaluating the safety and clinical effects of repifermin administered to reduce mucositis in patients undergoing autologous hematopoietic stem cell transplantation. Clin Cancer Res 10(24):8318–8324
74. Gebhard RL, Gerding DN, Olson MM et al (1985) Clinical and endoscopic findings in patients early in the course of clostridium difficile-associated pseudomembranous colitis. Am J Med 78(1):45–48
75. Manabe YC, Vinetz JM, Moore RD, Merz C, Charache P, Bartlett JG (1995) Clostridium difficile colitis: an efficient clinical approach to diagnosis. Ann Intern Med 123(11):835–840
76. Jones-Jackson L, Walker R, Purnell G et al (2005) Early detection of bone infection and differentiation from post-surgical inflammation using 2-deoxy-2-[18F]-fluoro-D-glucose positron emission tomography (FDG-PET) in an animal model. J Orthop Res 23(6):1484–1489
77. Miceli M, Atoui R, Thertulien R et al (2004) Deep septic thrombophlebitis: an unrecognized cause of relapsing bacteremia in patients with cancer. J Clin Oncol 22(8):1529–1531
78. Miceli MH, Jones Jackson LB, Walker RC, Talamo G, Barlogie B, Anaissie EJ (2004) Diagnosis of infection of implantable central venous catheters by [18F]fluorodeoxyglucose positron emission tomography. Nucl Med Commun 25(8):813–818
79. Mahfouz T, Miceli MH, Saghafifar F et al (2005) 18F-fluorodeoxyglucose positron emission tomography contributes to the diagnosis and management of infections in patients with multiple myeloma: a study of 165 infectious episodes. J Clin Oncol 23(31):7857–7863
80. Schaffel R, Portugal R, Maiolino A, Nucci M (2004) Strongyloidiasis pre and post autologous peripheral blood stem cell transplantation. Bone Marrow Transplant 33(1):117
81. Gentile G, Venditti M, Micozzi A et al (1991) Cryptosporidiosis in patients with hematologic malignancies. Rev Infect Dis 13(5):842–846

82. Schaffel R, Nucci M, Carvalho E et al (2001) The value of an immunoenzymatic test (enzyme-linked immunosorbent assay) for the diagnosis of strongyloidiasis in patients immunosuppressed by hematologic malignancies. Am J Trop Med Hyg 65(4):346–350
83. Maiolino A, Biasoli I, Lima J, Portugal AC, Pulcheri W, Nucci M (2003) Engraftment syndrome following autologous hematopoietic stem cell transplantation: definition of diagnostic criteria. Bone Marrow Transplant 31(5):393–397
84. Neufeld EJ (2006) Oral chelators deferasirox and deferiprone for transfusional iron overload in thalassemia major: new data, new questions. Blood 107(9):3436–3441

Chapter 8

Stem Cell Transplantation

John R. Wingard

Abstract Hematopoietic cell transplantation (HCT) is associated with profound compromises in host defenses. The patterns of immune compromise change over time. Infections are an important cause of serious morbidity and pose substantial threats to life. Thus, the challenges of infection facing the transplant clinician are both myriad and dynamic. Early after transplant, neutropenic infections are most important. Later herpesvirus and invasive fungal infections predominate. Even late after transplant, patients with chronic graft versus host disease remain susceptible to encapsulated bacterial, varicella zoster virus, and invasive fungal infections. Over time, with robust engraftment and control of GVHD, the risk of serious infections recedes with immune reconstitution.

Keywords Hematopoietic cell transplant • Antifungal prophylaxis • Antibiotic prophylaxis • Pneumonia • Diarrhea • Neutropenic fever • Cytomegalovirus • Respiratory viral infections • Varicella zoster virus infection

1. Hematopoietic Cell Transplantation

Hematopoietic cell transplant (HCT) is variously known as bone marrow transplant, stem cell transplant, or hematopoietic stem cell transplant. It is used to treat conditions that result in bone marrow failure (such as aplastic anemia or myelodysplastic syndromes), immunodeficiencies (such as severe combined immunodeficiency or chronic granulomatous disease), or congenital disorders that result in enzyme deficiencies in cells derived from hematopoietic precursors that result in metabolic disorders (such as mucopolysaccharidoses or glycogen storage diseases). These disorders are relatively rare in the general population. More commonly, HCT is used as a cancer therapy, primarily for hematologic malignancies (such as lymphomas, leukemias, and multiple myeloma). In this latter type of application, HCT is used to facilitate administration of intensive chemoradiotherapy. The intensive conditioning regimen suppresses and sometimes ablates the normal hematopoietic precursors. The graft is given to rescue the hematopoietic injury. In the case of allogeneic

From: *Managing Infections in Patients With Hematological Malignancies*: Contemporary Hematology, Edited by: M. Kleinberg, DOI 10.1007/978-1-59745-415-5_8,

HCT, the graft also provides adoptive immunotherapy targeting cancer cells that express novel antigens.

Autologous transplants do not require prolonged immunosuppressive therapy after the transplant and robust immune recovery typically occurs within 3–9 months. Allogeneic HCT necessitates stringent HLA matching to optimize engraftment and minimize the risk of graft versus host disease (GVHD). Immunosuppressive therapy is typically given posttransplant for 4–6 months and then tapered gradually and finally stopped after approximately 6 months. The occurrence of GVHD may necessitate a more prolonged course of immunotherapy and slow immune recovery. Immunodeficiency is more prolonged after allogeneic HCT (typically a year, sometimes longer) than after autologous transplant and the risk of infection is greater.

Each of the basic components of the transplant (the conditioning regimen, the graft, the posttransplant immunosuppressive therapy, and other supportive care regimens) influence the risk for infection and types of infectious syndromes that occur after transplant (Table 8-1).

Ablative conditioning regimens consisting of intensive chemotherapy or chemoradiotherapy have been the standard regimens used for decades. Ablative regimens have been associated with a number of toxicities to normal tissues (including mucosal injury) that are natural barriers against potential microbial pathogens. Mucosal injury allows easier entry of organisms that ordinarily colonize mucosal surfaces, leading to susceptibility to streptococcal organisms, enteric Gram negative organisms, anaerobes, and Candida.

In the past decade, transplant clinicians are increasingly using reduced intensity conditioning regimens in allogeneic HCT. Potent immunosuppressive

Table 8-1. Elements of the transplant procedure and their effects on infectious risk.

Component	Transplant role	Influence on infectious risk
Conditioning regimen	• Anticancer activity • Immunosuppression to facilitate engraftment	• Intensive conditioning regimens cause mucosal injury that increases susceptibility to bacteria and Candida infections • Myelosuppression poses risk for bacterial and Candida infections
Graft	• Hematopoietic reconstitution • B & T cell recovery	• Higher numbers of CD34+ cells associated with shorter neutropenia, fewer and less severe neutropenic infection • T cell depletion slows T cell reconstitution increasing susceptibility to viral and fungal infections • High T cell content increases risk for GVHD and susceptibility for viral and fungal infections • Histocompatibility differences between donor and recipient increases the risk for GVHD and susceptibility for viral and fungal infections
Immunosuppressive regimen	• Prevents graft rejection • Prevents GVHD	• Deficiency of T cell protective responses increases the risk for herpesvirus and fungal infections
Supportive care	• Central venous catheters permit administration of medications, transfusions, and blood sampling • HEPA filters in rooms	• Catheters breach the integument and increase risk for skin colonizing bacteria • Air filters reduce the exposure to air-borne mold pathogens

agents are used in the place of intensive chemoradiotherapy. Such regimens produce less acute toxicity sparing mucosal injury. In addition, myelosuppression is less and times to engraftment are typically shorter. With reduced intensity transplants, there is less susceptibility for neutropenia-associated bacterial and fungal infections. However, there still are substantial risks for later viral and fungal infections typically seen with GVHD and immunosuppressive therapy.

The graft used in HCT consists of a mixture of hematopoietic stem cells, more differentiated hematopoietic precursors, and mature immune cells. The grafts differ in several respects: peripheral blood grafts typically have higher numbers of hematopoietic precursors and also more lymphoid cells. Peripheral blood grafts are associated with faster neutrophil engraftment and more chronic GVHD. Cord blood grafts have fewer hematopoietic precursors and the lymphoid cells are more naïve immunophenotypically and functionally. Such cord blood grafts are associated with slower neutrophil recovery and less GVHD.

T lymphocytes in the donor graft are responsible for GVHD. The various immunosuppressive regimens used after transplant to prevent and treat GVHD suppress T cell function and increase the patient's vulnerability for infection. Fungal and herpesvirus infections are especially problematic. T cell depletion of the donor graft is sometimes used to reduce the risk for GVHD but T cell depletion increases the risk for graft rejection and slows B and T cell immune reconstitution, rendering the recipient vulnerable to opportunistic infections for a longer time after transplant. Several polymorphisms in immune response genes that affect the likelihood for both GVHD and infection have been identified.

2. Effects of HCT on Host Defenses: A Dynamic Scenario

There are three phases after HCT: early, mid, and late recovery. Each period is characterized by different kinds of deficits of host defenses and these differences account for varying susceptibilities to different kinds of infectious risks.

The early recovery phase is the interval from the start of the conditioning regimen to the time of engraftment, generally 3–4 weeks in duration. Compromises in host defenses during this interval are characterized by gut mucosal injury due to the cytotoxic effects of chemoradiotherapy and myelosuppression from the conditioning regimen. Tunneled central venous catheters are routinely used and these foreign bodies breach the integument, allowing invasion by skin colonizing organisms. The types of infectious syndromes commonly seen during the early phase are neutropenic infections due to enteric bacteria and Candida (discussed in more detail elsewhere), catheter-related infections, primarily due to skin colonizing bacteria, especially *Staphylococcus epidermidis* or less commonly *Staphylococcus aureus*, and organisms that colonize the oral mucosa, such as alpha streptococci. Reactivation of herpes simplex virus occurs in most patients treated with intensive conditioning regimens, with an average onset between 2 and 3 weeks after initiation of the conditioning regimen in the absence of prophylaxis.

Patients treated with a nonablative conditioning regimen have shorter times of neutropenia and also less mucosal injury. Typically, neutrophil counts do not fall until 7–10 days after graft infusion and the neutrophil count may not fall below 100 cells/μL. Thus, such patients are much less susceptible to early infections of all types. For that reason, nonablative transplant patients are generally managed in the outpatient clinic.

Upon engraftment, the transplant recipient enters the mid recovery phase. This phase spans the second and third month after transplant. With the restoration of neutrophils and healing of the damaged mucosal barriers, the overall risk for infection is less. The central venous catheter still poses a breach in the skin barrier and catheter-related infections remain a concern.

The mid recovery phase is characterized by a profound immunodeficiency of both B and T cell functions, which eventually recover later over a period of several months (after autologous HCT) or up to a year (for allogeneic HCT). *Pneumocystis jiroveci* (PCP), *Aspergillus*, and cytomegalovirus (CMV) infections can occur during this period. The risk for serious infection is greater after allogeneic HCT since GVHD or the use of high dose corticosteroids can intensify T cell immunodeficiency [1–4]. The use of anti-thymocyte globulin (or alemtuzumab) to prevent or treat GVHD or promote engraftment can have enduring effects on T cells (and NK cells in the case of alemtuzumab) and may render the patient vulnerable for a longer period of time. T cell depletion of the graft and HLA disparity between the donor and recipient delay T cell recovery. With nonablative transplants, the immunosuppressive regimen is frequently tapered more quickly (to provoke a graft-versus-tumor effect); this may increase the risk for GVHD. Various single center reports have suggested either an increase or decrease in infectious risk with nonablative transplants; as yet, the difference in conditioning regimens, case mix, and immunosuppressive regimens prevent a clear understanding of whether the risk of infection or timing of infection and epidemiology of infection is truly similar or different. Further study is needed.

The late recovery phase follows after the third month. The overall risk for infection recedes greatly as B and T cell immunity gradually improves. There remains some risk for PCP. There is also a risk for reactivation of varicella zoster virus (VZV) that occurs in approximately 40% of VZV seropositive patients. Patients who develop chronic GVHD require prolonged immunosuppressive therapy and are susceptible to fungal and viral infections due to T cell immunodeficiency. The need for prednisone at daily doses of 1 mg/kg/day for extended periods of time has been associated with a particularly high risk for aspergillosis. The use of infliximab renders the patient at even higher risk for aspergillosis. In patients with chronic GVHD, there is also a risk for infections by encapsulated bacteria (e.g., *S. pneumoniae*, *N. meningiditis*, and *H. influenzae*) due to poor opsonization.

Generally, by 1 year posttransplant, patients will recover their immune competence and will be no longer at risk for opportunistic infections except for patients who have developed chronic GVHD and who may have prolonged immunodeficiency extending for many months or years. At 1 year posttransplant, immunizations with the childhood vaccines should be given (see Chap. 13).

3. Major Infectious Syndromes: Clinical Manifestations and Diagnostic Approaches

3.1 Neutropenic Fever

Prior to engraftment, neutropenia lasts for a variable duration according to the transplant type: 10–14 days after autologous transplant, 17–21 days after myeloablative allogeneic transplant, and only 4–7 days after nonablative allogeneic transplant. Cord blood transplants often have longer durations of neutropenia that may extend up to 28–35 days. Neutropenic fever is common in the pre-engraftment period but is less problematic in nonablative transplants. Fever may be generally the only manifestation of infection and, operationally, infection should be approached as the likely cause since serious morbidity may ensue if untreated. Evaluation should include elicitation of symptoms suggestive of an infectious site and examination to look for an infectious site (especially skin, oral mucosa, lungs, catheter site, abdomen, and perianal area). Blood cultures should be obtained and cultures of any site suspected to be infected. A chest radiograph is generally done, but if the lungs are highly suspected from history or examination, then a CT scan is preferred since it would be more likely to yield useful information [6]. Persistent or recrudescent fever may be due to antibiotic-resistant Gram negative bacteria, Gram positive bacteria (especially *S. epidermidis*, less commonly an alpha streptococcus, or *S. aureus*), or fungus (especially *Candida* or *Aspergillus*). Evaluation and more specific diagnostic considerations for infections in the neutropenic host are addressed in Chap. 5 and have been delineated in consensus guidelines [7, 8].

3.2 Pneumonia

Pneumonia commonly occurs after HCT during all three phases of the postHCT period and may have both infectious and non-nfectious etiologies (Table 8-2) [9]. In the early recovery phase, bacterial and mold infections may be etiologic, and adult respiratory distress syndrome due to toxicity from the conditioning regimen may also occur. In the mid recovery phase, interstitial pneumonitis due to conditioning regimen toxicity or due to CMV may occur. Also, bacterial and fungal pneumonia due to Aspergillus or other molds may occur. During the late recovery phase, late-onset CMV pneumonia may occur, especially in patients with early CMV infection or a history of acute GVHD [10]. Late-onset Aspergillus pneumonia may also occur, especially in patients with chronic GVHD. In recent years, increasing instances of very late onset Aspergillus pneumonias occurring 6–12 months after HCT have been noted in

Table 8-2. Various etiologies of pneumonia after HCT.

Radiographic pattern	Early recovery	Mid recovery	Late recovery
Diffuse infiltrates	• ARDS • Hemorrhagic alveolitis • Respiratory virus	• Idiopathic interstitial pneumonitis • Hemorrhagic alveolitis • CMV • Respiratory virus • PCP	• Bronchiolitis obliterans or bronchiolitis obliterans with organizing pneumonia • CMV • Respiratory virus • PCP
Localized infiltrates	• Bacterial • Aspergillus • Zygomycete or other mold	• Bacterial • Aspergillus • Zygomycete or other mold • Nocardia	• Bacterial • Aspergillus • Zygomycete or other mold • Nocardia

patients with chronic persistent GVHD. PCP may occur during any of the 3 phases if prophylaxis is not given.

Respiratory viruses may occur during any of the 3 recovery phases. Influenza and respiratory syncytial virus (RSV) generally occur seasonally during the winter months [11–14]. Parainfluenza may occur at any time during the year. Adenovirus is an occasional pulmonary pathogen [15]. Upper respiratory symptoms generally precede lower tract involvement with respiratory viral infections, but not always.

Pneumonias may be caused by more than one pathogen; for example CMV may be accompanied by bacterial or Aspergillus infections. Thus, isolation of one pathogen may be an inadequate explanation for cause of pneumonia when the clinical syndrome suggests another etiology and further investigation is warranted.

Radiologic assessment by high resolution CT scan is key to the assessment of pneumonia [6, 16]. Pneumonias can generally be categorized radiographically into either diffuse infiltrates or localized infiltrates (Table 8-2). The diffuse infiltrates can be either non-specific alveolar ground glass, interstitial, mixed alveolar/interstitial, or diffuse micronodular patterns. The localized infiltrates may be macronodules (≥1 cm in diameter), consolidation, cavitary, or wedge-shaped.

The etiologies differ according to both the radiographic pattern and timing after transplant and evaluation and management strategies differ for each radiographic category and timepoint (Table 8-2). In the early recovery phase, diffuse infiltrates are most commonly due to noninfectious causes such as pulmonary edema, ARDS, or idiopathic interstitial pneumonitis. These are thought to be due mostly to toxicity related to the conditioning regimen and fluid balance. Occasionally, respiratory viruses may also be causative. Localized infiltrates during the early recovery period are usually due to bacterial pneumonia or mold pathogens (*Aspergillus* most commonly, or *Zygomycetes*, *Fusarium*, or *Scedosporium* less commonly).

During the mid recovery period, diffuse infiltrates are divided evenly between noninfectious and infectious etiologies. The potential etiologies are the same as in the early recovery period, but in addition, CMV becomes the major infectious etiology during this time interval. PCP assumes an important consideration but is effectively prevented by prophylaxis, which should be routinely given (see below). The diagnostic considerations for localized infiltrates are also the same as during the early period, but mold infections are more prominent concerns. In a large series of IA, macronodules with or without halos were present in 94% of cases of IA and 79% had multiple nodules [17]. Halo signs were present in 61%. In another small series, more than ten nodules or a pleural effusion tended to more likely in Zygomycosis compared to IA [18].

In the late recovery period, diffuse infiltrates have a more varied spectrum of etiologies [19]. CMV still is an important consideration as are PCP and respiratory viruses. Also important noninfectious considerations are bronchiolitis obliterans or bronchiolitis obliterans with organizing pneumonia. As for localized infiltrates, the same potential causes as during the earlier period are possible. Encapsulated bacteria are particularly important pathogens since opsonization is impaired in chronic GVHD. Also important is Nocardia, which can present in a similar manner as mold infections.

Prompt and thorough evaluation is crucial to treatment success. Elicitation of lower tract symptoms and evidence of consolidation on physical exam should alert the clinician to the possibility of pneumonia. However, even in the absence of any of these, fever of uncertain etiology may warrant investigation of pneumonia as the source of fever. Hemoptysis may occur with diffuse alveolar hemorrhage early after transplant. Hemoptysis, pleuritic pain, and the presence of pleural rub may suggest Aspergillosis. Upper respiratory tract symptoms suggest a respiratory viral infection. Lack of sputum is typical of respiratory virus, CMV, and PCP pneumonias. However, these manifestations are too insensitive and not sufficiently specific to indicate firmly the etiology. CT scans to determine the character of infiltrate is more useful. Prior to the onset of pneumonia symptoms, a number of tests may identify those at risk for or with incipient lower respiratory tract infection. Nasal viral cultures, shell vial centrifugation cultures using RSV-specific monoclonal antibodies, or rapid diagnostics using DFA or ELISA assays are important for diagnostic assessment of the respiratory viruses, and may be useful in the assessment of patients with symptoms of upper respiratory tract infection. CMV antigen assays or PCR assays of blood samples should be performed and often are positive 1–2 weeks in advance of CMV pneumonia. Serum galactomannan can be useful as an adjunct in the diagnosis of *Aspergillus* pneumonia [20–32].

For patients suspected to have pneumonia, CT examination, as noted above, is essential and should be done promptly. Bronchoscopic examination with bronchoalveolar lavage should be performed early in the assessment of pneumonia wherever feasible [33, 34]. The yield is high for agents that cause diffuse infiltrates (e.g., PCP, CMV, respiratory viruses), but tends to be low with agents that cause localized infiltrates, especially *Aspergillus*. Even in localized pneumonias where the yield is suboptimal, performance of bronchoscopy is advisable to exclude certain pathogens in order to narrow the use of agents in presumptive therapy and to identify co-infecting pathogens.

In many cases, treatment should be initiated presumptively for the most likely pathogen(s) while evaluation is proceeding since early initiation of therapy is crucial to optimize treatment success. Presumptive therapy, however, should not be given in order to justify the failure to perform a careful and thorough evaluation, since the spectrum of pathogens is large and the toxicities of prolonged "shot-gun" anti-infective therapies is considerable. Once the evaluation is complete, elimination of the presumptive therapies no longer justified is appropriate. In the case of a suspected mold infection, even with an extensive negative evaluation, continued therapy may be justified if the clinical suspicion remains high. If the etiology is not clear and the patient does not improve clinically and radiographically, further investigation should be undertaken. Typically, infiltrates may get worse early even in the face of clinical improvement and even though pneumonia ultimately responds. It generally requires 2 weeks at a minimum to see radiographic improvement. If a patient clinically deteriorates with empirical antimicrobial therapy, then additional evaluation should be considered, including a lung biopsy if the patient's condition permits.

3.3 Diarrhea

Diarrhea can occur at any time after HCT and there are a myriad of both infectious and noninfectious causes (Table 8-3). During or shortly after completion of the conditioning regimen, diarrhea may be caused by intestinal tract mucosal injury due to cytotoxicity from the conditioning regimen.

Table 8-3. Etiologies of diarrhea.

Early recovery	Mid recovery	Late recovery
• Chemotherapy	• GVHD	• GVHD
• Neutropenic enterocolitis	• *C. difficile* colitis	• *C. difficile*
• *C. difficile* colitis	• CMV	• CMV
• Enteric viruses	• Adenovirus	• Adenovirus
	• Enteric viruses	• Enteric viruses

Later during neutropenia, diarrhea is more likely to be infectious, due to either neutropenic enterocolitis or C. *difficile*. A highly virulent strain of *C. difficile* has been noted in outbreaks in Canada and northeastern US cities, and also in other locales in the US and Europe [35–39]. The use of fluoroquinolones (and other antibiotics as well) has been associated with predisposition to *C. difficile* infection. The use of gastric acid suppressants has also been implicated to add to the risk [40].

Neutropenic enterocolitis (typhlitis) is usually accompanied by abdominal pain [41–43]. Although there is a predilection for the ascending colon, other portions of the gut can also be involved. The microbiological etiology of neutropenic enterocolitis is rarely discerned but is presumed to be caused by gram-negative bacteria and anaerobic bacteria. In recent years, Candida has also been implicated as contributory [44, 45]. Toxic megacolon, perforation, and hypotension are complications of progressive enterocolitis and may result in death.

A variety of viruses are occasional causes of diarrhea in the HCT patient, such as the enteroviruses (including the coxsackieviruses), caliciviruses (including the Norwalk virus), and astroviruses [46–49]. These infections do not occur at specific times after HCT like the herpesviruses but rather may occur at different seasons of the year, tracking along with outbreaks in the general population of the local community. Also, adenovirus and CMV may be viral causes of diarrhea. Other infectious agents including enterobacteria, such as Salmonella, Shigella, *E. coli*, and protozoal and helminthic infections may also be rare causes of diarrhea.

GVHD may also present as diarrhea. Usually a skin rash is also present, but some cases of GVHD may present with gut involvement alone. This occurs mostly during the mid recovery phase, but in recent years late onset GVHD with features resembling acute GVHD have been noted with transplants performed with the use of peripheral blood as stem cell source, reduced intensity conditioning regimens, and donor lymphocyte infusions after transplant.

Evaluation should include stool assay for *C. difficile* antigen and toxin, viral cultures or ELISA assays, and CMV antigen or quantitative PCR testing. An abdominal CT scan should be performed to look for bowel thickening and/or dilatation. Serial KUB radiographs should be performed in patients with bowel wall thickening to screen for toxic megacolon. Colonoscopy should be performed for visual inspection, looking for pseudomembranes, and to perform biopsy for tissue examination and culture for the various infectious etiologies or GVHD.

3.4 Cytomegalovirus Infection

Historically, CMV was the most dangerous infectious pathogen and the cause of death in 15–20% of allogeneic HCT recipients. Although CMV infections (detected by detection of CMV pp65 antigen or quantitative PCR testing) occur frequently in autologous transplant recipients, CMV disease is generally infrequent. The chief risk factors identified for CMV symptomatic disease are allogeneic transplant type, older age, CMV seropositivity (of the recipient), and the occurrence of GVHD [4, 50]. Other factors that diminish T cell recovery also increase the risk for CMV disease, such as T cell depletion of the stem cell graft, HLA disparity between donor and recipient, and the use of certain immunosuppressive agents that produce profound and prolonged T cell deficiency such as antithymocyte globulin, alemtuzumab, or high doses of corticosteroids. Purine analogs, such as fludarabine, cladrabine, and pentostatin, given in the posttransplant period may also have prolonged immunosuppressive effects, but whether or not their more common use in the pretransplant conditioning regimen has any lingering posttransplant effects has not been studied.

The most common manifestation of CMV disease is pneumonia, but gastroenteritis can also occur. Rarely does CMV opthalmitis occur in HCT recipients in contrast to the situation with advanced HIV infection.

In past decades, most episodes of CMV pneumonia occurred during the mid recovery period, and only 10% occurred after 100 days. However, in recent years there has been a dramatic shift to later onset (beyond 100 days) [10]; this is particularly true in patients who develop acute GVHD or receive pre-emptive antiCMV therapy for CMV reactivation infection during the mid recovery period (see below).

The usual presentation of CMV pneumonia is low grade fever, a nonproductive cough, and dyspnea. Progressive worsening of symptoms occurs if untreated and the mortality untreated has ranged 80–90%. Chest radiographs show a mixed interstitial/alveolar infiltrate. Bronchoscopy with immunofluorescent stains for pp65 antigen of cytologic samples and shell vial cultures of BAL samples has a high diagnostic yield with sensitivity and specificity of at least 90%. Bronchoscopic biopsies are somewhat less sensitive than the BAL for CMV. Blood pp65 antigen and the PCR assay are usually positive before and at the onset of pneumonia, but since CMV viremia may be present without pneumonia, bronchoscopy is still required to determine if the lung process is due to the viremia. Co-infections with bacteria or *Aspergillus* may be present. Diarrhea is the chief manifestation of CMV enterocolitis. Colonoscopy with tissue biopsy is the diagnostic test of choice with immunofluorescent stains

3.5 Other Viral Infections

Adenovirus infections occasionally occur (generally in less than 5% of allogeneic HCT recipients) [15, 51, 52] and case fatality rates of 30–50% have been reported. As with CMV infections, factors that result in more profound T cell immunodeficiency pose greater susceptibility for adenovirus infection; in contrast to CMV, younger patients are at greater risk. Pneumonia, hepatitis, and gastrointestinal disease are the most common manifestations, but less frequent presentations include nephritis and cystitis. Viremia can be detected with PCR assays. Detection of virus in BAL or tissue samples can be achieved using rapid culture techniques or immunofluorescent antibody staining of cytologic or tissue specimens.

Community acquired respiratory viruses have been increasingly recognized as important respiratory pathogens as noted above [13, 53–56]. RSV, influenza, rhinovirus, and metapneumovirus infections have a seasonal pattern, mirroring occurrences in the community, whereas parainfluenza virus infections occur during all seasons. Upper tract symptoms typically occur before lower tract disease and this offers an opportunity for early diagnosis and potential intervention, although no studies have shown definitively that treatment of upper tract infection prevents lower tract disease. Nasal swabs are excellent means of detecting the virus in patients with upper tract symptoms by culture, immunofluorescent antibody staining, or PCR assays of specimens. BAL or tissue specimens can be assessed with the same diagnostic assays.

Herpesvirus 6 persists lifelong (like HSV, CMV and VZV) in most individuals after primary infection during infancy. Active infection can be detected in about one-third of HCT recipients. In most cases, it is asymptomatic, but it can be a cause of rash, encephalitis, and possibly pneumonitis [57, 58]. PCR assays can be useful in the diagnosis [57].

BK virus is a polyoma virus that infects many individuals early in life and persists lifelong in urogenital epithelial tissues. Reactivation may occur after allogeneic HCT, especially in patients with GVHD and is a cause of hemorrhagic cystitis [59, 60]. Cystitis generally occurs during the mid recovery period, but may occur at any time after HCT. Diagnosis is made generally by the use of immunofluorescent antibody staining or PCR assays of urine specimens. BK virus can also be detected in blood samples but its correlation with hemorrhagic cystitis has been less well documented.

3.6 Nonneutropenic Fever

At time of engraftment, fever occasionally occurs in the absence of infection (sometimes known as "engraftment syndrome"). After cultures are obtained with no growth after 24–48 h and CT scans of chest and abdomen are negative, a noninfectious etiology should be considered. A short course of corticosteroids is highly efficacious with rapid taper. Rash, elevation of transaminases or bilirubin, or dyspnea with an ARDS-like syndrome may accompany the fever.

After engraftment fever may present occasionally in the absence of other symptoms. A systemic evaluation strategy is necessary. Continued monitoring to elicit symptoms that may provide clues is needed. Careful examination of sinuses, oral cavity, catheter site and tunnel, skin, lungs, and perineal area is important and should be ongoing. Blood cultures for bacteria, fungi, and mycobacteria should be obtained. Urinalysis is useful. Blood sampling for CMV assays, galactomannan, or glucan assays may be useful. CT scans of sinuses, chest, and abdomen should be considered. If these do not provide an explanation after several days, removal of the venous catheter should be considered. Since drug fever may occur, careful consideration tof stopping any discretionary medications should be entertained.

3.7 Rash

Rashes are frequent and there are a myriad of causes. Erythema may be a prominent sign of GVHD. Involvement of palms, soles, and earlobes are especially seen in GVHD. Focal lesions may be seen with bacterial or fungal bloodstream infections. Paronychia should suggest the possibility of *Fusarium*. Vesicular lesions, especially in a dermatomal distribution, should suggest VZV infection. In most cases a biopsy should be done. Cultures should be performed if an infection is suggested. For lesions where a fungal etiology is suspected, fungal stains are necessary.

3.8 Hepatitis

The hepatic transaminases may be elevated for a variety of reasons, both infectious and noninfectious. Most commonly, this is a result of some drug reaction. Viral hepatitis, iron overload, sepsis, and GVHD may also be etiologic. Hepatic veno-occlusive disease (VOD) and GVHD more commonly have a cholestatic predominance rather than transaminemia. In the case of VOD, the onset is almost always before day 30; in the case of GVHD, onset is usually after engraftment. Hepatitis serologies and PCR assays, ferritin measurement should be performed. A liver biopsy should be considered if the patient is able to tolerate it.

In patients with chronic GVHD, a rare manifestation of VZV infection is fulminent hepatitis (with or without concomitant pancreatitis) antecedent to the cutaneous rash and which can pursue a virulent course leading rapidly to shock and death. Prompt presumptive antiVZV therapy is warranted.

4. Management Strategies

Specific management of the individual infections described above is discussed in other chapters. Only anti-infective strategies that pertain to HCT will be discussed below.

4.1 Bacterial Prophylaxis

A variety of antibacterial regimens have been evaluated in the HCT setting over the past decades. Indeed, several decontamination regimens have been advocated more as a way to reduce the release of proinflammatory cytokines, key contributors to GVHD, in order to reduce the risk for severe GVHD, rather than to reduce bacterial infections. Such regimens were difficult for patients to tolerate and definite benefits could not be discerned; over time, they have largely been abandoned.

Today, the fluoroquinolones have largely replaced other antibiotic regimens for the purpose of preventing bacterial infection during the pre-engraftment phase. The benefits of antibiotic prophylaxis after HCT have been debated and no firm recommendation was given in the HCT consensus guidelines in 2000 [5]. However, they are widely used in the pre-engraftment phase, and more recent studies suggest such benefits as reductions in febrile episodes, bacterial infections, and death (from any cause) in patients with neutropenia. Such benefits have been seen in patients with acute leukemia and HCT [61–63]. Ciprofloxacin and levofloxacin are the most suitable agents. Drawbacks include cost, toxicities, and the risk of antibiotic resistance. If antibiotic prophylaxis is elected, surveillance of isolates for resistance is important since various centers have reported the emergence of fluoroquinolone resistance [64]. Although most infections that are prevented are from gram-negative bacteria, there seems to also be some protection against alpha streptococcal and methicillin-sensitive *Staphylococcus aureus* infections as well [61]. Another concern is an increased susceptibility for *C. difficile* infection. Accordingly, centers that choose to use fluoroquinolone prophylaxis must monitor both resistance as well as *C. difficile* infection rates. The issues concerning antibiotic prophylaxis are discussed in greater detail in Chap. 10.

Severe infections by the encapsulated bacteria can occur in allogeneic HCT recipients with chronic GVHD. Although never tested in randomized trials, routine prophylaxis with antibiotics effective against this group of bacterial pathogens is advisable [5].

4.2 Fungal Prophylaxis

Several studies have demonstrated that the fluconazole is highly effective in the prevention of invasive Candida infections [65–67]. The use of fluconazole prophylaxis has been embraced by consensus guidelines for HCT [5] and the subject has been discussed widely [68, 69]. There are two HCT scenarios in which its use may not be necessary. After nonablative allogeneic HCT, the duration of neutropenia is short and the risk for invasive Candida infection is low; the need for routine prophylaxis in this situation has not been studied. Also, in autologous transplantation for solid tumors, some conditioning regimens do not cause significant mucosal injury and the risk for invasive Candida infections may be sufficiently low to not warrant routine prophylaxis. This has not been well studied.

Micafungin has also been found to be effective in the prevention of *Candida* infections after HCT [70] and caspofungin has been found to be effective in patients with neutropenia after treatment for hematologic malignancies [71]. Although the echinocandins do act against *Aspergillus* and have been studied as a salvage therapy for invasive aspergillosis (IA), they have not been adequately evaluated as prophylaxis against *Aspergillus*.

The lipid formulations of amphotericin B have been evaluated only in a limited manner as prophylaxis but they do offer protective effects [72, 73]. Both the echinocandins and polyenes will likely have limited roles for prophylaxis since they require parenteral administration, a major shortcoming for the prolonged period of risk for mold infections.

Most interest for antimold prophylaxis has been in the extended spectrum azoles, since oral formulations make them suitable for prolonged administration necessary to cover the protected risk period. Itraconazole, posaconazole, and voriconazole have been shown to offer protection against IA during neutropenia in nontransplant oncology settings [74–77]. Two studies of itraconazole prophylaxis in the allogeneic HCT setting suggest a potential for benefit to prevent IA [78, 79], but limitations include poor tolerability and concerns about toxicity. Posaconazole has been evaluated in HCT patients with acute and chronic GVHD and compared to fluconazole [80]. This "targeted" approach seems sensible since GVHD and its therapy are the major risk factors for IA. Although there was a decrease in breakthrough IA, there was no improvement in clinical success (defined as survival without IFI or use of systemic antifungal therapy). Voriconazole prophylaxis has also been studied in standard-risk allogeneic BMT patients in a randomized double-blind multicenter trial and is not found to be superior to fluconazole in terms of survival at 6 months free of invasive fungal infection although there were fewer IA infections and voriconazole was not associated with greater toxicity [81]. One potential concern with voriconazole is its lack of activity against *Zygomycetes*; its routine use has been associated with an apparent increase in zygomycosis in several single center studies [18, 82–84]. However, there were no increases in IA rates in the prospective randomized prophylaxis trial [81].

4.3 Neutropenic Fever

The management of neutropenic fever is a frequent challenge for the transplant clinician. The diagnostic considerations and approaches for evaluation and treatment in the HCT patient are similar to those in the nontransplant neutropenic patient and are discussed in detail elsewhere in Chap. 5.

4.4 CMV Management Strategies

The risks for serious morbidity and mortality from CMV disease are substantial. Technological advances have quelled this threat. Improvements in rapid diagnostics including the shell vial culture assay, pp65 antigen assay, and PCR assay, the validation of a high degree of accuracy in detection of CMV pneumonia by BAL to supplant the need for open lung biopsy [4, 10, 50]. The recognition that viremia generally precedes the onset of disease, the introduction of effective antiviral agents including ganciclovir, foscarnet, and cidofovir, and the testing of strategies to prevent or pre-empt CMV disease have all been major strides in reducing sequelae from CMV.

Prophylaxis with acyclovir, ganciclovir, and foscarnet has been shown to be effective [85–89]. Although acyclovir and its prodrug, valacyclovir, are well tolerated the relatively poor in vitro activity against CMV has led most clinicians to rely on ganciclovir which has much greater intrinsic anti-CMV activity. Unfortunately, ganciclovir is associated with myelosuppression. This toxicity has led to evaluation of serial monitoring of HCT patients with weekly testing of blood by the pp65 antigen or PCR assay, and institution of pre-emptive antiCMV therapy with ganciclovir (or foscarnet) in patients who become viremic [87, 90]. In general, there are advantages and disadvantages to both approaches. Prophylaxis is generally associated with fewer episodes of breakthrough CMV pneumonia, but more toxicity. Pre-emptive therapy is associated with more episodes of late-onset CMV pneumonia. Oral valganciclovir has good bioavailability and has been used in limited studies to replace intravenous ganciclovir. Although the toxicities are the same, there are obvious advantages in convenience and cost.

Most centers use the pre-emptive antiCMV strategies. Some centers stratify patients by risk: standard risk patients receive the pre-emptive strategy, while patients at high risk for CMV disease receive prophylaxis. Typical risks to consider include the use of a T cell depleted graft, HLA disparity between donor and recipient, use of antithymocyte globulin or alemtuzumab after transplant, or the use of steroids as prophylaxis. There are no data that suggest that nonablative transplant recipients should be monitored differently from ablative transplants.

A phase 2 trial of maribavir as CMV prophylaxis appears promising and a phase 3 trial is underway. This agent has the potential advantages of oral formulation and excellent tolerability and safety profiles.

Monitoring of patients beyond 100 days has assumed greater importance today with rising rates of late onset CMV disease. This is a challenge since most HCT patients are no longer receiving routine follow-up care at the transplant center after the mid recovery period and the knowledge level of community physicians of this threat is low and availability of the screening assays in the community setting is not good. A trial to evaluate the use of valganciclovir prophylaxis in patients at risk for late CMV disease is underway.

4.5 VZV Prophylaxis

VZV reactivation occurs in approximately 40% of HCT patients with a median onset of 5 months. Although acyclovir (or valacyclovir) treatment is effective, some patients can present with a life-threatening visceral infection (involving serosal intestinal wall, liver, or pancreas) without cutaneous lesions with a high fatality rate. This condition should be suspected in any HCT patient presenting with excruciating abdominal pain, even with a benign abdominal exam. Moreover, sequelae of VZV can pose significant compromises in quality of life in HCT survivors. Accordingly, there has been considerable interest in prevention. Acyclovir prophylaxis given for 6 months was associated with fewer VZV infections while the patient was receiving acyclovir, but relapses occurred shortly after cessation of drug abrogating the benefit. However, more recently, prophylaxis for 1 year has been shown to offer durable protection [91] and preservation of viral T cell helper responses but without rebound relapses after stopping prophylaxis.

4.6 Infection Control Measures

Infection control measures have not been well studied in HCT patients. Hospitalization in air filtered rooms with >12 air exchanges/hour is generally recommended [5]. This is particularly important during construction periods when air-borne pathogens (especially *Aspergillus*) pose threats to HCT patients [92]. Survival benefits of air filtration have been observed in allogeneic HCT patients given ablative conditioning regimens [93, 94]. Whether there is a demonstrable benefit for patients receiving nonablative conditioning regimens (whose treatment is mostly outpatient) or in patients undergoing autologous HCT is not known.

Handwashing has been recognized to be the single most important tool in infection prevention [95]. The use of alcohol-based rubs as a substitute for hand washing has become widely adopted. Although they have been shown to reduce the risk for antibiotic-resistant bacteria such as methicillin-resistant *S. aureus* and vancomycin-resistant enterococci [96], they lack activity against *C. difficile* and there is a potential for increased risk for nosocomial outbreaks from this organism. Guidelines for the prevention of nosocomial transmission of these infectious pathogens have been developed [97] and are discussed in detail in Chap. 12.

The occurrence of antibiotic resistance in bacteria continues to plague hospital environments and the HCT unit is no exception. HCT patients are at especially high risk due to immune compromise, the widespread use of multiple antibiotics, often for prolonged intervals, and the universal use of central venous catheters. Infections by methicillin-resistant *S. aureus* and vancomycin-resistant enterococci have been abundantly reported in HCT patients. Such resistant organisms are frequently associated with considerable morbidity and mortality. Handwashing and contact isolation of colonized patients is advocated to reduce the risk for nosocomial transmission [5].

Patients with respiratory viral infections should be placed under both contact and droplet precautions [5]. Prolonged shedding of virus can occur due to high viral burden and poor immune status and follow-up cultures are advisable to determine when isolation procedures may be discontinued. Infected health care workers (HCW) should avoid contact with patients until symptoms resolve.

References

1. Fukuda T, Boeckh M, Carter RA, Sandmaier BM, Maris MB, Maloney DG, Martin PJ, Storb RF, Marr KA (2003) Risks and outcomes of invasive fungal infections in recipients of allogeneic hematopoietic stem cell transplants after nonmyeloablative conditioning. Blood 102(3):827–833
2. De La Rosa GR, Champlin RE, Kontoyiannis DP (2002) Risk factors for the development of invasive fungal infections in allogeneic blood and marrow transplant recipients. Transpl Infect Dis 4(1):3–9
3. Marr KA, Carter RA, Boeckh M, Martin P, Corey L (2002) Invasive aspergillosis in allogeneic stem cell transplant recipients: changes in epidemiology and risk factors. Blood 100(13):4358–4366
4. Boeckh M, Nichols WG, Papanicolaou G, Rubin R, Wingard JR, Zaia J (2003) Cytomegalovirus in hematopoietic stem cell transplant recipients: Current status, known challenges, and future strategies. Biol Blood Marrow Transplant 9(9): 543–558
5. Dykewicz CA, Jaffe HW, Spira TJ, Jarvis WR, Kaplan JE, Edlin BR, Chen RT, Hibbs B, Bowden RA, Sullivan K, Emanuel D, Longworth DL, Rowlings PA, Rubin RH, Sepkowitz KA, Wingard JR, Modlin JF, Ambrosino DM, Baylor NW, Donnenberg AD, Gardner P, Giller RH, Halsey NA, Le CT, Molrine DC, Sullivan KM (2000) Guidelines for preventing opportunistic infections among hematopoietic stem cell transplant recipients. MMWR 49(RR-10):1–125
6. Heussel CP, Kauczor HU, Heussel G, Fischer B, Mildenberger P, Thelen M (1997) Early detection of pneumonia in febrile neutropenic patients: use of thin-section CT. AJR Am J Roentgenol 169(5):1347–1353
7. Hughes WT, Armstrong D, Bodey GP, Bow EJ, Brown AE, Calandra T, Feld R, Pizzo PA, Rolston KV, Shenep JL, Young LS (2002) 2002 guidelines for the use of antimicrobial agents in neutropenic patients with cancer. Clin Infect Dis 34(6):730–751
8. Friefeld AG, Baden LR, Brown AE, Elting L, Gelfand M, Greene JH, Ito JI, Karp JE, Kaul DR, King E, Marcucci G, Montoya JG, Morris A, Rolston K, Segal BH (2005) The NCCN fever and neutropenia clinical practice guidelines in oncology. Version 1
9. Gosselin MV, Adams RH (2002) Pulmonary complications in bone marrow transplantation. J Thorac Imaging 17(2):132–144
10. Boeckh M, Leisenring W, Riddell SR, Bowden RA, Huang ML, Myerson D, Stevens-Ayers T, Flowers ME, Cunningham T, Corey L (2003) Late cytomegalovirus disease and mortality in recipients of allogeneic hematopoietic stem cell transplants: importance of viral load and T-cell immunity. Blood 101(2): 407–414
11. Harrington RD, Hooton TM, Hackman RC, Storch GA, Osborne B, Gleaves CA, Benson A, Meyers JD (1992) An outbreak of respiratory syncytial virus in a bone marrow transplant center. J Infect Dis 165(6):987–993
12. Ljungman P (1997) Respiratory virus infections in bone marrow transplant recipients: the European perspective. Am J Med 102(3A):44–47
13. Whimbey E, Champlin RE, Couch RB, Englund JA, Goodrich JM, Raad I, Przepiorka D, Lewis VA, Mirza N, Yousuf H, Tarrand JJ, Bodey GP (1996)

Community respiratory virus infections among hospitalized adult bone marrow transplant recipients. Clin Infect Dis 22(5):778–782
14. Whimbey E, Englund JA, Couch RB (1997) Community respiratory virus infections in immunocompromised patients with cancer. Am J Med 102(3A):10–18
15. La Rosa AM, Champlin RE, Mirza N, Gajewski J, Giralt S, Rolston KV, Raad I, Jacobson K, Kontoyiannis D, Elting L, Whimbey E (2001) Adenovirus infections in adult recipients of blood and marrow transplants. Clin Infect Dis 32(6):871–876
16. Conces DJ Jr (1999) Noninfectious lung disease in immunocompromised patients. J Thorac Imaging 14(1):9–24
17. Greene RE, Schlamm HT, Oestmann JW, Stark P, Durand C, Lortholary O, Wingard JR, Herbrecht R, Ribaud P, Patterson TF, Troke PF, Denning DW, Bennett JE, de Pauw BE, Rubin RH (2007) Imaging findings in acute invasive pulmonary aspergillosis: clinical significance of the halo sign. Clin Infect Dis 44(3):373–379
18. Chamilos G, Marom EM, Lewis RE, Lionakis MS, Kontoyiannis DP (2005) Predictors of pulmonary zygomycosis versus invasive pulmonary aspergillosis in patients with cancer. Clin Infect Dis 41(1):60–66
19. Wingard JR, Santos GW, Saral R (1985) Late-onset interstitial pneumonia following allergenic bone marrow transplantation. Transplantation 39(1):21–23
20. Shao PL, Huang LM, Hsueh PR (2006) Invasive fungal infection – laboratory diagnosis and antifungal treatment. J Microbiol Immunol Infect 39(3):178–188
21. Maertens J, Theunissen K, Verhoef G, Verschakelen J, Lagrou K, Verbeken E, Wilmer A, Verhaegen J, Boogaerts M, Van Eldere J (2005) Galactomannan and computed tomography-based preemptive antifungal therapy in neutropenic patients at high risk for invasive fungal infection: a prospective feasibility study. Clin Infect Dis 41(9):1242–1250
22. Wheat LJ (2003) Rapid diagnosis of invasive aspergillosis by antigen detection. Transpl Infect Dis 5:158–166
23. Mennink-Kersten MA, Donnelly JP, Verweij PE (2004) Detection of circulating galactomannan for the diagnosis and management of invasive aspergillosis. Lancet Infect Dis 4:349–357
24. Maertens J, Van Eldere J, Verhaegen J, Verbeken E, Verschakelen J, Boogaerts M (2002) Use of circulating galactomannan screening for early diagnosis of invasive aspergillosis in allogeneic stem cell transplant recipients. J Infect Dis 186(9): 1297–1306
25. Herbrecht R, Letscher-Bru V, Oprea C, Lioure B, Waller J, Campos F, Villard O, Liu KL, Natarajan-Ame S, Lutz P, Dufour P, Bergerat JP, Candolfi E (2002) Aspergillus galactomannan detection in the diagnosis of invasive aspergillosis in cancer patients. J Clin Oncol 20(7):1898–1906
26. Maertens J, Verhaegen J, Van Eldere J, Boogaerts M (2001) Screening for circulating galactomannan as a noninvasive diagnostic tool for invasive aspergillosis in prolonged neutropenic patients and stem cell transplantation recipients: a prospective validation. Blood 97:1604–1610
27. Sulahian A, Boutboul F, Ribaud P, Leblanc T, Lacroix C, Derouin F (2001) Value of antigen detection using an enzyme immunoassay in the diagnosis and prediction of invasive aspergillosis in two adult and pediatric hematology units during a 4-year prospective study. Cancer 91(2):311–318
28. Pinel C, Fricker-Hidalgo H, Lebeau B, Garban F, Hamidfar R, Ambroise-Thomas P, Grillot R (2003) Detection of circulating Aspergillus fumigatus galactomannan: value and limits of the Platelia test for diagnosing invasive aspergillosis. J Clin Microbiol 41(5):2184–2186
29. Marr KA, Laverdiere M, Gugel A, Leisenring W (2005) Antifungal therapy decreases sensitivity of the Apsergillus galactomannan enzyme immunoassay. Clin Infect Dis 40:1762–1769
30. Marr KA, Balajee SA, McLaughlin L, Tabouret M, Bentsen C, Walsh TJ (2004) Detection of galactomannan antigenemia by enzyme immunoassay for the diagnosis

of invasive aspergillosis: variables that affect performance. J Infect Dis 190(3): 641–649
31. Hope WW, Walsh TJ, Denning DW (2005) Laboratory diagnosis of invasive aspergillosis. Lancet Infect Dis 5:609–622
32. Pfeiffer CD, Fine JP, Safdar N (2006) Diagnosis of invasive aspergillosis using a galactomannan assay: a meta-analysis. Clin Infect Dis 42:1417–1427
33. Dunagan DP, Baker AM, Hurd DD, Haponik EF (1997) Bronchoscopic evaluation of pulmonary infiltrates following bone marrow transplantation. Chest 111(1): 135–141
34. Feller-Kopman D, Ernst A (2003) The role of bronchoalveolar lavage in the immunocompromised host. Semin Respir Infect 18(2):87–94
35. Weiss K (2006) Poor infection control, not fluoroquinolones, likely to be primary cause of Clostridium difficile-associated diarrhea outbreaks in Quebec. Clin Infect Dis 42(5):725–727
36. McDonald LC, Killgore GE, Thompson A, Owens RC Jr, Kazakova SV, Sambol SP, Johnson S, Gerding DN (2005) An epidemic, toxin gene-variant strain of Clostridium difficile. N Engl J Med 353(23):2433–2441
37. Pepin J, Saheb N, Coulombe MA, Alary ME, Corriveau MP, Authier S, Leblanc M, Rivard G, Bettez M, Primeau V, Nguyen M, Jacob CE, Lanthier L (2005) Emergence of fluoroquinolones as the predominant risk factor for Clostridium difficile-associated diarrhea: a cohort study during an epidemic in Quebec. Clin Infect Dis 41(9):1254–1260
38. Kuijper EJ, van den Berg RJ, Debast S, Visser CE, Veenendaal D, Troelstra A, van der KT, van den HS, Notermans DW (2006) Clostridium difficile ribotype 027, toxinotype III, the Netherlands. Emerg Infect Dis 12(5):827–830
39. Loo VG, Poirier L, Miller MA, Oughton M, Libman MD, Michaud S, Bourgault AM, Nguyen T, Frenette C, Kelly M, Vibien A, Brassard P, Fenn S, Dewar K, Hudson TJ, Horn R, Rene P, Monczak Y, Dascal A (2005) A predominantly clonal multi-institutional outbreak of Clostridium difficile-associated diarrhea with high morbidity and mortality. N Engl J Med 353(23):2442–2449
40. Dial S, Delaney JA, Barkun AN, Suissa S (2005) Use of gastric acid-suppressive agents and the risk of community-acquired Clostridium difficile-associated disease. JAMA 294(23):2989–2995
41. Gorschluter M, Mey U, Strehl J, Ziske C, Schepke M, Schmidt-Wolf IG, Sauerbruch T, Glasmacher A (2005) Neutropenic enterocolitis in adults: systematic analysis of evidence quality. Eur J Haematol 75(1):1–13
42. Cardona AF, Ramos PL, Casasbuenas A (2005) From case reports to systematic reviews in neutropenic enterocolitis. Eur J Haematol 75(5):445–446
43. Aksoy DY, Tanriover MD, Uzun O, Zarakolu P, Ercis S, Erguven S, Oto A, Kerimoglu U, Hayran M, Abbasoglu O (2007) Diarrhea in neutropenic patients: a prospective cohort study with emphasis on neutropenic enterocolitis. Ann Oncol 18(1): 183–189
44. Cardona Zorrilla AF, Reveiz HL, Casasbuenas A, Aponte DM, Ramos PL (2006) Systematic review of case reports concerning adults suffering from neutropenic enterocolitis. Clin Transl Oncol 8(1):31–38
45. Gorschluter M, Mey U, Strehl J, Schmitz V, Rabe C, Pauls K, Ziske C, Schmidt-Wolf IG, Glasmacher A (2006) Invasive fungal infections in neutropenic enterocolitis: a systematic analysis of pathogens, incidence, treatment and mortality in adult patients. BMC Infect Dis 6:35
46. Yolken RH, Bishop CA, Townsend TR, Bolyard EA, Bartlett J, Santos GW, Saral R (1982) Infectious gastroenteritis in bone-marrow-transplant recipients. N Engl J Med 306(17):1010–1012
47. Townsend TR, Bolyard EA, Yolken RH, Beschorner WE, Bishop CA, Burns WH, Santos GW, Saral R (1982) Outbreak of Coxsackie A1 gastroenteritis: a complication of bone-marrow transplantation. Lancet 1(8276):820–823

48. Cox GJ, Matsui SM, Lo RS, Hinds M, Bowden RA, Hackman RC, Meyer WG, Mori M, Tarr PI, Oshiro LS (1994) Etiology and outcome of diarrhea after marrow transplantation: a prospective study. Gastroenterology 107(5):1398–1407
49. van Kraaij MG, Dekker AW, Verdonck LF, van Loon AM, Vinje J, Koopmans MP, Rozenberg-Arska M (2000) Infectious gastro-enteritis: an uncommon cause of diarrhoea in adult allogeneic and autologous stem cell transplant recipients. Bone Marrow Transplant 26(3):299–303
50. Boeckh M, Nichols WG (2004) The impact of cytomegalovirus serostatus of donor and recipient before hematopoietic stem cell transplantation in the era of antiviral prophylaxis and preemptive therapy. Blood 103(6):2003–2008
51. Shields AF, Hackman RC, Fife KH, Corey L, Meyers JD (1985) Adenovirus infections in patients undergoing bone-marrow transplantation. N Engl J Med 312(9):529–533
52. Hale GA, Heslop HE, Krance RA, Brenner MA, Jayawardene D, Srivastava DK, Patrick CC (1999) Adenovirus infection after pediatric bone marrow transplantation. Bone Marrow Transplant 23(3):277–282
53. Bowden RA (1997) Respiratory virus infections after marrow transplant: the Fred Hutchinson Cancer Research Center experience. Am J Med 102(3A):27–30
54. Nichols WG, Gooley T, Boeckh M (2001) Community-acquired respiratory syncytial virus and parainfluenza virus infections after hematopoietic stem cell transplantation: the Fred Hutchinson Cancer Research Center experience. Biol Blood Marrow Transplant 7(Suppl):11S–15S
55. Whimbey E, Vartivarian SE, Champlin RE, Elting LS, Luna M, Bodey GP (1993) Parainfluenza virus infection in adult bone marrow transplant recipients. Eur J Clin Microbiol Infect Dis 12(9):699–701
56. Ljungman P (2001) Respiratory virus infections in stem cell transplant patients: the European experience. Biol Blood Marrow Transplant 7(Suppl):5S–7S
57. Wang FZ, Linde A, Hagglund H, Testa M, Locasciulli A, Ljungman P (1999) Human herpesvirus 6 DNA in cerebrospinal fluid specimens from allogeneic bone marrow transplant patients: does it have clinical significance? Clin Infect Dis 28(3):562–568
58. Buchbinder S, Elmaagacli AH, Schaefer UW, Roggendorf M (2000) Human herpesvirus 6 is an important pathogen in infectious lung disease after allogeneic bone marrow transplantation. Bone Marrow Transplant 26(6):639–644
59. Leung AY, Suen CK, Lie AK, Liang RH, Yuen KY, Kwong YL (2001) Quantification of polyoma BK viruria in hemorrhagic cystitis complicating bone marrow transplantation. Blood 98(6):1971–1978
60. Azzi A, Cesaro S, Laszlo D, Zakrzewska K, Ciappi S, De Santis R, Fanci R, Pesavento G, Calore E, Bosi A (1999) Human polyomavirus BK (BKV) load and haemorrhagic cystitis in bone marrow transplantation patients. J Clin Virol 14(2):79–86
61. Leibovici L, Paul M, Cullen M, Bucaneve G, Gafter-Gvili A, Fraser A, Kern WV (2006) Antibiotic prophylaxis in neutropenic patients: new evidence, practical decisions. Cancer 107(8):1743–1751
62. Gafter-Gvili A, Fraser A, Paul M, Leibovici L (2005) Meta-analysis: antibiotic prophylaxis reduces mortality in neutropenic patients. Ann Intern Med 142(12 Pt 1): 979–995
63. Engels EA, Lau J, Barza M (1998) Efficacy of quinolone prophylaxis in neutropenic cancer patients: a meta-analysis. J Clin Oncol 16(3):1179–1187
64. Bucaneve G, Micozzi A, Menichetti F, Martino P, Dionisi MS, Martinelli G, Allione B, D'Antonio D, Buelli M, Nosari AM, Cilloni D, Zuffa E, Cantaffa R, Specchia G, Amadori S, Fabbiano F, Deliliers GL, Lauria F, Foa R, Del Favero A (2005) Levofloxacin to prevent bacterial infection in patients with cancer and neutropenia. N Engl J Med 353(10):977–987
65. Goodman JL, Winston DJ, Greenfield RA, Chandrasekar PH, Fox B, Kaizer H, Shadduck RK, Shea TC, Stiff P, Friedman DJ (1992) A controlled trial of fluconazole

to prevent fungal infections in patients undergoing bone marrow transplantation. N Engl J Med 326(13):845–851
66. Slavin MA, Osborne B, Adams R, Levenstein MJ, Schoch HG, Feldman AR, Meyers JD, Bowden RA (1995) Efficacy and safety of fluconazole prophylaxis for fungal infections after marrow transplantation – a prospective, randomized, double-blind study. J Infect Dis 171(6):1545–1552
67. Marr KA, Seidel K, Slavin MA, Bowden RA, Schoch HG, Flowers ME, Corey L, Boeckh M (2000) Prolonged fluconazole prophylaxis is associated with persistent protection against candidiasis-related death in allogeneic marrow transplant recipients: long-term follow-up of a randomized, placebo-controlled trial. Blood 96(6):2055–2061
68. Wingard JR (2002) Antifungal chemoprophylaxis after blood and marrow transplantation. Clin Infect Dis 34(10):1386–1390
69. Kanda Y, Yamamoto R, Chizuka A, Hamaki T, Suguro M, Arai C, Matsuyama T, Takezako N, Miwa A, Kern W, Kami M, Akiyama H, Hirai H, Togawa A (2000) Prophylactic action of oral fluconazole against fungal infection in neutropenic patients. A meta-analysis of 16 randomized, controlled trials. Cancer 89(7):1611–1625
70. van Burik JA, Ratanatharathorn V, Stepan DE, Miller CB, Lipton JH, Vesole DH, Bunin N, Wall DA, Hiemenz JW, Satoi Y, Lee JM, Walsh TJ (2004) Micafungin versus fluconazole for prophylaxis against invasive fungal infections during neutropenia in patients undergoing hematopoietic stem cell transplantation. Clin Infect Dis 39(10):1407–1416
71. Mattiuzzi GN, Alvarado G, Giles FJ, Ostrosky-Zeichner L, Cortes J, O'brien S, Verstovsek S, Faderl S, Zhou X, Raad II, Bekele BN, Leitz GJ, Lopez-Roman I, Estey EH (2006) Open-label, randomized comparison of itraconazole versus caspofungin for prophylaxis in patients with hematologic malignancies. Antimicrob Agents Chemother 50(1):143–147
72. Mattiuzzi GN, Estey E, Raad I, Giles F, Cortes J, Shen Y, Kontoyiannis D, Koller C, Munsell M, Beran M, Kantarjian H (2003) Liposomal amphotericin B versus the combination of fluconazole and itraconazole as prophylaxis for invasive fungal infections during induction chemotherapy for patients with acute myelogenous leukemia and myelodysplastic syndrome. Cancer 97(2):450–456
73. Peacock O, Reinwold M, Schmidt-Hieber M, Schwartz S, Martus P, Thiel E, Blau I (2005) Low dose liposomal amphotericin B (L-AmB) as prophylaxis of invasive fungal infections (IFI) in patients (pts) with prolonged neutropenia (N): results from a phase III trial. Abstract M-975. Interscience Conference on Antimicrobial Agents and Chemotherapy Annual Meeting in Washington, DC
74. Glasmacher A, Prentice A, Gorschluter M, Engelhart S, Hahn C, Djulbegovic B, Schmidt-Wolf IG (2003) Itraconazole prevents invasive fungal infections in neutropenic patients treated for hematologic malignancies: evidence from a meta-analysis of 3,597 patients. J Clin Oncol 21(24):4615–4626
75. Cornely OA, Maertens J, Winston DJ, Perfect J, Ullmann AJ, Walsh TJ, Helfgott D, Holowiecki J, Stockelberg D, Goh YT, Petrini M, Hardalo C, Suresh R, Angulo-Gonzalez D (2007) Posaconazole vs. fluconazole or itraconazole prophylaxis in patients with neutropenia. N Engl J Med 356(4):348–359
76. Rojas R, Serrano J, Martin C, Tabares S, Capote M, Fernandez M, Arqueros V, Molina JR, Martin V, Torres A (2005) Voriconazole in primary prophylaxis reduces the incidence of IFI in high risk hematologic patients. Abstract 5349. Presented at ASH Annual Meeting in Atlanta, GA
77. Mattiuzzi GN, Estey EH, Hernandez M, Cabanillas ME, Giles F, Cortes JE, O'Brien S, Verstovsek S, Kantarjian HM (2005) Voriconazole and liposomal amphotericin B (Ambisome) effectively prevent mold infections in patients (pts) with acute myelogenous leukemia (AML) following remission induction chemotherapy. Abstract 2773. Presented at ASH Annual Meeting in Atlanta, GA
78. Winston DJ, Maziarz RT, Chandrasekar PH, Lazarus HM, Goldman M, Blumer JL, Leitz GJ, Territo MC (2003) Intravenous and oral itraconazole versus intravenous

and oral fluconazole for long-term antifungal prophylaxis in allogeneic hematopoietic stem-cell transplant recipients. A multicenter, randomized trial. Ann Intern Med 138(9):705–713
79. Marr KA, Crippa F, Leisenring W, Hoyle M, Boeckh M, Balajee SA, Nichols WG, Musher B, Corey L (2004) Itraconazole versus fluconazole for prevention of fungal infections in patients receiving allogeneic stem cell transplants. Blood 103(4): 1527–1533
80. Ullmann AJ, Lipton JH, Vesole DH, Chandrasekar P, Langston A, Tarantolo SR, Greinix H, Morais dA, Reddy V, Boparai N, Pedicone L, Patino H, Durrant S (2007) Posaconazole or fluconazole for prophylaxis in severe graft-versus-host disease. N Engl J Med 356(4):335–347
81. Wingard JR, Carter SL, Walsh TJ, Kurtzberg J, Small TN, Gersten ID, Mendizabal AM, Leather H, Confer DL, Baden LR, Maziarz RT, Stadtmauer EA, Bolanos-Meade J, Brown J, DiPersio JF, Boeckh M, Marr KA (2007) Results of a randomized, double-blind trial of fluconazole (FLU) vs. Voriconazole (VORI) for the prevention of invasive fungal infections (IFI) in 600 allogeneic blood and marrow transplant (BMT) patients. Blood 110(11):55a Abstract #163
82. Marty FM, Cosimi LA, Baden LR (2004) Breakthrough zygomycosis after voriconazole treatment in recipients of hematopoietic stem-cell transplants. N Engl J Med 350(9):950–952
83. Kontoyiannis DP, Lionakis MS, Lewis RE, Chamilos G, Healy M, Perego C, Safdar A, Kantarjian H, Champlin R, Walsh TJ, Raad II (2005) Zygomycosis in a tertiary-care cancer center in the era of Aspergillus-active antifungal therapy: a case-control observational study of 27 recent cases. J Infect Dis 191(8):1350–1360
84. Siwek GT, Dodgson KJ, Magalhaes-Silverman M, Bartelt LA, Kilborn SB, Hoth PL, Diekema DJ, Pfaller MA (2004) Invasive zygomycosis in hematopoietic stem cell transplant recipients receiving voriconazole prophylaxis. Clin Infect Dis 39(4):584–587
85. Prentice HG, Gluckman E, Powles RL, Ljungman P, Milpied N, Fernandez Ranada JM, Mandelli F, Kho P, Kennedy L, Bell AR (1994) Impact of long-term acyclovir on cytomegalovirus infection and survival after allogeneic bone marrow transplantation. European Acyclovir for CMV Prophylaxis Study Group. Lancet 343(8900):749–753
86. Ljungman P, de La CR, Milpied N, Volin L, Russell CA, Crisp A, Webster A (2002) Randomized study of valacyclovir as prophylaxis against cytomegalovirus reactivation in recipients of allogeneic bone marrow transplants. Blood 99(8): 3050–3056
87. Boeckh M, Gooley TA, Myerson D, Cunningham T, Schoch G, Bowden RA (1996) Cytomegalovirus pp 65 antigenemia-guided early treatment with ganciclovir versus ganciclovir at engraftment after allogeneic marrow transplantation: a randomized double-blind study. Blood 88(10):4063–4071
88. Goodrich JM, Bowden RA, Fisher L, Keller C, Schoch G, Meyers JD (1993) Ganciclovir prophylaxis to prevent cytomegalovirus disease after allogeneic marrow transplant. Ann Intern Med 118(3):173–178
89. Winston DJ, Ho WG, Bartoni K, Du MC, Ebeling DF, Buhles WC, Champlin RE (1993) Ganciclovir prophylaxis of cytomegalovirus infection and disease in allogeneic bone marrow transplant recipients. Results of a placebo-controlled, double-blind trial. Ann Intern Med 118(3):179–184
90. Reusser P, Einsele H, Lee J, Volin L, Rovira M, Engelhard D, Finke J, Cordonnier C, Link H, Ljungman P (2002) Randomized multicenter trial of foscarnet versus ganciclovir for preemptive therapy of cytomegalovirus infection after allogeneic stem cell transplantation. Blood 99(4):1159–1164
91. Boeckh M, Kim HW, Flowers ME (2006) Long-term acyclovir for prevention of varicella zoster virus disease after allogeneic hematopoietic cell transplantation – a randomized double-blind placebo-controlled study. Blood 107:1800–1805

92. Sherertz RJ, Belani A, Kramer BS, Elfenbein GJ, Weiner RS, Sullivan ML, Thomas RG, Samsa GP (1987) Impact of air filtration on nosocomial Aspergillus infections. Unique risk of bone marrow transplant recipients. Am J Med 83(4):709–718
93. Storb R, Prentice RL, Buckner CD, Clift RA, Appelbaum F, Deeg J, Doney K, Hansen JA, Mason M, Sanders JE, Singer J, Sullivan KM, Witherspoon RP, Thomas ED (1983) Graft-versus-host disease and survival in patients with aplastic anemia treated by marrow grafts from HLA-identical siblings. Beneficial effect of a protective environment. N Engl J Med 308(6):302–307
94. Passweg JR, Rowlings PA, Atkinson KA, Barrett AJ, Gale RP, Gratwohl A, Jacobsen N, Klein JP, Ljungman P, Russell JA, Schaefer UW, Sobocinski KA, Vossen JM, Zhang MJ, Horowitz MM (1998) Influence of protective isolation on outcome of allogeneic bone marrow transplantation for leukemia. Bone Marrow Transplant 21(12):1231–1238
95. Garner JS (1996) Guideline for isolation precautions in hospitals. The Hospital Infection Control Practices Advisory Committee. Infect Control Hosp Epidemiol 17(1):53–80
96. Lai KK, Fontecchio S, Melvin Z, Baker SP (2006) Impact of alcohol-based, waterless hand antiseptic on the incidence of infection and colonization with methicillin-resistant Staphylococcus aureus and vancomycin-resistant enterococci. Infect Control Hosp Epidemiol 27(10):1018–1024
97. Muto CA, Jernigan JA, Ostrowsky BE, Richet HM, Jarvis WR, Boyce JM, Farr BM (2003) SHEA guideline for preventing nosocomial transmission of multidrug-resistant strains of Staphylococcus aureus and enterococcus. Infect Control Hosp Epidemiol 24(5):362–386

Special Topics

Chapter 9

Modulation of Immune Function

Nikolaos G. Almyroudis, Minoo Battiwalla, and Brahm H. Segal

Abstract Patients with hematologic malignancies and hematopoietic stem cell transplant recipients have a broad range of immune deficits that predispose to common and opportunistic infectious diseases. Infectious complications are a major cause of morbidity and mortality in these patients. Effective immune augmentation strategies used as prophylaxis and as adjunctive therapy represent an important unmet need. We discuss several immune-based strategies tailored to specific patient populations. These include strategies to augment neutrophil number, enhance function of neutrophils and macrophages, passive antibody therapy, and augmentation of cellular immunity. We evaluate immune-based therapies that are currently available and the evidence supporting their use. There is a large "pipeline" of novel and promising immunotherapies that are at preclinical and early stages of clinical development. These include augmentation of innate and antigen-specific immunity by stimulating pathogen recognition pathways, adoptive transfer of cellular immunity, and vaccine development. We review these more cutting-edge approaches, with an emphasis on opportunistic fungal and viral infections. We discuss gaps in knowledge and challenges in bringing promising immune-based therapies to clinical trials.

Keywords Immune modulation • Immune reconstitution • Growth factors • Adoptive transfer • Cellular immunity • Granulocyte transfusion • Colony-stimulating factors

1. Introduction

Patients with hematologic malignancies encompass a broad range of immunocompromised states. Important differences in both the degree and nature of the immunocompromise exist among different patients. Quantitative features of immune impairment are generally straightforward. For example, in neutropenic patients, the degree and duration of neutropenia predict the risk of life-threatening infections. Among allogeneic hematopoietic stem cell transplant recipients (HSCT), the early period of risk of infections corresponds to neutropenia and disruption of mucosal barriers following the conditioning regimen, and later

From: *Managing Infections in Patients With Hematological Malignancies*: Contemporary Hematology, Edited by: M. Kleinberg, DOI 10.1007/978-1-59745-415-5_9,

periods correspond to the intensity of immunosuppressive therapy required to control graft-vs.-host disease (GVHD). In severe GVHD, global immune impairment occurs that affects both innate phagocyte function and cellular and humoral immunity. The spectrum of opportunistic pathogens to which patients are susceptible is in fact broader in the setting of GVHD than in leukopenia from cytotoxic chemotherapy. Other agents, such as purine analogs and alemtuzumab disable host defense pathways that render patients susceptible to specific groups of pathogens. Indeed, multiple host defense pathways may be disabled by immunodeficiencies associated with the primary malignancy and cytotoxic and immunosuppressive agents (Tables 9-1 and 9-2).

Immunotherapy must be tailored to the specific immunodeficiency that exists in a given patient population (Table 9-3). This concept is straightforward for neutropenia in which the aim is to augment neutrophil number, for example, by colony-stimulating factors (CSFs) or granulocyte transfusions. In GVHD, the immune impairment is more complex; the immunotherapeutic strategy may at best ameliorate some features of the immunocompromised state, but would not reconstitute all of the disabled host defense pathways.

Major advances in preventing and treating life-threatening infectious complications in patients with hematologic malignancies have resulted from more

Table 9-1. Risk factors and infectious diseases associated with hematologic malignancies.

Risk factors	**Infection**	**Comment**
Malignancy-related factors		
Hematologic malignancies		
Myelodysplastic syndrome and acute leukemia	Bacteria, viruses, and fungi	Infectious risk related to prolonged neutropenia
CLL	Encapsulated bacteria	Infectious risk linked to hypogammaglobulinemia
Hairy cell leukemia	Mycobacteria, herpes viruses	Defective T cell immunity
Hodgkin's disease	Mycobacteria, herpes viruses	Defective T cell immunity
Adult T cell lymphoma/ leukemia	*Pneumocystis jiroveci* (formerly *Pneumocystis carinii*), *C. neoformans*, CMV, *Strongyloides stercoralis*	Defective T cell immunity
Multiple myeloma	Encapsulated bacteria, particularly *S. pneumoniae*	Impaired B-cell immunity
Treatment-related factors		
Neutropenia	Bacterial infections (Staphylococci., enterococci, viridans group streptococci, Enterobacteriaceae, *P. aeruginosa*) Fungal infections (candidiasis, aspergillosis, and other moulds)	
	Viral infections (herpes simplex virus, community respiratory viruses, e.g., influenza, parainfluenza, respiratory syncitial virus, adenovirus, and human metapneumoviruses)	
Mucositis	Bacterial infections caused by gastrointestinal bacterial flora, candidiasis	

(continued)

Table 9-1. (continued)

Risk factors	Infection	Comment
Corticosteroids	Bacteria, *Pneumocystis jiroveci*, *C. neoformans*, moulds, herpes viruses	Defects in phagocytosis and T-cell immunity. Decrease signs and symptoms of inflammation
Nucleoside analogues (e.g., fludarabine, 2-chlorodeoxyadenosine, and 2-deoxycoformycin)	Bacteria, *Pneumocystis jiroveci*, *C. neoformans*, herpes viruses	Defective T-cell immunity
Alemtuzumab	Opportunistic and nonopportunistic infections, including bacteria, viruses (e.g., herpes simplex virus, CMV, varicella zoster virus), *Pneumocystis jiroveci*, and other fungi	Defective cellular immunity and neutropenia
Rituximab	Rituximab, by itself, has modest immunosuppressive properties. Overall infectious risk dependent on coadministered chemotherapy cases of progressive multifocal leukoencephalopathy (PML) and fulminant reactivation of hepatitis B infection have occured	Impaired B-cell immunity
Daclizumab	Bacterial sepsis	Infections in the setting of steroid-refractory GVHD
Antibodies inhibiting cytokine signaling (e.g., infliximab)	Bacterial infections, Tuberculosis and other mycobacterial infections, mould infections in GVHD, other fungal infections (e.g., histoplasmosis)	Suppression of inflammation may allow infections to progress undetected
Calcineurin inhibitors	*Pneumocystis jiroveci*, VZV	
Radiation therapy	Local and systemic bacterial infections, mucosal candidiasis and HSV infection	Damages mucosal surfaces, marrow suppression
Asplenia	Encapsulated bacteria (*S. pneumoniae*, *H. influenzae*, and *Neisseria meningitidis*), *Salmonella*, *Capnocytophaga canimorsus*, *Babesia microti*, malaria	

effective and safer drugs. The development of antipseudomonal beta-lactams in the 1960s and 1970s and the routine use of empirical antibacterial therapy at the onset of neutropenic fever reduced mortality from bacterial infections [1]. Prophylactic and preemptive antiviral therapy for cytomegalovirus (CMV) has significantly reduced CMV disease, though not overall mortality, in allogeneic HSCT recipients [2–5]. Indeed, with improvements in antibacterial and antiviral therapy and the widespread use of fluconazole prophylaxis against invasive candidiasis [6–10], invasive mould infections became a leading cause of infection-related mortality among patients with acute leukemia and allogeneic HSCT recipients [11–17]. Recent developments in the antifungal armamentarium have translated into a reduction in the incidence and mortality due to invasive aspergillosis in randomized studies [18–20]. These important advances require us to look back at older trials of immunotherapy and ask what results are relevant today, and to look forward in asking what are the unmet needs that immunotherapy might address.

Our chapter focuses on immunotherapy to prevent and treat infectious diseases in patients with hematologic malignancies and allogeneic HSCT recipients,

Table 9-2. Time line of principal immune defects and infectious complications in allogeneic hematopoietic stem cell transplant recipients.

	Months after transplantation		
	<1	1–6	>6[a]
Principal immune defect	Neutropenia	T cell, humoral Phagocytic (qualitative)	Humoral
Bacterial pathogens	Staphylococci, enterococci, viridans group streptococci, Enterobacteriacea, *P. aeruginosa*	Bacterial infections encountered during neutropenia (e.g., Staphylococci, streptococci, gram-negative infections) are less common after neutrophil recovery. Encapsulated bacteria (generally 3 months or more after HSCT), *Listeria monocytogenes*, mycobacteria, nocardiosis are more common during the 1–6 month period than during neutropenia.	Encapsulated bacteria
Fungal pathogens	*Candida* species, *Aspergillus* species, and other moulds (e.g., zygomycetes, *Fusarium* species, *Scedosporium* species, dark-walled moulds)	Same as <1 month plus *Pneumocystis jiroveci*, *Candida* sp., *C. neoformans*, dimorphic fungi (e.g., histoplasmosis, coccidioidomycosis)	Risk of invasive fungal infections decreases after 6 months in absence of GVHD
Viral pathogens	Herpes simplex virus, community respiratory viruses (e.g., influenza, parainfluenza, RSV, adenovirus, metapneumoviruses)	CMV, varicella zoster virus, herpes simplex virus, EBV-associated lymphoproliferative disease,community respiratory viruses	Varicella zoster virus, community respiratory viruses. Risk of other opportunistic viral infections decreases after 6 months in absence of GVHD.
Parasitic infections		Toxoplasmosis, strongyloidiasis	

[a]Graft-vs.-host disease necessitating intensive immunosuppressive therapy leads to lack of reconstitution of phagocytic (qualitative) and cell-mediated immunity, thus prolonging the period of risk for infection with both common bacteria and opportunistic pathogens

with an emphasis on opportunistic fungal and viral infections. We discuss currently available modes of immunotherapy in the context of host factors and best practices for antimicrobial therapy. We also discuss novel experimental modes of immunotherapy that show promise at the preclinical level and pitfalls in paving the way from preclinical studies to early clinical trials.

2. Augmentation of Neutrophil Number

2.1. Colony-Stimulating Factors As Prophylaxis

Normal myelopoiesis requires myeloid stem cells. Under the influence of stem cell factor, interleukin-3 (IL-3), and granulocyte-macrophage colony-stimulating factor (GM-CSF), these give rise to the colony-forming

Table 9-3. Summary of immune augmentation strategies.

Aim	Strategy[a]
Increase neutrophil number	• Colony stimulating factors (CSFs)
	• Granulocyte transfusions
	• Experimental myeloid transfusion studies (see text)
Augment neutrophil and macrophage function	• Colony-stimulating factors (CSFs)
	• Cytokines (e.g., IFN-γ)
	• Toll-like receptor (TLR) ligands
	• Pentraxin-3
Augment T-cell immunity	• Vaccination
	• Adoptive transfer of T-cell populations
	• Cytokines (e.g., IFN-γ)
	• Toll-like receptor (TLR) ligands
	• Pentraxin-3
Augment humoral immunity	• Intravenous immunoglobulin
	• Yeast killer toxin antiidiotypic antibodies
	• Vaccination
Complement activation	• Mannose-binding lectin

[a]Several of the listed strategies are experimental (see text)

unit-granulocyte/macrophage (CFU-GM). Granulocyte-colony-stimulating factor (G-CSF) acts at a later stage in concert with other growth factors to specifically drive granulopoiesis. Primary administration of CSF has reduced the incidence of febrile neutropenia by approximately 50% in randomized trials in adults in whom the incidence of neutropenic fever was greater than 40% in the control group [21]. Multiple randomized clinical trials of prophylactic recombinant G-CSF and GM-CSF have shown the benefit of CSFs in reducing the time to neutrophil recovery and duration of fever and hospitalization in patients with acute myelogenous leukemia (AML) [22]. In one randomized study in patients receiving chemotherapy for AML with GM-CSF led to a lower frequency of fatal fungal infections compared with placebo and reduced overall early mortality [23].

A meta-analysis of randomized trials of prophylactic G-CSF and GM-CSF in autologous and allogeneic HSCT recipients showed that CSFs were associated with a small reduction in the risk of documented infections, but did not affect infection or treatment-related mortality [24]. In allogeneic HSCT recipients, G-CSF, but not GM-CSF, results in Th2 skewing of lymphocytes and promotes the development of T regulatory cells [25, 26]. G-CSF given after T-cell depleted haplotype-mismatched transplantation was associated with faster neutrophil recovery but prolonged cellular immune dysfunction [27]. A recent analysis of a large data registry from the Center for International Blood and Marrow Transplant Research (CIBMTR) found no risk or benefit of using G-CSF to promote myeloid recovery after allogeneic HSCT for myeloid leukemias with regard to GVHD, treatment-related mortality, leukemia-free survival, and overall survival [28].

The principal benefit of CSFs in patients receiving treatment for acute leukemia relates to modestly more rapid neutrophil recovery and fewer hospitalization days – which are important supportive care goals. In contrast, the benefit of CSFs in patients with solid tumors receiving cytotoxic regimens principally relates to prevention of neutropenic fever. The American Society of Clinical Oncology (ASCO) has established authoritative guidelines that expanded the use of prophylactic CSFs [29]. The panel considered the use of CSFs to be justified when the risk of neutropenic fever is approximately 20% and no other equally effective regimen is available. In the prior ASCO guidelines, the use of CSFs was advised when the risk of neutropenic fever was 40% or higher [21]. Reduction in the incidence of neutropenic fever is an important clinical outcome in terms of avoiding unnecessary use of antibiotics and potential hospitalization. An additional concern related to neutropenic fever is the potential for delay or dose-reduction of subsequent cycles of chemotherapy that can adversely affect the response to therapy. Whether CSFs in patients with solid tumors receiving cytotoxic regimens will translate into improved long-term outcomes is unknown.

ASCO guidelines also advise CSF prophylaxis in patients at increase risk for complications from prolonged neutropenia, even with regimens in which the expected frequency of neutropenic fever is less than 20% [29]. Examples include age >65 years, poor performance status, poor nutritional status, advanced cancer, bone marrow involvement by tumor with cytopenias, extensive prior treatment, and the presence of open wounds or active infections. Secondary prophylaxis with a CSF is advised in patients who experienced a neutropenic complication from a prior cycle of chemotherapy in which a reduced dose of chemotherapy may adversely affect treatment outcome.

2.2. Colony-Stimulating Factors As Adjunctive Therapy

The rationale for CSFs for established infections (as opposed to prophylaxis) stems from both the quantitative and qualitative effects of these agents on phagocytic cells. In neutropenic patients with life-threatening infections, survival is strongly influenced by the rapidity of neutrophil recovery [30]. Thus, CSFs may be used in these settings to augment the number of circulating neutrophils. CSFs should not routinely be used as adjunctive therapy for neutropenic fever. ASCO guidelines advise that CSFs can be considered in patients with neutropenic fever at high risk for infectious complications or prognostic factors predictive of poor clinical outcomes. Examples include age >65 years, uncontrolled malignancy, and prolonged (>10 days) and profound (absolute neutrophil count $<0.1 \times 10^9$/L) neutropenia [29]. Although the benefit of a CSF for established infections in neutropenic patients is unproven, ASCO guidelines reasonably advise that they can be considered in neutropenic patients with serious infections, such as pneumonia, hypotension, multiorgan dysfunction, and invasive fungal infection, and hospitalization at the time of development of fever [29].

There is significant interest in the potential for adjunctive CSFs in patients with invasive fungal infections, though the clinical database is limited. CSFs, in addition to augmenting leukocyte numbers, also augment phagocyte function. G-CSF, GM-CSF, and macrophage colony-stimulating factor (M-CSF) increase the fungicidal activity of phagocytes in vitro against *Candida* and *Aspergillus* species [31–34].

G-CSF influences survival, proliferation, and differentiation of all cells in the neutrophil lineage and augments the function of mature neutrophils.

M-CSF increases phagocytosis, chemotaxis, and secondary cytokine production in monocytes and macrophages [35], but has no effect on neutrophils. M-CSF was protective when given prophylactically in experimental aspergillosis in neutropenic animals [36], illustrating the potential for macrophages as a target for immunotherapy. A Phase I trial of rM-CSF in HSCT recipients with invasive fungal infections reported benefit in patients with invasive candidiasis (but not aspergillosis) and Karnofsy scores >20 compared with historical controls [37, 38].

GM-CSF stimulates various neutrophil effector functions and prolongs neutrophil survival in vitro, increases antibody-dependent cytotoxicity of eosinophils, accelerates the proliferation of the monocytes-macrophage system, and is a potent activator of monocytes and macrophages [35]. Thus, GM-CSF may have a theoretical advantage against pathogens such as *Candida* and *Aspergillus* species, for which host defense is dependent on both neutrophil and macrophage function.

Some studies in vitro [39] and in animal models [40, 41] show that G-CSF and GM-CSF have additive antifungal activity when combined with antifungal agents. A Phase II randomized study of G-CSF plus fluconazole for invasive candidiasis and candidemia in nonneutropenic patients showed the safety of G-CSF, but was not powered for efficacy [42]. Currently, the clinical database on CSFs as adjunctive therapy for fungal infections is inadequate to assess efficacy.

Another gap in knowledge is whether CSFs are safe and effective as either prophylaxis or adjunctive therapy in nonleukopenic patients with severe impairment in phagocyte function. Several studies have reported the predominance of invasive aspergillosis cases occurring in the postengraftment rather than in the neutropenic period in allogeneic HSCT recipients [13, 16, 43–48], with immunosuppressive therapy for GVHD and T-cell depletion being the principal risk factors. Intensive immunosuppressive corticosteroid-based regimens for GVHD cause global impairment of phagocyte effector functions and disable reconstitution of antigenspecific immunity, though circulating neutrophil counts are generally normal. In theory, the ability of GM-CSF to augment qualitative macrophage and neutrophil function may be of value as adjunctive therapy for severe invasive fungal infections in nonleukopenic, highly immunocompromised patients. The benefit vs. the risk of this approach, particularly with regard to exacerbating GVHD, is unknown; we therefore reserve adjunctive GM-CSF in nonleukopenic allogeneic HSCT recipients for treatment of life-threatening, refractory invasive fungal infections. There are no data to support prophylactic CSFs in nonneutropenic patients, and they should not be used as prophylaxis in this setting outside of a clinical trial.

2.3. Myeloid Progenitors

Hematopoietic progenitors committed to the myeloid lineage, the common myeloid and granulocyte-monocyte progenitors (CMP/GMP), have been identified. The addition of these progenitors to hematopoietic grafts in mice rendered neutropenic conferred protection against challenge with *Pseudomonas aeruginosa* and *Aspergillus fumigatus* [49]. Novel strategies such as this approach to accelerate neutrophil recovery merit further study.

2.4. Granulocyte Transfusions

The rationale for granulocyte transfusions is to provide supportive therapy for the neutropenic patient with a life-threatening infection by augmenting the number of circulating neutrophils until myeloid recovery occurs. In the 1970s, apheresis technology for harvesting large numbers of donor granulocytes became available. Controlled trials of granulocyte transfusions as adjunctive therapy in neutropenic patients with significant infections produced mixed results [50–53]. In the 1980s, the enthusiasm for granulocyte transfusions waned as more effective antibiotics became available, survival from serious bacterial infections improved, and recombinant growth factors reduced the duration of neutropenia. In addition, concerns about the toxicity of granulocyte transfusions, including acute pulmonary reactions, HLA alloimmunization (which could render patients refractory to platelet transfusions and potentially impair myeloid engraftment following HSCT), and transfusion-associated infections (particularly CMV) outweighed the perceived benefits.

Today, the impetus to reexamine the role of granulocyte transfusions stems largely from improvements in donor mobilization methods. Bensinger et al. [54] showed that G-CSF mobilization significantly increased the granulocyte yield, and resulted in improved circulating neutrophil levels in neutropenic recipients. Using a standard continuous flow centrifugation apparatus, the mean absolute neutrophil yield per collection is typically in the range of 8×10^{10} cells when both G-CSF and dexamethasone are used in the donor preparatory regimen. Higher numbers of harvested neutrophils correlated with higher posttransfusion neutrophil counts. Furthermore, the increase in circulating neutrophils tends to be sustained for 24–30 h following transfusion, as a consequence of prolonged circulating half-life of G-CSF mobilized granulocytes [55]. The qualitative functions of G-CSF- and steroid-mobilized neutrophils are intact based on in vitro bactericidal activity, respiratory burst, migration to experimental skin chambers, and localization to sites of inflammation.

Successful outcomes using granulocyte transfusions have been described in patients with life-threatening fungal infections in small series and in case reports. A phase I/II trial using G-CSF-mobilized granulocyte transfusions for refractory fungal infections in neutropenic patients with hematologic malignancies reported favorable responses in 11 of 15 patients [56]. Peters et al. [57] evaluated granulocyte transfusions (G-CSF- or prednisolone-mobilized) in 30 patients with neutropenia and life-threatening, refractory infections. Infections cleared in 20 of 30 patients, including 5 of 9 patients with invasive aspergillosis. No benefit of granulocyte transfusions was noted in neutropenic HSCT recipients with invasive mould infection in a retrospective series in which G-CSF donor granulocyte mobilization was not used [58].

Price et al. [59] conducted a phase I/II study of granulocyte transfusions derived from unrelated, non-HLA-matched, community donors, following G-CSF and dexamethasone mobilization. Chills, fever, and oxygen desaturation of $\geq 3\%$ occurred in association with 7% of transfusions, but did not limit therapy. Eight of the 11 patients with bacterial infections or candidemia survived, but all the 8 patients with invasive mould infection died. This study showed the safety and feasibility of using community donors for granulocytapheresis donations.

The Transfusion Medicine and Hemostasis network of the National Heart Lung and Blood Institute is currently in the planning stages of a randomized study of adjunctive granulocyte transfusions in neutropenic patients with severe bacterial and fungal infections. This study is expected to definitively evaluate the benefits and risks of adjunctive granulocyte transfusions.

In the absence of modern, prospective, randomized studies when might granulocyte transfusions be considered? Currently, there is no justification (outside of a clinical trial) to use granulocyte transfusions either as prophylaxis or in cases of documented infections that are likely to respond to conventional therapy. We reserve granulocyte transfusions for patients with prolonged neutropenia and life-threatening infections refractory to conventional therapy. Filamentous fungi are likely to constitute the majority of such refractory infections. Infusions of amphotericin B should be separated several hours from granulocyte transfusions to avoid pulmonary toxicity. In some highly alloimmunized patients, transfused granulocytes are rapidly consumed and are likely to have more toxicity than benefit. In allogeneic transplants in which the donor and recipient are CMV seronegative, using CMV seronegative granulocyte donors is advised [60].

3. Immunoglobulin Therapy

Dysfunctional humoral immunity can be a consequence of the underlying malignancy or result from therapy. Patients with chronic lymphocytic leukemia (CLL) frequently have hypogammaglobulinemia leading to increased susceptibility to encapsulated bacteria, principally *Streptococcus pneumoniae* [61]. Such patients may have recurrent sinopulmonary infections and septicemia. In patients with multiple myeloma, the repertoire of antibody production is restricted, predisposing to an increased risk of infection by encapsulated bacteria. Savage et al. [62] noted a biphasic pattern of infection among patients with multiple myeloma. Infections by *S. pneumoniae* and *Haemophilus influenzae* occurred early in the disease and in patients responding to chemotherapy, whereas infections by *Staphylococcus aureus* and gram-negative pathogens occurred more commonly in advanced disease and during neutropenia.

One randomized study showed that prophylactic intravenous immunoglobulin (IVIG) protected against serious infections in patients with multiple myeloma [63]. The patients who benefited most from immunoglobulin therapy were those with poor IgG antibody responses to pneumococcal vaccination. Today, more effective agents are available to treat multiple myeloma, notably thalidomide analogues and bortezomib. IVIG is not advised routinely in patients with CLL or multiple myeloma given the expense and lack of known benefit. IVIG should be considered in patients with refractory disease and recurrent sinopulmonary infections. Baseline and convalescent antibody titers following pneumococcal immunization will provide data on the patient's ability to respond to new bacterial antigens and may be useful in deciding whether to initiate IVIG.

Defective reconstitution of humoral immunity is a major factor contributing to increased infection susceptibility in the late transplant period. Winston et al. [64] noted a high frequency of pneumococcal infections between 7 and 36 months after transplantation, associated with serum opsonic deficiency for *S. pneumoniae*. Kulkarni et al. [65] reported that pneumococcal sepsis occurred in a median of 10 months after transplant (range, 3–187 months) and was significantly more frequent in patients with chronic GVHD.

Initial studies suggested that IVIG may decrease the incidence of infectious complications and GVHD in allogeneic HSCT recipients [66, 67]. However, a randomized, controlled study showed that monthly administration of IVIG given from day 90 to 360 did not reduce infectious complications or GVHD in allogeneic HSCT recipients and may impair long-term humoral immune reconstitution [68]. Thus, prophylactic IVIG should not be administered in HSCT recipients unless clinically significant hypogammaglobulinemia occurs. CMV immune globulin was ineffective in preventing acquisition of CMV infection or improving CMV disease in CMV-seronegative allogeneic HSCT recipients [69].

IVIG is used as adjunctive therapy (as opposed to prophylaxis) in specific viral diseases. Ganciclovir paired with CMV IVIG led to dramatically improved survival in allogeneic HSCT recipients with CMV pneumonia compared with historical patients with CMV pneumonia treated with other regimens (52% vs. 15%, respectively) [70]. Pilot studies suggest that ribavirin paired with IVIG with high neutralizing titers for respiratory syncytial virus (RSV) or [71, 72] RSV-specific monoclonal antibody (palivizumab) [72] is safe and may be associated with better outcomes than ribavirin alone as therapy for RSV infection in HSCT recipients. Machado et al. [73] reported high survival rates in allogeneic HSCT recipients with RSV infections treated with aerosolized ribavirin alone. Anaissie et al. [74] noted a high frequency of nasopharyngeal isolation of RSV in patients with cancer (mostly multiple myeloma) and HSCT recipients (mostly autologous) that did not correlate with serious morbidity or mortality in the absence of therapy.

Taken together, routine prophylaxis with IVII in the absence of symptomatic hypogammaglobulinemia is not supported in the literature. Pairing IVIG with antiviral agents is advised as the therapy for CMV pneumonia. The value of adjunctive IVIG as therapy for RSV and other community respiratory viruses is unknown.

4. Recombinant Interferon-γ

Interferons are immune modulators that regulate the expression of numerous genes that mediate inflammation. Interferon (IFN)-α is a cornerstone of therapy for chronic hepatitis C infection [75]. Several laboratories have shown that IFN-γ augments the antifungal activity of effector cells (macrophages and neutrophils) ex vivo against a variety of fungal pathogens, including *Candida albicans*, *Histoplasma capsulatum*, *Coccidiolides immitis*, *Cryptococcus neoformans*, and *Aspergillus* species [76]. Data in mouse models using cytokine depletion, gene knockout mice, and administration of exogenous cytokines have been instrumental in establishing the conceptual basis for immunotherapy in invasive mycoses and in paving the way to early clinical trials. Several cytokines, including, IL-12, IL-15 [77, 78], and TNF-α [79], and chemokines [80] hold promise as adjunctive therapeutics for invasive fungal infections. We will focus our discussion on rIFN-γ because the database is the most developed.

IFN-γ is produced by lymphocytes (CD4+, CD8+, NK cells) as well as macrophages and perhaps neutrophils [81]. It is induced by a number of signals, including IL-12 and IL-18 [82, 83] and in turn induces hundreds of genes, including its own inducers [84, 85]. Exposure to various pathogens can stimulate at least two patterns of cytokine production by CD4+ T cells. Th1 cells are defined by the production of IFN-γ, lymphotoxin and IL-2, and Th2 cells by the production of IL-4, IL-5, IL-9, IL-10, and IL-13. The antimicrobial activity induced by IFN-γ encompasses intracellular and extracellular parasites, bacteria, fungi, and viruses. In patients with hematologic malignancies, the use of rIFN-γ as adjunctive therapy for invasive fungal infections has attracted substantial interest.

Recombinant IFN- γ is licensed as a prophylactic agent in patients with CGD based on a randomized trial in which IFN- γ reduced the number and severity of infections in CGD by about 70%, regardless of antibiotic prophylaxis or genetic subtype of CGD [86]. Despite the widespread use of prophylactic rIFN- γ in CGD, invasive fungal infections have remained a persistent problem with an incidence of 0.1 fungal infections per patient in a year [87].

The value of rIFN- γ as adjunctive therapy for established fungal infection is unknown. Pappas et al. [88] conducted a phase II placebo-controlled study of adjunctive rIFN-γ in patients with AIDS-associated cryptococcal meningitis. Among 75 patients, negative CSF cultures at 2 weeks occurred in 13% of placebo recipients, 36% of rIFN-γ (100 μg subcutaneous thrice weekly) recipients, and 32% of rIFN-γ (200 μg subcutaneous thrice weekly) recipients. rIFN-γ was well tolerated, did not have an apparent effect on CD4 counts, and showed a trend toward an improved and combined clinical mycologic success.

Studies in vitro, in animal models [79], and limited patient data provide a rationale for adjunctive IFN-γ for invasive aspergillosis. rIFN-γ augmented human neutrophil oxidative response and killing of *A. fumigatus* hyphae in vitro and acted additively with G-CSF [31]. It prevented corticosteroid-mediated suppression of neutrophil killing of hyphae [89]. rIFN-γ also enhanced killing of *A. fumigatus* hyphae by human monocytes [32]. Administration of rIFN-γ to CGD patients augmented ex vivo neutrophil-mediated damage of *A. fumigatus* hyphae [90]. It was disappointing that a randomized trial evaluating rIFN- γ as adjunctive therapy for invasive aspergillosis was prematurely terminated before any patient was enrolled and before Institutional Review Board approval at most of the study sites.

Dignani et al. [91] reported successful outcomes using rIFN-g paired with CSFs in four patients with leukemia and refractory fungal disease. One concern about rIFN- γ in allogeneic HSCT recipients is the potential for worsening GVHD. Though preliminary results suggest that rIFN-γ may be safe in allogeneic HSCT recipients [92, 93], the safety of rIFN-γ cannot be predicted based on this limited database, and therefore merits evaluation in a clinical trial with safety as the primary endpoint.

We reserve rIFN-γ for patients with life-threatening invasive mould infections refractory to standard antifungal therapy. There is no standard dose as adjunctive rIFN-γ therapy. A dose of 100–200 μg subcutaneously thrice weekly was well tolerated in a preliminary trial in AIDS-associated cryptococcal meningitis (described above) [88]. Such decisions are necessarily based on retrospective analyses and anecdotal data. Pairing rIFN-γ with G-CSF or GM-CSF is another reasonable option in the setting of refractory fungal disease, though we emphasize that the clinical experience is anecdotal and that the efficacy of this approach is not established.

5. Innate Pathogen Recognition Receptors

5.1. Toll-Like Receptors

Toll-like receptors (TLR) are a conserved family of receptors that recognize common protein, carbohydrate, or DNA pattern motifs on microbes, leading to initiation of signaling for cytokine production and T-cell and dendritic cell (DC) maturation [94, 95]. Manipulation of TLR pathways has extraordinary potential as immunotherapy against bacteria, fungi, and viruses and as immune modulation in chronic inflammation relevant to the pathogenesis of diverse diseases, including cancer, inflammatory bowel disease, and atherosclerosis [96, 97]. We will focus our discussion on three classes of pathogen recognition receptors, TLRs, pentraxin 3, and mannose-binding lectin (MBL).

TLRs recognize motifs on *Candida* [98] and *Cryptococcus* species [99] and regulate the induced inflammatory responses. TLR4-defective mice are more susceptible to *C. albicans* infection, and this is associated with impaired chemokine expression and neutrophil recruitment [98]. *Aspergillus* conidia, but not hyphae, stimulate macrophages to produce the proinflammatory cytokines TNF-α and IL-1 in a TLR4-dependent fashion [100]. In contrast, *Aspergillus* hyphae, but not conidia, stimulate production of the antiinflammatory cytokine IL-10 through TLR2-dependent mechanisms. This switch from a proinflammatory to antiinflammatory signals during germination may help *Aspergillus* evade host defense. Wang et al. [101] reported that TLR4, but not TLR2, mediated activation of human monocytes by *A. fumigatus* hyphae. Other investigators found that both TLR 2 and 4 recognize *Aspergillus* hyphae stimulate proinflammatory cytokines in effector cells and neutrophil recruitment [102, 103].

Local delivery of CpG oligodeoxynucleotides (which signal through TLR 9) and the Asp f 16 *Aspergillus* allergen resulted in activation of airway DCs capable of inducing Th1 priming and resistance to the fungus [104]. Thymosin-α 1, a naturally occurring thymic peptide, induced maturation and IL-12 production in dendritic cells pulsed with *Aspergillus*, an effect mediated by distinct TLRs [105]. Thymosin-α 1 augmented Th1 immunity against *Aspergillus*, accelerated myeloid recovery in neutropenic mice and was protective against *Aspergillus* challenge in murine bone marrow transplant recipients.

Recognition of *Aspergillus* motifs and activation of neutrophils is coordinated by distinct members of the TLR family, each likely activating specialized antifungal effector functions and inflammatory responses [106]. Indeed, liposomal amphotericin B, in addition to its intrinsic antifungal activity, may activate antifungal resistance by activating TLR-4 in neutrophils [107]. These studies provide a rationale to stimulate or inhibit specific classes of TLRs as a means of enhancing both innate and antigen-specific immunity to fungi.

5.2. Pentraxin 3

Pentraxins are a superfamily of conserved proteins characterized by a cyclic multimeric structure. Pentraxin (PTX) 3 is an innate pathogen recognition protein that binds to specific motifs on *P. aeruginosa*, *Salmonella typhimurium*, and *A. fumigatus*. PTX3-deficient mice were highly susceptible to *Aspergillus* infection [108]. These mice demonstrated defective recognition of conidia by alveolar macrophages and dendritic cells, as well as inappropriate induction of type 2 cytokine responses. Administration of PTX3 protected against *Aspergillus* challenge in murine T-cell depleted allogeneic bone marrow transplant recipients [108] and potentiated the protective effect of subtherapeutic amphotericin B [109]. Recombinant pentraxin 3 is in early stages of clinical development.

5.3. Mannose-Binding Lectin

MBL is an innate pathogen recognitions receptor that recognizes carbohydrate motifs present on a broad range of pathogens, including certain bacteria, viruses, and fungi. MBL is a liver-derived protein and is secreted into the serum, where it can activate an immune response before the induction of antigen-specific immunity. MBL is able to activate to complement in the absence of antibodies. MBL-deficient mice are more susceptible to *S. aureus* [110] and herpes simplex virus-2 [111] infection than wild-type mice and have an altered immune response in experimental fungal asthma [112]. Epidemiological studies have suggested that allelic polymorphisms that affect MBL serum concentration influence the susceptibility to and the course of different types of infections, autoimmune, metabolic and cardiovascular diseases but this is still a subject of debate [113]. The fact that these allelic polymorphisms are common in the general population and that most individuals with low levels of serum MBL have no phenotype indicate that substantial redundancy exists in host defense and regulating inflammation.

A number of studies have reported an increased risk of infectious complications in patients with cancer receiving chemotherapy and in allogeneic HSCT recipients who harbor specific MBL polymorphisms [114–117], but this has not been a consistent finding [118–120]. One study reported that MBL deficiency increased the risk of childhood leukemia [121]. There is an interest in evaluating MBL replacement therapy in patients with cancer at a high risk for treatment-related infectious complications who have allelic polymorphisms that cause low endogenous serum MBL levels [122].

6. Adoptive Immunotherapy in HSCT Recipients

Intensive preparative regimens used in allogeneic HSCT result in a profound disruption of T-cell immunity. Reconstitution of T-cell immunity occurs over several months in uncomplicated cases and is further delayed in cases of GVHD requiring high-dose steroid therapy and antilymphocyte globulins. CMV and EBV establish latent infection in normal hosts, and control of reactivation is largely mediated by CD8+ cytotoxic T-lymphocytes (CTLs) [123]. CTLs recognize intracellular proteins that are presented by surface MHC class I molecules on antigen presenting cells. Viral antigen specific CD4+ T-cells may be required for long-term CD8+ T-cell persistence. Over the past decade, researchers have explored whether adoptive transfer of virus-specific CTLs may be protective.

In the first study evaluating the potential of CMV-specific CTLs to restore immunity, HLA-matched sibling allogeneic HSCT recipients received infusions of CD8+ CMV-specific CTL clones from their donors [124]. Such an approach led to early reconstitution of CMV-specific immunity, which persisted for at least 12 weeks after infusion, corresponding to the period of maximal risk for CMV disease. Dendritic cells and EBV-transformed cell lines transduced with a vector encoding the CMV early antigen pp65 and dendritic cells pulsed with pp65 also induce antigen-specific CTL responses.

While withdrawal of immunosuppression is often effective in controlling EBV-PTLD in solid organ transplant recipients, this approach is usually insufficient to generate adequate immune recovery in allogeneic HSCT recipients to control the disease. Infusions of unfractionated peripheral blood mononuclear cells from EBV-seropositive donors have been used to treat PTLD in allogeneic HSCT recipients [125]. However, alloreactive T-cells in such unfractionated preparations may induce GVHD. A potentially safer approach involves transfer of EBV-specific donor CTL clones which have been selectively enriched in vitro [126, 127]. This method has led to persistent cellular immune responses to EBV for as long as 18 months [127]. Adoptive transfer of EBV-specific CTLs has been generally safe and effective in controlling PTLD and in preventing EBV-LPD when used prophylactically.

The above studies establish a proof of principle with regard to the feasibility of adoptive transfer of viral antigen-specific CTLs. Additional research is focused on strategies to produce antigen presenting cells that display major antigens from multiple clinically relevant viruses to generate multispecific CTL populations [123].

7. Vaccine Development

Vaccine development is a priority for opportunistic fungal and viral pathogens that afflict patients with hematologic malignancies and allogeneic HSCT recipients. One impediment to vaccine development is that those patients who are most susceptible to opportunistic infections are least able to mount protective responses. Another impediment relates to the limited number of licensed vaccine adjuvants.

Candidate adjuvants that act on multiple innate and antigen-specific host defense pathways are likely to be the most effective in protecting against opportunistic fungal infections. The definition of adjuvants has mostly been restricted to those that stimulated antibody titers (e.g., pneumococcus) or, in the case of the Bacillus Calmette-Guerin (BCG) vaccine, delayed type hypersensitivity responses. More recently, the concept of adjuvants has been expanded to include soluble mediators and antigenic carriers (e.g., endotoxin, Flt3L, heat shock proteins) that activate antigen presenting cells and stimulate innate and cellular immunity [128].

Vaccine-based strategies have been effective in immunocompromised animal models. In mice, the importance of cell-mediated immunity against *Aspergillus* infection (an extracellular pathogen) has become well established [129, 130]. Immunization of immunocompetent mice with an *Aspergillus* crude filtrate resulted in memory responses mediated by antigen-specific, Th-1-committed CD4+ T-cells [131]. Adoptive transfer of these cells conferred protection to neutropenic mice – establishing a "proof of principle" regarding cellular immunity as a target for immune augmentation in invasive aspergillosis [131]. This study also showed that the dichotomy that host defense against extracellular pathogens (such as *Aspergillus*) is humoral while defense against intracellular pathogens that is cellular is overly simplistic. Torosantucci et al. [132] developed a fungal vaccine consisting of laminarin, a poorly immunogenic beta-glucan preparation (beta-glucan is a cell wall constituent in fungi, plants, and algae), conjugated to diphtheria toxoid. The vaccine was protective in experimental candidiasis and aspergillosis. Protection was, at least in part, mediated by anti-beta-glucan antibodies that could be adoptively transferred to naïve mice. Since beta-glucan is a ubiquitous cell wall constituent in fungi, this vaccine may be protective against a broad spectrum of fungal pathogens.

7.1. Cytomegalovirus

Although CMV exposure results in seroconversion, effective immunity is cellular. The immunodominant targets in CMV are the pp65 major matrix protein and the immediate early antigen [133]. There are several reasons why the development of effective CMV vaccination strategy is relevant and necessary in the HSCT setting. Antivirals, although effective in preventing CMV disease, may adversely affect immune reconstitution in allogeneic HSCT recipients through two possible mechanisms. First, suppressing CMV reactivation by antivirals may lead to reduced CMV antigenic stimulation and delayed reconstitution of CMV-specific cellular immunity that in turn predisposes to late CMV disease [134, 135]. Second, ganciclovir is marrow suppressive, leading to neutropenia in a significant minority of patients [3, 4, 136] and an increased risk of bacterial infections. Ganciclovir also inhibits lymphocyte proliferation [137]. Finally, CMV reactivation by itself has negative immunomodulatory effects that may increase the frequency of other infections and potentially inhibit the graft-vs.-leukemia effect [138].

Effective immunity is dependent on the frequency of CMV-specific CTLs in the graft [139]. Adoptive transfer of CTLs, although effective, is prohibitively expensive and labor intensive. To meet this need, several CMV-vaccines are in clinical development, including recombinant protein subunit vaccines, live-attenuated vaccines, poxvirus and alphavirus vectored subunit vaccines, and DNA vaccines [140–146]. Potential vaccine-based strategies to protect patients undergoing HSCT are pretransplant donor vaccination, pre- and/or posttransplant recipient vaccination, combined donor/recipient vaccination, or passive-vaccination.

The best studied vaccine is the live attenuated Towne vaccine. Towne vaccine is safe, well tolerated, and able to elicit humoral and cell-mediated immune responses in healthy seronegative individuals [147, 148]. The Towne vaccine was effective in preventing severe CMV disease in CMV-seronegative renal transplant recipients, but did not significantly affect the overall incidence of CMV infections [149]. Adjuvant IL-12 combined with the Towne vaccine augmented antibody and T cell immune responses to the CMV vaccine in CMV-seronegative health volunteers [150]. Another strategy to improve the immunogenicity involves generating recombinant chimera vaccines consisting of the Towne and virulent Toledo CMV strains [151].

8. Conclusions

There are a large number of promising immune-based strategies at the preclinical level and at early stages of clinical development. Most early studies focused on technology that was available, principally CSFs, granulocyte transfusions, and passive immunotherapy. Modern studies will involve strategies that refine older technologies (e.g., improved methods for donor granulocytapheresis for granulocyte transfusions). Trials that evaluate CSFs and cytokines as adjunctive therapy for severe infectious diseases are also required. Stimulation of innate pathogen recognition receptors is a promising experimental strategy to augment host defense against a number of opportunistic pathogens. Adoptive transfer of cellular immunity has been used to treat serious opportunistic viral infections in the clinic and this approach showed promise in experimental fungal infections. Finally, developing methods to enhance the efficacy of existing vaccines and developing novel vaccines against opportunistic fungal and viral infections are important priorities.

References

1. Schimpff S, Satterlee W, Young VM, Serpick A (1971) Empiric therapy with carbenicillin and gentamicin for febrile patients with cancer and granulocytopenia. N Engl J Med 284(19):1061–1065
2. Boeckh M, Gooley TA, Myerson D, Cunningham T, Schoch G, Bowden RA (1996) Cytomegalovirus pp 65 antigenemia-guided early treatment with ganciclovir versus ganciclovir at engraftment after allogeneic marrow transplantation: a randomized double-blind study. Blood 88(10):4063–4071
3. Goodrich JM, Bowden RA, Fisher L, Keller C, Schoch G, Meyers JD (1993) Ganciclovir prophylaxis to prevent cytomegalovirus disease after allogeneic marrow transplant. Ann Intern Med 118(3):173–178
4. Winston DJ, Ho WG, Bartoni K et al (1993) Ganciclovir prophylaxis of cytomegalovirus infection and disease in allogeneic bone marrow transplant recipients. Results of a placebo-controlled, double-blind trial. Ann Intern Med 118(3):179–184
5. Schmidt GM, Horak DA, Niland JC, Duncan SR, Forman SJ, Zaia JA (1991) A randomized, controlled trial of prophylactic ganciclovir for cytomegalovirus pulmonary infection in recipients of allogeneic bone marrow transplants; The City of Hope-Stanford-Syntex CMV Study Group [see comments]. N Engl J Med 324(15):1005–1011
6. Rotstein C, Bow EJ, Laverdiere M, Ioannou S, Carr D, Moghaddam N (1999) Randomized placebo-controlled trial of fluconazole prophylaxis for neutropenic cancer patients: benefit based on purpose and intensity of cytotoxic therapy. The Canadian Fluconazole Prophylaxis Study Group [In Process Citation]. Clin Infect Dis 28(2):331–340
7. Slavin MA, Osborne B, Adams R et al (1995) Efficacy and safety of fluconazole prophylaxis for fungal infections after marrow transplantation – a prospective, randomized, double-blind study. J Infect Dis 171(6):1545–1552
8. Goodman JL, Winston DJ, Greenfield RA et al (1992) A controlled trial of fluconazole to prevent fungal infections in patients undergoing bone marrow transplantation [see comments]. N Engl J Med 326(13):845–851
9. Marr KA, Seidel K, Slavin MA et al (2000) Prolonged fluconazole prophylaxis is associated with persistent protection against candidiasis-related death in allogeneic marrow transplant recipients: long-term follow-up of a randomized, placebo-controlled trial. Blood 96(6):2055–2061
10. Kanda Y, Yamamoto R, Chizuka A et al (2000) Prophylactic action of oral fluconazole against fungal infection in neutropenic patients. A meta-analysis of 16 randomized, controlled trials. Cancer 89(7):1611–1625
11. Segal BH, Walsh TJ (2006) Current approaches to diagnosis and treatment of invasive aspergillosis. Am J Respir Crit Care Med 173(7):707–717
12. van Burik JH, Leisenring W, Myerson D et al (1998) The effect of prophylactic fluconazole on the clinical spectrum of fungal diseases in bone marrow transplant recipients with special attention to hepatic candidiasis. An autopsy study of 355 patients. Medicine (Baltimore) 77(4):246–254

13. Shaukat A, Bakri F, Young P et al (2005) Invasive filamentous fungal infections in allogeneic hematopoietic stem cell transplant recipients after recovery from neutropenia: clinical, radiologic, and pathologic characteristics. Mycopathologia 159(2):181–188
14. Chamilos G, Luna M, Lewis RE et al (2006) Invasive fungal infections in patients with hematologic malignancies in a tertiary care cancer center: an autopsy study over a 15-year period (1989–2003). Haematologica 91(7):986–989
15. Marr KA, Carter RA, Crippa F, Wald A, Corey L (2002) Epidemiology and outcome of mould infections in hematopoietic stem cell transplant recipients. Clin Infect Dis 34(7):909–917
16. Marr KA, Carter RA, Boeckh M, Martin P, Corey L (2002) Invasive aspergillosis in allogeneic stem cell transplant recipients: changes in epidemiology and risk factors. Blood 100(13):4358–4366
17. Bhatti Z, Shaukat A, Almyroudis NG, Segal BH (2006) Review of epidemiology, diagnosis, and treatment of invasive mould infections in allogeneic hematopoietic stem cell transplant recipients. Mycopathologia 162(1):1–15
18. Herbrecht R, Denning DW, Patterson TF et al (2002) Voriconazole versus amphotericin B for primary therapy of invasive aspergillosis. N Engl J Med 347(6):408–415
19. Cornely OA, Maertens J, Winston DJ et al (2007) Posaconazole vs. fluconazole or itraconazole prophylaxis in patients with neutropenia. N Engl J Med 356(4):348–359
20. Ullmann AJ, Lipton JH, Vesole DH et al (2007) Posaconazole or fluconazole for prophylaxis in severe graft-versus-host disease. N Engl J Med 356(4):335–347
21. Ozer H, Armitage JO, Bennett CL et al (2000) 2000 update of recommendations for the use of hematopoietic colony-stimulating factors: evidence-based, clinical practice guidelines. American Society of Clinical Oncology Growth Factors Expert Panel. J Clin Oncol 18(20):3558–3585
22. Rowe JM (1998) Treatment of acute myeloid leukemia with cytokines: effect on duration of neutropenia and response to infections. Clin Infect Dis 26(6):1290–1294
23. Rowe JM, Andersen JW, Mazza JJ et al (1995) A randomized placebo-controlled phase III study of granulocyte-macrophage colony-stimulating factor in adult patients (>55 to 70 years of age) with acute myelogenous leukemia: a study of the Eastern Cooperative Oncology Group (E1490). Blood 86(2):457–462
24. Dekker A, Bulley S, Beyene J, Dupuis LL, Doyle JJ, Sung L (2006) Meta-analysis of randomized controlled trials of prophylactic granulocyte colony-stimulating factor and granulocyte-macrophage colony-stimulating factor after autologous and allogeneic stem cell transplantation. J Clin Oncol 24(33):5207–5215
25. Sloand EM, Kim S, Maciejewski JP et al (2000) Pharmacologic doses of granulocyte colony-stimulating factor affect cytokine production by lymphocytes in vitro and in vivo. Blood 95(7):2269–2274
26. Rutella S, Pierelli L, Bonanno G et al (2002) Role for granulocyte colony-stimulating factor in the generation of human T regulatory type 1 cells. Blood 100(7): 2562–2571
27. Volpi I, Perruccio K, Tosti A et al (2001) Postgrafting administration of granulocyte colony-stimulating factor impairs functional immune recovery in recipients of human leukocyte antigen haplotype-mismatched hematopoietic transplants. Blood 97(8):2514–2521
28. Khoury HJ, Loberiza FR Jr, Ringden O et al (2006) Impact of post-transplantation G-CSF on outcomes of allogeneic hematopoietic stem cell transplantation. Blood 107:1712–1716
29. Smith TJ, Khatcheressian J, Lyman GH et al (2006) 2006 update of recommendations for the use of white blood cell growth factors: an evidence-based clinical practice guideline. J Clin Oncol 24(19):3187–3205
30. Bodey GP, Buckley M, Sathe YS, Freireich EJ (1966) Quantitative relationships between circulating leukocytes and infection in patients with acute leukemia. Ann Intern Med 64(2):328–340

31. Roilides E, Uhlig K, Venzon D, Pizzo PA, Walsh TJ (1993) Enhancement of oxidative response and damage caused by human neutrophils to *Aspergillus fumigatus* hyphae by granulocyte colony-stimulating factor and gamma interferon. Infect Immun 61(4):1185–1193
32. Roilides E, Holmes A, Blake C, Venzon D, Pizzo PA, Walsh TJ (1994) Antifungal activity of elutriated human monocytes against *Aspergillus fumigatus* hyphae: enhancement by granulocyte-macrophage colony- stimulating factor and interferon-gamma. J Infect Dis 170(4):894–899
33. Roilides E, Sein T, Holmes A et al (1995) Effects of macrophage colony-stimulating factor on antifungal activity of mononuclear phagocytes against *Aspergillus fumigatus*. J Infect Dis 172(4):1028–1034
34. Roilides E, Holmes A, Blake C, Pizzo PA, Walsh TJ (1995) Effects of granulocyte colony-stimulating factor and interferon-gamma on antifungal activity of human polymorphonuclear neutrophils against pseudohyphae of different medically important *Candida* species. J Leukoc Biol 57(4):651–656
35. Nemunaitis J (1998) Use of macrophage colony-stimulating factor in the treatment of fungal infections. Clin Infect Dis 26(6):1279–1281
36. Gonzalez CE, Lyman CA, Lee S et al (2001) Recombinant human macrophage colony-stimulating factor augments pulmonary host defences against *Aspergillus fumigatus*. Cytokine 15(2):87–95
37. Nemunaitis J, Shannon-Dorcy K, Appelbaum FR et al (1993) Long-term follow-up of patients with invasive fungal disease who received adjunctive therapy with recombinant human macrophage colony-stimulating factor. Blood 82(5):1422–1427
38. Nemunaitis J, Meyers JD, Buckner CD et al (1991) Phase I trial of recombinant human macrophage colony-stimulating factor in patients with invasive fungal infections. Blood 78(4):907–913
39. Vora S, Purimetla N, Brummer E, Stevens DA (1998) Activity of voriconazole, a new triazole, combined with neutrophils or monocytes against *Candida albicans*: effect of granulocyte colony-stimulating factor and granulocyte-macrophage colony-stimulating factor [published erratum appears in Antimicrob Agents Chemother 1998 Aug;42(8):2152]. Antimicrob Agents Chemother 42(4):907–910
40. Sionov E, Mendlovic S, Segal E (2005) Experimental systemic murine aspergillosis: treatment with polyene and caspofungin combination and G-CSF. J Antimicrob Chemother 56(3):594–597
41. Sionov E, Segal E (2003) Polyene and cytokine treatment of experimental aspergillosis. FEMS Immunol Med Microbiol 39(3):221–227
42. Kullberg BJ, Vandewoude K, Herberecht R, Jacobs F, Aoun M, Kujath P (1998) A double-blind, randomized, placebo-controlled phase II study of filgrastim (recombinant granulocyte colony-stimulating factor) in combination with fluconazole for treatment of invasive candidiasis and candidemia in nonneutropenic patients. In: 38th Interscience Conference on Antimicrobial Agents and Chemotherapy, 1998. San Diego, CA. p. J-100
43. Wald A, Leisenring W, van Burik JA, Bowden RA (1997) Epidemiology of Aspergillus infections in a large cohort of patients undergoing bone marrow transplantation [see comments]. J Infect Dis 175(6):1459–1466
44. Baddley JW, Stroud TP, Salzman D, Pappas PG (2001) Invasive mold infections in allogeneic bone marrow transplant recipients. Clin Infect Dis 32(9):1319–1324
45. Grow WB, Moreb JS, Roque D et al (2002) Late onset of invasive aspergillus infection in bone marrow transplant patients at a university hospital. Bone Marrow Transplant 29(1):15–19
46. Jantunen E, Ruutu P, Niskanen L et al (1997) Incidence and risk factors for invasive fungal infections in allogeneic BMT recipients. Bone Marrow Transplant 19(8):801–808
47. McWhinney PH, Kibbler CC, Hamon MD et al (1993) Progress in the diagnosis and management of aspergillosis in bone marrow transplantation: 13 years' experience. Clin Infect Dis 17(3):397–404

48. Yuen KY, Woo PC, Ip MS et al (1997) Stage-specific manifestation of mold infections in bone marrow transplant recipients: risk factors and clinical significance of positive concentrated smears. Clin Infect Dis 25(1):37–42
49. BitMansour A, Burns SM, Traver D et al (2002) Myeloid progenitors protect against invasive aspergillosis and *Pseudomonas aeruginosa* infection following hematopoietic stem cell transplantation. Blood 100(13):4660–4667
50. Herzig RH, Herzig GP, Graw RG Jr, Bull MI, Ray KK (1977) Successful granulocyte transfusion therapy for gram-negative septicemia. A prospectively randomized controlled study. N Engl J Med 296(13):701–705
51. Vogler WR, Winton EF (1977) A controlled study of the efficacy of granulocyte transfusions in patients with neutropenia. Am J Med 63(4):548–555
52. Alavi JB, Root RK, Djerassi I et al (1977) A randomized clinical trial of granulocyte transfusions for infection in acute leukemia. N Engl J Med 296(13):706–711
53. Winston DJ, Ho WG, Gale RP (1982) Therapeutic granulocyte transfusions for documented infections. A controlled trial in ninety-five infectious granulocytopenic episodes. Ann Intern Med 97(4):509–515
54. Bensinger WI, Price TH, Dale DC et al (1993) The effects of daily recombinant human granulocyte colony-stimulating factor administration on normal granulocyte donors undergoing leukapheresis [see comments]. Blood 81(7):1883–1888
55. Dale DC, Liles WC, Llewellyn C, Rodger E, Price TH (1998) Neutrophil transfusions: kinetics and functions of neutrophils mobilized with granulocyte colony-stimulating factor and dexamethasone [see comments]. Transfusion 38(8):713–721
56. Dignani MC, Anaissie EJ, Hester JP et al (1997) Treatment of neutropenia-related fungal infections with granulocyte colony-stimulating factor-elicited white blood cell transfusions: a pilot study. Leukemia 11(10):1621–1630
57. Peters C, Minkov M, Matthes-Martin S et al (1999) Leucocyte transfusions from rhG-CSF or prednisolone stimulated donors for treatment of severe infections in immunocompromised neutropenic patients. Br J Haematol 106:689–696
58. Bhatia S, McCullough J, Perry EH, Clay M, Ramsay NK, Neglia JP (1994) Granulocyte transfusions: efficacy in treating fungal infections in neutropenic patients following bone marrow transplantation. Transfusion 34(3):226–232
59. Price TH, Bowden RA, Boeckh M et al (2000) Phase I/II trial of neutrophil transfusions from donors stimulated with G-CSF and dexamethasone for treatment of patients with infections in hematopoeitic stem cell transplantation. Blood 95:3302–3309
60. Nichols WG, Price T, Boeckh M (2002) Cytomegalovirus infections in cancer patients receiving granulocyte transfusions. Blood 99(9):3483–3484
61. Griffiths H, Lea J, Bunch C, Lee M, Chapel H (1992) Predictors of infection in chronic lymphocytic leukaemia (CLL). Clin Exp Immunol 89(3):374–377
62. Savage DG, Lindenbaum J, Garrett TJ (1982) Biphasic pattern of bacterial infection in multiple myeloma. Ann Intern Med 96(1):47–50
63. Chapel HM, Lee M, Hargreaves R, Pamphilon DH, Prentice AG (1994) Randomised trial of intravenous immunoglobulin as prophylaxis against infection in plateau-phase multiple myeloma. The UK Group for Immunoglobulin Replacement Therapy in Multiple Myeloma [see comments]. Lancet 343(8905):1059–1063
64. Winston DJ, Schiffman G, Wang DC et al (1979) Pneumococcal infections after human bone-marrow transplantation. Ann Intern Med 91(6):835–841
65. Kulkarni S, Powles R, Treleaven J et al (2000) Chronic graft versus host disease is associated with long-term risk fro pneumococcal infections in recipients of bone marrow transplants. Blood 95:3683–3686
66. Petersen FB, Bowden RA, Thornquist M et al (1987) The effect of prophylactic intravenous immune globulin on the incidence of septicemia in marrow transplant recipients. Bone Marrow Transplant 2(2):141–147
67. Sullivan KM, Kopecky KJ, Jocom J et al (1990) Immunomodulatory and antimicrobial efficacy of intravenous immunoglobulin in bone marrow transplantation [see comments]. N Engl J Med 323(11):705–712

68. Sullivan KM, Storek J, Kopecky KJ et al (1996) A controlled trial of long-term administration of intravenous immunoglobulin to prevent late infection and chronic graft-vs.-host disease after marrow transplantation: clinical outcome and effect on subsequent immune recovery. Biol Blood Marrow Transplant 2(1):44–53
69. Bowden RA, Sayers M, Flournoy N et al (1986) Cytomegalovirus immune globulin and seronegative blood products to prevent primary cytomegalovirus infection after marrow transplantation. N Engl J Med 314(16):1006–1010
70. Reed EC, Bowden RA, Dandliker PS, Lilleby KE, Meyers JD (1988) Treatment of cytomegalovirus pneumonia with ganciclovir and intravenous cytomegalovirus immunoglobulin in patients with bone marrow transplants. Ann Intern Med 109(10):783–788
71. Whimbey E, Champlin RE, Englund JA et al (1995) Combination therapy with aerosolized ribavirin and intravenous immunoglobulin for respiratory syncytial virus disease in adult bone marrow transplant recipients. Bone Marrow Transplant 16(3):393–399
72. Boeckh M, Berrey MM, Bowden RA, Crawford SW, Balsley J, Corey L (2001) Phase 1 evaluation of the respiratory syncytial virus-specific monoclonal antibody palivizumab in recipients of hematopoietic stem cell transplants. J Infect Dis 184(3):350–354
73. Machado CM, Boas LS, Mendes AV et al (2003) Low mortality rates related to respiratory virus infections after bone marrow transplantation. Bone Marrow Transplant 31(8):695–700
74. Anaissie EJ, Mahfouz TH, Aslan T et al (2004) The natural history of respiratory syncitial virus infection in cancer and transplant patients: implications for management. Blood 103:1611–1617
75. Schalm SW, Weiland O, Hansen BE et al (1999) Interferon-ribavirin for chronic hepatitis C with and without cirrhosis: analysis of individual patient data of six controlled trials. Eurohep Study Group for Viral Hepatitis. Gastroenterology 117(2):408–413
76. Stevens DA (1998) Combination immunotherapy and antifungal chemotherapy. Clin Infect Dis 26(6):1266–1269
77. Winn RM, Gil-Lamaignere C, Roilides E et al (2003) Selective effects of interleukin (IL)-15 on antifungal activity and IL-8 release by polymorphonuclear leukocytes in response to hyphae of Aspergillus species. J Infect Dis 188(4):585–590
78. Vazquez N, Walsh TJ, Friedman D, Chanock SJ, Lyman CA (1998) Interleukin-15 augments superoxide production and microbicidal activity of human monocytes against *Candida albicans*. Infect Immun 66(1):145–150
79. Nagai H, Guo J, Choi H, Kurup V (1995) Interferon-gamma and tumor necrosis factor-alpha protect mice from invasive aspergillosis. J Infect Dis 172(6):1554–1560
80. Mehrad B, Strieter RM, Moore TA, Tsai WC, Lira SA, Standiford TJ (1999) CXC chemokine receptor-2 ligands are necessary components of neutrophil-mediated host defense in invasive pulmonary aspergillosis. J Immunol 163(11):6086–6094
81. Wang J, Wakeham J, Harkness R, Xing Z (1999) Macrophages are a significant source of type 1 cytokines during mycobacterial infection. J Clin Invest 103(7):1023–1029
82. Mountford AP, Coulson PS, Cheever AW, Sher A, Wilson RA, Wynn TA (1999) Interleukin-12 can directly induce T-helper 1 responses in interferon-gamma (IFN-gamma) receptor-deficient mice, but requires IFN-gamma signalling to downregulate T-helper 2 responses. Immunology 97(4):588–594
83. Tomura M, Maruo S, Mu J et al (1998) Differential capacities of CD4+, CD8+, and CD4-CD8- T cell subsets to express IL-18 receptor and produce IFN-gamma in response to IL-18. J Immunol 160(8):3759–3765
84. Boehm U, Klamp T, Groot M, Howard JC (1997) Cellular responses to interferon-gamma. Annu Rev Immunol 15:749–795
85. Pien GC, Satoskar AR, Takeda K, Akira S, Biron CA (2000) Cutting edge: selective IL-18 requirements for induction of compartmental IFN-gamma responses during viral infection. J Immunol 165(9):4787–4791

86. (1991) A controlled trial of interferon gamma to prevent infection in chronic granulomatous disease. The International Chronic Granulomatous Disease Cooperative Study Group. N Engl J Med 324(8):509–516.
87. Winkelstein JA, Marino MC, RBJr J et al (2000) Chronic granulomatous disease: report on a national registry of 368 patients. Medicine (Baltimore) 79:155–169
88. Pappas PG, Bustamante B, Ticona E et al (2004) Recombinant interferon-gamma 1b as adjunctive therapy for AIDS-related acute cryptococcal meningitis. J Infect Dis 189(12):2185–2191
89. Roilides E, Uhlig K, Venzon D, Pizzo PA, Walsh TJ (1993) Prevention of corticosteroid-induced suppression of human polymorphonuclear leukocyte-induced damage of *Aspergillus fumigatus* hyphae by granulocyte colony-stimulating factor and gamma interferon. Infect Immun 61(11):4870–4877
90. Rex JH, Bennett JE, Gallin JI, Malech HL, DeCarlo ES, Melnick DA (1991) In vivo interferon-gamma therapy augments the in vitro ability of chronic granulomatous disease neutrophils to damage Aspergillus hyphae. J Infect Dis 163(4): 849–852
91. Dignani MC, Rex JH, Chan KW et al (2005) Immunomodulation with interferon-gamma and colony stimulating factors for refractory fungal infections in patients with leukemia. Cancer 104:199–204
92. Fleming RV, Anaissie EJ, Kantarjian HM, Savary C, Rex JH (1997) Safety of interferon-gamma plus G-CSF in cancer patients with refractory fungal infections. a pilot study. In: 37th Interscience Conference on Antimicrobial Agents and Chemotherapy, 1997. Toronto, CA. p. G-72
93. Safdar A, Rodriguez G, Ohmagari N et al (2005) The safety of interferon-gamma-1b for invasive fungal infections after hematopoietic stem cell transplantation. Cancer 103:731–739
94. Iwasaki A, Medzhitov R (2004) Toll-like receptor control of the adaptive immune responses. Nat Immunol 5(10):987–995
95. Blander JM, Medzhitov R (2004) Regulation of phagosome maturation by signals from toll-like receptors. Science 304(5673):1014–1018
96. Karin M, Greten FR (2005) NF-kappaB: linking inflammation and immunity to cancer development and progression. Nat Rev Immunol 5(10):749–759
97. Karin M, Lawrence T, Nizet V (2006) Innate immunity gone awry: linking microbial infections to chronic inflammation and cancer. Cell 124(4):823–835
98. Netea MG, Van Der Graaf CA, Vonk AG, Verschueren I, Van Der Meer JW, Kullberg BJ (2002) The role of toll-like receptor (TLR) 2 and TLR4 in the host defense against disseminated candidiasis. J Infect Dis 185(10):1483–1489
99. Shoham S, Huang C, Chen JM, Golenbock DT, Levitz SM (2001) Toll-like receptor 4 mediates intracellular signaling without TNF-alpha release in response to *Cryptococcus neoformans* polysaccharide capsule. J Immunol 166(7):4620–4626
100. Netea MG, Warris A, Van der Meer JW et al (2003) *Aspergillus fumigatus* evades immune recognition during germination through loss of toll-like receptor-4-mediated signal transduction. J Infect Dis 188(2):320–326
101. Wang JE, Warris A, Ellingsen EA et al (2001) Involvement of CD14 and toll-like receptors in activation of human monocytes by *Aspergillus fumigatus* hyphae. Infect Immun 69(4):2402–2406
102. Meier A, Kirschning CJ, Nikolaus T, Wagner H, Heesemann J, Ebel F (2003) Toll-like receptor (TLR) 2 and TLR4 are essential for Aspergillus-induced activation of murine macrophages. Cell Microbiol 5(8):561–570
103. Mambula SS, Sau K, Henneke P, Golenbock DT, Levitz SM (2002) Toll-like receptor (TLR) signaling in response to *Aspergillus fumigatus*. J Biol Chem 277(42):39320–39326
104. Bozza S, Gaziano R, Lipford GB et al (2002) Vaccination of mice against invasive aspergillosis with recombinant Aspergillus proteins and CpG oligodeoxynucleotides as adjuvants. Microbes Infect 4(13):1281–1290

105. Romani L, Bistoni F, Gaziano R et al (2004) Thymosin alpha 1 activates dendritic cells for antifungal Th1 resistance through toll-like receptor signaling. Blood 103(11):4232–4239
106. Bellocchio S, Moretti S, Perruccio K et al (2004) TLRs govern neutrophil activity in aspergillosis. J Immunol 173(12):7406–7415
107. Bellocchio S, Gaziano R, Bozza S et al (2005) Liposomal amphotericin B activates antifungal resistance with reduced toxicity by diverting Toll-like receptor signalling from TLR-2 to TLR-4. J Antimicrob Chemother 55(2):214–222
108. Garlanda C, Hirsch E, Bozza S et al (2002) Non-redundant role of the long pentraxin PTX3 in anti-fungal innate immune response. Nature 420(6912):182–186
109. Gaziano R, Bozza S, Bellocchio S et al (2004) Anti-*Aspergillus fumigatus* efficacy of pentraxin 3 alone and in combination with antifungals. Antimicrob Agents Chemother 48(11):4414–4421
110. Shi L, Takahashi K, Dundee J et al (2004) Mannose-binding lectin-deficient mice are susceptible to infection with *Staphylococcus aureus*. J Exp Med 199(10):1379–1390
111. Gadjeva M, Paludan SR, Thiel S et al (2004) Mannan-binding lectin modulates the response to HSV-2 infection. Clin Exp Immunol 138(2):304–311
112. Hogaboam CM, Takahashi K, Ezekowitz RA, Kunkel SL, Schuh JM (2004) Mannose-binding lectin deficiency alters the development of fungal asthma: effects on airway response, inflammation, and cytokine profile. J Leukoc Biol 75(5):805–814
113. Garred P, Larsen F, Seyfarth J, Fujita R, Madsen HO (2006) Mannose-binding lectin and its genetic variants. Genes Immun 7(2):85–94
114. Vekemans M, Robinson J, Georgala A et al (2007) Low mannose-binding lectin concentration is associated with severe infection in patients with hematological cancer who are undergoing chemotherapy. Clin Infect Dis 44(12):1593–1601
115. Mullighan CG, Bardy PG (2004) Mannose-binding lectin and infection following allogeneic hemopoietic stem cell transplantation. Leuk Lymphoma 45(2):247–256
116. Mullighan CG, Heatley S, Doherty K et al (2002) Mannose-binding lectin gene polymorphisms are associated with major infection following allogeneic hemopoietic stem cell transplantation. Blood 99(10):3524–3529
117. Peterslund NA, Koch C, Jensenius JC, Thiel S (2001) Association between deficiency of mannose-binding lectin and severe infections after chemotherapy. Lancet 358(9282):637–638
118. Bergmann OJ, Christiansen M, Laursen I et al (2003) Low levels of mannose-binding lectin do not affect occurrence of severe infections or duration of fever in acute myeloid leukaemia during remission induction therapy. Eur J Haematol 70(2):91–97
119. Lausen B, Schmiegelow K, Andreassen B, Madsen HO, Garred P (2006) Infections during induction therapy of childhood acute lymphoblastic leukemia – no association to mannose-binding lectin deficiency. Eur J Haematol 76(6):481–487
120. Choi EH, Taylor JG, Foster CB et al (2005) Common polymorphisms in critical genes of innate immunity do not contribute to the risk for chronic disseminated candidiasis in adult leukemia patients. Med Mycol 43(4):349–353
121. Schmiegelow K, Garred P, Lausen B, Andreassen B, Petersen BL, Madsen HO (2002) Increased frequency of mannose-binding lectin insufficiency among children with acute lymphoblastic leukemia. Blood 100(10):3757–3760
122. Summerfield JA (2003) Clinical potential of mannose-binding lectin-replacement therapy. Biochem Soc Trans 31(Pt 4):770–773
123. Gahn B, Hunt G, Rooney CM, Heslop HE (2002) Immunotherapy to reconstitute immunity to DNA viruses. Semin Hematol 39(1):41–47
124. Walter EA, Greenberg PD, Gilbert MJ et al (1995) Reconstitution of cellular immunity against cytomegalovirus in recipients of allogeneic bone marrow by transfer of T-cell clones from the donor [see comments]. N Engl J Med 333(16): 1038–1044

125. Papadopoulos EB, Ladanyi M, Emanuel D et al (1994) Infusions of donor leukocytes to treat Epstein-Barr virus-associated lymphoproliferative disorders after allogeneic bone marrow transplantation [see comments]. N Engl J Med 330(17):1185–1191
126. Rooney CM, Smith CA, Ng CY et al (1995) Use of gene-modified virus-specific T lymphocytes to control Epstein- Barr-virus-related lymphoproliferation. Lancet 345(8941):9–13
127. Heslop HE, Ng CY, Li C et al (1996) Long-term restoration of immunity against Epstein-Barr virus infection by adoptive transfer of gene-modified virus-specific T lymphocytes. Nat Med 2(5):551–555
128. Gamvrellis A, Leong D, Hanley JC, Xiang SD, Mottram P, Plebanski M (2004) Vaccines that facilitate antigen entry into dendritic cells. Immunol Cell Biol 82(5):506–516
129. Cenci E, Mencacci A, Del Sero G et al (1999) Interleukin-4 causes susceptibility to invasive pulmonary aspergillosis through suppression of protective type I responses. J Infect Dis 180(6):1957–1968
130. Cenci E, Perito S, Enssle KH et al (1997) Th1 and Th2 cytokines in mice with invasive aspergillosis. Infect Immun 65(2):564–570
131. Cenci E, Mencacci A, Bacci A, Bistoni F, Kurup VP, Romani L (2000) T cell vaccination in mice with invasive pulmonary aspergillosis. J Immunol 165(1):381–388
132. Torosantucci A, Bromuro C, Chiani P et al (2005) A novel glyco-conjugate vaccine against fungal pathogens. J Exp Med 202:597–606
133. Gibson L, Piccinini G, Lilleri D et al (2004) Human cytomegalovirus proteins pp 65 and immediate early protein 1 are common targets for CD8+ T cell responses in children with congenital or postnatal human cytomegalovirus infection. J Immunol 172(4):2256–2264
134. Nguyen Q, Champlin R, Giralt S et al (1999) Late cytomegalovirus pneumonia in adult allogeneic blood and marrow transplant recipients. Clin Infect Dis 28(3):618–623
135. Hakki M, Riddell SR, Storek J et al (2003) Immune reconstitution to cytomegalovirus after allogeneic hematopoietic stem cell transplantation: impact of host factors, drug therapy, and subclinical reactivation. Blood 102(8):3060–3067
136. Reusser P, Einsele H, Lee J et al (2002) Randomized multicenter trial of foscarnet versus ganciclovir for preemptive therapy of cytomegalovirus infection after allogeneic stem cell transplantation. Blood 99(4):1159–1164
137. Battiwalla M, Wu Y, Bajwa RPS et al (2007) Ganciclovir inhibits lymphocyte proliferation by impairing DNA synthesis. Biol Blood Marrow Transplant 13(7):765–770
138. Nakamura R, Battiwalla M, Solomon S et al (2004) Persisting posttransplantation cytomegalovirus antigenemia correlates with poor lymphocyte proliferation to cytomegalovirus antigen and predicts for increased late relapse and treatment failure. Biol Blood Marrow Transplant 10(1):49–57
139. Gratama JW, van Esser JW, Lamers CH et al (2001) Tetramer-based quantification of cytomegalovirus (CMV)-specific CD8+ T lymphocytes in T-cell-depleted stem cell grafts and after transplantation may identify patients at risk for progressive CMV infection. Blood 98(5):1358–1364
140. Daftarian P, Ali S, Sharan R et al (2003) Immunization with Th-CTL fusion peptide and cytosine-phosphate-guanine DNA in transgenic HLA-A2 mice induces recognition of HIV-infected T cells and clears vaccinia virus challenge. J Immunol 171(8):4028–4039
141. Schleiss M (2005) Progress in cytomegalovirus vaccine development. Herpes 12(3):66–75
142. La Rosa C, Wang Z, Brewer JC et al (2002) Preclinical development of an adjuvant-free peptide vaccine with activity against CMV pp 65 in HLA transgenic mice. Blood 100(10):3681–3689

143. Wang Z, La Rosa C, Lacey SF et al (2006) Attenuated poxvirus expressing three immunodominant CMV antigens as a vaccine strategy for CMV infection. J Clin Virol 35(3):324–331
144. Wang Z, La Rosa C, Mekhoubad S et al (2004) Attenuated poxviruses generate clinically relevant frequencies of CMV-specific T cells. Blood 104(3):847–856
145. Wang Z, Rosa CL, Li Z et al (2007) Vaccine properties of a novel marker gene-free recombinant modified vaccinia Ankara expressing immunodominant CMV antigens pp 65 and IE1. Vaccine 25(6):1132–1141
146. La Rosa C, Wang Z, Lacey SF et al (2006) In vitro expansion of polyclonal T-cell subsets for adoptive immunotherapy by recombinant modified vaccinia Ankara. Exp Hematol 34(4):497–507
147. Gonczol E, Ianacone J, Furlini G, Ho W, Plotkin SA (1989) Humoral immune response to cytomegalovirus Towne vaccine strain and to Toledo low-passage strain. J Infect Dis 159(5):851–859
148. Gehrz RC, Christianson WR, Linner KM, Groth KE, Balfour HH Jr (1980) Cytomegalovirus vaccine Specific humoral and cellular immune responses in human volunteers. Arch Intern Med 140(7):936–939
149. Plotkin SA, Higgins R, Kurtz JB et al (1994) Multicenter trial of Towne strain attenuated virus vaccine in seronegative renal transplant recipients. Transplantation 58(11):1176–1178
150. Jacobson MA, Sinclair E, Bredt B et al (2006) Safety and immunogenicity of Towne cytomegalovirus vaccine with or without adjuvant recombinant interleukin-12. Vaccine 24(25):5311–5319
151. Heineman TC, Schleiss M, Bernstein DI et al (2006) A phase 1 study of 4 live, recombinant human cytomegalovirus Towne/Toledo chimeric vaccines. J Infect Dis 193(10):1350–1360

Chapter 10

Prophylaxis

E.J. Bow

Abstract Neutropenic states are most often a function of haematopoietic failure secondary to myelophthisic disease or cytotoxic therapy for malignant and nonmalignant conditions. Patients so affected are susceptible to a rather wide spectrum of potentially life-threatening infections due to pathogens (bacterial fungal and viral) with a risk inversely proportional to the severity and duration of neutropenia. Strategies designed to prevent these infections have required an understanding of the normal human microbial ecology, the pathogenesis of the specific infection, and the pathogenesis of the neutropenic state. Fluroquinolone-based antibacterial chemoprophylaxis has been successful in reducing the incidence of febrile neutropenic episodes; documented bacterial infections, particularly gram-negative bacteraemia; infection-related mortality; and, all-cause mortality over the course of the neutropenic period. Success has been confounded by the prevalence of fluroquinolone resistance among gram-negative bacilli in the population at risk. Fluconazole-based antifungal prophylaxis has been successful in reducing invasive fungal infection, particularly due to fluconazole-susceptible *Candida* spp., but has had no effect on the incidence of filamentous fungal infections. Some studies have been able to demonstrate effects of reducing fungal infection-related mortality and all-cause mortality. Mold-active extended-spectrum azole antifungal agents such as posaconazole or voriconazole have been successful in reducing infections due to *Aspergillus* spp. Antiviral chemoprophylaxis targeting Herpes group viruses, particularly *Herpes simplex* virus and Human Cytomegalovirus, have been successful in reducing clinical disease in hematopoietic stem cell transplantation. The success of any given preventive strategy is directly related to the selection of the most appropriate risk group for application, the duration of time over which the risk applies, and the prevalence of resistance to the strategy among the pathogens of concern.

Keywords Prophylaxis • Prevention of infection • Barrier restrictions • Chemoprophylaxis • Protected environments • Neutropenic infections

From: *Managing Infections in Patients With Hematological Malignancies*: Contemporary Hematology, Edited by: M. Kleinberg, DOI 10.1007/978-1-59745-415-5_10,

1. Introduction

The desired outcome for antimicrobial prophylaxis strategies in neutropenic patients is to prevent infectious morbidity and all of its consequences including hospitalizations, impact upon quality of life, costs of treatment, treatment-related adverse effects, and death. Fever may represent the only manifestation of infection in the neutropenic host and, therefore, often represents the primary end-point for chemoprophylaxis strategies. It is also recognized that infection in the neutropenic patient may develop unassociated with fever. Moreover, fever may be a function of noninfectious processes including transfusion of blood products [1] or anticancer treatments, such as high-dose cytarabine [2]. Over 30 years ago it was recognized that the classical components of inflammation by which the clinician recognizes the presence of an infection may be muted or even absent as a function of the reduction in the absence of inflammatory cells [3]. Neither the pattern nor the magnitude of fever are predictive of the presence of infection relative to other noninfectious causes of fever [4].

The origins of the definition of normal body temperature are somewhat unclear [5]; however, the writings of Carl Wunderlich in 1868 suggested that any temperature above 38°C should be regarded as a febrile state [6]. However, a study of 148 healthy men and women at the University of Maryland demonstrated the mean of 700 baseline oral temperatures to be 36.8±0.4°C (98.2±0.7°F) [7]. While medical textbooks have varied with respect to the upper limit of normal (37.1–38°C) [5], published clinical guidelines, based upon clinical trial designs, have recommended that a single oral temperature ≥38.3°C or an oral temperature of ≥38.0°C sustained over at least 1 h be regarded as representing a febrile state [8–11]. The Japan Febrile Neutropenia Study Group recommended that a single oral temperature of ≥38.0°C or a single axillary temperature of ≥37.5°C be accepted as the definition of a febrile state.

Neutropaenia is defined by the number of segmented neutrophils and band neutrophils circulating in the bloodstream. As the absolute neutrophil cell count (ANC) falls below 1.0×10^9/L the risk of fever and pyogenic infection increases [12]. Moreover, over two-thirds of febrile episodes (70.1%) and documented infections (72.3%) occur when the ANC is $<0.5\times10^9$/L [12]. Bacteremic episodes tend to occur more often as the ANC falls below 0.1×10^9/L [13, 14]. In the context of fever and neutropaenia, risk may be defined in two broad ways. The infectious Diseases Working Party of the German Society of Hematology and Oncology define risk in terms of developing a potentially life-threatening infection [9]; whereas the Multinational Association of Supportive Care in Cancer (MASCC) and the Infectious Diseases Society of America (IDSA) define risk in terms of developing a medical complication such that admission to hospital or prolonged hospitalization is required [8, 15]. A scoring system has been developed and validated for use in segregating febrile neutropaenic patients into high- or low-risk for such complications [15–17]. This scoring system is useful for identifying risk in the context of febrile neutropaenic patients but not for identifying risk of febrile events for the purposes of allocating a preventive strategy.

Approximately, one-quarter of febrile neutropenic episodes represent bacteremia. Among neutropenic patients not receiving antibacterial chemoprophylaxis in one American study, the bacteremic isolates included coagulase-negative Staphylococci in 19%, viridans group Streptococci in 27%, other gram-positive bacteria in 16%, and gram-negative bacilli in 37% [18]. Only 8% of the febrile episodes were unexplained fevers and the remaining infections were clinical infections. The clinical site most involved was the gastrointestinal tract in 43% of cases, of which oropharyngitis (70%), oesophagitis (3%), enterocolitis (17%), and perirectal cellulitis (10%) comprised the major infected sites. Infections involving the skin and soft tissues occurred in 10% (venous access device-related infection 59%, cellulitis 35%, folliculitis 6%), pneumonias in 10%, and urinary tract in 6%. In another recent trial of fluoroquinolone-based antibacterial chemoprophylaxis unexplained fevers comprised 43%, clinical infections comprised 11%, bacteremias comprised 40%, and nonbacteremic microbiologically documented infections comprised 6% of febrile episodes, respectively, among placebo recipients [19]. The difference in these two studies appears to be in the proportion of cases in which clinical foci were identified. The former had significantly fewer unexplained fevers and more clinical infections despite having a very similar patient demographic. Not all investigators regard mucositis, oral or gastrointestinal, as clinical foci of infection [20] despite clear linkages to infection risk and febrile events [21, 22].

Prophylaxis strategies in neutropenic patients have focused upon prevention of exposure through management of patients in protected environments, augmentation of the damaged host defenses through hematopoietic growth factor-mediated stimulation of early myeloid reconstitution, suppression of reactivation of previously acquired viruses, and suppression of endogenous colonization and translocation by specified bacterial and fungal pathogens. This chapter will discuss each of these areas in light of newer understanding of pathogenesis and clinical trial-based experience.

2. Protected Environments

Comprehensive infection control procedures that include isolating patients within protective hospital environments have become accepted practices for certain patient groups during periods of particularly high risk. The objective for such procedures is to reduce the risk for nosocomial acquisition of infectious agents through contact (for example, vancomycin-resistant enterococci, VRE, or methicillin-resistant *Staphylococcus aureus*, MRSA) and air-borne (for example, some DNA viruses such as Varicella, or conidia of various molds such as *Aspergillus* spp.) transmission. Various authorities have recommended that patients receiving myelosuppressive and immunosuppressive therapy for acute leukemia or haematopoietic stem cell transplant (HSCT) be housed in hospital rooms equipped with high-efficiency particulate air filters (HEPA) with or without laminar air flow (LAF). A number of guidelines have been published regarding the use of such protected environments in high-risk patients [23–29]. A total of 211 recommendations applicable to HSCT recipients were graded by strength of recommendation (A to E) and quality of supportive evidence (I to III). Of these, 171 (81%) recommendations were level III (That is, expert opinion, consensus committee or descriptive studies), 33 (17%) were level II (that is, supported by at least one well-designed nonrandomized clinical trial, case-control or cohort study, multiple time-series studies, or dramatic results from uncontrolled studies), and only 7 (3%) were level I (supported by data from at least one randomized-controlled trial).

Table 10-1. Randomized-controlled trials evaluating the impact of protective environments on the incidence of pneumonia.

Reference	Subjects	Study	Control	PE event rate	Control event rate
[221]	AL	PE+PA	Ward	5/19 (26.3%)	19/33 (57.6%)
[222]	AL	PE+PA	Ward±PA	1/22 (4.5%)	11/66 (16.7%)
[223]	AL	LAF+PA	Ward±PA	3/24 (12.5%)	18/40 (45.0%)
[224]	AL	PE+PA	Ward±PA	17/86 (19.8%)	39/51 (76.5%)
[225]	AL	PE+PA+SA	Ward±PA/SA	8/63 (12.7%)	23/82 (28.0%)
[226]	AL	PE+PA	Ward±PA	0/11 (0)	6/31 (19.4%)
[227]	HSCT	LAF+PA	Ward±PA	0/56 (0)	3/45 (6.7%)
[228]	AL	PE+PA	Ward±PA	4/24 (16.7%)	4/21 (19.0%)
[229]	AL	PE	Ward	8/20 (40.0%)	10/23 (43.5%)
[230]	AL	PE+PA	Ward	2/47 (4.3%)	6/48 (12.5%)
[231]	HSCT	LAF+PA	Ward±PA	5/36 (13.9%)	15/64 (23.4%)
[232]	SCCL	PE+PA	Ward±PA	6/25 (24.0%)	12/30 (40.0%)
				60/433 (13.9%)[a]	166/534 (31.1%)[a]

AL acute leukemia; *HSCT* haematopoietic stem cell transplant; *PE* protective environment; *PA* prophylactic oral nonabsorbable antibiotics; *LAF* laminar air-flow; *SA* systemic antibiotics

[a]OR 0.29 (95% CI 0.20–0.41)

The bases for most of these recommendations are, therefore, uncontrolled studies, expert opinion, and only a handful of randomized controlled trials. This is the subject of a recent review [30]. A summary of randomized-controlled trials evaluating the impact of protective environments on incidence of pneumonia is shown in Table 10-1

The infections most prevalent during the premyeloid engraftment/reconstitution period include *Herpes simplex* virus, pyogenic bacterial infections due to gram-positive cocci, gram-negative bacilli, and *Candida* spp. colonizing mucosal surfaces, and opportunistic molds such as *Aspergillus* spp. [31]. Of these, only the opportunistic mold infection rate may be influenced by HEPA/LAF protective environments, and only while the patient is maintained within the environment. These facilities are expensive and are associated with significant psychological and emotional adverse effects as a function of social isolationism [32]. The overall value of these isolation strategies has been questioned [33].

Retrospective studies have demonstrated reduction in the number of airborne *Aspergillus* conidia in the air of clinical in-patient hospital wards equipped with HEPA filtration units as well as reduction in the event rate for invasive aspergillosis [34–36]. The efficacy of HEPA protected environments with or without LAF on outcome has been addressed in relatively few randomized-contolled clinical trials. A recent systematic review of the literature with meta-analysis, examined 16 trials with respect to two outcomes; all-cause mortality and proven infection due to *Aspergillus* spp. and non-*Candida* fungi [37]. Among six randomized-controlled trials which included death as an outcome, the all-cause mortality rate was 21% and 23% for the protective environments and unventilated control groups, respectively (Relative Risk [RR], 0.85, 95% confidence interval [CI] 0.65–1.14). Moreover, the event rates for invasive mold infection were similar, 4% and 7% for the protective environments and unventilated control groups in four trials reporting this outcome among 238 randomized subjects, respectively (RR 0.57, 95% CI 0.13–2.53). These analyses failed to document a protective effect for protective environments against invasive mold infections or an impact on all-cause mortality.

Despite these discouraging results, a further systematic review examining the efficacy of protective environments against undifferentiated clinical pneumonia syndromes (Table 10-1) suggested that the management of patients in protected environments can reduce the event rate for lower respiratory tract infections overall (OR 0.29, 95% CI 0.20–0.41). The potential impact of HEPA filtration units has been obviated to a great degree by transfer of much of the treatment of neutropenic patients and stem cell transplant recipients to an outpatient environment.

Strength of recommendations/quality of evidence regarding the use of HEPA-equipped protective environments has ranged from moderate evidence "for" based upon randomized-controlled trials (B-I) to moderate evidence "for" based upon expert opinion (B-III). The use of high-efficiency masks for acute leukemia and HSCT patients undergoing transport outside of the protective environment has been associated with as much as a 67% reduction in the incidence of nosocomial aspergillosis [38]. It seems prudent to recommend masking for such patients during transport within the hospital.

3. Antibacterial Chemoprophylaxis for Severely Neutropaenic Patients

Fluoroquinolones have emerged as popular choices for antibacterial chemoprophylaxis in the United States [39] and continental Europe [40], and the United Kingdom [41] with 59%, 61%, and 71% of centres, respectively, prescribing these agents for this indication. The start time for prophylaxis typically parallels that of the cytotoxic therapy. In Europe, 80–90% of physicians recommend that the course of chemoprophylaxis begin before the onset of neutropaenia until myeloid reconstitution (defined by recovery of the absolute neutrophil count to at least 0.5×10^9/L over two consecutive days). Approximately, two-thirds (70%) of European physicians tend to discontinue antibacterial prophylaxis with the onset of the febrile neutropaenic episode [40] whereas all centres surveyed in the USA recommended termination of the prophylaxis agent with onset of neutropenic fever [39].

A large database of published experience in this field has accumulated upon which policies and recommendations regarding antibacterial chemoprophylaxis might be based. There have been several recently published systematic reviews of antibacterial prophylaxis [42–52]. Two large clinical trials in high- [19] and lower-risk [53] patients have also been published. Several guidelines have been published that include recommendations for or against antibacterial prophylaxis strategies [8, 23, 54–60]. In addition, there have been recently published guidelines from Europe that have taken into account the experience contained in the published literature in this field [40].

3.1. Outcomes of Clinical Trials of Antibacterial Prophylaxis

There have been eight published systematic reviews encompassing 29 meta-analyses examining the role of antibacterial prophylaxis in neutropenic cancer patients [42, 44, 45, 47–50]. These analyses are reviewed in Table 10-2

Early observations over 30 years ago suggested that oral antibacterial agents such as trimethoprim/sulfamethoxazole (TMP/SMX) could reduce bacterial infections in children with acute lymphoblastic leukemia [61]. Subsequent tri-

Table 10-2. Summary of published systematic reviews and meta-analyses of antibacterial prophylaxis in neutropenic cancer patients.

Study	Meta-analyses	No. trials	No. randomized subjects	Outcomes measured	OR[a]/RR[b] (95% CI)	Study agent effect on outcome
Cruciani et al. (1996) [44]	FQ vs. TMP/SMX, NAA, or placebo	13	1,155	GNB-BSI	0.09[a] (0.05–0.16)	↓
				GPO-BSI	1.05[a] (0.76–1.45)	No effect
				Fever	0.76[a] (0.56–1.04)	No effect
				Mortality[c]	0.79[a] (0.47–1.34)	No effect
	FQ+GPP vs. FQ ($n=4$) or NAA ($n=2$)	6	957	GNB-BSI	0.80[a] (0.41–1.53)	No effect
				GPO-BSI	0.46[a] (0.33–0.63)	↓
				Fever	0.83[a] (0.62–1.13)	No effect
				Mortality[c]	0.74[a] (0.40–1.38)	No effect
Rotstein et al. (1997) [42]	FQ vs. placebo or no treatment	6	394	GNB-infection	0.20[a] (0.12–0.32)	↓
				GPO-infection	0.77[a] (0.49–1.20)	No effect
				Fungal infection	1.01[a] (0.40–2.54)	No effect
				Fever	0.37[a] (0.18–0.74)	↓
				Mortality[d]	0.96[a] (0.49–1.91)	No effect
				Side effects	2.00[a] (1.00–4.02)	↑
	FQ vs. TMP/ SMX±NAA or NAA	16	1,362	GNB-infection	0.22[a] (0.16–0.32)	↓
				GPO-infection	1.01[a] (0.76–1.35)	No effect
				Fungal infection	0.84[a] (0.55–1.30)	No effect
				Fever	0.81[a] (0.62–1.06)	No effect
				Mortality[d]	0.95[a] (0.64–1.41)	No effect
				Side effects	0.48[a] (0.35–0.65)	↓
	Ciprofloxacin vs. other FQ	3	902	GNB-infection	0.34[a] (0.21–0.57)	↓
				GPO-infection	0.91[a] (0.61–1.35)	No effect
				Fungal infection	0.69[a] (0.17–2.70)	No effect
				Fever	0.68[a] (0.51–0.91)	↓
				Mortality[d]	1.02[a] (0.68–1.51)	No effect
				Side effects	1.25[a] (0.72–2.19)	No effect
	FQ+GPP vs. FQ	6	922	GNB-infection	1.42[a] (0.61–3.30)	No effect
				GPO-infection	0.42[a] (0.30–0.58)	↓
				Fungal infection	0.90[a] (0.34–2.35)	No effect
				Fever	0.81[a] (0.61–1.09)	No effect
				Mortality[d]	1.27[a] (0.64–2.54)	No effect
				Side effects	1.17[a] (0.53–2.56)	No effect

Engels et al. (1998) [43]	FQ vs. placebo or no treatment	8	731	GNB-infection	0.21[b] (0.12–0.37)	↓
		6		GNB-BSI	0.23[b] (0.11–0.49)	↓
		8		GPO-infection	0.88[b] (0.65–1.18)	No effect
		5		GPO-BSI	0.69[b] (0.36–1.32)	No effect
		8		Fungal infection	1.11[b] (0.62–1.96)	No effect
		8		MDI	0.65[b] (0.50–0.85)	↓
		5		CDI	0.88[b] (0.71–1.08)	No effect
		5		Total infections	0.54[b] (0.31–0.95)	↓
		8		Fever	0.85[b] (0.73–0.99)	↓
		5		Mortality[c]	1.04[b] (0.40–2.70)	No effect
	FQ vs. TMP/SMX	8	677	GNB-infection	0.30[b] (0.17–0.54)	↓
		8		GNB-BSI	0.32[b] (0.16–0.64)	↓
		7		GPO-infection	1.10[b] (0.69–1.76)	No effect
		8		GPO-BSI	1.39[b] (0.88–2.20)	No effect
		8		Fungal infection	0.63[b] (0.29–1.36)	No effect
		9		MDI	0.72[b] (0.57–0.92)	↓
		9		CDI	1.05[b] (0.74–1.49)	No effect
		9		Total infections	0.83[b] (0.70–0.98)	↓
		8		Fever	0.89[b] (0.74–1.07)	No effect
		7		Mortality[c]	0.95[b] (0.45–2.02)	No effect
Cruciani et al. (2003) [45]	FQ+GPP vs. FQ	9	1,182	BSI-total	0.65[b] (0.53–0.79)	↓
		9	1,182	GNB-infections	1.00[b] (0.56–1.79)	No effect
		9	1,182	Staphylococcal infections	0.68[b] (0.49–0.96)	↓
		9	1,182	Streptococcal infections	0.45[b] (0.30–0.69)	↓
			1,055	CDI	1.12[b] (0.81–1.56)	No effect
			861	UF	0.96[b] (0.81–1.14)	No effect
		6	926	Fever	0.93[b] (0.86–1.00)	↓
		7	987	Mortality	1.06[b] (0.58–1.92)	No effect
		8	1,093	Side effects	2.17[b] (1.32–3.57)	↑

(continued)

Table 10-2. (continued)

Study	Meta-analyses	No. trials	No. randomized subjects	Outcomes measured	OR[a]/RR[b] (95% CI)	Study agent effect on outcome
Gafter-Gvili et al. (2005) [48]	Oral prophylaxis vs. placebo or no treatment	40	2,910	Mortality[d]	0.67[b] (0.55–0.81)	↓
	TMP/SMX vs. placebo or no treatment	14	870	Mortality[d]	0.71[b] (0.49–1.02)	No effect
		15	1,017	Mortality[c]	0.60[b] (0.41–0.87)	↓
		16	1,424	Fever	0.79[b] (0.69–0.90)	↓
		17	1,229	CDI	0.68[b] (0.56–0.82)	↓
		17	1,400	MDI	0.50[b] (0.38–0.65)	↓
				GNB-colonization	2.42[b] (1.35–4.36)	↑
				Side effects	3.63[b] (1.32–9.98)	↑
	FQ vs. placebo or no treatment	14	1,244	Mortality[d]	0.52[b] (0.35–0.77)	↓
		10	1,022	Mortality[c]	0.38[b] (0.21–0.69)	↓
		18	1,409	Fever	0.67[b] (0.56–0.81)	↓
		14	1,119	CDI	0.53[b] (0.36–0.80)	↓
		18	1,407	MDI	0.50[b] (0.35–0.70)	↓
				GNB-infection	0.26[b] (0.20–0.35)	↓
				GPO-infection	0.29[b] (0.22–0.77)	↓
				Fungal infection	0.83[b] (0.56–1.22)	No effect
				BSI-total	0.64[b] (0.52–0.77)	↓
				GNB-colonization	1.69[b] (0.73–3.92)	No effect
				Side effects	1.30[b] (0.61–2.67)	No effect
	FQ vs. TMP/SMX	10	917	Mortality[d]	1.07[b] (0.66–1.72)	No effect
		11	1,019	Mortality[c]	0.91[b] (0.54–1.54)	No effect
		10	931	Fever	0.95[b] (0.86–1.04)	No effect
		10	931	CDI	1.33[b] (1.06–1.66)	↑
		9	1,027	Side effects	0.74[b] (0.63–0.87)	↓

van de Wetering et al. (2005) [47]	TMP/SMX vs. placebo or no treatment	7	744	BSI-total	0.51[a] (0.33–0.79)	↓
			744	GNB-BSI	0.65[a] (0.36–1.17)	No effect
				GPO-BSI	0.47[a] (0.25–0.91)	↓
			405	Mortality[c]	0.51[a] (0.25–1.05)	No effect
	FQ vs. placebo or no treatment	6	561	BSI-total	0.44[a] (0.27–0.71)	↓
		5	466	GNB-BSI	0.16[a] (0.07–0.39)	↓
				GPO-BSI	1.10[a] (0.61–1.97)	No effect
			561	Mortality[c]	0.43[a] (0.15–1.27)	No effect
	Conventional chemotherapy: FQ or TMP/SMX vs. placebo or no treatment	9	712	BSI-total	0.47[a] (0.32–0.71)	↓
	Acute leukemia/HSCT: FQ or TMP/SMX vs. placebo or no treatment	3	436	BSI-total	0.52[a] (0.32–0.84)	↓
	FQ or TMP/SMX vs. placebo or no treatment	12	1,052	Fungemia	1.49[a] (0.65–3.43)	No effect
				Fungal mortality[c]	0.81[a] (0.35–1.86)	No effect
Leibovici et al. (2006) [50]	Acute leukemia/HSCT: FQ vs. placebo or no treatment	12	1,519	Fever	0.78[b] (0.74–0.83)	↓
		10	1,530	Mortality[d]	0.67[b] (0.46–0.98)	↓
	Solid tumor/Lymphoma: FQ vs. placebo or no treatment	5	1,933	Fever	0.67[b] (0.57–0.80)	↓
		4	1,892	Mortality[d]	0.51[b] (0.27–0.97)	↓
	FQ vs. placebo or no treatment	8	2,712	FQ-resistant MDI	1.04[b] (0.73–1.50)	No effect
		16	3,308	GPO-infection	0.37[b] (0.30–0.46)	↓
		5	2,529	*C. difficile*-associated diarrhea	1.44[b] (0.45–4.63)	No effect
	Levofloxacin vs. placebo or no treatment	2	2,301	Mortality[d]	0.60[b] (0.36–1.02)	No effect
	Ciprofloxacin vs. placebo or no treatment	6	521	Mortality[d]	0.32[b] (0.13–0.82)	↓
	Norfloxacin vs. placebo or no treatment	4	272	Mortality[d]	1.03[b] (0.58–1.81)	No effect
	Ofloxacin or perfloxacin or enoxacin vs. placebo or no treatment	3	346	Mortality[d]	0.44[b] (0.17–1.09)	No effect

(continued)

Table 10-2. (continued)

Study	Meta-analyses	No. trials	No. randomized subjects	Outcomes measured	OR[a]/RR[b] (95% CI)	Study agent effect on outcome
Gafter-Gvili et al. (2007) [49]	FQ vs. placebo or no treatment	3	161	Colonization by FQ-resistant bacteria	1.68[b] (0.71–4.00)	No effect
		8	2,712	MDI-FQ-resistant bacterial infection	1.04[b] (0.73–1.50)	No effect
				GNB-infection, FQ-resistant	1.30[b] (0.63–2.67)	No effect
				GPO-infection, FQ-resistant	0.93[b] (0.61–1.42)	No effect
	FQ vs. TMP/SMX	3	237	Colonization by bacteria resistant to study agent	0.49[b] (0.37–0.66)	↓
		6	366	MDI-infection, resistant to study agent	0.45[b] (0.27–0.74)	↓
	FQ vs. NAA	4	343	MDI-infection, resistant to study agent	1.19[b] (0.89–1.59)	No effect
	FQ+GPP vs. FQ	3	221	MDI-infection, resistant to study agent	0.11[b] (0.01–0.94)	↓

FQ fluoroquinolone (Norfloxacin, ciprofloxacin, perfloxacin, ofloxacin, enoxacin; *TMP/SMX* trimethoprim/sulfamethoxazole; *NAA* nonabsorbable antibiotics (Vancomycin, nystatin, gentamicin, tobramycin, colistin, polymyxin); *P* placebo; *GPP* Gram-positive prophylaxis (Vancomycin, penicillin G, penicillin V, amoxicillin, roxithromycin);*GNB* Gram-negative bacillus; *GPO* Gram-positive organism; *BSI* bloodstream infection; *MDI* microbiologically documented infection; *CDI* clinically documented infection; *UF* unexplained fever; *OR* odds ratio; *RR* relative risk; *CI* confidence interval; *HSCT* hematopoietic stem cell transplant.

[a]Odds ratio

[b]Relative risk

[c]Infection-related mortality

[d]Total (all-cause) patient mortality

[e]Weighted mean difference

Reduced event rate for the outcome

Increased event rate for the outcome

als further provided seminal evidence that antibacterial prophylaxis with TMP/SMX could reduce infectious morbidity in adults with acute leukemia [62, 63]. Among randomized, placebo or no treatment-controlled trials in neutropenic patients, TMP/SMX has been associated with reductions in febrile episodes (Relative risk reduction (RRR) 21%, number needed to treat (NNT) to prevent one febrile episode 7) [48], clinically documented infections (CDI; RRR 32%, NNT 6) [48], microbiologically documented infections (MDI; RRR 50%, NNT 5) [48], and bloodstream infections overall (RRR 49%, NNT 14) [47]. However the treatment effect was not consistent across all outcomes. Despite these encouraging observations, gram-negative bacteremia (RR 0.65, 95% CI 0.36–1.17) and all-cause mortality (RR 0.71, 95% CI 0.49–1.02) were not affected by TMP/SMX [48]. Moreover, two meta-analyses reported opposite observations for [48] and against [47] a treatment effect on infection-related mortality. Side effects were more common among TMP/SMX recipients compared to placebo or non treatment controls (RR 3.63, 95% CI 1.32–9.98) [48].

Fluoroquinolone-based (FQ) antibacterial prophylaxis has emerged as the preferred strategy to prevent pyogenic infection in neutropenic cancer patients [46]. The design of clinical trials examining this approach may be grouped as follows: FQ versus placebo or no treatment controls, FQ versus TMP/SMX or nonabsorbable oral antimicrobials (NAA), FQ versus other FQ, and FQ plus additional prophylactic agents with gram-positive activity (GPP) versus FQ alone. The outcomes studied in these trials include total infections overall, fever episodes; clinically documented infections; microbiologically documented infections including gram-negative infections overall, gram-negative bacteremia, gram-positive infections overall, gram-positive bacteremia, and invasive fungal infections; all-cause mortality, infection-related mortality, and side effects associated with therapy. These results of these study designs are reviewed in Table 10-2

The FQ versus placebo or no treatment trials have demonstrated protective treatment effects against bloodstream infections overall [47, 48], gram-negative infections overall [42, 43, 48], gram-negative bacteremia [43, 44, 47], gram-positive infection overall [48, 50], fever episodes [42, 43, 48, 50], clinically documented infections in some [48] but not all analyses [43], microbiologically documented infections [43, 48], infection-related mortality [48] (although other analyses failed to document similar effects [43, 44, 47]), and all-cause mortality [48, 50]. Side effects were more common among FQ recipients than placebo or no treatment recipients in some analyses [42] but not others [48]. FQ were associated with fewer side effects than TMP/SMX [42, 48]. Invasive fungal infections were not more likely to occur among FQ recipients compared to placebo or no treatment control recipients [42, 43, 47, 48]. Moreover, colonization by FQ-resistant bacteria, infection by FQ-resistant microorganisms, *Clostridium difficile*-associated diarrhea, did not occur more often among FQ recipients compared to their placebo or no treatment counterparts [48–50]. Of all the FQ studied compared to placebo or no treatment, ciprofloxacin has been associated with a reduction in all-cause mortality [50]. Protective effects of FQ for fever episodes and all-cause mortality have been demonstrated in both acute leukemia/HSCT and solid tumor/lymphoma patients [50]. FQ plus additional gram-positive agents such as roxithromycin or rifampin versus FQ alone have reduced gram-positive infections but not gram-negative infections [42, 44, 45].

These observations have led to recommendations for the use of FQ prophylaxis by the Infectious Diseases Working Party of the European Blood and Marrow Transplant Group, the European Leukemia Net, the Infectious Diseases Group of the European Organisation for the Treatment and Research in Cancer, and the International Immunocompromised Host Society [40]. FQ (levofloxacin [A-I], ciprofloxacin [A-I], ofloxacin [B-I], or norfloxacin [B-I]), are being recommended for the prevention of bacterial infections, primarily gram-negative infections, among acute leukemia patients and HSCT recipients starting with the initiation of the cytotoxic therapy until myeloid reconstitution or the onset of a febrile neutropaenic episode (A-II) [40]. The National Comprehensive Cancer Network (NCCN) guidelines have made recommendations regarding antibacterial prophylaxis on the basis of infection risk; low, intermediate, or high [9, 60, 64–67]. Prophylaxis is not recommended for those at low-risk defined as recipients of conventional chemotherapy regimens for solid tumors and those wherein the expected duration of neutropenia (ANC $<0.5 \times 10^9$/L) is less than 7 days [60]. The NCCN panel recommended that FQ prophylaxis be considered for intermediate-risk patients defined as autologous HSCT recipients or patients with lymphoma, chronic lymphocytic leukemia, myeloma, recipients of purine analog therapy (fludarabine or 2-doxyadenosine), and those with an anticipated duration of neutropenia of 7–10 days [60]. FQ prophylaxis should also be considered for high-risk patients such as those undergoing allogeneic HSCT, intensive cytotoxic therapy for acute leukemia or myelodysplastic syndromes wherein the expected duration of neutropenia is more than 10 days [60]. The Infectious Diseases Working Party of the German Society of Hematology and Oncology recommend the use of FQ prophylaxis for the prevention of gram-negative infections primarily during the pre-engraftment period among allogeneic HSCT recipients [56]. Other organizations have not yet adopted these recommendations [8, 23, 57].

Despite this experience and these recommendations there remains considerable controversy. Concerns regarding cost, drug-related toxicities, selection, emergence of antibiotic-resistant bacteria, and overgrowth of fungi prevent universal applicability [8]. Moreover, there is controversy regarding the patient populations most likely to benefit from antibacterial chemoprophylaxis when balanced against the cost of the chemoprophylaxis strategy, the drug-related toxicities, and the development of antimicrobial resistance.

3.2. Fluoroquinolone Prophylaxis and Antimicrobial Resistance

One of the main arguments against the wider application of antibacterial prophylaxis in neutropenic patients, has been based upon the concern for the emergence of antimicrobial resistance [68]. This may be considered on three levels; namely, colonization by and then infection with resistant microorganisms in the individual neutropenic patient, the change in the microflora of the in-patient unit where the policy of chemoprophylaxis has been adopted, and change in resistance profiles to the chemotherapeutic agent in the population at large [50].

The rise in bacterial antimicrobial resistance is directly related to resource expenditures such as prolonged hospital stays (US Congress, Office of Technology Assessment. Impacts of antibiotic resistant bacteria. Document no. OTA-H-629. Washington, DC: US Government Printing Office, 1995). Increased FQ use in the community is associated with increased risk of FQ-resistance among gram-negative bacilli [69]. Observational studies have reported that routine use of antibacterial prophylaxis is often followed by colonization by prophylactic agent-resistant bacteria; however, this has not predictably resulted in infection by these resistant bacteria [70–73]. Despite this, concerns remain about the possibility of an increased risk for FQ-resistant gram-negative bacteremia among neutropaenic cancer patients receiving FQ prophylaxis [70, 74].

A retrospective study from Ulm, Germany, examined the effect of discontinuing a policy of FQ-based (levofloxacin) chemoprophylaxis in neutropenic patients on infectious morbidity and mortality over three time periods; a baseline period of levofloxacin prophylaxis (1 year), a period of discontinuance of the policy (3 weeks), and a period of reintroduction of the policy (3 months) [75]. During the first period the rates of gram-negative bacteremia and overall mortality were 4.8% (15 of 310 patients, of which 9 isolates, 60%, were FQ-resistant) and 2.9% (9 of 310 patients), respectively. During the second period, the rates of gram-negative bacteremia and overall mortality were 44.4% (4 of 9 patients, of which all were susceptible to FQ) and 33.3% (3 of 9 patients), respectively. During the third period, following the reintroduction of the FQ-prophylaxis policy, the rates of gram-negative bacteremia and overall mortality rate were 5.7% (4 of 70 patients, of which 3 of 4 isolates, 75%, were FQ-resistant) and 1.4% (1 of 70 patients), respectively. It is noteworthy that the mortality rates during periods one and three were low despite the numbers of FQ-resistant gram-negative bacteremias. The authors concluded that levofloxacin prophylaxis had a beneficial protective effect upon infectious morbidity and overall mortality despite increased gram-negative FQ resistance [75]. This, among few others [76], was one of the earliest observations of a possible FQ prophylaxis-related effect on all-cause mortality.

A more systematic examination of this question has been undertaken. Colonization by FQ-resistant bacteria was observed in only 9 (11%) of 82 FQ-prophylaxis recipients compared to 6 (8%) of 79 placebo or no treatment controls (RR 1.68, 95% CI 0.71–4.00, P=0.461) in the three trials reporting this outcome [49]. A systematic review of eight studies demonstrated that patients receiving FQ were no more likely to develop an infection due to an FQ-resistant microorganism than a placebo recipient (54 of 1,358 subjects vs. 51 of 1,354 subjects, respectively, OR 1.06, 95% CI 0.72–1.56) [50]. Moreover, FQ-recipients were no more likely to develop fungal infections than placebo or untreated controls (RR 1.07, 95% CI 0.83–1.37) [48]. However, approximately one-third (54 of 154, 35%) of all microbiologically documented infections occurring among FQ recipients have been due to FQ-resistant organisms; accordingly, it seems appropriate to recommend that FQ should not be administered as a treatment for the febrile episode.

It seems reasonable to speculate that a high prevalence of gram-negative bacterial FQ-resistance would reduce the potential efficacy of FQ prophylaxis in neutropenic patients. This begs the question of the existence of a threshold prevalence above which the protective effects are lost [50]. In a large randomized placebo-controlled study among higher-risk neutropenic cancer patients, levofloxacin prophylaxis reduced the number of gram-negative infections by 56% (NNT=13) despite a prevalence of FQ-resistance in gram-negative bacilli of 17% in the placebo control group [19]. These observations suggest that a protective treatment effect can be demonstrable even under circumstances of gram-negative FQ resistance of at least that magnitude.

Taken together, these observations suggest that in neutropenic cancer patients infections due to FQ-resistant bacteria may be expected; however, these events are relatively uncommon and do not appear to affect the overall efficacy of the strategy for the important outcomes.

3.4. Who Should Receive Antibacterial Prophylaxis: High- or Low-Risk?

The majority of the recommendations for the application of antibacterial prophylaxis strategies have focused upon the patients with the highest risk of developing infection during the neutropenic period, predominantly those undergoing allogeneic HSCT and intensive induction or reinduction therapy for acute leukemia [60] wherein the neutropenic fever event rate has been reported to be in the order of 87% (95% CI 83–89%) [50]. In contrast, the event rates of patients with solid tumors and lymphomas having neutropenic fever is approximately 70% lower (25%, 95% CI 22–28%) [50].

However, this latter group of patients is very heterogeneous with respect to the risk for febrile neutropenic episodes.[64]. The risk factors cited for neutropenic fever in this group have included older age, poor performance status, underlying disease for which cytotoxic therapy is being administered (testicular carcinoma 28%, small cell lung cancer 17%, non-Hodgkin's lymphoma 14%, breast cancer 12%), low serum albumin (<35 g/L), elevated lactate dehydrogenase, bone marrow involvement with lymphoma, lymphopenia (ALC $<0.7\times10^9$/L) at day 5 of the treatment regimen, and choice of cytotoxic regimen [52, 64, 67, 77]. The incidence of neutropenic fevers is highest within the first one to two cycles of chemotherapy [52, 64].

Arguments for the use of antibacterial chemoprophylaxis in solid tumor and lymphoma patients have been based upon the results of clinical trials. The largest clinical trial, the SIGNIFICANT trial, included 1,565 subjects with solid tumors or lymphoma randomly allocated to receive oral levofloxacin (500 mg) or placebo prophylaxis once daily for 7 days beginning on day 8 for all 14- and 21-day cycles and on day 15 for all 28-day cycles [53]. While all-cause mortality in this study was unaffected by the prophylaxis (RR 0.67, 95% CI 0.32–1.38), the event rates for fever and bacterial infection were reduced (RR 0.71, 95% CI 0.55–0.92, NNT 23; and, RR 0.82, 95% CI 0.73–0.94, NNT 13, respectively). The need to admit patients to hospital for the treatment of suspected infection during the first cycle was reduced by 36% with prophylaxis (NNT 27). Despite these positive outcomes, there were no effects upon the incidence of severe infection or death from severe infection and there was a 92% increase in side effects [78].

The role of prophylactic ciprofloxacin plus roxithromycin for reducing febrile neutropaenic episode in small cell lung cancer patients receiving an intensified chemotherapeutic regimen of cyclophosphamide, doxorubicin, and etoposide (CDE) plus filgrastim compared to standard-dose CDE without filgrastim has been explored in a randomized placebo-controlled trial using a 2×2 factorial design [79]. Among the standard CDE recipients, the antibiotic prophylaxis had no effect upon the febrile neutropaenic episode rate (24% vs. 29%, $\chi^2=0.210$, $P=0.647$) whereas among the intensified CDE plus filgrastim recipients, the prophylaxis strategy reduced the FNE rate by 57% from 56% to 24% ($\chi^2=8.570$, $P=0.003$, NNT=3). Among the placebo recipients, the febrile neutropaenic episode rate was significantly higher (56%) in the intensified CDE plus filgrastim group compared to the standard CDE group (29%, $\chi^2=5.93$, $P=0.015$). However, among ciprofloxacin plus roxithromycin recipients, the febrile neutropaenic episode rates for the intensified CDE plus filgrastim group were the same as for the standard CDE group (24%). While the prophylactic antibiotic strategy appeared effective for controlling neutropenic fevers in the intensified CDE plus filgrastim group, it is disconcerting that the febrile neutropaenic episode rates were the same (24%) for the prophylaxis recipients independent of whether standard or intensified CDE was administered and that these rates were similar to that for the placebo group receiving standard CDE (29%). Lastly, overall mortality was not affected in any arm of the trial.

A second study from the same group addressed the question of the role of the haematopoietic growth factor support [80]. The overall febrile neutropaenic episode rate was reduced by 44% (NNT=7) from 32% to 18% among filgrastim recipients. It is to be noted that the event rate among control patients receiving standard CDE and prophylactic antibiotics in this study (32%) was similar to that (24%) in the previous trial ($P=0.394$) [79]. Moreover, the treatment effect was observed predominantly in the first cycle of chemotherapy. Despite a baseline febrile neutropaenic episode event rate of 24% and the 58% relative risk reduction, a follow-up pharmacoeconomic analysis failed to demonstrate that the addition of filgrastim was cost-effective [81].

An analysis of four trials [53, 79, 82, 83] comparing FQ to placebo in this same patient population was able to demonstrate an effect upon all-cause mortality (first cycle) in 30-days (RR 0.51, 95% CI 0.27–0.97, NNT 72) [50]. Approximately 50–60% of all the deaths associated with these treatments occur during the first cycle [50, 64].

The available evidence suggests that patients undergoing cyclical chemotherapy for solid tumors or lymphoma glean a survival benefit from FQ-based antibacterial prophylaxis during at least the first cycle of anticancer treatment [50, 52]. The effects of prophylaxis on febrile event rates and hospitalization are also most pronounced over the first cycle of chemotherapy [52]. Moreover, febrile episodes during the first cycle of anticancer treatment appear to predict circumstances wherein, FQ-based prophylaxis should be considered for the reduction of febrile events during subsequent cycles [52].

The design of the SIGNIFICANT study drug administration protocol [53] could conceivably improve compliance, reduce expense, and exposure-related side effects and bacterial resistance by the intermittent short duration of drug exposure rather than the more usual continuous administration protocols employed in other trials. Despite this design, almost one-fifth (19%) of subjects in the SIGNIFICANT study [53] declined to take the study drug over all the cycles of anticancer treatment. In order to obtain the protective benefits described in the trial, almost 18,000 doses had to be administered. For example, in order to prevent one febrile episode over a mean of 4.4 cycles per patient for 7 days per cycle, 23 patients would require the administration of just over 700 doses of prophylaxis.

FQ has become an important part of the empirical antibiotic management of neutropenic fevers in low-risk cancer patient populations [9, 60]. A systematic review of clinical trials examining the efficacy of oral FQ-based empirical antibiotic therapy compared to standard intravenous antibiotic regimens, demonstrated that regimens containing FQ alone or FQ plus additional oral agents such as amoxicillin/clavulanic acid, phenoxymethyl penicillin, or clindamycin had similar outcomes (all-cause mortality, RR 0.7, 95% CI 0.37–1.35; and, treatment failure, RR 0.91, 95% CI 0.75–1.11) as for intravenous antibiotic regimens [84]. Use of FQ-based prophylaxis precludes use of a FQ as part of the empirical treatment for neutropenic fever in this group of patients. The reported all-cause mortality rates for patients receiving chemotherapy for solid tumor and lymphoma in clinical trials of FQ prophylaxis (1.4% and 2.7% for FQ and placebo recipients, respectively) [50] are very similar to those in clinical trials of oral FQ empirical antibiotic therapy for neutropenic fever (1.7% and 2.5% for oral FQ treatment and intravenous antibiotic recipients, respectively (84), $\chi^2=5.708$, df=3, $P=0.127$). This consideration suggests that for the group of low-risk patients receiving chemotherapy for solid tumors or lymphoma there appears to be no survival advantage for the FQ-based prophylaxis strategy compared to the FQ-based treatment strategy. Accordingly, an argument may be made for reserving FQ for treatment rather than prophylaxis.

4. Role of Hematopoietic Growth Factors for the Prevention of Infection in Neutropenic Cancer Patients

Chemotherapy-induced neutropenia is a major risk for infection-related morbidity and mortality for patients undergoing sequential therapy for solid tumors and lymphoma [64]. It is also a major factor governing clinical decisions to attenuate subsequent chemotherapy dose-intensity which, in turn, has an impact upon overall survival [85]. Hematopoietic growth factors, granulocyte colony-stimulating factor (G-CSF) and granulocyte-macrophage colony-stimulating factor (GM-CSF), have been administered as a prophylactic strategy to reduce chemotherapy-induced neutropenia and, thereby, neutropenic fevers.

At least six systematic reviews with meta-analyses have been published evaluating the efficacy of hematopoietic growth factors in randomized, placebo- or no treatment controlled clinical trials for a variety of outcomes including neutropenic fevers, documented infections, use of amphotericin B, duration (in days) of neutropenia (ANC $<0.5\times10^9$/L), duration (in days) of hospitalization, duration (in days) of parenteral antibiotic therapy, duration (in days) of chemotherapy delay due to neutropenia, and infection-related and all-cause mortality [86–91]. Not all of these examined the same outcomes or performed the same meta-analyses. These reviews are summarized in Table 10-3. Five of these studies were able to demonstrate significant reductions in the event rate for neutropenic fevers (RRR 37%) and for documented infections (RRR 30%), respectively. One pediatric study reported a 50% reduction in the need to prescribe amphotericin B (RR 0.5, 95% CI 0.28–0.87) [87]. There were consistent reductions demonstrable in the duration of neutropenia, duration of intravenous antibiotic therapy, and duration of hospitalization across studies [87, 90, 91]. Infection-related mortality was unaffected by hematopoietic growth factors in four reviews [86, 87, 91]. All-cause mortality in lymphoma patients and HSCT recipients was similarly uninfluenced by hematopoietic growth factors (RR 0.93, 95% CI 0.60–1.43, and RR 0.93, 95% CI 0.82–1.04, respectively) [89, 91]. Although there were noted increases in dose-intensity among lymphoma patients receiving hematopoietic growth factors, there was no increase in complete response rate (RR 1.02, 95% CI 0.94–1.11) [89]. It is noteworthy that in the lymphoma population, antibiotic prophylaxis reduced the risk of neutropenic fevers and documented infections by 26% independent of the hematopoietic growth factors (RR 0.74, 95% CI 0.62–0.89, and RR

Table 10-3. Summary of published systematic reviews and meta-analyses of haematopoietic growth factors for preventing infection in neutropenic cancer patients.

Study	Meta-analyses	No. trials	No. randomized subjects	Outcomes measured	OR[a]/RR[b]/WMD[c] (95% CI)	Study Agent Effect on outcome
Lyman et al. (2002) [86]	HGF vs. placebo or no treatment (8 trials, 1,144 randomized subjects)	NS	NS	Fever	0.38[a] (0.29–0.49)	↓
		NS	NS	Documented infection	0.51[a] (0.36–0.73)	↓
		NS	NS	Mortality[d]	0.60[a] (0.30–1.22)	No effect
		NS	NS	Side effects: bone pain	2.90[a] (1.60–4.80)	↑
Lyman and Kuderer (2004) [88]	Pegylated filgrastim vs. filgrastim	4	NS	Febrile neutropenia	0.66[b] (0.44–1.00)	↓
Sung et al. (2004) [87]	HGF vs. Placebo or no treatment in pediatric cancer patients (16 trials, 1,183 randomized subjects)	11	NS	Febrile neutropenia	0.80[a] (0.67–0.95)	↓
		11	NS	Documented infection	0.78[a] (0.62–0.97)	↓
		2	NS	Amphotericin B use	0.50[a] (0.28–0.87)	↓
		9	NS	Mortality[d]	1.02[a] (0.34–3.06)	No effect
		11	NS	Days to ANC $\geq 0.5 \times 10^9$/L[c]	−3.9 (−5.2 to −2.6)	↓
		8	NS	Days to hospital discharge[c]	−1.9 (−2.7 to −1.1)	↓
		6	NS	Days of IV antibiotics[c]	−0.8 (−2.3–0.7)	No effect
		4	NS	Days of chemotherapy delay[c]	−4.3 (−10.6–2.02)	No effect
Bohlius et al. (2004) [89]	HGF vs. Placebo or no treatment	8	1,013	Neutropenia	0.67[a] (0.60–0.73)	↓
		5	360	Febrile neutropenia	0.74[a] (0.62–0.89)	↓
		11	1,292	Documented infection	0.74[a] (0.64–0.85)	↓
		9	1,051	Mortality[d]	1.37[a] (0.66–2.82)	No effect
		10	1,170	Mortality[e]	0.93[a] (0.60–1.43)	No effect
		10	1,584	Complete tumor response	1.02[a] (0.94–1.11)	No effect
		8	1,204	Bone pain	3.57[a] (2.09–6.12)	↑
		2	232	Rash (GM-CSF)	7.69[a] (2.84–20.82)	↑
		2	337	Injection site reaction (GM-CSF)	6.55[a] (3.01–14.25)	↑
	G-CSF vs. GM-CSF	8	1,013	Neutropenia	0.67[a] (0.60–0.73)	↓
		11	1,292	Documented infection	0.74[a] (0.64–0.85)	↓
	Use of prophylactic antibiotics	5	360	Febrile neutropenia	0.74[a] (0.62–0.89)	↓
		11	1,292	Documented infection	0.74[a] (0.64–0.85)	↓

(continued)

Table 10-3. (continued)

Study	Meta-analyses	No. trials	No. randomized subjects	Outcomes measured	OR[a]/RR[b]/WMD[c] (95% CI)	Study Agent Effect on outcome
Dekker et al. (2006) [91]	HGF vs. placebo or no treatment in HSCT recipients (34 trials, 2 ,669 randomized subjects)	12	NS	Documented infection	0.87[b] (0.76–1.00)	↓
		11	NS	MDI	0.78[b] (0.58–1.03)	No effect
		6	NS	CDI	0.80[b] (0.59–1.08)	No effect
		11	NS	Days of fever[c]	−0.22 (−1.36–0.93)	No effect
		16	NS	Days of IV antibiotics[c]	−1.39 (−2.56 to −0.22)	↓
		23	NS	Days to ANC $\geq 0.5 \times 10^9$/L[c]	−3.98 (−4.74 to −3.22)	↓
		20	NS	Days to hospital discharge[c]	−2.94 (−3.81 to −2.06)	↓
		13	NS	Mortality[d]	0.76 (0.41–1.44)	No effect
		8	NS	Mortality[e]	0.93[b] (0.82–1.04)	No effect
Wittman et al. (2006) [90]	HGF vs. placebo or no treatment in pediatric cancer patients	12	804	Febrile neutropenia	0.59[a] (0.43–0.81)	↓
		7	501	Documented infections	0.66[a] (0.43–1.01)	No effect
		10	624	Days of IV antibiotics[c]	−1.97 (−3.59 to −0.35)	↓
		13	867	Days to ANC $\geq 0.5 \times 10^9$/L[c]	−3.40 (−4.96 to −1.85)	↓
		13	931	Days to hospital discharge[c]	−1.72 (−2.52 to −0.92)	↓

MDI microbiologically documented infection; *CDI* clinically documented infection; *OR* odds ratio; *RR* relative risk; *CI* confidence interval; *HSCT* hematopoietic stem cell transplant; *HGF* hematopoietic growth factor; *WMD* weighted mean difference; *ANC* absolute count; *NS* not stated

[a] Odds ratio

[b] Relative risk

[c] Weighted mean difference

[d] Infection-related mortality

[e] Total (all-cause) patient mortality

↓ Reduced event rate for the outcome

↑ Increased event rate for the outcome

0.74, 95% CI 0.64–0.85, respectively) [89]. Despite this, no impact upon the numbers of subjects requiring intravenous antibiotics was observed (RR 0.82, 95% CI 0.57–1.18) [89]. G-CSF may have an advantage over GM-CSF with regard to documented infection. Adverse effects such as bone pain, skin rash, and local reactions at the injection sites were more common among hematopoietic growth factors recipients. There was considerable heterogeneity in the study populations, supportive care protocols, underlying diseases, and in the study drug used (G-CSF, pegylated G-CSF, GM-CSF). Despite the limitations of heterogeneity, these studies suggest that primary prophylaxis with hematopoietic growth factors can significantly affect the risk for neutropenia, febrile neutropenia and infections in adult and pediatric patients undergoing treatment for solid tumors, patients undergoing conventional chemotherapy for malignant lymphoma, and patients undergoing HSCT. There is no evidence that these products improve tumor control, overall survival, or quality of life [92, 93].

The 2005 Update Committee of the American Society of Clinical Oncology (ASCO) have revised the 1996 and 2000 ASCO Guidelines for the use of hematopoietic growth factors [92]. Primary prophylaxis is recommended for the prevention of neutropenic fevers in high-risk patients wherein the risk for such events is 20% or more based on age, medical history, disease characteristics, and myelotoxicity of the chemotherapy regimen. Most commonly used regimens have risks of neutropenic fevers of less than 20% [67, 92]. For example, these recommendations would include patients undergoing intensive cytotoxic therapy, including CHOP-based regimens, for aggressive non-Hodgkin's lymphoma who are 65 years of age or more, in order to reduce infectious complications. Secondary prophylaxis is recommended for those patients experiencing a neutropenia-related complication during previous cycles of chemotherapy [92]. Hematopoietic growth factors permit a modest increase in dose-density and dose-intensity; however, an effect upon survival has been observed in the context of dose-dense treatment regimens only [93, 94]. Primary prophylaxis with hematopoietic growth factors following autologous HSCT is recommended because of the effects of reduced length of stay in hospital and associated medical costs [95]. Similar economic benefits have not been observed among allogeneic HSCT recipients of hematopoietic growth factors [96]. Moreover, hematopoietic growth factor-associated increase in graft-versus-host reactions and lower overall survival has been reported [97]. While the Update Panel felt that the use of hematopoietic growth factors for induction therapy in AML may be reasonable, particularly in patients 55 years of age or older, there appears to be no significant impact upon outcomes such as response or survival [92]. Hematopoietic growth factors are recommended for administration to AML patients undergoing postremission consolidation [98, 99]. The routine long-term, continuous administration of hematopoietic growth factors to patients with myelodysplastic syndromes is not recommended. In contrast, hematopoietic growth factors are recommended for patients undergoing induction or postremission consolidation for acute lymphoblastic leukemia to reduce the duration of neutropenia; however, the impact on infectious morbidity has been minimal.

In these groups the impact of the interaction between hematopoietic growth factors and FQ-based antibacterial prophylaxis is unclear. The major role for hematopoietic growth factors in primary prophylaxis appears to be in the solid tumor and lymphoma patient populations, particularly in the first cycle of chemotherapy among those in whom the neutropenic fever risk is at least 20%. However, the addition of hematopoietic growth factors to antibacterial prophylaxis has not resulted in significant cost savings [81]. Given these observations and the lack of consistent effects upon survival outcomes, prudence in the prescription of hematopoietic growth factors for primary prophylaxis should be exercised. It may be appropriate to consider primary hematopoietic growth factors prophylaxis without antibacterial prophylaxis for the out-patient populations receiving first cycles of chemotherapy for solid tumors or lymphoma. Combined hematopoietic growth factors and antibacterial prophylaxis may be best reserved for those patients receiving intensive postremission consolidation for acute leukemia or autologous HSCT. FQ-based antibacterial prophylaxis alone without hematopoietic growth factors may be reserved for patients undergoing remission-induction therapy for acute leukemia or allogeneic HSCT during the pre-engraftment period.

5. Antifungal Chemoprophylaxis

Opportunistic invasive fungal infections have emerged as major complications among high-risk patients undergoing intensive cytotoxic therapy for acute leukemia or haematopoietic stem cell transplantation. Most of these infections (up to 75% in some institutions (100)) remain undiagnosed antemortem. The prevalence of invasive mold infection appears to be increasing [100]. Since the late 1980s the incidence of invasive aspergillosis among Italian acute leukemia patients has risen from 4.7% in the years 1987–1998 to 12.6% in 2006 [101–103]. The incidence of invasive fungal infection (IFI), particularly invasive mold infections, among allogeneic HSCT recipients has also been increasing [104–106]. The pathogens associated with invasive fungal infections (IFI) in HSCT recipients have included *Candida* spp. (25%), *Aspergillus* spp. (71%), non-*Aspergillus* molds (4%) [106]. Ninety percent of the invasive infections due to yeasts were candidaemia, and over 90% of mold infections were due to *Aspergillus* spp. [102, 106].

An understanding of the event rates for IFI is important of estimating the effectiveness and likelihood of any given chemoprophylaxis strategy to prevent these infections would be effective. The lowest IFI event rates among untreated patients for which statistically significant prophylactic treatment effects have been reported are of the order of 5–6% [107, 108]. Chemoprophylaxis strategies to patient groups with IFI event rates of less than 5%, are less likely to be demonstrably effective without large sample sizes. The ability of any given antifungal agent to produce a detectable protective treatment effect is also important. The effect size may be based upon the relative risk reduction for IFI relative to a comparator.

The event rates of IFI among control subjects reported in clinical trials of antifungal prophylaxis in allogeneic HSCT recipients have been about double that for acute leukemia patients (12.4% vs. 5.9%) [108]. Among HSCT patients at high-risk for IFI, because of advanced grade III/IV acute graft versus host disease (GvHD), event rates as high as 35% have been reported [109]. The reported event rates for invasive candidiasis and invasive aspergillosis in a general population of acute myeloid leukemia patients has been 4.4% and 7.9%, respectively [102]. With the more widespread use of fluconazole-based antifungal prophylaxis, the frequency of invasive candidiasis has been eclipsed by invasive mold infections [102, 106].

There have been numerous clinical trials of antifungal prophylaxis in immunocompromised and neutropenic patient populations. Oral nonabsorbable antifungal agents such as nystatin have not been helpful in controlling fungal colonization (RR 0.85, 95% CI 0.65–1.13) or infection (RR 0.40, 95% CI 0.17–0.93) compared to placebo or to azole antifungal agents in these higher risk patient populations [110]. Despite the lack of evidence for clinical efficacy, oral nonabsorbable antifungal agents have been used in practice and have often been deployed in the control arms of clinical trials evaluating the prophylaxis efficacy of azoles such as fluconazole, itraconazole, or ketoconazole in neutropenic cancer patients [107] (Table 10-4).

There have been at least eight systematic reviews of published randomized-controlled clinical trials of antifungal chemoprophylaxis, encompassing at least 28 meta-analyses in this patient population [107, 108, 111–116]. Outcomes examined have included prophylaxis success (defined as the completion of the study without the administration of parenteral full-dose antifungal therapy for suspected or proven IFI), total invasive fungal infection, invasive yeast infection, invasive aspergillosis, invasive mold infection, superficial fungal infection, empirical antifungal therapy, withdrawals for intolerance, fungal infection-related mortality, and all-cause mortality. One of the earlier publications included both prophylaxis trials and trials of empirical antifungal therapy for the persistent neutropenic fever syndrome [111]; accordingly, the results of the analyses from that study have been difficult to interpret. A summary of the published meta-analyses are presented in Table 10-4.

Current evidence from systematically reviewed randomized-controlled clinical trials support the efficacy of fluconazole, itraconazole oral suspension, and posaconazole antifungal prophylaxis for a variety of outcomes and under specified conditions [108].

It has been argued that all-cause mortality is one of the more clinically important end-points. Overall, no treatment effects on all-cause mortality have been demonstrated for fluconazole, itraconazole, ketoconazole, or low-dose intravenous amphotericin B [107, 111, 113], with the exception of the study from Israel [108]. Patients from 31 studies (n=5,881 randomized subjects) receiving systemic antifungal prophylaxis with azoles or low-dose amphotericin B had a 16% lower all-cause mortality rate than control patients receiving placebo, no treatment, or oral polyenes (RR 0.84, 95% CI 0.74–0.95) [108]. In contrast, in an earlier Canadian study of 31 trials involving 7,014 randomized subjects, an overall reduction in all-cause mortality was not demonstrable (OR 0.87, 95% CI 0.74–1.02) [107]. However, in subset analyses, a prophylaxis-related 24% reduction in all-cause mortality was observed in patients with prolonged durations of neutropenia of >15 days (OR 0.76, 95% CI 0.62–0.94) [107]. Antifungal prophylaxis-related reductions in all-cause mortality have been observed in other subgroup analyses including allogeneic HSCT recipients (RR 0.62, 95% CI 0.45–0.85), autologous HSCT recipients (RR 0.27, 95% CI 0.08–0.95), in patients receiving concomitant antibacterial prophylaxis (RR 0.08, 95% CI 0.67–0.96), and in HSCT recipients receiving low-dose intravenous amphotericin B as the antifungal prophylaxis (RR0.31, 95% CI 0.14–0.72) [108]. The effect seems to be greatest when assessed at 30 days post-treatment. Based upon these analyses, it appears that antifungal prophylaxis

Table 10-4. Summary of the systematic reviews and meta-analyses for antifungal prophylaxis.

Study	Meta-analyses	No. trials	No. randomized subjects	Outcomes measured	OR[a]/RR[b,c] (95% CI)	Study agent effect on outcome
KandaY et al. (2000) [112]	FLU vs. placebo or no treatment or nonabsorbable antifungal agents (16 trials, 3,734 randomized subjects)	16	3,734	IFI	0.42[a] (0.31–0.57)	↓
		6	1,373	IFI, non-BMT trials	0.85[a] (0.47–1.55)	No effect
		NS	NS	IFI, event rate <15%	0.78[a] (0.50–1.21)	No effect
		NS	NS	IFI, event rate >15%	0.23[a] (0.15–0.36)	↓
		NS	NS	IFI, C. *krusei/glabrata*	0.88[a] (0.46–1.68)	No effect
		NS	NS	Colonization, *C. krusei*	2.01[a] (1.30–3.12)	↑
		NS	NS	Colonization, *C. glabrata*	2.18[a] (1.17–4.08)	↑
		16	3,734	Mortality[d]	0.45[a] (0.29–0.72)	↓
		6	1,373	Mortality[d], non-BMT trials	0.91[a] (0.30–2.82)	No effect
		16	3,734	SFI	0.23[a] (0.17–0.31)	↓
		6	1,373	SFI, non-BMT trials	0.44[a] (0.24–0.80)	↓
		16	3,734	AMB	0.76[a] (0.60–0.96)	↓
		6	1,373	AMB, non-BMT trials	0.90[a] (0.56–1.45)	No effect
		16	3,734	IA	1.24[a] (0.71–2.18)	No effect
		6	1,373	IA, non-BMT trials	1.81[a] (0.61–5.36)	No effect
		8	1,539	IA, HD-FLU	1.49[a] (0.69–3.22)	No effect
		8	2,195	IA, LD-FLU	1.02[a] (0.45–2.32)	No effect
BowEJ et al. (2002) [107]	FLU vs. placebo or no treatment	8	1,520	Prophylaxis success	1.91[a] (1.49–2.37)	↑
		5	1,336	SFI	0.18[a] (0.12–0.27)	↓
		8	1,520	IFI	0.30[a] (0.21–0.45)	↓
		7	1,450	IA	1.18[a] (0.53–2.62)	No effect
		7	1,450	Mortality[e]	0.92[a] (0.70–1.20)	No effect
		7	1,450	Mortality[d]	0.48[a] (0.28–0.81)	↓
	FLU vs. oral polyenes	9	2,542	Prophylaxis success	1.45[a] (1.21–1.73)	↑
		8	2,412	SFI	0.28[a] (0.16–0.49)	↓
		9	2,542	IFI	0.60[a] (0.36–0.99)	↓
		9	2,542	IA	1.08[a] (0.46–2.53)	No effect
		7	1,956	Mortality[e]	0.89[a] (0.62–1.29)	No effect
		5	1,365	Mortality[d]	0.70[a] (0.28–1.76)	No effect
	ITR vs. placebo or no treatment	3	815	Prophylaxis success	1.67[a] (1.24–2.25)	↑
		2	615	SFI	0.67[a] (0.31–1.44)	No effect
		3	815	IFI	0.54[a] (0.28–1.04)	No effect

	3	815	IA	1.65[a] (0.51–5.35)	No effect
	3	815	Mortality[e]	0.85[a] (0.55–1.32)	No effect
	3	815	Mortality[d]	0.83[a] (0.34–2.05)	No effect
ITR vs. oral polyenes	2	834	Prophylaxis success	1.42[a] (1.08–1.87)	↑
	2	834	SFI	0.24[a] (0.09–0.59)	↓
	2	834	IFI	0.71[a] (0.36–1.41)	No effect
	2	834	IA	0.64[a] (0.26–1.59)	No effect
	2	834	Mortality[e]	0.83[a] (0.48–1.43)	No effect
	2	834	Mortality[d]	0.73[a] (0.24–2.22)	No effect
KET vs. placebo or no treatment	5	473	Prophylaxis success	2.02[a] (1.27–3.24)	↑
	4	348	SFI	0.36[a] (0.20–0.66)	↓
	5	473	IFI	0.86[a] (0.44–1.70)	No effect
	5	473	IA	0.87[a] (0.18–4.17)	No effect
	3	310	Mortality[e]	0.94[a] (0.49–1.80)	No effect
	3	310	Mortality[d]	0.96[a] (0.39–2.33)	No effect
KET vs. oral polyenes	5	246	Prophylaxis success	2.41[a] (1.29–4.50)	↑
	4	210	SFI	0.27[a] (0.13–0.53)	↓
	5	246	IFI	0.18[a] (0.08–0.44)	↓
	4	210	IA	0.85[a] (0.13–5.73)	No effect
	5	246	Mortality[e]	0.46[a] (0.18–1.14)	No effect
	5	246	Mortality[d]	0.39[a] (0.09–1.70)	No effect
AMB vs. placebo	4	454	Prophylaxis success	1.87[a] (1.20–2.91)	↑
	3	378	SFI	0.87[a] (0.54–1.42)	No effect
	4	454	IFI	0.23[a] (0.09—0.61)	↓
	4	454	IA	1.35[a] (0.20–9.01)	No effect
	3	419	Mortality[e]	0.82[a] (0.46–1.45)	No effect
	3	378	Mortality[d]	0.79[a] (0.18–3.44)	No effect
Systemic antifungals vs. placebo or no treatment, duration of neutropenia >15 days			Prophylaxis success	0.55[a] (0.45–0.68)	↓
			SFI	0.54[a] (0.44–0.74)	↓
			IFI	0.51[a] (0.38–0.69)	↓
			IA	0.95[a] (0.57–1.59)	No effect
			Mortality[e]	0.76[a] (0.62–0.94)	↓

(continued)

Study	Meta-analyses	No. trials	No. randomized subjects	Outcomes measured	OR[a]/RR[b,c] (95% CI)	Study agent effect on outcome
				Mortality[d]	0.65[a] (0.44–0.95)	↓
Glasmacher et al. (2003) [113]	ITR vs. placebo, no treatment, FLU, or oral polyenes	13	3,597	IFI	0.60[a] (0.43–0.83)	↓
		12	3,320	IYI	0.47[a] (0.28–0.79)	↓
				IYI, *C. albicans*	0.43[a] (0.16–1.11)	No effect
				IYI, non-*albicans Candida*	0.47[a] (0.25–0.89)	↓
		12	3,320	IA	0.67[a] (0.41–1.10)	No effect
		13	3,597	Mortality[d]	0.65[a] (0.43–0.98)	↓
		13	3,597	Mortality[e]	0.98[a] (0.79–1.22)	No effect
	ITR oral solution vs. placebo, no treatment, FLU, or oral polyenes	8	2,862	IFI	0.51[a] (0.35–0.75)	↓
		7	2,585	IYI	0.40[a] (0.21–0.76)	↓
		7	2,585	IA	0.52[a] (0.30–0.90)	↓
				Mortality[d]	0.58[a] (0.36–0.91)	↓
	ITR capsules vs. placebo, no treatment, FLU, or oral polyenes	5	735	IFI	0.92[a] (0.49–1.74)	No effect
		5	735	IYI	0.63[a] (0.26–1.55)	No effect
		5	735	IA	1.75[a] (0.61–5.07)	No effect
				Mortality[d]	1.01[a] (0.43–2.39)	No effect
	ITR (BDD > 200 mg/day) vs placebo, no treatment, FLU, or oral polyenes	7	2,585	IFI	0.47[a] (0.31–0.70)	↓
	ITR (BDD < 110 mg/day) vs. placebo, no treatment, FLU, or oral polyenes	6	1,012	IFI	0.92[a] (0.54–1.59)	No effect
	ITR vs. FLU		1,769	IFI	0.60[a] (0.37–0.97)	↓
				Withdrawal/(intolerance)	1.95[a] (1.57–2.44)	↑
	ITR vs. oral polyenes		1,731	IFI	0.60[a] (0.38–0.95)	↓
Vardakas et al. (2005) [115]	ITR vs. FLU (5 trials, 1,279 randomized subjects)	5	1,279	DFI	1.51[a] (0.97–2.35)	No effect
		4	NS	IFI	1.44[a] (0.96–2.17)	No effect
		4	NS	IMI	1.36[a] (0.83–2.24)	No effect
		4	NS	IYI	2.28[a] (0.92–5.66)	No effect
		5	1,279	SFI	1.49[a] (0.67–3.31)	No effect
		5	1,279	Mortality[d]	1.30[a] (0.75–2.25)	No effect
		5	1,279	Mortality[e]	0.89[a] 0.63–1.24)	No effect
		5	1,279	Withdrawals (intolerance)	0.27[a] (0.18–0.41)	↓

Robenshtok et al. (2007) [108]	Systemic anti-fungals vs. placebo or no treatment or non-systemic agents	39	7,001	IFI	0.50[b] (0.41–0.61)	↓
				IYI, *Candida* sp	0.31[b] (0.23–0.41)	↓
				IYI, non-*albicans Candida* sp	0.46[b] (0.31–0.47)	↓
		31	5,881	Mortality[e]	0.84[b] (0.74–0.95)	↓
		31	5,881	Mortality[d]	0.55[b] (0.41–0.74)	↓
				Empirical antifungal therapy	0.83[b] (0.73–0.88)	↓
	Systemic antifungals vs. placebo or no treatment or nonsystemic agents, allogeneic HSCT	4	552	Mortality[e]	0.62[b] (0.45–0.85)	↓
		4	552	Mortality[d]	0.52[b] (0.27–0.99)	↓
		4	552	IFI	0.33[b] (0.18–0.63)	↓
	Systemic antifungals vs. placebo or no treatment or nonsystemic agents, autologous HSCT	1	182	Mortality[e]	0.27[b] (0.08–0.95)	↓
		4	298	Mortality[d]	0.28[b] (0.06–1.28)	No effect
		4	233	IFI	0.36[b] (0.13–1.01)	No effect
	Systemic antifungals vs. placebo or no treatment or nonsystemic agents, acute leukemia	24	3,430	Mortality[e]	0.88[b] (0.74–1.06)	No effect
		24	3,430	Mortality[d]	0.66[b] (0.44–1.00)	No effect
		24	4,206	IFI	0.69[b] (0.53–0.90)	↓
	Systemic antifungals vs. placebo or no treatment or nonsystemic agents, with antibacterial prophylaxis	16	2,654	Mortality[e]	0.80[b] (0.67–0.96)	↓
		17	2,705	IFI	0.50[b] (0.37–0.68)	↓
	FLU vs. placebo or no treatment or nonsystemic agents	15	3,371	Mortality[e]	0.88[b] (0.75–1.02)	No effect
		13	2,554	Mortality[d]	0.49[b] (0.32–0.75)	↓
	ITR capsules vs. placebo or no treatment or nonsystemic agents	3	357	Mortality[e]	0.97[b] (0.57–1.64)	No effect

(continued)

Table 10-4. (continued)

Study	Meta-analyses	No. trials	No. randomized subjects	Outcomes measured	OR[a]/RR[b,c] (95% CI)	Study agent effect on outcome
		3	357	Mortality[d]	1.00[b] (0.40–2.49)	No effect
	ITR oral solution vs. placebo or no treatment or nonsystemic agents	4	1,345	Mortality[e]	0.85[b] (0.60–1.21)	No effect
		4	1,345	Mortality[d]	0.44[b] (0.20–0.99)	↓
	IV AMB vs. placebo	2	217	Mortality[e]	0.31[b] (0.14–0.72)	↓
		3	377	Mortality[d]	0.29[b] (0.10–0.87)	↓
	FLU vs. IV AMB	3	NS	IFI	0.49[b] (0.29–0.86)	↓
		3	NS	Intolerance/withdrawal	0.15[a] (0.06–0.38)	↓
	POS vs. FLU or ITR	2	NS	Proven/Probable IFI	0.47[b] (0.30–0.74)	↓
		2	NS	Mortality[e]	0.77[b] (0.59–1.01)	No effect
		2	NS	Mortality[d]	0.25[b] (0.11–0.57)	↓
		2	NS	IA	0.22[b] (0.11–0.42)	↓

Abbreviations: *FLU* fluconazole; *ITR* itraconazole; *IV* intravenous; *AMB* amphotericin B; *KET* ketoconazole; *POS* posaconazole; *IFI* proven invasive fungal infection; *event rate <15%*, IFI event rate in the control group of <15%; *event rate >15%*, IFI event rate in the control group >15%; *HD-FLU* high-dose FLU of at least 400 mg/day; *LD-FLU* low-dose FLU of less than 400 mg/day; *BMT* bone marrow transplant; *IFI C krusei/glabrata*, invasive fungal infection due to *Candida krusei* or *C. glabrata*; *SFI* superficial fungal infection; *BDD* bioavailable daily dose; *AMB* empirical amphotericin B; *IA*, invasive aspergillosis; *DFI*, documented fungal infection (sum of IFI+SFI); *IMI*, invasive mold infection; *IYI*, invasive yeast infection; *OR* odds ratio; *RR* relative risk; *CI*, confidence interval; *HSCT*, hematopoietic stem cell transplant.

[a] Odds ratio

[b] Relative risk

[c] Weighted mean difference

[d] Fungal infection-related mortality

[e] Total (all-cause) patient mortality

↓ Reduced event rate for the outcome

↑ Increased event rate for the outcome

can have a demonstrable effect upon all-cause mortality in specific subgroups of patients at higher risk due to prolonged neutropenia and during the pre-engraftment period in allogeneic HSCT recipients. Moreover, an overall 62% survival benefit of fluconazole-based antifungal prophylaxis has been demonstrable over an 8-year follow-up period in HSCT recipients [117].

Fungal infection-related mortality, as an end-point, is arguable, subject to the bias of the investigator trying to judge whether or not a death was due to the fungal infection. Several analyses have demonstrated reductions in fungal infection-related mortality of approximately 40–50% among fluconazole recipients (Table 10-4) [107, 108, 112] and itraconazole oral solution recipients [108, 113]. No differences were observed in this regard in comparisons of fluconazole and itraconazole (OR 1.30, 95% CI 0.75–2.25) [115]; however, posaconazole, an extended-spectrum azole, appeared to have an advantage over either (RR 0.25, 95% CI 0.11–0.57) [108].

Azole-based antifungal prophylaxis with fluconazole or itraconazole oral solution in comparison to placebo, no treatment, or oral polyenes also reduces the incidence of overall IFI by approximately 50% (Table 10-4) [107, 108, 112, 113]. The largest effects are observed under the following conditions (Table 10-4): where the expected event rate for IFI is >15% [107, 112]; where the prescribed daily doses of fluconazole or itraconazole are higher than 200 mg [107, 113]; if itraconazole is being prescribed, where the oral solution formulation is administered rather than the oral capsules [113]; where prophylaxis is prescribed to patients undergoing allogeneic HSCT [107, 108] or autologous HSCT who are not receiving HGF support [118]; among patients with a prolonged duration of neutropenia of >15 days [107] and, among acute leukemia patients receiving induction therapy [108], but not postremission consolidation [118]. Under circumstances where the risk for mold infection is higher than 5% [119, 120], extended-spectrum azoles such as posaconazole are superior to fluconazole or itraconzole for preventing overall IFI (RR 0.47, 95% CI 0.30–0.74) and invasive aspergillosis (RR 0.22, 95% CI 0.11 and 0.42), but not for invasive candidiasis (RR 0.83, 95% CI 0.46–1.52) [108]. Withdrawal of prophylaxis due to intolerance is observed much less frequently with fluconazole than either itraconazole (RR 0.27–0.51, 95% CI 0.18–0.41 to 0.41–0.63) [113, 115] or amphotericin B (RR 0.15, 95% CI 0.06–0.38) [108].

Voriconazole, another extended-spectrum azole with proven antimold activity [121, 122], has being studied in leukemia and allogeneic HSCT recipients. Employed as an empirical antifungal regimen for the persistent neutropenic fever syndrome, voriconazole recipients had fewer breakthrough invasive fungal infections than those receiving the liposomal amphotericin B comparator (1.9% vs. 5.0%; RR 0.39, 95% CI 0.17–0.82; RRR=61%, NNT=33) [123]. These observations suggested that voriconazole would be an effective agent in a prophylaxis strategy. In a multicentred European trial of voriconazole prophylaxis in patients with acute myeloid leukemia [124], 25 patients were randomly allocated to receive voriconazole ($n=10$) or placebo ($n=15$). The trial was terminated early upon publication of the posaconazole experience [119]. Although there were no cases of IFI in the trial, there was a difference in the incidence of pulmonary infiltrates, none versus five among voriconazole and placebo recipients, respectively ($\chi^2=4.167$, $P=0.041$) [124]. Furthermore, there were four cases of hepatosplenic candidiasis in the placebo group and none in the voriconazole group ($\chi^2=3.175$, $P=0.075$) [124]. Voriconazole was compared to fluconazole in allogeneic HSCT recipients [125]. There were fewer cases of invasive aspergillosis in the voriconazole group (7 of 305, 2.3%, vs. 16 of 279, 5.4%, $\chi^2=3.982$, $P=0.046$, NNT=32) [125]. Three patients developed invasive candidiasis in each group (1%), indicating similar efficacy against opportunistic yeast infections. Taken together, these observations suggest that voriconazole is a reasonable alternative for antimold prophylaxis in high risk patient groups.

The echinocandin agents, micafungin and caspofungin, have also been studied for antifungal prophylaxis [126, 127] and for the prevention of breakthrough of IFI during empirical antifungal therapy for the persistent neutropenic fever syndrome [128]. These agents were compared to fluconazole, itraconazole, and liposomal amphotericin B, respectively. There were no demonstrable differential treatment effects in pooled analyses for overall rates of IFI (OR 1.04, 95% CI 0.67–1.63), invasive aspergillosis (OR 0.85, 95% CI 0.39–1.88), or all-cause mortality (OR 0.78, 95% CI 0.58–1.05). Although there was a 29% reduction in the use of empirical antifungal therapy for suspected IFI among micafungin recipients compared to fluconazole recipients (NNT=16) [126], this review provides no compelling evidence for the use of these agents for prophylaxis.

The available evidence supports the use of fluconazole, itraconazole oral solution, or extended-spectrum azoles such as posaconazole or voriconazole for antifungal prophylaxis under defined circumstances. Numerous guidelines regarding the use of antifungal prophylaxis in defined patient groups have been published [8, 25, 27, 30, 57, 60, 114, 129, 130]. There is no evidence to support the use of antifungal prophylaxis in patients undergoing conventional chemotherapy for solid tumors or lymphoma (A-III). Moreover, there is poor evidence to support inhalational or aerosolized amphotericin B to prevent invasive mold infections [130]. Guidelines from the American Society of Blood and Marrow Transplantation, Immunocompromised Host Society, and the European Blood and Marrow Transplantation Society have recommended in the setting of allogeneic HSCT, the use of fluconazole (A-I), posaconazole (A-I), or itraconazole oral solution (B-I) for the prevention of IFI during the pre-engraftment period, through engraftment to at least day +75 or until the end of immunosuppression (B-III) [129]. The recommendations for micafungin or intravenous low-dose amphotericin B were less enthusiastic (C-I). In the setting of acute leukemia induction or re-induction therapy, posaconazole (A-I), fluconazole (C-I), or itraconazole oral solution (C-I) may be considered. Other groups have been more positive about the recommendations for prophylactic fluconazole administration from the onset of induction therapy until myeloid reconstitution in acute leukemia patients [8, 57, 60]. The evidence in Table 10-4 would further support a more robust recommendation for fluconazole or itraconazole oral solution during induction therapy for acute leukemia (A-I).

6. Antiviral Chemoprophylaxis

Most of the viral infections that complicate the course of patients with haematologic malignancies, those undergoing HSCT or receiving intermittent cytotoxic therapy for solid tissue malignancies, are a function of re-activation of latent virus acquired earlier in life, primarily the Herpesviruses. In the majority of cases, the presence of latent virus or evidence of past infection can be determined from the detection of virus-specific IgG antibody in serum. In the setting of cytotoxic therapy-induced neutropaenia, mucocutaneous infection due to Herpes simplex virus is the most common [131]. Severe, community-acquired respiratory virus infection appear to be less common overall except during periods of a community outbreak [132]. Several sets of guidelines regarding the preventions of these infections have been published [10, 23, 131, 133]. This topic has been recently reviewed [134]. A summary of the recommendations discussed herein for antiviral prophylaxis is shown in Table 10-5.

Table 10-5. Summary of recommendations pertaining to antiviral prophylaxis.

Pathogen	Conventional chemotherapy[a]	Acute leukemia[b]	Autologous HSCT[c]	Allogeneic HSCT[d]	T-cell depletional therapy[e]
HSV[f]	NR	R[g,h]	R[g,h,i]	R[g,h,j]	R[g,k]
VZV[f]	NR	NR[l]	NR[l]	R/NR[l,m,n]	R/NR[l,m]
CMV[f]	NR	NR	R[o]	R[o,p]	NR
HHV-6, HHV-7	NR	NR	NR	NR	NR
EBV[f]	NR	NR	NR	NR[q]	NR
HAV	NR[r]	NR[r]	NR[r]	NR[r]	NR[r]
HBV	R[s,t]	R[s,t]	R[s,t]	R[s,t]	R[s,t]
HCV	NR[u]	NR[u]	NR[u]	NR[u]	NR[u]
Influenza A, B	R[v,w]	R[v,w]	R[v,w]	R[v,w]	R[v,w]
RSV	NR	NR	NR	NR	NR
PIV, Adenovirus, hMPV	NR	NR	NR	NR	NR

NR Not recommended/No recommendations; *R* Recommended; *HSV* Herpes simplex virus; *VZV* Varicella-zoster virus; *CMV* Cytomegalovirus; *EBV* Epstein Barr virus; *RSV* Respiratory syncytial virus; *PIV* Parainfluenza viruses; *HHV* Human herpes virus; *HAV* Hepatitis A virus; *HBV* Hepatitis B virus; *HCV* Hepatitis C virus; *hMPV* human metapneumovirus; HB_sAg Hepatitis B surface antigen; HB_cAg Hepatitis B core antigen; $Anti\text{-}HB_c$ Antibody to Hepatitis B core antigen; *PTLD* Post-transplant lymphoproliferative disorder; *ANC* Absolute neutrophil count; *Auto-HSCT* Autologous haematopoietic stem cell transplant; *HSCT* Haematopoietic stem cell transplant; *GvHD* Graft-versus-host disease; *GCV* ganciclovir; *PCR* polymerase chain reaction; *ACV* acyclovir; *CMV-DNA* cytomegalovirus deoxyribonucleic acid

[a]Conventional regimens for solid tissue malignancies or first-line treatments for lymphoreticular malignancies

[b]Intensive cytotoxic chemotherapy for remission-induction, re-induction, or postremission consolidation

[c]Haematopoietic stem cell autografts with or without CD34 selection/T-cell depletion and with or without haematopoietic growth factor support

[d]Haematopoietic stem cell allografts from matched-related, mismatched-related, or unrelated donors, or cord blood transplants

[e]Purine analog therapy (e.g., fludarabine, 2-deoxyadenosine) in patients with additional risk factors (eg. second-line therapy, concomitant corticosteroid therapy, peripheral CD4 T-lymphocyte counts <0.05×10^9/L, older age >65 years, ANC <0.5×10^9/L) or alemtuzumab therapy recipients

[f]Patients who are IgG antibody sero-positive

[g]HSV- and VZV-active nucleoside analogs including acyclovir, valacyclovir, and famiciclovir; although data on valacyclovir or famiciclovir under these circumstances are limited (C-III). Patients unable to tolerate oral antiviral agents may receive intravenous acyclovir 250 mg/m^2 every 8 h (B-III)

[h]Duration of prophylaxis: from day 1 of cytoxic therapy or conditioning therapy throughout the neutropenic period until myeloid reconstitution (ANC >0.5×10^9/L over 2 consecutive days) and resolution of mucositis [23, 60, 131]

[i]Auto-HSCT with CD34 selection/T-cell depletion

[j]Prolonged periods of prophylaxis for HSV beyond engraftment may be prudent in the setting of GvHD and a history of repeated episodes of reactivation

[k]Duration of prophylaxis: from the first week of treatment until at least 2 months after cessation of treatment or until the peripheral CD4 T-lymphyocyte count is >0.2×10^9/L

(continued)

Table 10-5. (continued)

[l]Postexposure prophylaxis (within 96 h) in a susceptible (VZV sero-negative or adult or adolescent HSCT recipient <24 months from HSCT or who are receiving augmented immunosuppressive therapy post HSCT for GvHD) patient with Varicella-zoster immune globulin (125 units/10 kg to a maximum of 625 units administered intramuscularly) (A-II) [23]. Note that treatment can extend the incubation period from 10 to 21 days to 10–28 days. Varicella vaccine is contraindicated in VZV sero-negative immunocompromised patients such as those undergoing HSCT (A-III) [233]

[m]Long-term chemoprophylaxis has been recommended by some [60] but not others [23, 133]

[n]Varicella vaccination of VZV seronegative family members no later than 4 weeks before HSCT conditioning is scheduled is recommended (B-III) [131]

[o]Pre-emptive CMV therapy in allogeneic HSCT recipients or CD34 selected autologous HSCT recipients [234] at onset of CMV pp65 antigenemia or ≥2 consecutive positive CMV-DNA PCR tests: GCV 5 mg/kg IV every 12 h for 7–14 days then 5 mg/kg/day for 5 days/week until day+100 or for 3 weeks (whichever is longer) (A-I), or, alternatively, for 3–6 weeks if the CMV-DNA PCR test becomes negative (B-I)

[p]CMV prophylaxis for HSCT centres where CMV surveillance is unavailable: GCV 5 mg/kg/dose intravenously (IV) every 12 h for 5–7 days then 5–6 mg/kg/day IV 5 days/week from engraftment until d+100 (A-I) [23]. Foscarnet 60 mg/kg IV every 12 h for 7 days, then 90–120 mg/kg IV daily may be an alternative (C-III)

[q]EBV sero-positive patients with ≥3 risk factors for PTLD should be offered active surveillance for EBV and a single pre-emptive dose of anti-CD20 monoclonal antibody, rituximab (375 mg/m^2 IV) [131] if the serum viral load is >1,000 copies/mL (C-III) [169]

[r]Postexposure prophylactic or pre-emptive therapy against HAV with immune globulin (0.02 mL/kg) administered within 2 weeks of exposure is recommended (A-I) [192]

[s]Patients who are in an inactive chronic carrier state (HB_sAg sero-positive >6 months, HB_cAg sero-negative, anti-HB_c sero-positive, HBV viral load <2,000 copies/mL, normal transaminases, liver biopsy confirming absence of hepatitis) should receive lamivudine 100 mg/day orally throughout chemotherapy until 3 months following cessation of chemotherapy [197]

[t]Cancer patients who are HB_sAg sero-negative but anti-HB_c sero-positive are regarded as having had prior HBV infection. Such individuals may be offered lamivudine prophylaxis throughout chemotherapy or close monitoring for evidence of reactivation with targeted therapy (C-III) [197]

[u]Patients who are HCV sero-positive who are free of immunosuppressive therapy for >6 months and who have no evidence of myelosuppression or GvHD may be considered for pegylated interferon therapy with or without ribavirin (C-III) [197]

[v]Influenza chemoprophylaxis or pre-emptive therapy (following exposure to a confirmed case) during an established community or healthcare facility outbreak (amantidine or rimantidine 100 mg twice daily orally; or oseltamivir 75 mg daily orally) (A-I) [29]. No recommendation is available governing the prophylactic use of zanamivir. Amantidine and rimantidine are not effective for Influenza B

[w]Influenza vaccination (life-long, annual) is recommended for cancer patients (B-III) [60, 131, 178, 233]

6.1. Herpes Group Viruses

This group of DNA viruses consists of eight members including Herpes simplex virus (HSV) types 1 and 2, Varicella-Zoster virus (VZV), Cytomegalovirus (CMV), Epstein–Barr virus (EBV), and Human Herpesviruses (HHV) 6–8.

Mucositis is an important complication of cytotoxic therapy in neutropaenic cancer patients [135]. Herpes simplex virus (HSV) is responsible for a significant proportion of the oral morbidity observed among cancer patients receiving intensive cytotoxic chemo-radiotherapy [136–139]. The HSV reactivation rate among patients receiving intensive cancer chemotherapy has been reported to be high in the range of 37–57% [140] and even higher (68–90%) among myeloablative allogeneic HSCT recipients [141–143]. Nucleoside analogs such as acyclovir have proven activity for the treatment of HSV infections [144, 145]. Multiple studies have demonstrated the efficacy of these agents in the prevention of HSV re-activation and disease in cancer patients [141–143, 146–149]. In a single center experience of remission-induction therapy of acute myeloid leukemia in elderly patients, acyclovir prophylaxis, 800 mg orally administered twice daily, reduced the event rate for HSV mucositis by 88% (number needed to treat, 3) [150]. In contrast, no significant treatment effect-related impact upon the need for antibiotic therapy, duration of neutropaenia, or on the incidence of other opportunistic infections has been observed [131, 140, 151]. Despite this, different groups have generated recommendations for or against the prophylactic administration of nucleoside analogs (acyclovir, valacyclovir, or famciclovir) to high-risk HSV seropositive individuals [8, 10, 23, 131, 133].

In general, antiviral prophylaxis is not recommended for patients receiving conventional chemotherapy for solid tissue malignancies or lymphoma [8, 10, 131]. The National Comprehensive Cancer Network (NCCN) [10] recommends the administration of acyclovir or valacyclovir for HSV seropositive patients who are undergoing allogeneic HSCT or acute leukemia induction or reinduction therapy, in those autologous HSCT recipients at high risk for mucositis during the neutropaenic period, and those receiving T-cell depleting therapy such as fludarabine- or alemtuzumab-based regimens. Prophylaxis is recommended for administration throughout the neutropaenic period and until 30 days post-transplant. For those receiving T-cell depleting therapy, prophylaxis is recommended for administration until a minimum of 2 months after alemtuzumab therapy and until the circulating CD4 T-lymphocyte count is $\geq 0.2 \times 10^9$/L [10, 131]. HSV prophylaxis is not recommended for HSV seronegative patients, except under the circumstances in allogeneic HSCT, wherein the donor may be HSV seropositive.

While the re-activation rate for VZV among HSCT recipients is more than 30% after 1 year from transplant [152–158], these infections typically occurs in the postengraftment period rather than during the neutropaenic period [159]. The antiviral effect of prophylactic acyclovir on HSV during periods of myelosuppression appears to extend to a suppressive effect on VZV [155, 159]. Re-activation of VZV appears more linked to the degree of immunosuppression rather than to the degree of myelosuppression. Although long-term acyclovir prophylaxis (800 mg twice daily orally) from 1 to 2 months until 1 year postallogeneic HSCT, reduced the relative risk of re-activation of VZV by 81% (number needed to treat, 5) [159], the incidence of postprophylaxis VZV disease was unaffected. The Centers for Disease Control does not recommend routine long-term VZV chemoprophylaxis [160]. In contrast, the NCCN panel recommends the administration of acyclovir-based VZV prophylaxis in VZV seropositive allogeneic HSCT recipients from the 1st to the 12th post-transplant month [60]. The German guidelines recommend that VZV seronegative family members and significant others of HSCT patients be vaccinated with live attenuated Varicella vaccine at a time no later than 4 weeks before conditioning begins [131]. Neither the German nor the British guidelines make any recommendations regarding VZV prophylaxis [131, 133]. For those allogeneic HSCT recipients who are exposed to varicella or zoster while receiving immunosuppressive therapy for graft-versus-host disease (or who are less than 2 years from transplant), pre-emptive treatment with Varicella-zoster immune globulin (125 units/10 kg to a maximum of 625 units IM) is recommended for administration within 96 h of exposure [131, 160].

HHV-6 and HHV-7 have a prevalence approaching 100% in adults. While these related viruses have been linked to pneumonitis, hepatitis, encephalitis, and prolonged time-to-engraftment among HSCT recipients [161], they have not been associated with neutropaenic fever syndromes [162, 163]. The role of nucleoside analog-based antiviral prophylaxis for HHV6 or 7 is not clear. Since the IC_{50} values of acyclovir for HHV-6 and HHV-7 are significantly higher than for HSV (66–106 μM vs. 0.1–3.0 μM, respectively) [163], the standard acyclovir regimens recommended for HSV prophylaxis during neutropaenia may not be as effective for HHV. No recommendations for prophylaxis can be made at this time [131].

The risks of CMV re-activation and developing CMV disease have been reported as 45–86% and 20–30%, respectively among CMV seropositive allogeneic HSCT recipients [164–166]. The risk for CMV re-activation for autologous HSCT recipients is significantly lower, 4.2% [167]. The re-activation risk of alemtuzumab recipient (50%) appears to be significantly higher than for rituximab recipients (2.6%, $P=0.001$) [167]. In patients with T-cell lymphomas treated with CHOP (cyclophosphamide, hydroxydaunorubicin, vincristine, and prednisone) and alemtuzumab, the CMV re-activation rate of 25% was associated with pyrexia and with CMV disease syndromes (retinitis and pneumonitis) that required antiviral therapy after a median of 12 weeks of anticancer therapy [168]. Fludarabine-related CMV re-activation has been approximately only 5% [167], half of which have tended to occur after the completion of chemotherapy treatment [131]. In contrast with the above circumstances, CMV viraemia has been detected in up to 25% of neutropaenic patients with unexplained fevers [163], the clinical significance of which remains unclear. Routine CMV antiviral chemoprophylaxis or CMV DNA or antigen monitoring is not currently recommended for neutropaenic patients, including those undergoing autologous HSCT [131]. CMV chemoprophylaxis or monitoring is not recommended in the German guidelines for alemtuzumab recipients given the lack of robust clinical trial-based evidence of efficacy under these circumstances [131]. However, the NCCN guidelines do recommend active surveillance using genomic or antigen detection methods for those at high-risk for CMV disease (allogeneic HSCT or alemtuzumab recipients) and pre-emptive therapy with ganiclovir, valganciclovir, or foscarnet for at least 2 weeks or until CMV is no longer detectable [60]. The British guidelines also support this approach for allogeneic HSCT recipients [133]. Chemoprophylaxis for CMV has largely been supplanted by the pre-emptive approach based upon CMV re-activation surveillance [160]. For those CMV seronegative donor/recipient combinations (including CMV seronegative autologous HSCT recipients), the British guidelines advocate the use of CMV-negative or leukodepleted blood products to prevent the acquisition of CMV [133].

The major threat of Epstein–Barr virus (EBV) re-activation is post-transplant lymphoproliferative disorder (PTLD), which applies primarily to allogeneic HSCT recipients and which occurs well after engraftment. HSCT candidates who are EBV seronegative should be counseled regarding behaviors that could decrease the likelihood of EBV exposure [160]. Antiviral chemotherapy for prophylaxis or pre-emptive therapy is not recommended, given the lack of data about efficacy [131, 133, 160]. The German guidelines [131] recommend that those EBV seropositive patients who have three or more risk factors for PTLD (including T-cell depleted grafts, treatment with antithymocyte globulin or anti-CD3 antibodies, or unrelated or HLA-mismatched transplants) should receive active surveillance for EBV and be offered a single pre-emptive dose of rituximab (375 mg/m^2 intravenously) where the viral load is >1,000 copies/mL or where there is a rising titre [169]. The value of this approach remains controversial.

6.2. Respiratory Viruses

Community-acquired respiratory viruses such as Influenza A and B viruses, Respiratory Syncytial virus (RSV), the Parainfluenzaviruses (PIV) Types I-IV, Human Metapneumovirus (hMPV), Adenoviruses, and the Picornaviruses are common causes of a symptom complex characterized by rhinorrhoea, nasal or sinus congestion, sore throat, and cough commonly referred to in normal hosts as an upper respiratory tract infection. This topic has been recently reviewed [134].

Infection with these viruses in the setting of hematological malignancy may be associated with prolonged viral shedding and a higher risk for nosocomial transmission. Moreover, these viruses may be associated with more serious sequelae including pneumonia and death in immunocompromised patients undergoing HSCT or cytotoxic therapy for haematologic malignancies [132, 170–173]. With the exception of PIV infections which are observed year round, these infections have a typical seasonal pattern of onset between November and May. Influenza season typically follows RSV season with peak onset in December and January. Among patients with pre-existing serious comorbidities such as cancer, influenzavirus infection is approximately six times as likely to result in hospital admission [174].

Strategies of prevention, focus upon interrupting the person to person spread of infected secretions through aerosol droplet or contact transmission. Such strategies include contact isolation of infected patients, handwashing with soap and water or with alcohol-based gels prior to and after each patient contact, educational programs targeting not only families but also health care workers, avoidance of contact with secretions from infected patients by family and health care workers, and programs of annual influenzavirus immunizations for families and health care workers [160, 175, 176].

A proportion of myelosuppressed and immunosuppressed patients who develop a viral URTI may progress to pneumonia and even death. Among patients with acute leukemia that proportion may be as high as 43% with a case-fatality rate of approximately 1:5 (18%) [177]. Among allogeneic HSCT recipients the progression to pneumonia may be of the order of 1:3 (33%) with a case-fatality rate of 17% [177]. Almost 1:2 neutropaenic patients may show progression with a case-fatality rate almost 1:4 (23%) [177]. Early therapy of influenzavirus infection or RSV at the time of onset of the URTI can reduce the rate of progression by 66–75% [177]. The success of this approach is largely dependent upon making a rapid virological diagnosis based upon nasopharyngeal and throat swabs, or sputum and bronchoalveolar lavage specimens, and applying appropriate treatment plans.

The most effective strategy for preventing influenzavirus infections in health care settings is through annual immunization [178]. Recommendations have advocated immunization of target patient groups at risk, including cancer patients [176, 178]. Experience suggests that patients with lymphoproliferative disorders given influenza vaccine do have effective immune responses to the vaccine [179–181]. Antiviral drugs, while effective for chemoprophylaxis and treatment of influenza, are not substitutes for annual vaccination [178].

There are four agents licensed for use in the United States for influenza; amantidine, ramantidine, zanamivir, and oseltamivir. Influenza A virus may develop resistance to amantidine and ramantidine rapidly during treatment.

Zanamivir and oseltamivir are neuraminidase inhibitors that are effective against both Influenza A virus and Influenza B virus and have prevented influenza illness with reported efficacies of 68–89% among persons administered chemoprophylaxis after contact with a household member with influenza [178]. The number of subjects requiring treatment in order to prevent a single case in immunocompetant subjects has been quite high ($n = 89$), however [182, 183]. The efficacy of antiviral agents in preventing influenza among severely immunocompromised persons is unclear [178]. Accordingly, chemoprophylaxis may be considered for persons at high risk from the time of vaccination until immunity has developed, approximately 2 weeks, or those high risk persons considered likely to have an inadequate antibody response to influenza vaccine. Zanamivir may be administered in inhaled doses of 10 mg once daily, and oseltamivir may be administered in oral doses of 75 mg daily for subjects aged 13 years or more. The dosing for the latter agent in children <13 years is based upon weight (≤15 kg, 30 mg daily; >15 kg but <23 kg, 45 mg daily; 23–40 kg, 60 mg once daily; and >40 kg, 75 mg daily) [178]. Outside the circumstances of exposure or an outbreak, routine anti-influenza chemoprophylaxis is not recommended [60, 131, 160].

Immunization of health care providers has been associated with reductions in influenza, influenza-like illnesses, and all-cause mortality in long-term care facilities [184–186]. Despite this, approximately only 10–40% of those eligible are immunized [187]. Nevertheless, vaccination of healthcare providers is recommended [60, 131, 160]. The intranasal attenuated influenza vaccine is not recommended for immunosuppressed patients given the theoretical risk of severe infection in these patients [60].

No recommendations regarding immuno-prophylaxis, chemoprophylaxis, or pre-emptive therapy can be made for adenoviruses or parainfluenzaviruses, given the lack of availability of effective agents [131, 160].

Respiratory syncytial virus (RSV) pneumonia has a high case-fatality rate of approximately 1:3 in leukemia and HSCT patients [134]. Treatment may include aerosolized ribavirin with or without palivizumab [188]. There are no compelling data to support any recommendations regarding the optimal method for RSV prophylactic and preemptive therapy [131, 160].

6.3. Hepatitis A Virus Infection

It is known that viral hepatitis may be associated with transient myelosuppression [189]. Neutropaenia itself, however, does not appear to be a risk factor for viral hepatitis [190]. It is possible that exposure to Hepatitis A virus (HAV) during periods of neutropaenia may permit greater viral replication that enhance the likelihood of a more fulminate disease process as has been observed in animal models [191]. Perhaps the most relevant question in this context is how to manage a neutropaenic patient who has been exposed to HAV (as well as for other hepatitis viruses, HBV and HCV) even though the event rate for such an occurrence is expected to be very low. Currently, immune globulin (0.02 mL/kg body weight administered within 2 weeks of exposure) is the only product recommended for post exposure prophylaxis [192]. Patients who have received a single dose of HAV vaccine within 4 weeks of exposure may not require immune globulin. HAV vaccine is not licensed for postexposure prophylaxis. In a recent study, postexposure HAV vaccinated patients had a

30% higher rate of HAV compared to immune globulin recipients [193]. Some have advocated use of both approaches, HAV vaccine and immune globulin, postexposure [194].

6.4. Hepatitis B Virus Infection

The relationship between administration of chemotherapy with subsequent decrease in anti-HBsAG titre, followed by reactivation of hepatitis B virus infection among chronic carriers was recognized in 1975 [195]. Patients with hematological malignancies undergoing intensive cytotoxic therapy have a high risk of reactivation of hepatitis B virus infection with a range of rates of 20–50% being reported [196, 197]. HBsAg-positive carriers receiving anthracycline-based regimens for malignant lymphoma may reactivate in up to one in four cases [198]. Among HBsAG-positive patients undergoing haematopoietic stem cell transplantation the risk for graft-versus-host disease and veno-occlusive disease appears to be increased [199]. Reactivation following allogeneic HSCT appears to differ depending upon serostatus at the time of transplant; 2–3 months for HBsAg-positive subjects and much later (median 19 months) for anti-HBs-positive subjects [200]. Among patients with chronic or previous HBV infection, reactivation may best be defined by the development of acute hepatitis in association with newly detected or a greater than tenfold increase in HBV viral load [201].

Three distinct, previously exposed groups at risk for re-activation have been recognized [197]. One is a group of chronically infected viraemic patients who develop increased serum HBV DNA levels and clinical disease. A second is a group of chronic inactive carriers (HBsAgpositivee, HBV DNA-negative) who after chemotherapy begin to show evidence of re-activation. A third is a group of patients with evidence of immunity to HBV (HBsAg-negative, anti-HBs-positive, anti-HBc-positive) but who re-activate with increases in HBsAg and HBV DNA in plasma. The risk factors reported to be associated with increased risk of disease include male sex, younger age, prechemotherapy elevations in the serum alanine transferase, and prechemotherapy HBV DNA titres of $>3 \times 10^5$ copies/mL [202–205].

The risks of re-activation and significant consequent clinical disease among HBV-positive patients with hematological malignancies have warranted the development of strategies designed to prevent these complications associated with cytotoxic anticancer therapy. In chronic HBV carriers, corticosteroid therapy has long been known to increase the titres of HBsAg, HBcAg, viral loads, and clinical hepatitis [206–210]. Accordingly, avoidance of steroid-containing anticancer therapies seems prudent. The administration of steroid-free antilymphoma regimens for chronic HBV-positive lymphoma patients reduced HBV re-activation by up to 48%; however, this strategy was also associated with reduced tumor response rates and overall survivals by similar magnitudes [211]. Pre-emptive interferon therapy, while promising, has been associated with unacceptable toxicities [212]. Prophylactic or pre-emptive nucleoside analog therapy with lamivudine among high-risk chronic HBV carrier patients receiving chemotherapy has been extensively studied [198, 212–217]. Such approaches have reduced the re-activation event rate from 24–53% to 0–5% [197] and have improved the hepatitis-free survival [198, 217]. Accordingly, it has been recommended that all patients scheduled to receive chemotherapy or undergo a HSCT be screened for HBV infection prior to initiation of immunosuppressive therapy [197, 218]. HBV test positive subjects should receive nucleoside analog-based therapy (lamivudine 100 mg orally daily) throughout the treatment period beginning 1 week before treatment until 3–6 months following the completion of treatment [197, 218]. Adefovir or entecavir may be useful alternative agents in the setting of lamivudine resistance [218]. Nucleoside analog prophylaxis may be discontinued only if there is no biochemical or serological evidence of HBV activation (disappearance of HBsAg, appearance of anti-HBe antibody, and a reduction in viral lead to $<10^4$ copies/mL). Thereafter, patients at risk should be monitored for post-prophylaxis re-activation.

The Infectious Diseases Working Party of the German Society for Hematology/Oncology has recommended the daily administration of lamivudine 100 mg orally for all those patients who are HBsAg-positive or who are HBsAg-negative and anti-HBs-negative but anti-HBc positive and who are receiving conventional cytotoxic therapy (A-II) or autologous HSCT (A-II) [131]. Moreover, the recommendations have been extended to those patients receiving immunosuppressive therapy with alemtuzumab or rituximab, or have risk factors including a circulating CD4 T-lymphocyte count of $<0.05 \times 10^9$/L, age >65 years, or severe neutropaenia ($<0.5 \times 10^9$/L) (C-II) [131]. Based upon the current literature, the guideline committee was unable to provide clearer recommendation with regard to duration of prophylaxis; however, a minimum duration of 2–3 months following the completion of antitumor therapy was proposed, as well as postprophylaxis monitoring for high-risk subjects [131].

6.5. Hepatitis C Virus Infection

The prevalence of HCV infection among European patients with non-Hodgkin's lymphoma has been estimated to be in the range of 8–32% [219]. Moreover the range of prevalence of HCV infection among HSCT recipients is very wide, 5–70% [197]. While HCV infection can adversely affect outcomes in ztion upon the outcomes of patients undergoing intensive cytotoxic therapy or haematopoietic stem cell transplantation remains unclear. Circumstantial evidence suggests that augmented immunosuppression may promote HCV-related disease progression [197]. The results of anti-HCV chemotherapy in immunocompromised patients has been disappointing and there are insufficient data on which to base recommendations for chemoprophylaxis.

References

1. Henderson RA, Pinder L (1990) Acute transfusion reactions. N Z Med J 103(900):509–511
2. Gonen C, Celik I, Cetinkaya YS, Haznedaroglu I (2005) Cytarabine-induced fever complicating the clinical course of leukemia. Anticancer Drugs 16(1):59–62
3. Sickles EA, Greene WH, Wiernik PH (1975) Clinical presentation of infection in granulocytopenic patients. Arch Intern Med 135(5):715–719
4. Pizzo PA (1999) Fever in immunocompromised patients. N Engl J Med 341(12): 893–900
5. Mackowiak PA, Bartlett JG, Borden EC, Goldblum SE, Hasday JD, Munford RS et al (1997) Concepts of fever: Recent advances and lingering dogma. Clin Infect Dis 25(1):119–138

6. Wunderlich CA, Seguin E (1871) Medical Thermometry and Human Temperature. William Wood & Co., New York
7. Mackowiak PA, Wasserman SS, Levine MM (1992) A critical appraisal of 98.6 degrees F, the upper limit of the normal body temperature, and other legacies of Carl Reinhold August Wunderlich. JAMA 268(12):1578–1580
8. Hughes WT, Armstrong D, Bodey GP, Bow EJ, Brown AE, Calandra T et al (2002) 2002 guidelines for the use of antimicrobial agents in neutropenic patients with cancer. Clin Infect Dis 34(6):730–751
9. Link H, Bohme A, Cornely OA, Hoffken K, Kellner O, Kern WV et al (2003) Antimicrobial therapy of unexplained fever in neutropenic patients – guidelines of the Infectious Diseases Working Party (AGIHO) of the German Society of Hematology and Oncology (DGHO), Study Group Interventional Therapy of Unexplained Fever, Arbeitsgemeinschaft Supportivmassnahmen in der Onkologie (ASO) of the Deutsche Krebsgesellschaft (DKG-German Cancer Society). Ann Hematol 82(Suppl 2):S105–S117
10. Freifeld AG, Baden LR, Brown AE, Elting L, Gelfand M, Greene JN et al (2004) Fever and neutropenia. J Natl Compr Canc Netw 2(5):390–432
11. (2005) Guidelines for the use of antimicrobial agents in patients with febrile neutropenia in Taiwan. J Microbiol Immunol Infect 38(6):455–7.
12. Bodey GP, Rodriguez V, Chang HY, Narboni G (1978) Fever and infection in leukemic patients: A study of 494 consecutive patients. Cancer 41(4):1610–1622
13. Bodey GP, Buckley M, Sathe YS, Freireich EJ (1966) Quantitative relationships between circulating leukocytes and infection in patients with acute leukemia. Ann Intern Med 64(2):328–340
14. Schimpff SC (1995) Infections in the Cancer Patient. In: Mandell GL, Bennet JE, Dolin R (eds) Principles and Practice of Infectious Diseases, 4th edn. Churchill Livingston, New York, pp 2666–2675
15. Klastersky J, Paesmans M, Rubenstein EB, Boyer M, Elting L, Feld R et al (2000) The Multinational Association for Supportive Care in Cancer risk index: A multinational scoring system for identifying low-risk febrile neutropenic cancer patients. J Clin Oncol 18(16):3038–3051
16. Klastersky J, Paesmans M, Georgala A, Muanza F, Plehiers B, Dubreucq L et al (2006) Outpatient oral antibiotics for febrile neutropenic cancer patients using a score predictive for complications. J Clin Oncol 24(25):4129–4134
17. Uys A, Rapoport BL, Anderson R (2004) Febrile neutropenia: A prospective study to validate the Multinational Association of Supportive Care of Cancer (MASCC) risk-index score. Support Care Cancer 12(8):555–560
18. Peacock JE, Herrington DA, Wade JC, Lazarus HM, Reed MD, Sinclair JW et al (2002) Ciprofloxacin plus piperacillin compared with tobramycin plus piperacillin as empirical therapy in febrile neutropenic patients. A randomized, double-blind trial. Ann Intern Med 137(2):77–87
19. Bucaneve G, Micozzi A, Menichetti F, Martino P, Dionisi MS, Martinelli G et al (2005) Levofloxacin to prevent bacterial infection in patients with cancer and neutropenia. N Engl J Med 353(10):977–987
20. Rubenstein EB, Peterson DE, Schubert M, Keefe D, McGuire D, Epstein J et al (2004) Clinical practice guidelines for the prevention and treatment of cancer therapy-induced oral and gastrointestinal mucositis. Cancer 100(9 Suppl):2026–2046
21. Bochud P-Y, Eggiman P, Calandra T, Van Melle G, Saghafi L, Francioli P (1994) Bacteremia due to viridans streptococcus in neutropenic patients with cancer: Clinical spectrum and risk factors. Clin Infect Dis 18:25–31
22. Sonis ST, Oster G, Fuchs H, Bellm L, Bradford WZ, Edelsberg J et al (2001) Oral mucositis and the clinical and economic outcomes of hematopoietic stem-cell transplantation. J Clin Oncol 19(8):2201–2205
23. Centers for Disease Control and Prevention (2000) Guidelines for preventing opportunistic infections among hematopoietic stem cell transplant recipients. MMWR Recomm Rep 49(RR-10):1–7

24. Centers for Disease Control and Prevention (1997) Guidelines for Prevention of Nosocomial Pneumonia. MMWR Morb Mortal Wkly Rep 46:1–79
25. Dykewicz CA, Jaffe HA, Kaplan JE (2000) Guidelines for preventing opportunistic infections among hematopoietic stem cell transplant recipients. Biol Blood Marrow Transplant 6(6a):659–713
26. Dykewicz CA (2001) Hospital infection control in hematopoietic stem cell transplant recipients. Emerg Infect Dis 7(2):263–267
27. Dykewicz CA (2001) Summary of the Guidelines for Preventing Opportunistic Infections among Hematopoietic Stem Cell Transplant Recipients. Clin Infect Dis 33(2):139–144
28. Sehulster L, Chinn RY (2003) Guidelines for environmental infection control in health-care facilities. Recommendations of CDC and the Healthcare Infection Control Practices Advisory Committee (HICPAC). MMWR Recomm Rep 52(RR-10):1–42
29. Tablan OC, Anderson LJ, Besser R, Bridges C, Hajjeh R (2004) Guidelines for preventing health-care associated pneumonia, 2003: Recommendations of CDC and the Healthcare Infection Control Practices Advisory Committee. MMWR Recomm Rep 53(RR-3):1–36
30. Sullivan KM, Dykewicz CA, Longworth DL, Boeckh M, Baden LR, Rubin RH, et al. (2001) Preventing opportunistic infections after hematopoietic stem cell transplantation: The Centers for Disease Control and Prevention, Infectious Diseases Society of America, and American Society for Blood and Marrow Transplantation Practice Guidelines and beyond. Hematology Am Soc Hematol Educ Program 392–421.
31. Bow EJ (2003) Infectious complications in patients receiving cytotoxic therapy for acute leukemia: History, background and approaches to managment. In: Wingard JR, Bowden RA (eds) Management of Infection in Oncology Patients. Martin Dunitz, London, pp 71–104
32. Sasaki T, Akaho R, Sakamaki H, Akiyama H, Yoshino M, Hagiya K et al (2000) Mental disturbances during isolation in bone marrow transplant patients with leukemia. Bone Marrow Transplant 25(3):315–318
33. Hayes-Lattin B, Leis JF, Maziarz RT (2005) Isolation in the allogeneic transplant environment: How protective is it? Bone Marrow Transplant 36(5):373–381
34. Sherertz RJ, Belani A, Kramer BS, Elfenbein GJ, Weiner RS, Sullivan ML et al (1987) Impact of air filtration on nosocomial Aspergillus infections. Unique risk of bone marrow transplant recipients. Am J Med 83(4):709–718
35. Cornet M, Levy V, Fleury L, Lotholary J, Barquins S, Coureul M-H et al (1999) Efficacy of prevention by high-efficiency particulate air filtration or laminar airflow against Aspergillus airborne contamination during hospital renovation. Infect Control Hosp Epidemiol 20(7):508–513
36. Passweg JR, Rowlings PA, Atkinson KA, Barrett AJ, Gale RP, Gratwohl A et al (1998) Influence of protective isolation on outcome of allogeneic bone marrow transplantation for leukemia. Bone Marrow Transplant 21(12):1231–1238
37. Eckmanns T, Ruden H, Gastmeier P (2006) The influence of high-efficiency particulate air filtration on mortality and fungal infection among highly immunosuppressed patients: A systematic review. J Infect Dis 193(10):1408–1418
38. Raad I, Hanna H, Osting C, Hachem R, Umphrey J, Tarrand J et al (2002) Masking of neutropenic patients on transport from hospital rooms is associated with a decrease in nosocomial aspergillosis during construction. Infect Control Hosp Epidemiol 23(1):41–43
39. Trifilio S, Verma A, Mehta J (2004) Antimicrobial prophylaxis in hematopoietic stem cell transplant recipients: Heterogeneity of current clinical practice. Bone Marrow Transplant 33(7):735–739
40. Bucaneve G, Castagnola E, Viscoli C, Leibovici L, Menichetti F (2007) Quinolone prophylaxis for bacterial infections in afebrile high risk neutropenic patients. Eur J Cancer Suppl 5(2):5–12

41. Ziglam HM, Gelly KJ, Olver WJ (2005) A survey of the antibiotic treatment of febrile neutropenia in haematology units in the United Kingdom. Clin Lab Haematol 27(6):374–378
42. Rotstein C, Mandell L, Goldberg N (1997) Fluoroquinolone prophylaxis for profoundly neutropenic cancer patients: A meta-analysis. Curr Oncol 4(Suppl 2):S2–S7
43. Engels EA, Lau J, Barza M (1998) Efficacy of quinolone prophylaxis in neutropenic cancer patients: A meta-analysis. J Clin Oncol 16(3):1179–1187
44. Cruciani M, Rampazzo R, Malena M, Lazzarini L, Todeschini G, Messori A et al (1996) Prophylaxis with fluoroquinolones for bacterial infections in neutropenic patients: A meta-analysis. Clin Infect Dis 23(4):795–805
45. Cruciani M, Malena M, Bosco O, Nardi S, Serpelloni G, Mengoli C (2003) Reappraisal with meta-analysis of the addition of Gram-positive prophylaxis to fluoroquinolone in neutropenic patients. J Clin Oncol 21(22):4127–4137
46. Bow EJ (2004) Point: Fluoroquinolone-based antibacterial chemoprophylaxis in neutropenic cancer patients works for defined populations, but must be used wisely. J Natl Compr Canc Netw 2(5):433–444
47. van de Wetering MD, de Witte MA, Kremer LC, Offringa M, Scholten RJ, Caron HN (2005) Efficacy of oral prophylactic antibiotics in neutropenic afebrile oncology patients: A systematic review of randomised controlled trials3. Eur J Cancer 41(10):1372–1382
48. Gafter-Gvili A, Fraser A, Paul M, Leibovici L (2005) Meta-analysis: Antibiotic prophylaxis reduces mortality in neutropenic patients. Ann Intern Med 142(12 Pt 1):979–995
49. Gafter-Gvili A, Paul M, Fraser A, Leibovici L (2007) Effect of quinolone prophylaxis in afebrile neutropenic patients on microbial resistance: Systematic review and meta-analysis. J Antimicrob Chemother 59(1):5–22
50. Leibovici L, Paul M, Cullen M, Bucaneve G, Gafter-Gvili A, Fraser A et al (2006) Antibiotic prophylaxis in neutropenic patients: New evidence, practical decisions. Cancer 107(8):1743–1751
51. Timmer-Bonte JN, Tjan-Heijnen VC (2006) Febrile neutropenia: Highlighting the role of prophylactic antibiotics and granulocyte colony-stimulating factor during standard dose chemotherapy for solid tumors. Anticancer Drugs 17(8):881–889
52. Cullen MH, Billingham LJ, Gaunt CH, Steven NM (2007) Rational selection of patients for antibacterial prophylaxis after chemotherapy. J Clin Oncol 25(30):4821–4828
53. Cullen M, Steven N, Billingham L, Gaunt C, Hastings M, Simmonds P et al (2005) Antibacterial prophylaxis after chemotherapy for solid tumors and lymphomas. N Engl J Med 353(10):988–998
54. Kern WV, Beyer J, Bohme A, Buchheidt D, Cornely O, Einsele H et al (2000) Prophylaxis of infection in neutropenic patients. Guidelines of the Working Party on Infections in Hematology and Oncology. Dtsch Med Wochenschr 125(51–52):1582–1588
55. Yoshida M (2004) Guidelines for the management of deep mycosis in neutropenic patients. Nippon Ishinkin Gakkai Zasshi 45(4):209–215
56. Kruger WH, Bohlius J, Cornely OA, Einsele H, Hebart H, Massenkeil G et al (2005) Antimicrobial prophylaxis in allogeneic bone marrow transplantation. Guidelines of the infectious diseases working party (AGIHO) of the german society of haematology and oncology. Ann Oncol 16(8):1381–1390
57. Santolaya ME, Rabagliati R, Bidart T, Paya E, Guzman AM, Morales R et al (2005) Consensus: Rational approach towards the patient with cancer, fever and neutropenia. Rev Chilena Infectol 22(Suppl 2):S79–S113
58. Graubner UB, Boos J, Creutzig U, Dorffel W, Lakomek M, Niemeyer C et al (1999) Antiinfectious prophylaxis in pediatric oncology. Work group "Quality Assurance" of Society for Pediatric Oncology and Hematology (GPOH). Klin Padiatr 211(4):347–352

59. Tamura K (2005) Clinical guidelines for the management of neutropenic patients with unexplained fever in Japan: Validation by the Japan Febrile Neutropenia Study Group. Int J Antimicrob Agents 26(Suppl 2):S123–S127
60. Freifeld AG, Segal BH, Baden LR, Brown AE, Caspar C, deShazzo M, et al. (2007) Prevention and treatment of cancer-related infections. National Comprehensive Cancer Network – Clinical practice Guidelines in Oncology 2007 Available at: http://www.nccn.org/professionals/physician_gls/PDF/infections.pdf
61. Hughes WT, Kuhn S, Chaudhary S, Feldman S, Verzosa M, Aur RJ et al (1977) Successful chemoprophylaxis for Pneumocystis carinii pneumonitis. N Engl J Med 297(26):1419–1426
62. Enno A, Catovsky D, Darrell J, Goldman JM, Hows J, Galton DA (1978) Co-trimoxazole for prevention of infection in acute leukaemia. Lancet 2(8086): 395–397
63. Gurwith MJ, Brunton JL, Lank BA, Harding GKM, Ronald AR (1979) A prospective controlled investigation of prophylactic trimethoprim/sulfamethoxazole in hospitalized granulocytopenic patients. Am J Med 66:248–256
64. Crawford J, Dale DC, Lyman GH (2004) Chemotherapy-induced neutropenia: Risks, consequences, and new directions for its management. Cancer 100(2):228–237
65. Kern WV (2001) Risk assessment and risk-based therapeutic strategies in febrile neutropenia. Curr Opin Infect Dis 14(4):415–422
66. Kern WV (2006) Risk assessment and treatment of low-risk patients with febrile neutropenia. Clin Infect Dis 42(4):533–540
67. Aapro MS, Cameron DA, Pettengell R, Bohlius J, Crawford J, Ellis M et al (2006) EORTC guidelines for the use of granulocyte-colony stimulating factor to reduce the incidence of chemotherapy-induced febrile neutropenia in adult patients with lymphomas and solid tumours. Eur J Cancer 42(15):2433–2453
68. Kleinberg M (2004) Counterpoint: Routine anti-bacterial prophylaxis is not indicated in neutropenic patients with hematological maligancies. J Natl Compr Canc Netw 2(5):445–451
69. Pena C, Albareda JM, Pallares R, Pujol M, Tubau F, Ariza J (1995) Relationship between quinolone use and emergence of ciprofloxacin-resistant Escherichia coli in bloodstream infections. Antimicrob Agents Chemother 39(2):520–524
70. Cometta A, Calandra T, Bille J, Glauser MP (1994) Escherichia coli resistant to fluoroquinolones in patients with cancer and neutropenia. N Engl J Med 330(17):1240–1241
71. Kern WV, Andriof E, Oethinger M, Kern P, Hacker J, Marre R (1994) Emergence of fluoroquinolone-resistant Escherichia coli at a cancer center. Antimicrob Agents Chemother 38(4):681–687
72. Baum HV, Franz U, Geiss HK (2000) Prevalence of ciprofloxacin-resistant Escherichia coli in hematologic-oncologic patients. Infection 28(5):278–281
73. Razonable RR, Litzow MR, Khaliq Y, Piper KE, Rouse MS, Patel R (2002) Bacteremia due to viridans group Streptococci with diminished susceptibility to Levofloxacin among neutropenic patients receiving levofloxacin prophylaxis. Clin Infect Dis 34(11):1469–1474
74. Carratala J, Fernandez-Sevilla A, Tubau F, Callis M, Gudiol F (1995) Emergence of quinolone-resistant Escherichia coli bacteremia in neutropenic patients with cancer who have received prophylactic norfloxacin. Clin Infect Dis 20(3):557–560
75. Reuter S, Kern WV, Sigge A, Dohner H, Marre R, Kern P et al (2005) Impact of fluoroquinolone prophylaxis on reduced infection-related mortality among patients with neutropenia and hematologic malignancies. Clin Infect Dis 40(8):1087–1093
76. Delarive P, Baumgartner JD, Glauser MP, Cometta A (2000) Evaluation of antibiotic prophylaxis in neutropenic patients with hematologic malignancies. Schweiz Med Wochenschr 130(48):1837–1844

77. Lyman GH, Morrison VA, Dale DC, Crawford J, Delgado DJ, Fridman M (2003) Risk of febrile neutropenia among patients with intermediate-grade non-Hodgkin's lymphoma receiving CHOP chemotherapy. Leuk Lymphoma 44(12):2069–2076
78. Baden LR (2005) Prophylactic antimicrobial agents and the importance of fitness. N Engl J Med 353(10):1052–1054
79. Tjan-Heijnen VC, Postmus PE, Ardizzoni A, Manegold CH, Burghouts J, van Meerbeeck J et al (2001) Reduction of chemotherapy-induced febrile leucopenia by prophylactic use of ciprofloxacin and roxithromycin in small-cell lung cancer patients: An EORTC double-blind placebo-controlled phase III study. Ann Oncol 12(10):1359–1368
80. Timmer-Bonte JN, de Boo TM, Smit HJ, Biesma B, Wilschut FA, Cheragwandi SA et al (2005) Prevention of chemotherapy-induced febrile neutropenia by prophylactic antibiotics plus or minus granulocyte colony-stimulating factor in small-cell lung cancer: A Dutch Randomized Phase III Study. J Clin Oncol 23(31): 7974–7984
81. Timmer-Bonte JN, Adang EM, Smit HJ, Biesma B, Wilschut FA, Bootsma GP et al (2006) Cost-effectiveness of adding granulocyte colony-stimulating factor to primary prophylaxis with antibiotics in small-cell lung cancer. J Clin Oncol 24(19):2991–2997
82. Schroeder M, Schadeck-Gressel C, Selbach J, Westerhausen M (1992) Antibiotic prophylaxis with gyrase inhibitors during cytostatically induced granulocytopenias in patients with solid tumors: A double-blind prospective randomized study. Onkologie 15:476–479
83. Carlson JW, Fowler JM, Mitchell SK, Carson LF, Mayer AR, Copeland LJ (1997) Chemoprophylaxis with ciprofloxacin in ovarian cancer patients receiving paclitaxel: A randomized trial. Gynecol Oncol 65(2):325–329
84. Vidal L, Paul M, Ben Dor I, Soares-Weiser K, Leibovici L (2004) Oral versus intravenous antibiotic treatment for febrile neutropenia in cancer patients: A systematic review and meta-analysis of randomized trials. J Antimicrob Chemother 54(1):29–37
85. Chrischilles EA, Link BK, Scott SD, Delgado DJ, Fridman M (2003) Factors associated with early termination of CHOP therapy and the impact on survival among patients with chemosensitive intermediate-grade non-Hodgkin's lymphoma. Cancer Control 10(5):396–403
86. Lyman GH, Kuderer NM, Djulbegovic B (2002) Prophylactic granulocyte colony-stimulating factor in patients receiving dose-intensive cancer chemotherapy: A meta-analysis. Am J Med 112(5):406–411
87. Sung L, Nathan PC, Lange B, Beyene J, Buchanan GR (2004) Prophylactic granulocyte colony-stimulating factor and granulocyte-macrophage colony stimulating factor decrease febrile neutropenia after chemotherapy in children with cancer: A meta-analysis of randomized controlled trials. J Clin Oncol 22(16):3350–3356
88. Lyman GH, Kuderer NM (2004) The economics of the colony-stimulating factors in the prevention and treatment of febrile neutropenia. Crit Rev Oncol Hematol 50(2):129–146
89. Bohlius J, Reiser M, Schwarzer G, Engert A. (2004) Granulopoiesis-stimulating factors to prevent adverse effects in the treatment of malignant lymphoma. Cochrane Database Syst Rev (1):CD003189.
90. Wittman B, Horan J, Lyman GH (2006) Prophylactic colony-stimulating factors in children receiving myelosuppressive chemotherapy: A meta-analysis of randomized controlled trials. Cancer Treat Rev 32(4):289–303
91. Dekker A, Bulley S, Beyene J, Dupuis LL, Doyle JJ, Sung L (2006) Meta-analysis of randomized controlled trials of prophylactic granulocyte colony-stimulating factor and granulocyte-macrophage colony-stimulating factor after autologous and allogeneic stem cell transplantation. J Clin Oncol 24(33):5207–5215

92. Smith TJ, Khatcheressian J, Lyman GH, Ozer H, Armitage JO, Balducci L et al (2006) 2006 update of recommendations for the use of white blood cell growth factors: An evidence-based clinical practice guideline. J Clin Oncol 24(19): 3187–3205
93. Thatcher N, Girling DJ, Hopwood P, Sambrook RJ, Qian W, Stephens RJ (2000) Improving survival without reducing quality of life in small-cell lung cancer patients by increasing the dose-intensity of chemotherapy with granulocyte colony-stimulating factor support: Results of a British Medical Research Council Multicenter Randomized Trial. Medical Research Council Lung Cancer Working Party. J Clin Oncol 18(2):395–404
94. Citron ML, Berry DA, Cirrincione C, Hudis C, Winer EP, Gradishar WJ et al (2003) Randomized trial of dose-dense versus conventionally scheduled and sequential versus concurrent combination chemotherapy as postoperative adjuvant treatment of node-positive primary breast cancer: First report of Intergroup Trial C9741/Cancer and Leukemia Group B Trial 9741. J Clin Oncol 21(8):1431–1439
95. McQuaker IG, Hunter AE, Pacey S, Haynes AP, Iqbal A, Russell NH (1997) Low-dose filgrastim significantly enhances neutrophil recovery following autologous peripheral-blood stem-cell transplantation in patients with lymphoproliferative disorders: Evidence for clinical and economic benefit. J Clin Oncol 15(2):451–457
96. Stinson TJ, Adams JR, Bishop MR, Kruse S, Tarantolo S, Bennet CL (2000) Economic analysis of a phase III study of G-CSF vs placebo following allogeneic blood stem cell transplantation. Bone Marrow Transplant 26(6):663–666
97. Ringden O, Labopin M, Gorin NC, Le BK, Rocha V, Gluckman E et al (2004) Treatment with granulocyte colony-stimulating factor after allogeneic bone marrow transplantation for acute leukemia increases the risk of graft-versus-host disease and death: A study from the Acute Leukemia Working Party of the European Group for Blood and Marrow Transplantation. J Clin Oncol 22(3):416–423
98. Harousseau JL, Witz B, Lioure B, Hunault-Berger M, Desablens B, Delain M et al (2000) Granulocyte colony-stimulating factor after intensive consolidation chemotherapy in acute myeloid leukemia: Results of a randomized trial of the Groupe Ouest-Est Leucemies Aigues Myeloblastiques. J Clin Oncol 18(4):780–787
99. Heil G, Hoelzer D, Sanz MA, Lechner K, Liu Yin JA, Papa G et al (1997) A randomized, double-blind, placebo-controlled, phase III study of filgrastim in remission induction and consolidation therapy for adults with de novo acute myeloid leukemia. The International Acute Myeloid Leukemia Study Group. Blood 90(12):4710–4718
100. Chamilos G, Luna M, Lewis RE, Bodey GP, Chemaly R, Tarrand JJ et al (2006) Invasive fungal infections in patients with hematologic malignancies in a tertiary care cancer center: An autopsy study over a 15-year period (1989–2003). Haematologica 91(7):986–989
101. Pagano L, Girmenia C, Mele L, Ricci P, Tosti ME, Nosari A et al (2001) Infections caused by filamentous fungi in patients with hematologic malignancies. A report of 391 cases by GIMEMA Infection Program. Haematologica 86(8):862–870
102. Pagano L, Caira M, Candoni A, Offidani M, Fianchi L, Martino B et al (2006) The epidemiology of fungal infections in patients with hematologic malignancies: The SEIFEM-2004 study. Haematologica 91(8):1068–1075
103. Pagano L, Caira M, Picardi M, Candoni A, Melillo L, Fianchi L et al (2007) Invasive Aspergillosis in patients with acute leukemia: Update on morbidity and mortality – SEIFEM-C Report. Clin Infect Dis 44(11):1524–1525
104. Marr KA, Carter RA, Boeckh M, Martin P, Corey L (2002) Invasive aspergillosis in allogeneic stem cell transplant recipients: Changes in epidemiology and risk factors. Blood 100(13):4358–4366

105. Marr KA, Carter RA, Crippa F, Wald A, Corey L (2002) Epidemiology and outcome of mould infections in hematopoietic stem cell transplant recipients. Clin Infect Dis 34(7):909–917
106. Pagano L, Caira M, Nosari A, Van Lint MT, Candoni A, Offidani M et al (2007) Fungal infections in recipients of hematopoietic stem cell transplants: Results of the SEIFEM B-2004 study – Sorveglianza Epidemiologica Infezioni Fungine Nelle Emopatie Maligne. Clin Infect Dis 45(9):1161–1170
107. Bow EJ, Laverdiere M, Lussier N, Rotstein C, Cheang MS, Ioannou S (2002) Antifungal prophylaxis for severely neutropenic chemotherapy recipients: A meta analysis of randomized-controlled clinical trials. Cancer 94(12):3230–3246
108. Robenshtok E, Gafter-Gvili A, Goldberg E, Weinberger M, Yeshurun M, Leibovici L et al (2007) Antifungal prophylaxis in cancer patients after chemotherapy or hematopoietic stem-cell transplantation: Systematic review and meta-analysis. J Clin Oncol 25(34):5471–5489
109. Jantunen E, Ruutu P, Niskanen L, Volin L, Parkkali T, Koukila-Kahkola P et al (1997) Incidence and risk factors for invasive fungal infections in allogeneic BMT recipients. Bone Marrow Transplant 19(8):801–808
110. Gotzsche PC, Johansen HK. (2002) Nystatin prophylaxis and treatment in severely immunodepressed patients. Cochrane Database Syst Rev (2):CD002033.
111. Gotzsche PC, Johansen HK (1997) Meta-analysis of prophylactic or empirical antifungal treatment versus placebo or no treatment in patients with cancer com plicated by neutropenia. BMJ 314(7089):1238–1244
112. Kanda Y, Yamamoto R, Chizuka A, Hamaki T, Suguro M, Arai C et al (2000) Prophylactic action of oral fluconazole against infection in neutropenic patients - a meta-analysis of 16 randomized, controlled trials. Cancer 89:1611–1625
113. Glasmacher A, Prentice A, Gorschluter M, Engelhart S, Hahn C, Djulbegovic B et al (2003) Itraconazole prevents invasive fungal infections in neutropenic patients treated for hematologic malignancies: Evidence from a meta-analysis of 3, 597 patients. J Clin Oncol 21(24):4615–4626
114. Glasmacher A, Prentice AG (2005) Evidence-based review of antifungal prophylaxis in neutropenic patients with haematological malignancies. J Antimicrob Chemother 56(Suppl 1):i23–i32
115. Vardakas KZ, Michalopoulos A, Falagas ME (2005) Fluconazole versus itraconazole for antifungal prophylaxis in neutropenic patients with haematological malignancies: A meta-analysis of randomised-controlled trials. Br J Haematol 131(1):22–28
116. Cornely OA, Ullmann AJ, Karthaus M (2003) Evidence-based assessment of primary antifungal prophylaxis in patients with hematologic malignancies. Blood 101(9):3365–3372
117. Marr KA, Seidel K, Slavin MA, Bowden RA, Schoch HG, Flowers MED et al (2000) Prolonged fluconazole prophylaxis is associated with persistent protection against candidiasis-related death in allogeneic marrow transplant recipients: Long-term follow-up of a randomized, placebo-controlled trial. Blood 96(6):2055–2061
118. Rotstein C, Bow EJ, Laverdiere M, Ioannou S, Carr D, Moghaddam N (1999) Randomized placebo-controlled trial of fluconazole prophylaxis for neutropenic cancer patients: Benefit based on purpose and intensity of cytotoxic therapy. The Canadian Fluconazole Prophylaxis Study Group. Clin Infect Dis 28(2):331–340
119. Cornely OA, Maertens J, Winston DJ, Perfect J, Ullmann AJ, Walsh TJ et al (2007) Posaconazole vs. fluconazole or itraconazole prophylaxis in patients with neutropenia. N Engl J Med 356(4):348–359
120. Ullmann AJ, Lipton JH, Vesole DH, Chandrasekar P, Langston A, Tarantolo SR et al (2007) Posaconazole or fluconazole for prophylaxis in severe graft-versus-host disease. N Engl J Med 356(4):335–347

121. Herbrecht R, Denning DW, Patterson TF, Bennett JE, Greene RE, Oestmann JW et al (2002) Voriconazole versus amphotericin B for primary therapy of invasive aspergillosis. N Engl J Med 347(6):408–415
122. Herbrecht R, Fluckiger U, Gachot B, Ribaud P, Thiebaut A, Cordonnier C (2007) Treatment of invasive Candida and invasive Aspergillus infections in adult haematological patients. Eur J Cancer Suppl 5(2):49–59
123. Walsh TJ, Pappas P, Winston DJ, Lazarus HM, Petersen F, Raffalli J et al (2002) Voriconazole compared with liposomal amphotericin B for empirical antifungal therapy in patients with neutropenia and persistent fever. N Engl J Med 346(4):225–234
124. Vehreschild JJ, Bohme A, Buchheidt D, Arenz D, Harnischmacher U, Heussel CP et al (2007) A double-blind trial on prophylactic voriconazole (VRC) or placebo during induction chemotherapy for acute myelogenous leukaemia (AML). J Infect 55(5):445–449
125. Wingard JR, Carter CL, Walsh TJ, Kurtzberg J, Small TN, Gersten ID et al (2007) Results of a Randomized, Double-Blind Trial of Fluconazole (FLU) vs. Voriconazole (VORI) for the Prevention of Invasive Fungal Infections (IFI) in 600 Allogeneic Blood and Marrow Transplant (BMT) Patients (Abstract #163). Blood 110(11):55a
126. van Burik JA, Ratanatharathorn V, Stepan DE, Miller CB, Lipton JH, Vesole DH et al (2004) Micafungin versus fluconazole for prophylaxis against invasive fungal infections during neutropenia in patients undergoing hematopoietic stem cell transplantation. Clin Infect Dis 39(10):1407–1416
127. Mattiuzzi GN, Alvarado G, Giles FJ, Ostrosky-Zeichner L, Cortes J, O'Brien S et al (2006) Open-Label, Randomized Comparison of Itraconazole versus Caspofungin for Prophylaxis in Patients with Hematologic Malignancies. Antimicrob Agents Chemother 50(1):143–147
128. Walsh TJ, Teppler H, Donowitz GR, Maertens JA, Baden LR, Dmoszynska A et al (2004) Caspofungin versus liposomal amphotericin B for empirical antifungal therapy in patients with persistent fever and neutropenia. N Engl J Med 351(14):1391–1402
129. Maertens JA, Frere P, Lass-Florl C, Heinz W, Cornely OA (2007) Primary antifungal prophylaxis in leukaemia patients. Eur J Cancer Suppl 5(2):43–48
130. Cornely OA, Bohme A, Buchheidt D, Glasmacher A, Kahl C, Karthaus M et al (2003) Prophylaxis of invasive fungal infections in patients with hematological malignancies and solid tumors – guidelines of the Infectious Diseases Working Party (AGIHO) of the German Society of Hematology and Oncology (DGHO). Ann Hematol 82(Suppl 2):S186–S200
131. Sandherr M, Einsele H, Hebart H, Kahl C, Kern W, Kiehl M et al (2006) Antiviral prophylaxis in patients with haematological malignancies and solid tumours: Guidelines of the Infectious Diseases Working Party (AGIHO) of the German Society for Hematology and Oncology (DGHO). Ann Oncol 17(7):1051–1059
132. Hicks KL, Chemaly RF, Kontoyiannis DP (2003) Common community respiratory viruses in patients with cancer: More than just "common colds". Cancer 97(10):2576–2587
133. British Society for Antimicrobial Chemotherapy Working Party on Antiviral Therapy (2000) Management of herpes virus infections following transplantation. J Antimicrob Chemother 45(6):729–748
134. Wade JC. (2006) Viral infections in patients with hematological malignancies. Hematology Am Soc Hematol Educ Program 368–74.
135. Sonis ST, Elting LS, Keefe D, Peterson DE, Schubert M, Hauer-Jensen M et al (2004) Perspectives on cancer therapy-induced mucosal injury: Pathogenesis, measurement, epidemiology, and consequences for patients. Cancer 100(9 Suppl):1995–2025
136. Redding SW. (1990) Role of herpes simplex virus reactivation in chemotherapy-induced oral mucositis. NCI Monogr (9):103–5.

137. Seto BG, Kim M, Wolinsky L, Mito RS, Champlin R (1985) Oral mucositis in patients undergoing bone marrow transplantation. Oral Surg Oral Med Oral Pathol 60(5):493–497
138. Rand KH, Kramer B, Johnson AC (1982) Cancer chemotherapy associated symptomatic stomatitis: Role of Herpes simplex virus (HSV). Cancer 50(7): 1262–1265
139. Montgomery MT, Redding SW, LeMaistre CF (1986) The incidence of oral herpes simplex virus infection in patients undergoing cancer chemotherapy. Oral Surg Oral Med Oral Pathol 61(3):238–242
140. Woo SB, Sonis ST, Sonis AL (1990) The role of herpes simplex virus in the development of oral mucositis in bone marrow transplant recipients. Cancer 66(11):2375–2379
141. Wade JC, Newton B, Flournoy N, Meyers JD (1984) Oral acyclovir for prevention of herpes simplex virus reactivation after marrow transplantation. Ann Intern Med 100(6):823–828
142. Saral R, Burns WH, Laskin OL, Santos GW, Lietman PS (1981) Acyclovir prophylaxis of herpes-simplex-virus infections. N Engl J Med 305(2):63–67
143. Gluckman E, Lotsberg J, Devergie A, Zhao XM, Melo R, Gomez-Morales M et al (1983) Oral acyclovir prophylactic treatment of herpes simplex infection after bone marrow transplantation. J Antimicrob Chemother 12(Suppl B): 161–167
144. Wade JC, Newton B, McLaren C, Flournoy N, Keeney RE, Meyers JD (1982) Intravenous acyclovir to treat mucocutaneous herpes simplex virus infection after marrow transplantation: A double-blind trial. Ann Intern Med 96(3):265–269
145. Redding SW, Montgomery MT (1989) Acyclovir prophylaxis for oral herpes simplex virus infection in patients with bone marrow transplants. Oral Surg Oral Med Oral Pathol 67(6):680–683
146. Anderson H, Scarffe JH, Sutton RN, Hickmott E, Brigden D, Burke C (1984) Oral acyclovir prophylaxis against herpes simplex virus in non-Hodgkin lymphoma and acute lymphoblastic leukaemia patients receiving remission induction chemotherapy. A randomised double blind, placebo controlled trial. Br J Cancer 50(1):45–49
147. Bergmann OJ, Ellermann-Eriksen S, Mogensen SC, Ellegaard J (1995) Acyclovir given as prophylaxis against oral ulcers in acute myeloid leukaemia: Randomised, double blind, placebo controlled trial. BMJ 310(6988):1169–1172
148. Bergmann OJ, Mogensen SC, Ellermann-Eriksen S, Ellegaard J (1997) Acyclovir prophylaxis and fever during remission-induction therapy of patients with acute myeloid leukemia: A randomized, double-blind, placebo-controlled trial. J Clin Oncol 15(6):2269–2274
149. Hann IM, Prentice HG, Blacklock HA, Ross MGR, Brigden D, Rosling AE et al (1983) Acyclovir prophylaxis against herpes simplex virus infections in severely immunocompromised patients: A randomised double blind trial. Br Med J 287:384–388
150. Moltzan C, Bow EJ, Loewen R, Freed B (1996) Acyclovir prophylaxis against herpes simplex mucositis in elderly patients receiving induction therapy for untreated acute myeloid leukemia. Blood 88(Suppl):82a Abstract #316
151. Lonnqvist B, Palmblad J, Ljungman P, Grimfors G, Jarnmark M, Lerner R et al (1993) Oral acyclovir as prophylaxis for bacterial infections during induction therapy for acute leukaemia in adults. The Leukemia Group of Middle Sweden. Support Care Cancer 1(3):139–144
152. Locksley RM, Flournoy N, Sullivan KM, Meyers JD (1985) Infection with varicella-zoster virus after marrow transplantation. J Infect Dis 152(6):1172–1181
153. Koc Y, Miller KB, Schenkein DP, Griffith J, Akhtar M, DesJardin J et al (2000) Varicella zoster virus infections following allogeneic bone marrow transplantation: Frequency, risk factors, and clinical outcome. Biol Blood Marrow Transplant 6(1):44–49

154. Han CS, Miller W, Haake R, Weisdorf D (1994) Varicella zoster infection after bone marrow transplantation: Incidence, risk factors and complications. Bone Marrow Transplant 13(3):277–283
155. Tomonari A, Iseki T, Takahashi S, Ooi J, Takasugi K, Shimohakamada Y et al (2003) Varicella-zoster virus infection in adult patients after unrelated cord blood transplantation: A single institute experience in Japan. Br J Haematol 122(5):802–805
156. Leung TF, Chik KW, Li CK, Lai H, Shing MM, Chan PK et al (2000) Incidence, risk factors and outcome of varicella-zoster virus infection in children after haematopoietic stem cell transplantation. Bone Marrow Transplant 25(2):167–172
157. Arvin AM (2000) Varicella-Zoster virus: Pathogenesis, immunity, and clinical management in hematopoietic cell transplant recipients. Biol Blood Marrow Transplant 6(3):219–230
158. Berman JN, Wang M, Berry W, Neuberg DS, Guinan EC (2006) Herpes zoster infection in the post-hematopoietic stem cell transplant pediatric population may be preceded by transaminitis: An institutional experience. Bone Marrow Transplant 37(1):73–80
159. Boeckh M, Kim HW, Flowers ME, Meyers JD, Bowden RA (2006) Long-term acyclovir for prevention of varicella zoster virus disease after allogeneic hematopoietic cell transplantation – a randomized double-blind placebo-controlled study. Blood 107(5):1800–1805
160. (2000) Guidelines for preventing opportunistic infections among hematopoietic stem cell transplant recipients. Biol Blood Marrow Transplant 6(6a):659–713.
161. Chan PK, Peiris JS, Yuen KY, Liang RH, Lau YL, Chen FE et al (1997) Human herpesvirus-6 and human herpesvirus-7 infections in bone marrow transplant recipients. J Med Virol 53(3):295–305
162. Michalek J, Horvath R, Benedik J, Hrstkova H (1999) Human herpesvirus-6 infection in children with cancer. Pediatr Hematol Oncol 16(5):423–430
163. Persson L, Dahl H, Linde A, Engervall P, Vikerfors T, Tidefelt U (2003) Human cytomegalovirus, human herpesvirus-6 and human herpesvirus-7 in neutropenic patients with fever of unknown origin. Clin Microbiol Infect 9(7):640–644
164. Ruutu T, Ljungman P, Brinch L, Lenhoff S, Lonnqvist B, Ringden O et al (1997) No prevention of cytomegalovirus infection by anticytomegalovirus hyperimmune globulin in seronegative bone marrow transplant recipients. The Nordic BMT Group. Bone Marrow Transplant 19(3):233–236
165. Ljungman P, De La CR, Milpied N, Volin L, Russell CA, Crisp A et al (2002) Randomized study of valacyclovir as prophylaxis against cytomegalovirus reactivation in recipients of allogeneic bone marrow transplants. Blood 99(8):3050–3056
166. Goodrich JM, Bowden RA, Fisher L, Keller C, Schoch G, Meyers JD (1993) Ganciclovir prophylaxis to prevent cytomegalovirus disease after allogeneic marrow transplant. Ann Intern Med 118(3):173–178
167. Ng AP, Worth L, Chen L, Seymour JF, Prince HM, Slavin M et al (2005) Cytomegalovirus DNAemia and disease: Incidence, natural history and management in settings other than allogeneic stem cell transplantation. Haematologica 90(12):1672–1679
168. Kim JG, Sohn SK, Chae YS, Cho YY, Yang DH, Lee JJ et al (2007) Alemtuzumab plus CHOP as front-line chemotherapy for patients with peripheral T-cell lymphomas: A phase II study. Cancer Chemother Pharmacol 60(1):129–134
169. van Esser JW, Niesters HG, van der Holt B, Meijer E, Osterhaus AD, Gratama JW et al (2002) Prevention of Epstein-Barr virus-lymphoproliferative disease by molecular monitoring and preemptive rituximab in high-risk patients after allogeneic stem cell transplantation. Blood 99(12):4364–4369
170. Whimbey E, Englund JA, Couch RB (1996) Community respiratory virus infections in immunocompromised patients with cancer. Am J Med 102(3A):10–18

171. Whimbey E, Champlin RE, Couch RB, Englund JA, Goodrich JM, Raad I et al (1996) Community respiratory virus infections among hospitalized adult bone marrow transplant recipients. Clin Infect Dis 22(5):778–782
172. Hohenthal U, Nikoskelainen J, Vainionpaa R, Peltonen R, Routamaa M, Itala M et al (2001) Parainfluenza virus type 3 infections in a hematology unit. Bone Marrow Transplant 27(3):295–300
173. Ebbert JO, Limper AH (2005) Respiratory syncytial virus pneumonitis in immunocompromised adults: Clinical features and outcome. Respiration 72(3):263–269
174. Whitley RJ, Monto AS (2006) Prevention and treatment of influenza in high-risk groups: Children, pregnant women, immunocompromised hosts, and nursing home residents. J Infect Dis 194(Suppl 2):S133–S138
175. (1997) Immunization of health-care workers: recommendations of the Advisory Committee on Immunization Practices (ACIP) and the Hospital Infection Control Practices Advisory Committee (HICPAC). MMWR Recomm Rep 46(RR-18): 1–42.
176. (1996) Prevention and control of influenza: Recommendations of the Advisory Committee on Immunization Practices (ACIP). Centers for Disease Control and Prevention. MMWR Recomm Rep 45(RR-5):1–24.
177. Chemaly RF, Ghosh S, Bodey GP, Rohatgi N, Safdar A, Keating MJ et al (2006) Respiratory viral infections in adults with hematologic malignancies and human stem cell transplantation recipients: A retrospective study at a major cancer center. Medicine (Baltimore) 85(5):278–287
178. Fiore AE, Shay DK, Haber P, Iskander JK, Uyeki TM, Mootrey G et al (2007) Prevention and control of influenza. Recommendations of the Advisory Committee on Immunization Practices (ACIP), 2007. MMWR Recomm Rep 56(RR-6):1–54
179. Hsieh YC, Lu MY, Kao CL, Chiang BL, Lin DT, Lin KS et al (2002) Response to influenza vaccine in children with leukemia undergoing chemotherapy. J Formos Med Assoc 101(10):700–704
180. Rapezzi D, Sticchi L, Racchi O, Mangerini R, Ferraris AM, Gaetani GF (2003) Influenza vaccine in chronic lymphoproliferative disorders and multiple myeloma. Eur J Haematol 70(4):225–230
181. Porter CC, Edwards KM, Zhu Y, Frangoul H (2004) Immune responses to influenza immunization in children receiving maintenance chemotherapy for acute lymphoblastic leukemia. Pediatr Blood Cancer 42(1):36–40
182. Lyles A (2007) Influenza chemoprophylaxis: The relative utility of number needed to treat and cost-effectiveness analyses. Clin Ther 29(8):1577–1578
183. Laforce C, Man CY, Henderson FW, McElhaney JE, Hampel FC Jr, Bettis R et al (2007) Efficacy and Safety of Inhaled Zanamivir in the Prevention of Influenza in Community-Dwelling, High-Risk Adult and Adolescent Subjects: A 28-day, Multicenter, Randomized, Double-Blind, Placebo-Controlled Trial. Clin Ther 29(8):1579–1590
184. Wilde JA, McMillan JA, Serwint J, Butta J, O'Riordan MA, Steinhoff MC (1999) Effectiveness of influenza vaccine in health care professionals: A randomized trial. JAMA 281(10):908–913
185. Carman WF, Elder AG, Wallace LA, McAulay K, Walker A, Murray GD et al (2000) Effects of influenza vaccination of health care workers on mortality of elderly people in long-term care: A randomised controlled trial. Lancet 355(9198):93–97
186. Potter J, Stott DJ, Roberts MA, Elder AG, O'Donnell B, Knight PV et al (1997) Influenza vaccination of health care workers in long-term-care hospitals reduces the mortality of elderly patients. J Infect Dis 175(1):1–6
187. Harper SA, Fukuda K, Uyeki TM, Cox NJ, Bridges CB (2005) Prevention and control of influenza. Recommendations of the Advisory Committee on Immunization Practices (ACIP). MMWR Recomm Rep 54(RR-8):1–40

188. Nichols WG, Gooley T, Boeckh M (2001) Community-acquired respiratory syncytial virus and parainfluenza virus infections after hematopoietic stem cell transplantation: The Fred Hutchinson Cancer Research Center experience. Biol Blood Marrow Transplant 7(Suppl):11S–15S
189. Firkin FC, Nicholls K, Whelan G (1978) Transient myeloid and erythroid aplasia associated with infectious hepatitis. Br Med J 2(6151):1534
190. Cooper CL, Al-Bedwawi S, Lee C, Garber G (2006) Rate of infectious complications during interferon-based therapy for hepatitis C is not related to neutropenia. Clin Infect Dis 42(12):1674–1678
191. Zhou J, Stohlman SA, Hinton DR, Marten NW (2003) Neutrophils promote mononuclear cell infiltration during viral-induced encephalitis. J Immunol 170(6):3331–3336
192. Fiore AE, Wasley A, Bell BP (2006) Prevention of hepatitis A through active or passive immunization: Recommendations of the Advisory Committee on Immunization Practices (ACIP). MMWR Recomm Rep 55(RR-7):1–23
193. Victor JC, Monto AS, Surdina TY, Suleimenova SZ, Vaughan G, Nainan OV et al (2007) Hepatitis A vaccine versus immune globulin for postexposure prophylaxis. N Engl J Med 357(17):1685–1694
194. Betz TG (2008) Hepatitis A vaccine versus immune globulin for postexposure prophylaxis. N Engl J Med 358(5):531
195. Wands JR, Chura CM, Roll FJ, Maddrey WC (1975) Serial studies of hepatitis-associated antigen and antibody in patients receiving antitumor chemotherapy for myeloproliferative and lymphoproliferative disorders. Gastroenterology 68(1):105–112
196. Rossi G, Pelizzari A, Motta M, Puoti M (2001) Primary prophylaxis with lamivudine of hepatitis B virus reactivation in chronic HbsAg carriers with lymphoid malignancies treated with chemotherapy. Br J Haematol 115(1):58–62
197. Firpi RJ, Nelson DR (2006) Viral Hepatitis: Manifestations and Management Strategy. Hematology 2006(1):375–380
198. Yeo W, Chan PK, Ho WM, Zee B, Lam KC, Lei KI et al (2004) Lamivudine for the prevention of hepatitis B virus reactivation in hepatitis B s-antigen seropositive cancer patients undergoing cytotoxic chemotherapy. J Clin Oncol 22(5): 927–934
199. Liang R, Lau GK, Kwong YL (1999) Chemotherapy and bone marrow transplantation for cancer patients who are also chronic hepatitis B carriers: A review of the problem. J Clin Oncol 17(1):394–398
200. Knoll A, Boehm S, Hahn J, Holler E, Jilg W (2004) Reactivation of resolved hepatitis B virus infection after allogeneic haematopoietic stem cell transplantation. Bone Marrow Transplant 33(9):925–929
201. Xunrong L, Yan AW, Liang R, Lau GK (2001) Hepatitis B virus (HBV) reactivation after cytotoxic or immunosuppressive therapy – pathogenesis and management. Rev Med Virol 11(5):287–299
202. Lok AS, Liang RH, Chiu EK, Wong KL, Chan TK, Todd D (1991) Reactivation of hepatitis B virus replication in patients receiving cytotoxic therapy. Report of a prospective study. Gastroenterology 100(1):182–188
203. Yeo W, Chan PK, Zhong S, Ho WM, Steinberg JL, Tam JS et al (2000) Frequency of hepatitis B virus reactivation in cancer patients undergoing cytotoxic chemotherapy: A prospective study of 626 patients with identification of risk factors. J Med Virol 62(3):299–307
204. Yeo W, Johnson PJ (2006) Diagnosis, prevention and management of hepatitis B virus reactivation during anticancer therapy. Hepatology 43(2):209–220
205. Zhong S, Yeo W, Schroder C, Chan PK, Wong WL, Ho WM et al (2004) High hepatitis B virus (HBV) DNA viral load is an important risk factor for HBV reactivation in breast cancer patients undergoing cytotoxic chemotherapy. J Viral Hepat 11(1):55–59

206. Sagnelli E, Manzillo G, Maio G, Pasquale G, Felaco FM, Filippini P et al (1980) Serum levels of hepatitis B surface and core antigens during immunosuppressive treatment of HBsAg-positive chronic active hepatitis. Lancet 2(8191):395–397
207. Scullard GH, Smith CI, Merigan TC, Robinson WS, Gregory PB (1981) Effects of immunosuppressive therapy on viral markers in chronic active hepatitis B. Gastroenterology 81(6):987–991
208. Lam KC, Lai CL, Trepo C, Wu PC (1981) Deleterious effect of prednisolone in HBsAg-positive chronic active hepatitis. N Engl J Med 304(7):380–386
209. Hoofnagle JH, Davis GL, Pappas SC, Hanson RG, Peters M, Avigan MI et al (1986) A short course of prednisolone in chronic type B hepatitis. Report of a randomized, double-blind, placebo-controlled trial. Ann Intern Med 104(1):12–17
210. Lee SD, Tong MJ, Wu JC, Lin HC, Tsai YT, Lo KJ (1991) A randomised double-blind placebo-controlled trial of prednisolone therapy in HBeAg and HBV DNA positive Chinese patients with chronic active hepatitis B. J Hepatol 12(2): 246–250
211. Cheng AL, Hsiung CA, Su IJ, Chen PJ, Chang MC, Tsao CJ et al (2003) Steroid-free chemotherapy decreases risk of hepatitis B virus (HBV) reactivation in HBV-carriers with lymphoma. Hepatology 37(6):1320–1328
212. Leaw SJ, Yen CJ, Huang WT, Chen TY, Su WC, Tsao CJ (2004) Preemptive use of interferon or lamivudine for hepatitis B reactivation in patients with aggressive lymphoma receiving chemotherapy. Ann Hematol 83(5):270–275
213. Dai MS, Chao TY (2005) Lamivudine therapy in HBsAg-carrying breast cancer patients undergoing chemotherapy: Prophylactic or preemptive? Breast Cancer Res Treat 92(1):95–96
214. Hui CK, Cheung WW, Au WY, Lie AK, Zhang HY, Yueng YH et al (2005) Hepatitis B reactivation after withdrawal of pre-emptive lamivudine in patients with haematological malignancy on completion of cytotoxic chemotherapy. Gut 54(11):1597–1603
215. Idilman R, Arat M, Soydan E, Toruner M, Soykan I, Akbulut H et al (2004) Lamivudine prophylaxis for prevention of chemotherapy-induced hepatitis B virus reactivation in hepatitis B virus carriers with malignancies. J Viral Hepat 11(2):141–147
216. Nagamatsu H, Itano S, Nagaoka S, Akiyoshi J, Matsugaki S, Kurogi J et al (2004) Prophylactic lamivudine administration prevents exacerbation of liver damage in HBe antigen positive patients with hepatocellular carcinoma undergoing transhepatic arterial infusion chemotherapy. Am J Gastroenterol 99(12):2369–2375
217. Lau GK, Yiu HH, Fong DY, Cheng HC, Au WY, Lai LS et al (2003) Early is superior to deferred preemptive lamivudine therapy for hepatitis B patients undergoing chemotherapy. Gastroenterology 125(6):1742–1749
218. Mindikoglu AL, Regev A, Schiff ER (2006) Hepatitis B virus reactivation after cytotoxic chemotherapy: The disease and its prevention. Clin Gastroenterol Hepatol 4(9):1076–1081
219. Zuckerman E, Zuckerman T, Levine AM, Douer D, Gutekunst K, Mizokami M et al (1997) Hepatitis C virus infection in patients with B-cell non-Hodgkin lymphoma. Ann Intern Med 127(6):423–428
220. Charlton M, Seaberg E, Wiesner R, Everhart J, Zetterman R, Lake J et al (1998) Predictors of patient and graft survival following liver transplantation for hepatitis C. Hepatology 28(3):823–830
221. Yates JW, Holland JF (1973) A controlled study of isolation and endogenous microbial suppression in acute myelocytic leukemia patients. Cancer 32(6): 1490–1498
222. Levine AS, Siegel SE, Schreiber AD, Hauser J, Preisler H, Goldstein IM et al (1973) Protected environments and prophylactic antibiotics. A prospective controlled study of their utility in acute leukemia. N Engl J Med 288(10):477–487

223. Schimpff SC, Greene WH, Young VM, Fortner CL, Jepsen L, Cusack N et al (1975) Infection prevention in acute nonlymphocytic leukemia - laminar air flow room reverse isolation with oral nonabsorbable antibiotic prophylaxis. Ann Intern Med 82(3):351–358
224. Dietrich M, Gaus W, Vossen J, van der Waaij D, Wendt F, EORTC International Antimicrobial Therapy Cooperative Project Group (1977) Protective isolation and antimicrobial decontamination in patients with high susceptibility to infection: A prospective cooperative study of gnotobiotic care in acute leukemia patients. 1. Clinical results. Infection 5:107–114
225. Rodriguez V, Bodey GP, Freireich EJ, McCredie KB, Gutterman JU, Keating MJ et al (1978) Randomized trial of protected environment-prophylactic antibiotics in 145 adults with acute leukemia. Medicine 57(3):253–266
226. Schimpff SC, Hahn DM, Brouillet MD, Young VM, Fortner CL, Wiernik PH (1978) Comparison of basic infection prevention techniques, with standard room reverse isolation or with reverse isolation plus added air filtration. Leuk Res 2(3):231–240
227. Buckner CD, Clift RA, Sanders JE, Meyers JD, Counts GW, Farewell VT et al (1978) Protective environment for marrow transplant recipients - a prospective study. Ann Intern Med 89:893–901
228. Lohner D, Debusscher L, Prévost JM, Klastersky J (1979) Comparative randomized study of protected environment plus oral antibiotics versus oral antibiotics alone in neutropenic patients. Cancer Treatment Reports 63:363–368
229. Nauseef WM, Maki DG (1981) A study of the value of simple protective isolation in patients with granulocytopenia. N Engl J Med 304(8):448–453
230. Ribas-Mundo M, Granena A, Rozman C (1981) Evaluation of a protective environment in the management of granulocytopenic patients: A comparative study. Cancer 48:419–424
231. Navari RM, Buckner CD, Clift RA, Storb R, Sanders JE, Stewart P et al (1984) Prophylaxis of infection in patients with aplastic anemia receiving allogeneic marrow transplants. Am J Med 76(4):564–572
232. Valdivieso M, Cabanillas F, Keating M, Barkley HT, Murphy WK, Burgess MA et al (1984) Effects of intensive induction chemotherapy for extensive-disease small cell bronchogenic carcinoma in protected environment-prophylactic antibiotic units. Am J Med 76:405–412
233. Centers for Disease Control and Prevention (2006) Recommended Adult Immunization Schedule - United States, October 2006-September 2007. MMWR Morb Mortal Wkly Rep Quickguide 55(40):Q1–Q4
234. Holmberg LA, Boeckh M, Hooper H, Leisenring W, Rowley S, Heimfeld S et al (1999) Increased incidence of cytomegalovirus disease after autologous CD34-selected peripheral blood stem cell transplantation. Blood 94(12):4029–4035

Chapter 11

Infection Control and Prevention

Kerri Thom and Mary-Claire Roghmann

Abstract Cancer center patients are frequently immune suppressed and are, therefore, at risk for a wide range of opportunistic pathogens in addition to common nosocomial pathogens that are a problem for patients throughout the hospital. A good infection control program is extremely important in this setting to reduce the risks of community- and hospital-acquired infections among patients. In addition to protecting patients, it is also important to protect health care workers, other employees, and visitors. This chapter focuses on general infection control measures, as well as infection control measures specific to patients, health care workers, and visitors in the cancer center setting. In addition, we discuss infection control measures directed at specific nosocomial infections that are of particular risk in this population. Finally, guidelines and examples for starting an infection control program will be given. The role for antimicrobial prophylaxis in infection prevention is discussed in chapter 10.

Keywords Infection control • Prevention • Hand hygiene • Bacterial resistance • Patient isolation • Health care worker immunizations • Pregnant health care worker • Quality assurance

1. General Infection Control Measures

1.1. Hand Hygiene

Proper hand hygiene is a critical step in preventing nosocomial infection. Everyone, especially health care workers (HCW), should be trained to perform hand hygiene before and after entering the room of an immunocompromised patient, even if they used gloves or did not touch the patient. In addition, it is also important to repeat hand hygiene after examining different contaminated body sites, for example, after changing a dressing. Hand hygiene will not be effective in the presence of artificial nails or natural nails longer than 1/4 in. On the basis of the 2003 Hand Hygiene Guidelines [1], most health care facilities have restricted the wearing of artificial nails to workers without direct patient contact.

From: *Managing Infections in Patients With Hematological Malignancies*: Contemporary Hematology, Edited by: M. Kleinberg, DOI 10.1007/978-1-59745-415-5_11,

Hand hygiene can be performed by "handwashing" with or without water. Alcohol-based hand rubs, containing 60–95% ethanol or isopropanolol, have superior antimicrobial activity over handwashing with plain soap and water. In addition, alcohol-based hand rubs are less drying to the skin [1] and importantly are faster to use than plain soap and water [2]. Thus, alcohol-based hand rubs are the preferred method for the routine decontamination of the hands. Handwashing with soap and water is recommended if the hands are visibly dirty or soiled. Alcohol has poor activity against bacterial spores, protozoan oocysts, and certain nonenveloped viruses such as Norwalk virus. Therefore, after leaving the room of a patient with diarrhea, HCWs should wash hands with soap and water.

Access to hand hygiene facilities (i.e., sinks or alcohol-based hand rub dispensers) can impact compliance with hand washing [1]. Sinks should be easily accessible and remain free of clutter to encourage proper hand hygiene. Placement of dispensers for alcohol-based hand rubs does not require plumbing and, therefore, is more flexible than sink placement. Dispensers should be placed in convenient, easy to access locations such as adjacent to the patient's bed or at the entrance to the room. Individual pocket-sized containers for alcohol-based hand rubs carried by HCWs may also improve compliance. Care should be taken to ensure that all dispensers remain full and are functioning properly.

1.2. Isolation Precautions

Standard Precautions are infection control precautions, in addition to hand hygiene, to be used for all patients regardless of their diagnoses. Standard Precautions are a combination of Universal Precautions and Body Substance Isolation [3]. HCWs should wear gloves for anticipated contact with blood or any body fluid contaminated with blood, urine, saliva, or non-intact skin of patients. HCWs should wear gowns, and don masks with a face shield and/or goggles for situations in which splashes of these bodily fluids could occur.

Transmission based precautions are for patients with specific conditions or syndromes suspicious for specific conditions. There are three major types: Contact Precautions, Droplet Precautions, and Airborne Precautions.

- Contact Precautions are used for patients who are infected or colonized with pathogens transmitted by physical contact either directly (patient-to-patient) or indirectly (patient-to-fomite-to-health care worker). HCWs must wear gloves and a gown to enter the room and dispose of both upon exiting. Disposable or dedicated equipment (e.g., stethoscopes, thermometers, and blood pressure cuffs) should be used whenever possible. Patients on Contact Precautions should be placed in a single room or cohorted with other patients infected or colonized with the same transmissible pathogens.
- Droplet Precautions are used for patients infected or colonized with pathogens such as influenza where large respiratory droplets are the dominant route of transmission. HCWs should don a surgical mask before entering the room and dispose of upon exiting. Patients on Droplet Precautions should also be placed in a single room or cohorted with other patients infected or colonized with the same organism. Patients on Droplet Precautions should be restricted to their rooms except for necessary procedures and tests.
- Airborne Precautions are used to prevent spread of pathogens such as tuberculosis where small respiratory droplets/particles are the dominant

route of transmission. Surgical-style masks are not sufficient to prevent inhalation of these small respiratory droplets/particles. Therefore, respiratory protection of HCWs should be more stringent, requiring the use of approved respiratory protection on entering the room wearing a powered air purifying respirator or a fit-tested N95 face mask. The N95 masks filter >95% of small respiratory droplets/particles and require individualized fitting of masks as mandated by OSHA regulations. Patients on Airborne Precautions must be placed in single rooms, known as Airborne Infection Isolation Rooms (AIIR), with special air-handling requirements where the patient's room air pressure is negative relative to the hallway. In addition, these rooms must have 6–12 air exchanges per hour and which are exhausted outside the building. Patients on Airborne Precautions should be restricted to their rooms except for necessary procedures.

Patients on any of the above isolation precautions should have movements outside their rooms limited whenever possible. When patient transport is necessary, care should be taken to minimize opportunities for transmission of pathogens. Patients should wear appropriate barriers (gowns and gloves for Contact Precautions or a surgical mask for Droplet and Airborne Precautions) when outside their rooms. HCWs and patients should be educated regarding the risk of potential transmission, as well as ways to prevent transmission of the infectious pathogen to others. When patients are transported to other areas of the hospital, receiving personnel should be aware of the patient's isolation status, and the above recommendations should be followed.

1.3. Shared Equipment/Devices and Common Areas

Standard Precautions require that all reusable patient care equipment is adequately cleaned between each patient use [3]. For patients placed under Contact Precautions, patient care equipment should be restricted to the use of a single patient whenever possible. If the use of shared equipment is unavoidable, then it should be thoroughly disinfected by EPA-registered disinfectants such as alcohols, sodium hypochlorites, quaternary ammonium compounds, phenolics, and iodophors before use with another patient [3, 4].

Common areas, particularly pediatric play areas, should be kept clean [5]. These areas should be cleaned and disinfected at least once per week. Any shared toys, including videos and electronic equipment, should be disinfected prior to placement on the unit and at least weekly thereafter and as often as needed. Cloth or plush toys can be cleaned in a washing machine using the hot cycle. Hard toys can be cleaned in a dishwasher on the hot cycle or scrubbed and disinfected by hand. Nontoxic disinfectants registered by the Food and Drug Administration or the Environmental Protection Agency are recommended.

2. Rules for Health Care Workers and Visitors

2.1. Immunizations

HCWs are at the unique risk of both exposure to and transmission of many infectious diseases, including vaccine preventable diseases. The U.S. Public Health Service's Advisory Committee on Immunization Practices (ACIP) recommends that any health care facility involved in direct patient care develop an immunization policy for HCWs [6]. A lengthy discussion regarding all ACIP recommended vaccinations is beyond the scope of this chapter. For specific recommendations regarding vaccinations and vaccine schedules in HCWs, please refer to the CDC Guideline for Infection Control in Health Care Personnel [6]. Based on nosocomial transmission rates and vaccine availability, the ACIP strongly recommends vaccination for the following infections: hepatitis B, influenza, measles, mumps, rubella, varicella, and pertussis [7]. The Tdap, or combined tetanus, diphtheria, and pertussis, vaccine is now recommended instead of the Td (tetanus-diphtheria) booster for adults [7]. In general, those persons born before 1957 are considered immune to measles and rubella. However, given the potential risk of infection and transmission in the health care setting, the ACIP recommends that all HCWs should be vaccinated with the Measles-Mumps-Rubella (MMR) vaccine or have documented immunity.

The use of live-attenuated vaccines in persons who care for or are in close contact with immunocompromised patients deserves special mention due to the theoretical risk of transmission of the vaccine strain pathogens. The vaccine strain polio virus in oral polio vaccine is known to have the potential for person-to-person transmission and is absolutely contraindicated in HCWs, family members, and friends who may be caring for immunocompromised patients [8]. In the U.S., however, live-attenuated polio vaccine is rarely indicated and has largely been replaced by the inactivated polio vaccine. On the opposite spectrum, there is no evidence that the live-attenuated vaccine strain viruses in the MMR vaccine are transmitted from person-to-person and this vaccine is generally considered safe for all immunocompetent HCWs [9].

Of particular interest in the cancer center is the risk of transmission of vaccine virus due to the live-attenuated influenza and varicella vaccines. The live-attenuated influenza vaccine (LAIV) has been shown to shed vaccine virus at very low levels for some time after administration and person-to-person transmission of the vaccine strain virus is theoretically possible [10, 11]. On the basis of this information, the CDC does not recommend the use of the LAIV in any persons who may have close contact with "severely" immunosuppressed patients (i.e., patients who have recently had a bone marrow transplant and require a protected environment). The vaccine, however, can be used for HCWs who do not have contact with the severely immunosuppressed populations. Cancer centers within larger health care systems should be aware of their system's policy on use of LAIV and instruct cancer center HCWs, who work with bone marrow and stem cell recipients, to avoid LAIV and receive the killed influenza vaccine instead. Although theoretically possible, no cases of person-to-person transmission of LAIV have been documented, and at this time no recommendations exist to exclude LAIV in populations other than HCWs who have close contact with "severely" immunosuppressed patients. Transmission of varicella-vaccine virus has been documented but is thought to be a rare occurrence [12]. Recommendations state that any HCW who develops a rash, which cannot be covered, within the first 42 days of receiving the varicella vaccine should avoid any contact with immunosuppressed patients [6]. Contact should be avoided until the rash has crusted over.

2.2. Transmissible Diseases

Leukemia patients and hematopoietic stem cell recipients often have prolonged hospitalizations. They may have a large number of visitors both in hospital and at home while still profoundly immunosuppressed. All visitors should be instructed on basic infection prevention including hand hygiene techniques and isolation procedures. In the hospital, a system should be established whereby all visitors can be screened for potential transmissible diseases [5]. The CDC recommends that any visitor with an upper respiratory tract infection, a flu-like illness, a herpes zoster rash (whether it is covered or not), or recent known exposure to any transmittable disease should not be allowed access to the unit or at least should be restricted from visiting severely immunosuppressed patients [5]. Likewise, visitors should be asked about recent vaccinations. Any visitor with a recent history of receiving the oral polio vaccine or those who develop a rash within 6 weeks or receiving the live-attenuated varicella zoster virus (VZV) vaccination should also be restricted [8, 12]. Any HCW with a disease transmitted by air, droplet, or direct contact should be restricted from direct patient contact [5]. Details regarding specific infections will be covered in Sect. III – Specific Transmissible Diseases.

3. Patient Measures

3.1. Device Associated Infections

Intravascular catheters are common throughout the hospital and catheter related infections contribute to significant morbidity and mortality. Because of the unique needs of cancer patients, intravascular catheters are used more often and for longer durations compared with other hospitalized patients. As such, these patients are at increased risk for catheter related complications such as insertion site infection, septic thrombophlebitis, blood stream infection, endocarditis, and disseminated infections. Catheter related bloodstream infections (CR-BSI), in particular, are feared complications due to their high incidences and associated morbidity and mortality. A total of 250,000 cases of CR-BSI are estimated to occur annually [13]. Blood stream infections represent approximately 15% of all nosocomial infections [14] and lead to adverse patient outcomes, such as increased mortality, prolonged hospital course and increased heath care costs [15–20]. Weinstock et al. evaluated CR-BSI in cancer patients at their institution and found an incidence of 7.31 per 1,000 catheter days [21].

Catheter related infections are more common with the use of non-tunneled central venous catheters (CVC). More permanent, tunneled catheters are thought to have a decreased risk of infectious complications (Table 11-1). These catheters, however, are not without risk. Rotstein et al. showed an incidence of Hickman-catheter related blood stream infections of 3.05 per 1,000 catheter days in cancer patients [22].

The best way to prevent catheter related complications is to minimize the use of intravascular catheters. In many cases, this is not a feasible option and the use of catheters, particularly non-tunneled CVCs, should be reassessed on a regular basis, and they should be removed when no longer needed.

3.1.1. Site of Insertion for Non-tunneled Catheters

The preferred site for non-tunneled catheter insertion in adults is the subclavian vein [13]. Studies suggest that catheters inserted into the internal jugular and femoral veins are associated with a higher risk for infection than those

Table 11-1. Catheter types and infection risk (adapted from Guidelines for the Prevention of Intravascular Catheter-Related Infections [78]).

Catheter type	Entry site	Comments
Non-tunneled CVC	Percutaneously inserted into central veins	Account for majority of CR-BSI
Peripherally inserted central venous catheters (PICC)	Inserted into cephalic or brachial veins and enter the subclavian vein	Lower rate of infection than non-tunneled CVC
Tunneled CVC (such as Hickman catheters, PICC)	Implanted into brachial, subclavian, internal jugular or femoral veins	Lower rate of infection than non-tunneled CVC
Totally implantable (such as Mediports)	Tunneled beneath the skin, with subcutaneous port accessed with a needle; implanted in subclavian or internal jugular vein	Lowest risk of CR-BSI; no need for local catheter site care; surgery required for catheter removal

CVC central venous catheter, *CR-BSI* catheter-related bloodstream infection

inserted into a subclavian vein [23–25]. When choosing a site for catheter insertions, factors other than risk of infection should be considered, such as patient comfort, safety, and the risk for mechanical complications. The femoral site is known to have a greater risk of deep vein thrombosis and generally should be avoided in adults [13, 24].

3.1.2. Sterile Techniques

The use of maximal sterile precautions (cap, mask, sterile gown, sterile glove, and large sterile drape) during insertion has been shown to reduce the incidence of CR-BSI compared with the use of sterile gloves and small drapes alone [23, 26]. Although no studies exist, the use of maximal sterile precautions is extended to the insertion of PICC lines and other tunneled catheters [13]. Disinfection of the skin at the site of insertion with 2% aqueous chlorhexidine gluconate is recommended over 10% povidone-iodine or 70% alcohol [27].

3.1.3. Site Care

The use of either sterile gauze or transparent semipermeable dressing to cover the catheter site is accepted [13]. These dressings should be changed at least weekly and possibly more frequently depending on the circumstances. The skin at the catheter site should be disinfected with an antiseptic containing 2% chlorhexidine at the time of dressing change. Catheters should not be submerged underwater and precautions (such as the use of an impermeable cover) should be taken when bathing and showering. Vancomycin-based antibiotic lock prophylaxis has been shown to reduce the rate of CR-BSI with vancomycin susceptible organisms. However, this practice is recommended only for selected patients because of the increased risk of acquisition of vancomycin-resistant enterococci (VRE) [13].

3.1.4. Antimicrobial Impregnated Non-tunneled Catheters

Although more expensive, antimicrobial impregnated non-tunneled catheters may decrease both the cost and risk of CR-BSI [28]. Several randomized controlled trials have demonstrated a decrease in microbial colonization of the catheter with the use of either antiseptic (chlorhexidine/silver-sulfadiazine) or antibiotic (minocycline/rifampin) impregnated catheters when compared with non-coated catheters [29–33]. Despite this, a reduction of CR-BSI has not been demonstrated consistently. Two recent meta-analyses, however, do show a decrease in CR-BSI with the use of antimicrobial impregnated catheters and cite inadequate power of the individual trials to evaluate the true differences in incidence rates of CR-BSI. Veenstra et al. found antiseptic-impregnated catheters to be effective in reducing both catheter colonization and CR-BSI in high risk patients with short-term CVC [34]. In a separate meta-analysis by Walder et al. and others, both antiseptic and antibiotic-impregnated catheters were compared with non-coated catheters; and both were effective in reducing colonization and CR-BSIs when compared with non-coated catheters [35]. Darouiche et al. compared antiseptic and antibiotic-impregnated catheters head with head and showed that the catheters coated with minocycline/rifampin were less likely to become colonized or complicated by CR-BSI than antiseptic coated catheters [36]. Catheters impregnated with platinum and silver remain under investigation. At this time, there are no published data to suggest platinum and silver have an antimicrobial effect [13]. Importantly, these trials have only shown benefit for short-term use of non-tunneled CVCs. Currently, antimicrobial impregnated catheters are not available for tunneled CVCs.

3.2. Hygiene

Proper hygiene is important in preventing infection in any person and especially those patients with prolonged neutropenia. Daily showers or baths, with mild soap, are recommended. Complete skin inspection should be done on a daily basis. Particular attention should be given to sites of possible infection, such as intravascular catheter sites and the perineum. Perineal care should be gentle but thorough. Female patients should clean the area from the front to the back to prevent contamination of the urethra. Experts recommend avoiding digital rectal examinations and the use of rectal thermometers, enemas, and suppositories during periods of neutropenia in order to prevent mucosal breakdown which may lead to infection [5].

Since the oral cavity is an important source of potentially pathogenic bacteria, stringent periodontal health is important. A complete periodontal examination followed by necessary treatment is recommended before management of head and neck cancers, high dose chemotherapy, hematopoietic stem cell transplants, and any cancer regimen that is expected to lead to significant myelosuppression [5]. Routine oral hygiene is also important to minimize infections and may improve healing of mucositis. Oral rinses with sterile water or normal saline are recommended 4–6 times per day. Patients should brush their teeth at least twice daily with a soft, regular toothbrush.

3.3. Low Microbial Diet

The Center for Disease Control and Prevention recommends a low microbial diet for hematopoietic stem cell transplant recipients [5]. There are no specific guidelines for the use of a low microbial diet in cancer center patients who do not receive stem cell transplants; however, many centers will prescribe one for patients with hematologic malignancies during periods of neutropenia.

Theoretically, reducing exposure to bacteria in foods such as unpasteurized cheeses, raw fruits, and vegetables and undercooked meats during periods of neutropenia may decrease the incidence of infection. However, to date, there is no scientific evidence to suggest the effectiveness of low microbial diets in any patient population.

4. Specific Nosocomial Infections

4.1. Conjunctivitis

Conjunctivitis describes any inflammatory condition of the conjunctiva and is most commonly due to bacterial or viral infections. Adenovirus has been identified as the primary cause of nosocomial conjunctivitis. The typical incubation period ranges from 5 to 12 days and viral shedding may continue for 14 days after the onset of disease. Transmission occurs via contaminated hands and fomites. Routine handwashing and glove use, as well as disinfection of contaminated equipment, may prevent spread. Health care personnel and visitors with infectious conjunctivitis should be restricted from direct patient contact until drainage resolves [5].

4.2. Respiratory Syndromes

4.2.1. Acute Respiratory Disease: Community Respiratory Viruses

Infection with common community respiratory viruses can lead to serious disease and significant morbidity and mortality among patients with cancer, especially allogeneic stem cell recipients. Given the potential adverse outcomes and the relative ease of spread of infection, nosocomial transmission is a serious concern. Significant effort to prevent and control the spread of these infections should be made.

Acute, viral respiratory infections are most commonly due to respiratory syncytial virus (RSV), influenza viruses, rhinoviruses, parainfluenza viruses, and adenoviruses [37]. In healthy adults, infection with these organisms typically leads to the "common cold" or acute upper respiratory tract infection. Immunosuppressed patients may present with typical upper respiratory tract disease or atypical lower tract disease. Studies suggest that more than half of cancer patients (bone marrow transplant recipients and leukemia patients) infected with these viruses progress to viral pneumonia with a mortality rate of greater than 50% [37]. The highest risk of morbidity and mortality has been described with RSV and influenza viruses. Because of limited effective treatments, prevention is essential in control of infection with these organisms.

An effective infection control strategy against community respiratory viruses includes the following: vaccination (for influenza); surveillance for community outbreaks; surveillance for nosocomial transmission and hospital outbreaks; patient and personnel education regarding disease recognition and modes of transmission; rapid diagnosis and early isolation for suspected and confirmed cases; and finally restriction of potentially infected visitors and HCWs from the cancer center (CDC Website).

Annual inactivated influenza vaccination is currently recommended by the CDC for all patients with chronic medical diseases, including persons with cancer, HSCT recipients, and otherwise immunosuppressed patients [11]. All health care personnel should be vaccinated yearly. Vaccination is also recommended for close contacts of immunosuppressed patients, including HCWs and house-hold contacts [11]. In these instances, the use of LAIV should be avoided if possible. If LAIV is administered to these persons, they should avoid contact with "severely" immunosuppressed patients (recent HSCT recipients) for 7 days [11]. Currently, there are no licensed vaccines against RSV, parainfluenza viruses or adenoviruses.

Infection with the common respiratory viruses in cancer patients tends to reflect disease activity in the community [37]. As such community surveillance through a local health department is an important infection control tool to alert cancer center staff of the possibility of infection in their patients. A useful resource is found at the CDC website (http://www.cdc.gov/flu/weekly/usmap.htm), which provides weekly updates of influenza activity by geographic region. Once patients are admitted to the hospital, nosocomial surveillance is necessary to identify cases or outbreaks and interrupt transmission.

Prompt diagnosis and implementation of appropriate infection control measures are essential to the prevention and control of nosocomial spread. Whenever possible, all patients who present with acute respiratory symptoms, including rhinorrhea, nasal congestion, pharyngitis, cough and fever, during winter months should be placed on both Contact and Droplet Precautions until a diagnosis is made. If a particular etiology is determined, isolation precautions can be geared to each specific virus (Table 11-2). Despite these guidelines, some experts believe that Droplet Precautions should be combined with Contact Precautions for most respiratory viruses due to the potential of hand to mucous membrane transmission.

During the winter months (RSV and influenza season), visitors and health care personnel should be screened specifically for signs and symptoms of acute viral respiratory infection. No specific recommendations exist for the best method of screening. Examples of screening methods include the use of posted signs to alert visitors with signs or symptoms of respiratory disease not to visit patients or a questionnaire to gauge current symptoms [3]. To minimize the risk of transmission, persons with viral symptoms should be restricted

Table 11.2. Community respiratory viruses: modes of transmission and isolation requirements.

Virus	Seasonality	Mode of transmission	Isolation precautions[h]
Respiratory syncytial virus	Winter	Close contact[a] Large droplets Fomites/hands	Contact
Influenza virus	Winter	Small aerosols[b,c] Large droplets Fomites/hands	Droplet
Parainfluenza virus	Year-round	Close contact[d,e] Large droplet	Contact

[a]Falsey AR, Walsh EE (2000) Clin Microbiol Rev 13:371–384
[b]Hayden FG (1997) Am J Med 102:55–60
[c]Small aerosols are more common
[d]Henrickson KJ. Human parainfluenza viruses. In Gorbach SL, Bartlett JG, Blacklow NR (eds) Infectious Diseases, 3rd ed
[e]Little is know regarding transmission of parvovirus; data based on RSV
[f]Horwitz MS. Adenoviruses. In Knipe DM and Howley PM (eds) Fields Virology, 4th ed
[g]Sporadic cases via close contact, epidemic cases via aerosols
[h]Garner, HICPAC Isolation Guidelines

from the cancer center and any contact with immunosuppressed patients [5]. Specifically, the CDC recommends restriction of HCWs with acute respiratory syndromes from the care of immunosuppressed patients during community outbreaks of RSV and Influenza [6].

4.2.2. Legionella Pneumonia

Legionella pneumophila should be considered in the differential diagnosis of both community acquired and hospital acquired pneumonias, especially in high risk immunocompromised patients. Diagnosis is typically made by respiratory culture or detection of *Legionella* antigen in the urine. The use of culture to detect Legionella requires selective media, and the clinical laboratory should be alerted when this is considered in the differential diagnosis. The urinary antigen test detects only serotype 1, the most common serotype in community acquired *Legionella* pneumonia. When investigating nosocomial outbreaks, the urinary antigen test will not be useful for serotypes other than serotype 1. Transmission occurs through inhalation of infected aerosols in the environment, or potentially, from drinking water. Hospital acquired transmission is often linked to an environmental source, most commonly water supplies, and therefore a single case may represent a potential outbreak. The incubation period of Legionnaires' disease is estimated to be between 2 and 10 days [38]. Therefore, patients who develop Legionnaires' disease after being hospitalized for 10 consecutive days are considered to have definite nosocomial *Legionella* infection. Those who develop disease between 2 and 9 days are considered to have possible nosocomial *Legionella* infection. In the case of either definite or possible Legionnaires' disease, infection control should be contacted and a thorough epidemiologic investigation should be undertaken [39]. In addition, *Legionella* is a reportable disease in most states.

Stem cell transplant recipients in particular are at increased risk for disease and mortality due to *Legionella* infections compared to other patients. Many centers have decided to perform periodic surveillance cultures for *Legionella* from water samples to identify risk of nosocomial transmission of hospital water supplies. The cost-effectiveness of this strategy has not been determined, and methodologies such as frequency of surveillance are unknown. As a result, the CDC does not provide specific recommendations at this time. If *Legionella* is detected from water supplies, either as a result of routine surveillance or during the course of a potential outbreak investigation, the water supply should be decontaminated and measures should be taken to protect patients. Showers and faucets contaminated with *Legionella* should not be used to prevent generation of aerosols. Patients should receive sponge baths with non-contaminated water instead of showering. Sterile water should be used for drinking, brushing teeth, flushing nasogastric tubes, and rinsing or cleaning respiratory equipment including nebulizers.

4.2.3. Fungal Pneumonia

Invasive pulmonary aspergillosis and other fungal pneumonias are a serious concern, particularly in those patients with prolonged neutropenia or hematopoietic stem cell transplant recipients [40, 41]. The rate of invasive pulmonary infections has increased over the last several decades, and the mortality rate remains high [42–44]. *Aspergillus* species are ubiquitous in the environment, and infection occurs through inhalation of conidia in the air. These properties make it difficult to distinguish between community acquired and nosocomial transmission.

The Center for Disease Control (CDC) and Prevention recommends active surveillance of microbiologic, histological, and post mortem data to identify cases and potential trends [39]. Infection control should be notified when *Aspergillus* species are cultured from a respiratory tract source (i.e., sputum or bronchial cultures). When there is an increase in positive clinical cultures above the baseline detected from routine surveillance, an epidemiologic investigation should be done to determine and eliminate the source [39].

High-efficiency particulate air (HEPA) filters have been used to maintain ultraclean air in areas where patients may be at high risk for aspergillosis. Studies have reported a decrease in *Aspergillus* conidia counts from 2 to 15 colony forming units per cubic meter to approximately 0.01 cfu/mm^3 [45, 46]. HEPA filtration has been shown to decrease nosocomial infection with *Aspergillus* in stem cell transplant recipients by 19%, and the CDC currently recommends them for all HSCT patients [39, 46]. HEPA filtration also been shown to decrease nosocomial infection during outbreak situations in patients with hematologic malignancies; however, there is not enough information at this time for the CDC to make an official recommendation in these patients in the endemic setting [39, 47]. For HSCT recipients, rooms should also have directed air flow and positive air pressure relative to the corridor, be properly ventilated (≥12 air changes per hour), be well sealed, and be designed to minimize dust (i.e., avoid carpets and upholstery) in addition to HEPA filtration [3].

Several *Aspergillus* outbreaks have been linked to hospital construction or renovation [48]. A hospital plan should be made during all times of construction to prevent *Aspergillus* exposures, including the construction of an impermeable barrier between the construction and patient care areas [39].

Aspergillus species have been isolated from both dried and fresh flowers as well as potted plants. Although exposure to flowers and plants has not been directly linked to fungal pneumonia, there remains a theoretical risk of transmission following exposure. As a result, HSCT recipients should not be exposed to these items [5].

4.2.4. Mycobacterium tuberculosis

Transmission of *Mycobacterium tuberculosis* (MTB) in the health care setting poses a significant risk to both patients and HCWs. An increase in nosocomial outbreaks of MTB in the mid-1980s highlighted the need for a heightened awareness of disease (especially in immunocompromised patients) and stringent infection control practices [49, 50]. An intact cellular immune response is essential in the control of active MTB infection [51]. Impairments in cellular immunity may increase the likelihood of infection after exposure and the risk for developing active disease once infected [52, 53]. Cancer has long been considered a risk factor for MTB infection, but in recent years, the potential risk in patients with cancer is thought to be increasing [54, 55]. This concern for risk is due to the development and increased use of specific chemotherapeutics, which alter cellular immunity (purine analogs, anti-lymphocyte monoclonal antibodies and corticosteroids), increased number of stem cell transplant recipients, and an increase in foreign-born patients seeking care in the US [55]. According to a recent report, MTB infection in foreign-born persons accounts for more than one-half of all US cases, with prevalence and incidence varying by birth country [56]. Researchers at Memorial Sloan Kettering Cancer Center recently found similar results in their patient population [55].

The Advisory Council for the Elimination of Tuberculosis recommends screening for latent MTB infection based on risk [54]. Among the cancer center population, persons considered at risk include those with hematologic malignancies (leukemias and lymphomas), carcinoma of the head and neck and conditions requiring prolonged high dose corticosteroid therapy (>15 mg/day Prednisone equivalent for >1 month), and other immunosuppressive therapy (including bone marrow transplant recipients). Screening consists of a complete history and physical and tuberculin skin testing (TST). In this risk group, a positive reaction is considered to be an induration of 10 mm or more at the injection site [54]. Patients with a current or past history of a positive TST or those with recent exposure to active, infectious cases (pulmonary or laryngeal) or other strong epidemiological evidence of TB infection (i.e., raised in country with high TB prevalence) should be treated for latent tuberculosis with a 9 month course of isoniazid [54].

Diagnosis of active MTB infection is sometimes difficult, especially in immunosuppressed patients who may have atypical presentations. A review of 31 cases of mycobacterial infection among HSCT recipients showed the lung to be the most common site; however, 45% of patients presented with extrapulmonary disease. Among those with pulmonary disease, a diffuse interstitial or alveolar pattern was most commonly seen on chest radiograph [57]. In addition, there was a delay of 19 days from onset of symptoms to time of diagnosis in HSCT recipients [57]. This is critical, since delays in diagnosis are thought to be responsible, at least in part, for nosocomial transmission and outbreaks of disease [51]. Transmission of disease is largely via inhalation of aerosolized droplets, and hospitalized patients with known or suspected pulmonary or laryngeal MTB infection should be isolated according to Airborne Precautions [49]. Patients with suspected TB infections should be placed in a single patient room with negative pressure relative to the surrounding areas under Airborne Precautions (see above) [49]. All persons entering the room should wear approved respiratory protection designed to protect against inhalation of small respiratory droplets/particles [49].

4.3. Acute GI Infections

Many bacterial, viral, and protozoan pathogens can cause acute gastrointestinal infections; however, *Clostridium difficile*, rotavirus, and toxigenic *Staphylococcus aureus* have been most commonly reported in cases of nosocomial transmission [6]. Transmission occurs via consumption of contaminated food or water as well as contact with infected patients, objects, or equipment [6, 58]. Adequate handwashing is essential to prevent the spread of these pathogens. It should be noted that there is a theoretical decreased activity of alcohol-based hand rubs against spore forming organisms, including *C. difficile*, and non-enveloped viruses, such as Norwalk virus [1]. Therefore, HCWs should be instructed to thoroughly wash hands with soap and water after caring for patients with suspected infectious diarrhea. Contact Precautions are also important in preventing transmission. Current guidelines recommend Contact Precautions for *C. difficille* colitis and rotavirus infection for the duration of the illness. For all other enteric pathogens, contact isolation is only recommended for care of those patients who are incontinent or wear diapers [3]. HCWs who develop symptoms of acute gastroenteritis, vomiting or diarrhea, should be restricted from patient care duties [1].

The duration of restriction will depend on the causative agent but at a minimum will cover the length of symptoms.

4.4. Rash

Rash is a common physical finding among patients with cancer and can have multiple etiologies. Determining the etiology of the rash is often difficult and requires cooperation between oncology, dermatology, and infectious disease practitioners. Communicable infections that may present with rash include viruses such as herpes simplex virus (HSV), varicella, parvovirus B19, bacteria such as meningococcus, and parasites such as scabies.

Nosocomial transmission of HSV is considered uncommon but can occur patient-to-patient or between patients and health care personnel. Transmission occurs through direct contact with infectious lesions or though exposure to virus containing secretions such as saliva or vaginal fluid. Persons with active lesions are considered the most infectious; however, viral shedding has been demonstrated in asymptomatic persons as well [59–64]. The risk of transmission can be minimized with adherence to Standard Precautions [3]. Patients with severe cutaneous infection or those with disseminated disease should be maintained on Contact Precautions for the duration of their illness [3]. Health care personnel with active herpetic lesions on their fingers and hands should be excluded from active patient care until all lesions are crusted and dry. Those with orofacial lesions should be limited from contact with persons considered high risk including the severely malnourished, patients with burns or defects in the integrity of the skin and immunocompromised patients [3]. All personnel who continue to work should cover lesions completely.

Chickenpox caused by VZV is considered highly contagious. Nosocomial transmission can occur in all patient populations, but certain groups are considered at particular risk for severe disease including pregnant women, premature infants, and immunocompromised patients. Transmission in chickenpox is thought to occur via respiratory droplet secretions. Transmission of VZV via direct contact with cutaneous lesions, either from chickenpox infection or herpes zoster, can also occur. Reports of nosocomial transmission and outbreaks among persons without direct contact to the index case suggest airborne transmission may also occur [65–67]. To prevent nosocomial spread, any person with chickenpox should be placed on Airborne Precautions until all lesions are crusted over. Patients with chickenpox should be discharged as soon as medically feasible to minimize potential nosocomial spread. For immunocompetent patients with localized herpes zoster, Standard Precautions are considered sufficient. However, most authors recommend only staff considered immune to VZV to care for these patients. For immunocompromised patients with herpes zoster or others with severe disease, the CDC recommends both Airborne and Contact Precautions for the duration of their illness [3]. VZV is both highly contagious and carries great risk of morbidity and mortality in certain patient populations, and therefore, any suspected case of hospital acquired varicella infection should be reported to your hospital's infection control practitioner.

Scabies is caused by the highly infectious mite, *Sarcoptes scabei.* Transmission is common in the health care setting from undiagnosed infections. Typical scabies presents as an itchy macular-papular rash in warm moist areas of the body. Atypical or Norwegian scabies, which occurs in immune compromised patients, presents with a psoriasis-like rash. Because of the high infectivity, patients with suspected scabies should be placed preemptively in Contact Precautions [3]. Diagnosis of a single patient with scabies on a unit should trigger an outbreak investigation.

4.5. Antimicrobial Resistant Organisms

Over the past 20 years, the incidence of infections caused by multi-drug-resistant organisms (MDRO) such as methicillin-resistant *S. aureus*, VRE, and multi-drug-resistant gram-negative bacteria has increased dramatically [68], especially in immunocompromised populations such as cancer patients. Infections due to multi-drug-resistant pathogens are a significant problem in cancer patients [69–71], regardless of whether they are cared for in specialized units or centers. These patients are at risk for acquisition of MDROs because of frequent hospital visits and antibiotic use. Morbidity and mortality of MDRO infections in cancer patients has not specifically been measured; however, multiple studies in other populations have shown that these infections increase mortality and morbidity in general [72, 73]. Thus, preventing MDRO infections is paramount.

Most MDROs are opportunistic pathogens and colonize patients prior to causing an infection. Thus, prevention can occur at two levels: preventing initial colonization and preventing progression to infection after patients are colonized.

Preventing the acquisition of MDROs requires identifying MDRO-colonized patients in the cancer center and preventing spread to other patients. Identification of MDRO-colonized patients is best accomplished through a program of active surveillance cultures. Surveillance cultures from rectal, nares, and/or throat swabs, when used for infection control purposes, can identify colonized patients before any manifestation of clinical infection. MDRO-colonized patients are then placed on Contact Precautions. The use of surveillance cultures is important because clinical cultures only identify 20% of patients with an MDRO. Surveillance cultures are best performed on admission, weekly, and at discharge. Positive admission cultures assure that patients are isolated promptly. However, colonization with MDRO may not be detected until treatment with anti-infectives amplifies low level MDRO colonization; hence the importance of weekly monitoring. Many centers have chosen to use preemptive Contact Precautions for patients new to their center or unit while waiting for surveillance culture results to return. Cultures during hospitalization allow for calculation of an acquisition rate as well as identifying patients who now need to be placed on Contact Precautions [74].

The body sites cultured depends on the MDRO. Cultures of the anterior nares or throat and any area of skin breakdown are sensitive tests for MRSA colonization. Cultures of the perirectal or perineal skin are sensitive tests for VRE and multi-resistant gram-negative rods. The prevalence of these organisms should be used to determine the culture sites and the frequency of culturing. Although the concept of "decolonization" is attractive, it has not worked well in practice for either VRE [75] or MRSA [76].

4.6. The Pregnant Health Care Worker

Infection with VZV, Parvovirus B19, or Cytomegalovirus (CMV) is of particular concern to the pregnant HCW due to the potential adverse effects on the fetus such as congenital abnormalities and fetal death. Pregnant personnel and women of child bearing age should be counseled regarding the risk to the fetus during infection with these viruses as well as prevention of transmission [6, 77].

4.6.1. *Cytomegalovirus*

The exact risk of nosocomial transmission of CMV is unknown. Studies have suggested only minimal risk of patient-to-staff transmission, which appears to be no different from that of the general population. In addition, there appears to be no increased risk of HCWs who care for high risk patients [77–81]. Transmission is thought to occur through close and intimate contact with persons shedding virus or through contact with contaminated body fluids. The risk of transmission is decreased with the use of Standard Precautions; thus, patients with CMV infection or disease are not placed on Contact Precautions. HCWs with active CMV infection should not be restricted from duties [6]. Recommendations regarding the nosocomial transmission of CMV in the pregnant HCW are controversial due to potential risks to the fetus following primary CMV infection of the mother; however, given that the risk of transmission among HCWs does not appear higher than the general public, there are no current recommendations regarding transfer of pregnant HCWs to lower risk areas [6, 77].

4.6.2. *Parvovirus B19*

Parvovirus B19 is a small DNA virus in the family Parvoviridae. Infection occurs most commonly in children as erythema infectiosum or fifth disease. In adults, infection is often asymptomatic; however, a variety of syndromes can be encountered depending on the host. Occasionally, healthy adults (most commonly women) develop an acute symmetrical polyarthropathy that mimics rheumatoid arthritis. Infection in persons with hemolytic disorders may lead to transient aplastic crisis, while immunocompromised patients may develop persistent infection and chronic anemia or pure red cell aplasia.

Transmission of the virus is via close contact with infected persons or infected respiratory secretions [6]. Nosocomial transmission is felt to be rare, but has been reported [6]. Patients with erythema infectiosum or polyarthropathy are considered infectious before the onset of their symptoms, and therefore isolation is not routinely recommended [3, 6]. Patients with aplastic crisis are typically infectious for 7 days after onset of illness, and isolation using droplet precautions for the first 7 days of their hospitalization is recommended. Those with pure red cell aplasia may be infectious for years and should be placed on droplet precautions for the entire duration of their hospitalization. Pregnant personnel are not considered to have an increased risk of transmission; however, they should be counseled regarding potential risks and prevention of transmission. Current guidelines do not recommend work restrictions for infected health care personnel, however, if infection is known it seems reasonable to restrict them from the active care of immunosuppressed patients [6].

4.7. Continued Infection Control in the Outpatient

Some patients, particularly HSCT recipients, may remain immunosuppressed and are therefore at increased risk for development of infection after discharge from the cancer center. These patients, and their families, should be educated regarding ways to decrease their personal risk of transmission and infection with microorganisms. Detailed guidelines for continued infection control in the outpatient are available from the CDC [5]. Emphasis should be placed on continued hand hygiene in the home. To prevent common respiratory infection, in addition to scrupulous hand hygiene, patients should avoid contacts with persons who have respiratory symptoms (including rhinorrhea, nasal congestion, pharyngitis, cough and fever). If at all possible, they should also avoid crowded places where respiratory diseases may be easily transmissible; if this is not possible, they should consider wearing a surgical mask. Food preparers should wash hands frequently, and food preparation areas and utensils should be kept clean. Raw meats should be handled separately and should not contaminate other food. Meat should be properly cooked. Patients who are neutropenic should avoid high risk foods as discussed above. Patients should avoid gardening or direct contact with soil or plants while immune suppressed to reduce the risk of infection with organisms such as *Toxoplasma, Histoplasma, Cryptococcus, Nocardia* or *Aspergillus*. Patients should be advised to limit their contact with their pets while immune suppressed and to be diligent regarding the pet's health maintenance. Patients should avoid contact with animal saliva, urine, and feces. Immune suppressed patients should not have contact with exotic pets or wild animals. Patients should be instructed to avoid sexual practices that result in oral exposure to feces. Given the risk of infection among international travelers, patients should consult their physician before travel to developing countries.

4.8. Developing an Infection Control Program

Cancer centers vary in their scope of care in terms of the type of cancer population served (e.g., pediatric vs. adult; hematologic malignancies vs. solid tumors) and procedures performed (e.g., types of hematopoietic stem cell transplants performed). Hospital-wide infection control programs perform an annual risk assessment to set their goals for the year. This is a useful exercise that is also required by JCAHO standards. An infection control program for a cancer center or unit should use similar methodologies. A risk assessment incorporates three elements: how common the type of infection is, the impact of those infections, and the "preventability" of the infection.

There are a number of ways to measure how common certain infections are in a cancer center population. Most infection control programs have abandoned "whole house" surveillance (following every patient for every type of infection) in favor of targeted surveillance (targeting specific types of infections in certain high risk populations). However, a center-wide or unit-wide surveillance for a limited period of time may be extremely helpful for a risk assessment snapshot. Depending on the size of the cancer center, this can involve a 1 day point prevalence survey of every patient for target infections for a large center or an incidence study over 90 days for a smaller center. Accounting for seasonal variations (e.g., respiratory viruses such as influenza), this data may provide important information on the relative frequencies of different infections.

The impact of each infection is measured by mortality and morbidity attributable to the infection. The distinction between overall and attributable mortality is important as more effort should be placed into preventing those infections with a high attributable mortality, especially in those infected patients who otherwise are expected to have an excellent response in their hematological malignancies.

Table 11-3.

Types of infection	Infection volume	Infection impact on patient	Infection preventability	Priority score
	1 = Low	1 = Increased length of stay	1 = Difficult	Preventability
	2 = Medium	2 = Disability	2 = Moderate	Impact x
	3 = High	3 = Life threatening	3 = Easy	= Infection volume x
Viral respiratory syndromes – RSV, influenza	3	3	2	18
HSV	3	2	3	18
Catheter related BSI	2	3	3	18
VZV-zoster	2	2	3	12
VRE	3	2	2	12
MRSA	2	3	2	12
VZV-varicella	1	3	3	9
Legionella pneumonia	1	3	3	9
Fungal pneumonia	2	3	1	6
Clostridium difficile	2	1	3	6
Multi-antibiotic resistant gram-negative bacteria	1	3	2	6
Mycobacterium tuberculosis	1	3	1	3
Conjunctivitis	1	1	2	2

The "preventability" of an infection is a measure of the ease by which an infection control program can reduce incidence and transmission of a target infection. It often makes sense to institute infection control measures that are easy and inexpensive to implement even if the target infection is relatively uncommon or causes less morbidity and mortality than other infections. Some infections are extremely difficult or expensive to prevent. Decisions on how to use limited resources should be guided by the frequencies of these difficult-to-prevent infections and their impact on patients.

Table 11-3 shows a hypothetical risk assessment for a 60 bed cancer center that serves adults with both solid and hematological malignancies and performs all types of stem cell transplants.

References

1. Boyce JM, Pittet D (2002) Guideline for Hand Hygiene in Health-Care Settings. Recommendations of the Healthcare Infection Control Practices Advisory Committee and the HICPAC/SHEA/APIC/IDSA Hand Hygiene Task Force. Society for Healthcare Epidemiology of America/Association for Professionals in Infection Control/Infectious Diseases Society of America. MMWR Recomm Rep 51:1–45 quiz CE1–4
2. Voss A, Widmer AF (1997) No time for handwashing!? Handwashing versus alcoholic rub: can we afford 100% compliance? Infect Control Hosp Epidemiol 18:205–208
3. Siegel JD, Rhinehart E, Jackson M, Chiarello L (2007) 2007 Guidelines for isolation precautions: preventing transmission of infectious agents in healthcare settings.

4. Sehulster L, Chinn RY (2003) Guidelines for environmental infection control in health-care facilities. Recommendations of CDC and the Healthcare Infection Control Practices Advisory Committee (HICPAC). MMWR Recomm Rep 52:1–42
5. (2000) Guidelines for preventing opportunistic infections among hematopoietic stem cell transplant recipients. MMWR Recomm Rep 49:1–125, CE1–7
6. Bolyard EA, Tablan OC, Williams WW, Pearson ML, Shapiro CN, Deitchmann SD (1998) Guideline for infection control in healthcare personnel, 1998. Hospital Infection Control Practices Advisory Committee. Infect Control Hosp Epidemiol 19:407–463
7. Broder KR, Cortese MM, Iskander JK, Kretsinger K, Slade BA, Brown KH, Mijalski CM, Tiwari T, Weston EJ, Cohn AC, Srivastava PU, Moran JS, Schwartz B, Murphy TV (2006) Preventing tetanus, diphtheria, and pertussis among adolescents: use of tetanus toxoid, reduced diphtheria toxoid and acellular pertussis vaccines recommendations of the Advisory Committee on Immunization Practices (ACIP). MMWR Recomm Rep 55:1–34
8. Prevots DR, Burr RK, Sutter RW, Murphy TV (2000) Poliomyelitis prevention in the United States. Updated recommendations of the Advisory Committee on Immunization Practices (ACIP). MMWR Recomm Rep 49:1–22 quiz CE1–7
9. Watson JC, Hadler SC, Dykewicz CA, Reef S, Phillips L (1998) Measles, mumps, and rubella–vaccine use and strategies for elimination of measles, rubella, and congenital rubella syndrome and control of mumps: recommendations of the Advisory Committee on Immunization Practices (ACIP). MMWR Recomm Rep 47:1–57
10. Pearson ML, Bridges CB, Harper SA (2006) Influenza vaccination of healthcare personnel: recommendations of the Healthcare Infection Control Practices Advisory Committee (HICPAC) and the Advisory Committee on Immunization Practices (ACIP). MMWR Recomm Rep 55:1–16
11. Smith NM, Bresee JS, Shay DK, Uyeki TM, Cox NJ, Strikas RA (2006) Prevention and Control of Influenza: recommendations of the Advisory Committee on Immunization Practices (ACIP). MMWR Recomm Rep 55:1–42
12. (1999) Prevention of varicella. Update recommendations of the Advisory Committee on Immunization Practices (ACIP). MMWR Recomm Rep 48:1–5
13. O'Grady NP, Alexander M, Dellinger EP, Gerberding JL, Heard SO, Maki DG, Masur H, McCormick RD, Mermel LA, Pearson ML, Raad II, Randolph A, Weinstein RA (2002) Guidelines for the prevention of intravascular catheter-related infections. Centers for Disease Control and Prevention. MMWR Recomm Rep 51:1–29
14. NNIS System (2003) National Nosocomial Infections Surveillance (NNIS) System Report, data summary from January 1992 through June 2003, issued August 2003. Am J Infect Control 31:481–98
15. Kim PW, Perl TM, Keelaghan EF, Langenberg P, Perencevich EN, Harris AD, Song X, Roghmann MC (2005) Risk of mortality with a bloodstream infection is higher in the less severely ill at admission. Am J Respir Crit Care Med 171:616–620
16. Pittet D, Tarara D, Wenzel RP (1994) Nosocomial bloodstream infection in critically ill patients. Excess length of stay, extra costs, and attributable mortality. JAMA 271:1598–1601
17. Rosenthal VD, Guzman S, Migone O, Crnich CJ (2003) The attributable cost, length of hospital stay, and mortality of central line-associated bloodstream infection in intensive care departments in Argentina: A prospective, matched analysis. Am J Infect Control 31:475–480
18. Smith RL, Meixler SM, Simberkoff MS (1991) Excess mortality in critically ill patients with nosocomial bloodstream infections. Chest 100:164–167
19. Soufir L, Timsit JF, Mahe C, Carlet J, Regnier B, Chevret S (1999) Attributable morbidity and mortality of catheter-related septicemia in critically ill patients: a matched, risk-adjusted, cohort study. Infect Control Hosp Epidemiol 20:396–401
20. Weinstein MP, Murphy JR, Reller LB, Lichtenstein KA (1983) The clinical significance of positive blood cultures: a comprehensive analysis of 500 episodes of

bacteremia and fungemia in adults. II. Clinical observations, with special reference to factors influencing prognosis. Rev Infect Dis 5:54–70
21. Weinstock DM, Rogers M, Eagan J, Malak SA, Sepkowitz KA (2002) Nosocomial central venous catheter infections among patients with different types of cancer. Infect Control Hosp Epidemiol 23:234–235
22. Rotstein C, Brock L, Roberts RS (1995) The incidence of first Hickman catheter-related infection and predictors of catheter removal in cancer patients. Infect Control Hosp Epidemiol 16:451–458
23. Mermel LA, McCormick RD, Springman SR, Maki DG (1991) The pathogenesis and epidemiology of catheter-related infection with pulmonary artery Swan-Ganz catheters: a prospective study utilizing molecular subtyping. Am J Med 91:197S–205S
24. Merrer J, De Jonghe B, Golliot F, Lefrant JY, Raffy B, Barre E, Rigaud JP, Casciani D, Misset B, Bosquet C, Outin H, Brun-Buisson C, Nitenberg G (2001) Complications of femoral and subclavian venous catheterization in critically ill patients: a randomized controlled trial. JAMA 286:700–707
25. Richet H, Hubert B, Nitemberg G, Andremont A, Buu-Hoi A, Ourbak P, Galicier C, Veron M, Boisivon A, Bouvier AM et al (1990) Prospective multicenter study of vascular-catheter-related complications and risk factors for positive central-catheter cultures in intensive care unit patients. J Clin Microbiol 28:2520–2525
26. Raad DC II, Hohn BJ, Gilbreath NS, Hill LA, Bruso PA, Marts K, Mansfield PF, Bodey GP (1994) Prevention of central venous catheter-related infections by using maximal sterile barrier precautions during insertion. Infect Control Hosp Epidemiol 15:231–238
27. Maki DG, Ringer M, Alvarado CJ (1991) Prospective randomised trial of povidone-iodine, alcohol, and chlorhexidine for prevention of infection associated with central venous and arterial catheters. Lancet 338:339–343
28. Veenstra DL, Saint S, Sullivan SD (1999) Cost-effectiveness of antiseptic-impregnated central venous catheters for the prevention of catheter-related bloodstream infection. JAMA 282:554–560
29. Brun-Buisson C, Doyon F, Sollet JP, Cochard JF, Cohen Y, Nitenberg G (2004) Prevention of intravascular catheter-related infection with newer chlorhexidine-silver sulfadiazine-coated catheters: a randomized controlled trial. Intensive Care Med 30:837–843
30. Maki DG, Stolz SM, Wheeler S, Mermel LA (1997) Prevention of central venous catheter-related bloodstream infection by use of an antiseptic-impregnated catheter. A randomized, controlled trial. Ann Intern Med 127:257–266
31. Raad I, Darouiche R, Dupuis J, Abi-Said D, Gabrielli A, Hachem R, Wall M, Harris R, Jones J, Buzaid A, Robertson C, Shenaq S, Curling P, Burke T, Ericsson C (1997) Central venous catheters coated with minocycline and rifampin for the prevention of catheter-related colonization and bloodstream infections. A randomized, double-blind trial. The Texas Medical Center Catheter Study Group. Ann Intern Med 127:267–274
32. Rupp ME, Lisco SJ, Lipsett PA, Perl TM, Keating K, Civetta JM, Mermel LA, Lee D, Dellinger EP, Donahoe M, Giles D, Pfaller MA, Maki DG, Sherertz R (2005) Effect of a second-generation venous catheter impregnated with chlorhexidine and silver sulfadiazine on central catheter-related infections: a randomized, controlled trial. Ann Intern Med 143:570–580
33. Sheng WH, Ko WJ, Wang JT, Chang SC, Hsueh PR, Luh KT (2000) Evaluation of antiseptic-impregnated central venous catheters for prevention of catheter-related infection in intensive care unit patients. Diagn Microbiol Infect Dis 38:1–5
34. Veenstra DL, Saint S, Saha S, Lumley T, Sullivan SD (1999) Efficacy of antiseptic-impregnated central venous catheters in preventing catheter-related bloodstream infection: a meta-analysis. JAMA 281:261–267
35. Walder B, Pittet D, Tramer MR (2002) Prevention of bloodstream infections with central venous catheters treated with anti-infective agents depends on catheter type

and insertion time: evidence from a meta-analysis. Infect Control Hosp Epidemiol 23:748–756
36. Darouiche RO, Raad SO II, Heard JI, Thornby OC, Wenker AG, Berg J, Khardori N, Hanna H, Hachem R, Harris RL, Mayhall G (1999) A comparison of two antimicrobial-impregnated central venous catheters. Catheter Study Group. N Engl J Med 340:1–8
37. Whimbey E, Englund JA, Couch RB (1997) Community respiratory virus infections in immunocompromised patients with cancer. Am J Med 102:10–18 discussion 25–6
38. Fraser DW, Tsai TR, Orenstein W, Parkin WE, Beecham HJ, Sharrar RG, Harris J, Mallison GF, Martin SM, McDade JE, Shepard CC, Brachman PS (1977) Legionnaires' disease: description of an epidemic of pneumonia. N Engl J Med 297:1189–1197
39. Tablan OC, Anderson LJ, Besser R, Bridges C, Hajjeh R (2004) Guidelines for preventing health-care-associated pneumonia, 2003: recommendations of CDC and the Healthcare Infection Control Practices Advisory Committee. MMWR Recomm Rep 53:1–36
40. Allam MF, Del Castillo AS, Diaz-Molina C, Navajas RF (2002) Invasive pulmonary aspergillosis: identification of risk factors. Scand J Infect Dis 34:819–822
41. Gerson SL, Talbot GH, Hurwitz S, Strom BL, Lusk EJ, Cassileth PA (1984) Prolonged granulocytopenia: the major risk factor for invasive pulmonary aspergillosis in patients with acute leukemia. Ann Intern Med 100:345–351
42. Groll AH, Shah PM, Mentzel C, Schneider M, Just-Nuebling G, Huebner K (1996) Trends in the postmortem epidemiology of invasive fungal infections at a university hospital. J Infect 33:23–32
43. Pagano L, Caira M, Candoni A, Offidani M, Fianchi L, Martino B, Pastore D, Picardi M, Bonini A, Chierichini A, Fanci R, Caramatti C, Invernizzi R, Mattei D, Mitra ME, Melillo L, Aversa F, Van Lint MT, Falcucci P, Valentini CG, Girmenia C, Nosari A (2006) The epidemiology of fungal infections in patients with hematologic malignancies: the SEIFEM-2004 study. Haematologica 91:1068–1075
44. Patterson TF, Kirkpatrick WR, White M, Hiemenz JW, Wingard JR, Dupont B, Rinaldi MG, Stevens DA, Graybill JR (2000) Invasive aspergillosis. Disease spectrum, treatment practices, and outcomes. 13 Aspergillus Study Group. Medicine (Baltimore) 79:250–260
45. Rhame FS (1989) Nosocomial aspergillosis: how much protection for which patients? Infect Control Hosp Epidemiol 10:296–298
46. Sherertz RJ, Belani A, Kramer BS, Elfenbein GJ, Weiner RS, Sullivan ML, Thomas RG, Samsa GP (1987) Impact of air filtration on nosocomial Aspergillus infections. Unique risk of bone marrow transplant recipients. Am J Med 83:709–718
47. Hahn T, Cummings KM, Michalek AM, Lipman BJ, Segal BH, McCarthy PL Jr (2002) Efficacy of high-efficiency particulate air filtration in preventing aspergillosis in immunocompromised patients with hematologic malignancies. Infect Control Hosp Epidemiol 23:525–531
48. Vonberg RP, Gastmeier P (2006) Nosocomial aspergillosis in outbreak settings. J Hosp Infect 63:246–254
49. (1994) Guidelines for preventing the transmission of Mycobacterium tuberculosis in health-care facilities, 1994. Centers for Disease Control and Prevention. MMWR Recomm Rep 43:1–132
50. Paolo WF Jr, Nosanchuk JD (2004) Tuberculosis in New York city: recent lessons and a look ahead. Lancet Infect Dis 4:287–293
51. Fitzergald D, Haas DW (2005) Mycobacterium tuberculosis, vol. 2, 6th edn. Elsevier Churchill Livingstone, Philadelphia, PA
52. (2000) Diagnostic Standards and Classification of Tuberculosis in Adults and Children. This official statement of the American Thoracic Society and the Centers for Disease Control and Prevention was adopted by the ATS Board of Directors,

July 1999. This statement was endorsed by the Council of the Infectious Disease Society of America, September 1999. Am J Respir Crit Care Med 161:1376–1395
53. Malone JL, Ijaz K, Lambert L, Rosencrans L, Phillips L, Tomlinson V, Arbise M, Moolenaar RL, Dworkin MS, Simoes EJ (2004) Investigation of healthcare-associated transmission of Mycobacterium tuberculosis among patients with malignancies at three hospitals and at a residential facility. Cancer 101:2713–2721
54. (1995) Essential components of a tuberculosis prevention and control program. Recommendations of the Advisory Council for the Elimination of Tuberculosis. MMWR Recomm Rep 44:1–16
55. Kamboj M, Sepkowitz KA (2006) The risk of tuberculosis in patients with cancer. Clin Infect Dis 42:1592–1595
56. Centers for Disease Control and Prevention (CDC) (2004) Trends in tuberculosis-United States, 1998-2003. MMWR Morb Mortal Wkly Rep 53:209–14
57. Cordonnier C, Martino R, Trabasso P, Held TK, Akan H, Ward MS, Fabian K, Ullmann AJ, Wulffraat N, Ljungman P, Alessandrino EP, Pretnar J, Gmur J, Varela R, Vitek A, Sica S, Rovira M (2004) Mycobacterial infection: a difficult and late diagnosis in stem cell transplant recipients. Clin Infect Dis 38:1229–1236
58. Sepkowitz KA (1996) Occupationally acquired infections in health care workers. Part II. Ann Intern Med 125:917–928
59. da Silva LM, Guimaraes AL, Victoria JM, Gomes CC, Gomez RS (2005) Herpes simplex virus type 1 shedding in the oral cavity of seropositive patients. Oral Dis 11:13–16
60. Kameyama T, Sujaku C, Yamamoto S, Hwang CB, Shillitoe EJ (1988) Shedding of herpes simplex virus type 1 into saliva. J Oral Pathol 17:478–481
61. Knaup B, Schunemann S, Wolff MH (2000) Subclinical reactivation of herpes simplex virus type 1 in the oral cavity. Oral Microbiol Immunol 15:281–283
62. Koelle DM, Wald A (2000) Herpes simplex virus: the importance of asymptomatic shedding. J Antimicrob Chemother 45(Suppl T3):1–8
63. Scott DA, Coulter WA, Lamey PJ (1997) Oral shedding of herpes simplex virus type 1: a review. J Oral Pathol Med 26:441–447
64. Wolff MH, Schmitt J, Rahaus M, Dudda H, Hatzmann W (2002) Clinical and subclinical reactivation of genital herpes virus. Intervirology 45:20–23
65. Gustafson TL, Lavely GB, Brawner ER Jr, Hutcheson RH Jr, Wright PF, Schaffner W (1982) An outbreak of airborne nosocomial varicella. Pediatrics 70:550–556
66. Josephson A, Gombert ME (1988) Airborne transmission of nosocomial varicella from localized zoster. J Infect Dis 158:238–241
67. Menkhaus NA, Lanphear B, Linnemann CC (1990) Airborne transmission of varicella-zoster virus in hospitals. Lancet 336:1315
68. National Nosocomial Infections Surveillance System (2004) National Nosocomial Infections Surveillance (NNIS) System Report, data summary from January 1992 through June 2004, issued October 2004. Am J Infect Control 32:470–85
69. Henning KJ, Delencastre H, Eagan J, Boone N, Brown A, Chung M, Wollner N, Armstrong D (1996) Vancomycin-resistant Enterococcus faecium on a pediatric oncology ward: duration of stool shedding and incidence of clinical infection. Pediatr Infect Dis J 15:848–854
70. Montecalvo MA, Horowitz H, Gedris C, Carbonaro C, Tenover FC, Issah A, Cook P, Wormser GP (1994) Outbreak of vancomycin-, ampicillin-, and aminoglycoside-resistant Enterococcus faecium bacteremia in an adult oncology unit. Antimicrob Agents Chemother 38:1363–1367
71. Roghmann MC, Qaiyumi S, Johnson JA, Schwalbe R, Morris JG Jr (1997) Recurrent vancomycin-resistant Enterococcus faecium bacteremia in a leukemia patient who was persistently colonized with vancomycin-resistant enterococci for two years. Clin Infect Dis 24:514–515
72. Cosgrove SE, Sakoulas G, Perencevich EN, Schwaber MJ, Karchmer AW, Carmeli Y (2003) Comparison of mortality associated with methicillin-resistant and methi-

cillin-susceptible Staphylococcus aureus bacteremia: a meta-analysis. Clin Infect Dis 36:53–59
73. DiazGranados CA, Zimmer SM, Klein M, Jernigan JA (2005) Comparison of mortality associated with vancomycin-resistant and vancomycin-susceptible enterococcal bloodstream infections: a meta-analysis. Clin Infect Dis 41:327–333
74. Hachem R, Graviss L, Hanna H, Arbuckle R, Dvorak T, Hackett B, Gonzalez V, Perego C, Tarrand J, Raad I (2004) Impact of surveillance for vancomycin-resistant enterococci on controlling a bloodstream outbreak among patients with hematologic malignancy. Infect Control Hosp Epidemiol 25:391–394
75. Wong MT, Kauffman CA, Standiford HC, Linden P, Fort G, Fuchs HJ, Porter SB, Wenzel RP (2001) Effective suppression of vancomycin-resistant Enterococcus species in asymptomatic gastrointestinal carriers by a novel glycolipodepsipeptide, ramoplanin. Clin Infect Dis 33:1476–1482
76. Laupland KB, Conly JM (2003) Treatment of Staphylococcus aureus colonization and prophylaxis for infection with topical intranasal mupirocin: an evidence-based review. Clin Infect Dis 37:933–938
77. Mirza A, Wyatt M, Begue RE (1999) Infection control practices and the pregnant health care worker. Pediatr Infect Dis J 18:18–22
78. Balfour CL, Balfour HH Jr (1986) Cytomegalovirus is not an occupational risk for nurses in renal transplant and neonatal units. Results of a prospective surveillance study. JAMA 256:1909–1914
79. Demmler GJ, Yow MD, Spector SA, Reis SG, Brady MT, Anderson DC, Taber LH (1987) Nosocomial cytomegalovirus infections within two hospitals caring for infants and children. J Infect Dis 156:9–16
80. Dworsky ME, Welch K, Cassady G, Stagno S (1983) Occupational risk for primary cytomegalovirus infection among pediatric health-care workers. N Engl J Med 309:950–953
81. Gerberding JL (1994) Incidence and prevalence of human immunodeficiency virus, hepatitis B virus, hepatitis C virus, and cytomegalovirus among health care personnel at risk for blood exposure: final report from a longitudinal study. J Infect Dis 170:1410–1417

Chapter 12

Immunizations

Alan Cross

Abstract Immunization is the most effective means of preventing infections; yet the oncology population is poorly capable of responding to vaccines because of either the underlying disease or immunocompromising therapy received. Patients may safely receive either the killed or subunit vaccines; however, since live attenuated vaccines rely on limited replication, in the absence of a fully functional immune system, such vaccines pose a significant morbidity risk. Novel strategies are now being evaluated to improve the poor response to immunization in this patient population.

Keywords Immunization • Vaccines • Stem cell transplantation • Acute lymphocytic leukemia • Oncology

1. Recommendations for Immunization of the Oncology Patient

Immunization is the most effective means of preventing infections; yet the hematological malignancy in patient population, that is most susceptible to infections, is poorly capable of responding to immunization because of either the underlying disease and/or the anti-neoplastic therapy. Oncology patients comprise a heterogeneous population with varying immune defects (e.g., patients with lymphoma, leukemia, stem cell transplantation [SCT] recipients). It is beyond the scope of this chapter to review how the specific immune deficits of each oncology subpopulation relate to either their susceptibility to specific infections or responses to each vaccine. The proposed recommendations for patients undergoing bone marrow transplantation (BMT) and SCT, as well as the conclusions drawn from the many small studies of vaccine safety and efficacy performed in patients treated for malignancies in a non-transplant setting, are reviewed.

From: *Managing Infections in Patients With Hematological Malignancies*: Contemporary Hematology, Edited by: M. Kleinberg, DOI 10.1007/978-1-59745-415-5_12,

1.2. General Principles

Following chemotherapy and bone marrow and/or SCT, there is a loss of pre-existing antibodies to vaccine-preventable infections. Immunocompromised patients can be administered safely killed or subunit vaccines in a manner similar to vaccination of immunocompetent people. In general, it is desirable to immunize at least 2 weeks or more before the anticipated initiation of either chemotherapy or immunosuppressive therapy. Immunization should be avoided during chemotherapy, graft-versus-host disease (GVHD), receipt of immunosuppressives (including treatment for acute GVHD), or irradiation. SCT recipients are presumed to be immunocompetent at ≥24 months after SCT if they do not receive immunosuppressive therapy and do not have GVHD. Immunodeficiency is considered less profound after autologous SCT compared to allogeneic SCT.

2. Bone Marrow and Stem Cell Transplantation

During transplantation, the immune system becomes compromised by the conditioning regimens (radiation and chemotherapy) and the ensuing myelosuppression. While the neutrophil count recovers shortly after engraftment, the decrease in cellular immunity persists for months even in the absence of GVHD or immunosuppressive medications. After both autologous and allogeneic SCT, there is a decline in specific pre-treatment antibody levels and a delay in B- and T-cell recovery and natural killer cell function. Even though the total immunoglobulin level may appear "normal," there is likely to be deficiencies in the immunoglobulin G subclasses required to defend against encapsulated bacteria, and an impaired ability to switch immunoglobulin classes. Further, since the CD8 T cells recover more rapidly than the CD4 T cells, there is a reversal in the CD4/CD8 T cell ratio that may persist for 12 months. This change in T cell levels may alter the immune response to administered vaccines [1, 2]. During this time, physicians may monitor the CD4 cell counts and gamma globulin levels to gauge the recovery of immune system capability.

2.1. Infectious Risks

The most common infections documented with BMT and SCT are caused by *Varicella zoster* virus (VZV), cytomegalovirus (CMV), Epstein Barr virus (EBV), *Pneumococcus*, *Pneumocystis*, *Aspergillus*, *Pseudomonas*, toxoplasmosis, and *Nocardia* [3, 4]. In BMT and SCT, the well-established loss of pre-existing protective antibody to vaccine-preventable infections has led to the recommendation of vaccination for all transplantation recipients in the post-transplant period. While data has established the safety and efficacy of many vaccines administered after BMT, vaccines have been underutilized in the post-transplant period, and immunization practices vary widely among US transplant centers [5]. Consensus guidelines for the immunization of transplant recipients have been developed in the last few years, both in Europe [6] and in the United States [7].

2.2. Immunization Recommendations (Table 12-1)

The ability to respond to immunization post-SCT depends on the time elapsed since transplantation, the nature of the donor cells, the presence of GVHD, and

Table 12-1. Recommended vaccinations for hematopoietic stem cell transplant (HSCT) recipients, including both allogeneic and autologous recipients.

Vaccine	Timing relative to SCT or GVHD	Comments
Tetanus-diphtheria toxoid (Td)	12, 14 and 24 months	If <7 years old, include pertussis (DTP). Revaccinate every 10 years.
Hemophilus influenzae type b conjugate (Hib)	12, 14 and 24	Recommended for HSCT recipients of any age.
Hepatitis B (Hep B)	12, 14, 24	Recommended for all susceptible persons ≤18 years and for adults with risk factors for hepatitis B infection. May need high (40 μg/dose) dose. Test after last dose.
Pneumococcal polysaccharide, 23-valent	12, 24	24 month dose not a booster, but to catch non-responders to 12 month dose
Influenza type A	Lifelong, seasonal	Begin before HSCT and resume after 6 months. If ≤9 years, need two doses.
Inactivated polio vaccine (IPV)	12, 14 and 24 months	Immunogenic but no data on efficacy in HSCT recipients.
Measles-mumps-rubella	24 months; second dose 6–12 months later.	Administer only if HSCT recipient considered immunocompetent.

HSCT recipients are presumed immunocompetent at >24 months after HSCT if they are not on immunosuppressive therapy and do not have graft-versus-host disease (GVHD). Live vaccines contraindicated for patients, not considered for patients, not considered immunocompetent. All non-live vaccines should be administered to HSCT recipients, regardless of HSCT type or presence of GVHD. Live attenuated vaccines (e.g., measles-mumps-rubella, varicella, Bacillus Calmette-Guerin, yellow fever and oral typhoid vaccines) should not be administered to any HSCT recipient with active GVHD or immunosuppression. To date, no adverse events have been reported (e.g., exacerbation of any GVHD) among vaccinated HSCT recipients. No contraindications to simultaneous administration of any vaccines exist, except cholera and yellow fever.

also whether serial immunizations are employed. As a general rule, patients with a compromised immune system should not receive any live attenuated vaccines (e.g., oral polio, live attenuated measles or varicella) until after 24 months, at which time the immune system is considered competent (in the absence of GVHD or continued immunosuppressive therapy). Live attenuated vaccines rely on limited replication within the immunocompetent host; however, in the absence of a fully functional immune system, even the attenuated vaccine organisms may disseminate and cause significant morbidity and even mortality.

2.3. Pneumococcus and *Haemophilus influenzae* Type B

The highest risk for both *S. pneumoniae* and *Haemophilus influenzae* type b (HIB) infections appear to be beyond 6 months after transplantation when pre-existing levels of protective antibody have declined, but the patient has an impaired ability to respond to infection. In a 3.5-year prospective study, 51 episodes of invasive pneumococcal infection were diagnosed in patients, with more occurring following BMT than peripheral SCT (43 vs. 8), and allogeneic rather than autologous grafts (35 vs. 16). Most of the episodes (44) occurred ≥100 days after transplantation [8]. A 23-valent pneumococcal polysaccharide vaccine (PPV) has been licensed for the prevention of pneumococcal infections in the general adult population; however, the inability of pediatric populations to respond to polysaccharide antigens has led to the development of a pneumococcal conjugate vaccine (PCV) whereby pneumococcal oligosaccharides from different serotypes are conjugated to protein carriers. Because the protein carriers require T cell help, pediatric patients mount an effective serum antibody response to the pneumococcal serotypes included in the vaccine. Currently, a 7-valent conjugate vaccine is licensed in the United States, and conjugate vaccines with broader serotype coverage are under development.

Early studies noted little (<20%) antibody response in adults if the 23-valent PPV was administered ≤24 months post-transplantation [9, 10]. Despite poor antibody responses, the CDC recommends that all allogeneic SCT patients should receive the PPV at 12 months after transplantation [7]. A second dose of vaccine is recommended at 24 months to "capture" any subject who did not respond to the 12-month immunization (i.e., not considered a "booster" dose). One study found that the PCV is immunogenic in the autologous SCT setting when administered at 3, 6 and 12 months after transplantation [11]. In a recent study of children with autologous SCT, immunization with a PCV resulted in seroconversion of all the serotypes in over 80% of subjects [12]. Since preliminary data show that immunization of allogeneic stem cell donors with various vaccines enhances vaccine responses in allogeneic stem cell graft recipients, it is not surprising that immunization of allogeneic donors with either the PPV or PCV primes the recipient to respond better to these vaccines in the post-transplant period [13, 14].

HIB can be a significant pathogen in individuals who lack antibody to the polysaccharide capsule. Natural antibody immunity to HIB usually develops by adulthood. The transplant-associated decline in pre-existing protective levels of antibody to HIB exposes the transplant patients to the risk of serious HIB infection. Widespread vaccination with the HIB conjugate vaccine has markedly reduced serious infection in children. Studies in children with autologous SCT showed that vaccination against HIB induced protective antibody levels in 100% of subjects [12], while the HIB conjugate vaccine induces protective levels of antibodies in allogeneic transplant recipients, with >80% response rate after the second dose of vaccine [10, 15]. Protective levels of antibody are achieved earlier in patients receiving peripheral blood SCT compared to BMT patients. Consequently, the CDC recommends that this vaccine be given at 12, 14 and 24 months post-transplant (Table 12-1).

2.4. Tetanus, Diphtheria, Pertussis

Antibody levels against tetanus, diphtheria and pertussis decline post-transplantation as well. Since immunization can restore protective antibody levels in transplant recipients, the CDC recommends that the combined tetanus/diphtheria toxoid/pertussis vaccine be given at 12, 14 and 24 months to children <7 years if there is no contraindication to the pertussis vaccine; however, only the tetanus-diphtheria toxoid vaccine is recommended for children ≥7 years and adults. Immunization of children receiving autologous SCT with tetanus resulted in the induction of protective antibodies in 100% of subjects [12]. While there are relatively little data available on the use of the acellular pertussis vaccine in the SCT setting, it has fewer adverse effects than the cellular pertussis vaccine, and should be considered for administration in children <7 years.

2.5. Influenza

Given the increased morbidity and mortality of influenza infection in transplant recipients, annual immunization with influenza vaccine is recommended regardless of the transplantation stage. While vaccine provided protective titers in <20% of subjects immunized in the first 2 years post-transplant, higher rates of seroconversion were reported for those immunized 2 years after transplantation [16, 17]. Annual influenza vaccination should also be provided routinely to all family members and close household contacts during each influenza season (Table 12-2). Given the poor antibody response to influenza immunization within the first 2 years of transplantation, chemoprophylaxis should be considered in addition to immunization during outbreaks of influenza in the community. The intranasally-administered live attenuated influenza vaccine (FluMist®) is indicated only for healthy individuals between 2 and 49 years of age. Since its administration to children <24 months resulted in increased rates of wheezing and hospitalization, it should not be given to patients whose immune systems are compromised.

2.6. Hepatitis B

Hepatitis B vaccination is recommended for all susceptible persons <18 years of age and for adults who have risk factors for hepatitis B virus infection. While there are little data on the response of immunocompromised hosts to hepatitis B vaccine, the Advisory Committee on Immunization Practices (ACIP) recommends that a high dose vaccine (40 mcg) be given to immunocompromised hosts. Hepatitis B vaccine is given as a 3-dose regimen to individuals <18 years of

Table 12-2. Immunization of family and healthcare workers of HSCT recipients.

Vaccine	Comments
Varicella	Should be administered to all susceptible HCW, household contacts who are not pregnant or immunocompromised.
Measles-mumps-rubella	Recommended for all persons ≥12 months and who are not pregnant or immunocompromised.
Polio	Not routinely recommended for adults, but if indicated IPV should be used.
Influenza	All household contacts of immunocompromised HSCT recipients should be immunized annually. Little data on safety of intranasally-administered live attenuated influenza vaccine (FluMist®) to family members of immunocompromised patients.
Rotavirus	No data on safety of this vaccine in setting of household contacts of immunocompromised patients.

Adapted from Goldberg et al [2]

age and in those with risk factors. Hepatitis B vaccine should be given at 12, 14 and 24 months post-transplantation. Testing for hepatitis B surface antigen antibody should be performed 1–2 months after the third dose of vaccine.

2.7. Polio

While poliomyelitis is a rare infection in the United States, polio may be acquired from visitors to the United States coming from those countries with endemic polio. In addition, there is the potential for contracting vaccine-related infection from children following receipt of the oral live attenuated vaccine. Following SCT, there is a continuous loss of antibody for up to 3 years with 25% of autologous patients and 100% of allogeneic SCT patients lacking protective levels of antibodies to the three polio serotypes [18]. Patients should receive three doses of inactivated polio vaccine (IPV) at 12, 14 and 24 months after transplantation which induces protective levels of antibody >80% of vaccines [12, 18]. In the absence of GVHD, immunization with IPV will provide protective levels to all three serotypes for up to 10 years [19]. Importantly, healthy children in the household of an immunocompromised patient should be immunized with IPV instead of the live attenuated polio vaccine (Table 12-2).

2.8. Measles, Mumps, Rubella

Following allogeneic SCT, most patients become seronegative for measles antibodies and vulnerable to measles infection. Immunization with live attenuated Measles, Mumps, Rubella (MMR) vaccine is recommended at 24 months post-transplant even though immunization in allogeneic transplant recipients without GVHD prior to 24 months appears to be safe [3, 12]. All pediatric subjects with allo- or autoSCT developed protective antibodies to measles following immunization [12]. MMR vaccination of close contacts is not contraindicated [7] (Table 12-2).

2.9. Additional Immunizations

Several vaccines are not recommended for routine administration, but should be considered in individual circumstances.

2.9.1. Hepatitis A

Routine hepatitis A vaccination is not recommended, either for the general population or for those with transplants, unless such individuals engage in high risk behavior or travel frequently to developing countries.

2.9.2. Meningococcus

There is limited data on their use in the allogeneic BMT/SCT population. Routine administration of the meningococcal vaccine is not indicated but should be considered for hematopoietic stem cell transplant (HSCT) recipients who live in or will travel to endemic areas. In one study, all pediatric recipients of allo- or autoSCT developed protective levels to meningococcal C conjugate vaccine [12].

2.9.3. Varicella

Although SCT recipients are at an increased risk of acquiring varicella infections, the use of this live attenuated vaccine is not recommended among SCT recipients until >24 months after SCT. Varicella-zoster reactivations occur in 20–50% of patients and require prompt antiviral therapy to avoid dissemination and post-herpetic neuralgia. Consequently, novel immunization strategies have been examined (see below).

2.10. Additional Considerations

HSCT recipients traveling to endemic areas for selected vaccine-preventable diseases may require additional immunizations; however, live attenuated vaccines (yellow fever, oral typhoid, and Bacillus Calmette-Guerin [BCG]) are contraindicated. Little data exists either on safety or efficacy of non-viable vaccines such as those for hepatitis A, Japanese B encephalitis, rabies, intramuscular typhoid, plague, or Lyme. Booster dose of IPV can be administered to those traveling to endemic areas.

2.10.1. Novel Immunization Strategies

Despite recommendations from various authorities, immunizations following SCT according to recommended guidelines often fail to induce protective antibody levels. Consequently, investigators have attempted novel strategies in an attempt to improve the immune response. One such approach in allogeneic transplantation is to immunize the donor at least 2 weeks prior to stem cell collection. Following the infusion of the allogeneic stem cells, immunization of recipients with the same vaccine may promote a better immune response; however, both the optimal timing and the number of immunizations have to be studied [13]. For autologous transplant patients, a markedly improved anti-pneumococcal antibody response was observed if the patient was immunized with PCV before stem cell collection and the harvested, vaccine-sensitized lymphocytes were activated and expanded ex vivo. These autologous lymphocytes were then administered before immunization with PCV 30 and 90 days post-transplant. These patients had a greatly enhanced antibody response compared to subjects similarly administered, activated, expanded before booster doses, but who were not immunized prior to lymphocyte harvest. [21].

Given both the frequency and morbidity of *Varicella zoster* infections after transplantation, preventive strategies are highly desirable. An effective varicella vaccine is available; however, since it is a live attenuated virus vaccine, it is not recommended for SCT within the first 24 months post-transplantation. Using a heat-inactivated version of the live attenuated vaccine with apparently preserved immunogenic epitopes, Hata and colleagues demonstrated that an intensive course of immunization in the first 90 days after transplantation led to a decrease in infection and attenuation of symptoms in those with breakthrough disease. Furthermore, there was in vitro evidence of a cellular immune response. [20].

3. Immunization in the Non-transplant Setting

3.1. Acute Lymphoblastic Leukemia

Most studies of immunization in non-SCT patients focus on children with leukemia, particularly those with acute lymphoblastic leukemia (ALL). While leukemia itself may modify the adaptive immune response, chemotherapy leads to a decrease in B and T lymphocyte numbers and a decrease in the IgM and IgG levels (particularly IgG2). Recovery of lymphocyte function usually occurs within 6 months.

Eight studies published since 1980 reported vaccination data of children with ALL. These studies generally observed that while pre-existing antibody levels to vaccine-preventable diseases declined during chemotherapy [22], some vaccine-induced antibody levels were preserved [23]. These differences are likely due to the severity of the underlying disease and the intensity of chemotherapy regimen. As >80% of ALL patients respond to immunization following chemotherapy [23, 24], revaccination is warranted. Current US guidelines recommend initiation of a multi-dose revaccination at 3 months after completion of chemotherapy, while British guidelines recommend revaccination with a single dose of vaccine at 6 months after completion of therapy [24]. These recommendations are based primarily on expert opinion and data from relatively few studies.

Since safety of toxoids and inactivated vaccines in the pediatric ALL population is well-documented, several immunogenicity studies have been undertaken. After vaccination of children with ALL against HIB, tetanus and diphtheria, high risk patients (leukocyte count $>50 \times 10^9\,L^{-1}$ with either CNS and/or testicular involvement or T cell leukemia) had poor antibody responses which correlated with low numbers of memory B cells after marrow recovery [25]. All standard (leukocyte count $<10 \times 10^9\,L^{-1}$ and absence of high risk criteria) and intermediate risk (leukocyte count between 10 and $50 \times 10^9\,L^{-1}$ and lacking high risk criteria) patients developed fully protective antibody levels. In general, children treated for leukemia had less robust responses to re-immunization with childhood vaccines than patients treated for solid tumors [23]. In contrast to HIB, tetanus, and diphtheria vaccines, immune responses to measles and mumps vaccination has been more variable. Responses to DPT and/or measles/mumps vaccines were studied in 37 newly diagnosed childhood ALL patients and in 14 healthy controls [26]. After vaccination, all 37 ALL patients either on maintenance chemotherapy or off therapy for 3–6 months developed anti-diphtheria and anti-tetanus toxoid antibody responses, but only 66% developed significantly lower antibody levels to pertussis compared to healthy controls. Responses to measles and mumps vaccinations were not different from the control subjects. Variably protective responses to measles and mumps vaccines may be due to the high prevalence of humoral immune defects, unrelated to specific chemotherapeutic regimens in ALL patients in remission at least 1 year after completion of chemotherapy [27]. In a study of hepatitis B immunization, approximately one-third of children undergoing maintenance chemotherapy for ALL developed a protective response after three doses [28].

A large number of studies have been published on the safety and efficacy of influenza and pneumococcal vaccines in ALL patients, even for those undergoing anti-neoplastic treatment. Trivalent influenza subunit vaccine is safe in children with ALL and produces a significant response in about 50–60% of immunized children [29–31]. In a recent study of influenza immunization, children receiving maintenance chemotherapy for ALL responded with a lower geometric mean antibody titer (GMT) than healthy children. However, most children with ALL showed a fourfold rise in hemagglutination inhibition (HAI) antibody titers, which is considered protective [32]. In another study [33], children with ALL had a higher seroconversion rate to influenza vaccination when off chemotherapy for at least 1 month (and with a peripheral white blood cell count of >1,000). The antibody seroconversion rate was less if ALL patients were immunized during chemotherapy administration rather than between courses [34].

Children with ALL have a 10-fold higher risk for invasive pneumococcal infection than the general pediatric population. Much of this risk occurs during maintenance chemotherapy [35]. These children have suboptimal responses to 14-valent PPV [36]. To date, there are few reports of PCV in children with ALL.

For the purpose of live virus vaccines, patients with leukemia in remission and off chemotherapy for 3 months or longer are not considered to be severely immunocompromised [7]. With the availability of IPV, concern for live attenuated virus vaccines is limited largely to the Oka strain varicella vaccine. Interestingly, the Oka vaccine for varicella was licensed originally for use in immunocompromised children in Japan, Korea, and some European countries. FDA indications allowed the vaccine to be used in leukemic children in remission for at least 1 year on an individual basis. The child should have a total peripheral lymphocyte count of ≥700 cells per mm^3 on the day of immunization, and anti-leukemic chemotherapy should be withheld for 1 week prior to and 1 week after immunization. Further, no steroid therapy should be given for 2 weeks after vaccination. While two doses of vaccine are administered at 3-month interval, it is not necessary to withhold chemotherapy after the first dose. If children develop ≥50 skin lesions after immunization, they should be treated with acyclovir. Live attenuated varicella vaccine has approximately 90% efficacy in leukemic children [3]. In an analysis of 511 children with ALL who were vaccinated against chicken pox, the risk of subsequent development of zoster was decreased [37].

The timing of immunization is a critical factor in inducing an antibody response. Patel et al [24] immunized 59 children 6 months after completion of standard chemotherapy for ALL with HIB, tetanus, diphtheria, acellular pertussis, meningococcus C, polio, measles, vaccines (a pneumococcal vaccine was not given). A single revaccination resulted in significant increase in the antibody levels to each vaccine antigen. Optimal antibody titers were achieved against tetanus in 100%, 93% for HIB, 94% for measles, 96% for meningococcus C, 85% for all three polioviruses, A decline in antibody levels was observed at 12 months following immunization with all vaccines; however, the levels remained in the protective range for all patients with HIB, tetanus, measles immunization, but in only 47% for all three serotypes with polio immunization.

4. Immunization in Other Oncology Patient Populations

There are far fewer studies conducted on immunization responses in oncology patients other than stem cell transplant recipients and children with ALL. Because of the relative frequency of invasive pneumococcal disease in both the general and in the immunocompromised patients, and the potentially life-threatening consequences of these infections, much attention has been focused on the ability of pneumococcal vaccines to induce potentially protective antibody responses in the oncology population. PPV is effective in preventing infection caused by vaccine serotypes in non-oncology patients with asplenia, an established risk factor for invasive pneumococcal disease, but was not protective in adult patients with lymphoma, leukemia or multiple myeloma [38]. In contrast, patients with solid tumors respond with antibody levels similar to healthy controls. [39]. Adult lymphoma patients treated with chemotherapy have poor antibody responses to 23-valent PPV. Patients with chronic lymphocytic leukemia (CLL) have even lower antibody levels.

In adult patients with B-cell CLL, immunization raised the antibody levels to the protective range from 38% pre-immunization to 50% with the 23-valent PPV, and from 35% pre-immunization to 48% with the conjugated HIB vaccine. Response was correlated with less advanced diseases [40]. Adult patients with either solid tumors or lymphoreticular neoplasms had a decreased frequency of greater than fourfold response to inactivated influenza vaccine and lower levels of antibody compared to healthy controls [41]. Influenza vaccine is also effective and well-tolerated in adult patients with chronic lymphoproliferative disorders and multiple myeloma [41].

5. Future Directions

Studies to date demonstrate that revaccination of patients following either chemotherapy for malignant diseases or following HSCT will induce increases in antibody levels that appear to persist over time. Few studies of vaccine efficacy have been reported, however. These data along with the safety profile of these vaccines suggest that universal immunization may be a more cost-effective approach than testing of individual patients for specific antibody levels. Current immunization guidelines, particularly for HSCT patients, recommend initiation relatively late following therapy, thereby exposing the patient to potential risks of infection in the early post-transplantation period. Recent studies have investigated novel and often more intensive immunization regimens early in the post-HSCT period. Although new vaccine adjuvants are being rapidly developed, there are no studies assessing their ability to enhance the immune response to vaccines in the oncology population. Further studies are needed to determine whether increasing the antigenic dose(s) of vaccines for routine immunization of immunocompromised hosts may lead to an improved antibody response, as has been suggested for hepatitis B. In the coming years, studies using simplified immunization schedules or novel immunization strategies in combination with new adjuvants may lead to more effective immunization practices in this patient population. These efforts must be accompanied by an examination of the impact of newer oncologic therapeutic regimens on the immune response, particularly those agents that modulate the immune system such as fludarabine and lenalidomide. For example, treatment of patients with relapsed, low-grade lymphoma with the chimeric CD20 monoclonal antibody (rituximab) resulted in a decreased humoral immune response to primary and recall antigens (42). Thus, as therapies improve patient survival, considerably more studies will be required to determine the optimal strategies for restoring antibody levels for vaccine-preventable diseases.

References

1. Avigan D, Pirofski L-A, Lazarus HM (2001) Vaccination against infectious disease following hematopoietic stem cell transplantation. Biol Blood Marrow Transplant 7:171–183
2. Antin JH (2002) Long-term care after hematopoietic-cell transplantation in adults. N Engl J Med 347:36–42
3. Ambrosino DM, Molrine DC (1993) Critical appraisal of immunization strategies for prevention of infection in the compromised host. In infectious complications in the immunocompromised host II. Hematol Oncol Clin North Am 7:1027–1050
4. Goldberg SL, Cicogna CE, Rowley SD, Pecora AL (2003) Vaccinations against infectious diseases in hematologic stem cell transplant recipients. Oncology 17: 539–559
5. Henning KJ, White MH, Sepkowitz KA, Armstrong D (1997) A national survey of immunization practices following allogeneic bone marrow transplantation. JAMA 277:1148–1151
6. Ljungman P, Engelhard D, de la Camara R, Einsele H, Locasciulli A, Martino R, Ribaud P, Ward K, Cordonnier C, Infectious Diseases Working Party of the European Group for Blood and Bone Marrow Transplantation (2005) Vaccination of stem cell transplant recipients: recommendations of the Infectious Diseases Working Party of the EBMT. Bone Marrow Transplant 35:737–746
7. (2000) Guidelines for preventing opportunistic infections among hematopoietic stem cell transplant recipients: recommendations of Centers for Disease Control and Prevention, the Infectious Disease Society of America, and the American Society of Blood and Marrow Transplantation. MMWR Recomm Rep 49(RR-10):1–125, CE-17
8. Engelhard D, Cordonnier C, Shaw PJ et al (2002) Early and late invasive pneumococcal infection following stem cell transplantation: a European Bone Marrow Transplant survey. Br J Haematol 117:444–450
9. Avanzini MA, Carra AM, Maccario R, Zecca M, Pignatti P, Marconi M, Comoli P, Bonetti F, DeStefano P, Locatelli F (1995) Antibody response to pneumococcal vaccine in children receiving bone marrow transplantation. J Clin Immunol 15:137–144
10. Guinan EC, Molrine DC, Antin JH, Lee MC, Weinstein HJ, Sallan SE, Parsons SK, Wheeler C, Gross W, McGarigle C et al (1994) Polysaccharide conjugate vaccine responses in bone marrow transplant patients. Transplantation 57:677–684
11. Antin JH, Guinan EC, Avigan D, Soiffer RJ, Joyce RM, Martin VJ, Molrine DC (2005) Protective antibody responses to pneumococcal conjugate vaccine after autologous hematopoietic stem cell transplantation. Biol Blood Marrow Transplant 11:213–222
12. Patel SR, Ortin M, Cohen BJ, Borrow R, Irving D, Sheldon J, Heath PT (2007) Revaccination with measles, tetanus, poliovirus, Haemophilus influenzae type B, meningococcus C, and pneumococcus vaccines in children after hematopoietic stem cell transplantation. Clin Infect Dis 44:625–634
13. Gottlieb DJ, Cryz SJ Jr, Furer E, Que J, Prentice HG, Duncombe AS, Brenner MK (1990) Immunity against *Pseudomonas aeruginosa* adoptively transferred to bone marrow transplant recipients. Blood 76:2470–2475
14. Kumar D, Chen MH, Welsh B, Siegal D, Cobos I, Messner HA, Lipton J, Humar A (2007) A randomized, double-blind trial of pneumococcal vaccination in adult allogeneic stem cell transplant donors and recipients. Clin Infect Dis 45:1576–1582
15. Barra A, Cordonnier C, Presiosi MP, Intrator L, Hessel L, Fritzell B, Preud'homme JL (1992) Immunogenicity of Haemophilus influenzae type b conjugate vaccine in allogeneic bone marrow recipients. J Infect Dis 166:1021–1028

16. Engelhard D, Nagler A, Hardan I, Morag A, Aker M, Baciu H, Strauss N, Parag G, Naparstek E, Ravid Z et al (1993) Antibody response to a two-dose regimen of influenza vaccine in allogeneic T cell-depleted and autologous BMT recipients. Bone Marrow Transplant 11:1–5
17. Gandhi MK, Egner W, Sizer L, Inman I, Zambon M, Craig JIO, Marcus RE (2001) Antibody responses to vaccinations given within the first two years after transplant are similar between autologous peripheral blood stem cell and bone marrow transplant recipients. Bone Marrow Transplant 28:775–781
18. Pauksen K, Hammarstrom V, Ljungman P, Sjolin J, Oberg G, Lonnerholm L, Mangius L, Simonsson B (1994) Immunity to poliovirus and immunization with inactivated poliovirus vaccine after autologous bone marrow transplantation. Clin Infect Dis 18:547–552
19. Ljungman P, Aschan J, Gustafsson B, Lewensohn-Fuchs I, Winiarski J, Ringden O (2004) Long-term immunity to poliovirus after vaccination of allogeneic stem cell transplant recipients. Bone Marrow Transplant 34:1067–1069
20. Rapoport AP, Stadtmauer EA, Aqui N, Badros A, Cotte J et al (2005) Restoration of immunity in lymphopenic individuals with cancer by vaccination and adoptive T-cell transfer. Nat Med 11:1230–1237
21. Hata A, Asanuma H, Rinki M, Sharp M, Wong RM, Blumek K, Arvin AM (2002) Use of inactivated varicella vaccine in recipients of hematopoietic stem cell transplantation. N Engl J Med 347:26–34
22. Van Tilburg CM, Sanders EA, Rovers MM, Wolfs TF, Bierings MB (2006) Loss of antibodies and response to (re)-vaccination in children after treatment for acute lymphocytic leukemia: a systematic review. Leukemia 20:1717–1722
23. Ridgway D, Wolff LJ (1993) Active immunization of children with leukemia and other malignancies. Leuk Lymphoma 9:177–192
24. Patel SR, Ortin M, Choen BJ, Borrow R, Irving D, Sheldon J, Heath PT (2007) Revaccination of children after completion of standard chemotherapy for acute leukemia. Clin Infect Dis 44:635–642
25. Ek T, Mellander L, Hahn-Zoric M, Abrahamsson J (2004) Intensive treatment for chilhood acute lymphoblastic leukemia reduces immune responses to diphtheria, tetanus, and Haeumophilus influenzae type b. J Pediatr Hematol Oncol 26: 727–734
26. Ercan TE, Soycan LYm Apak H, Celkan T, Ozkan A, Akdenizli E, Kasapcopur O, Yildiz I (2005) Antibody titers and immune response to diphtheria-tetanus-pertussis and measles-mumps-rubella vaccination in children treated for acute lymphoblastic leukemia. J Pediatr Hematol Oncol 27:273–277
27. Brodtman DH, Rosenthal DW, Redner A, Lanzkowsky P, Bonagura VR (2005) Immunodeficency in children with acute lymphoblastic leukemia after completion of modern aggressive chemotherapeutic regimens. J Pediatr 146:654–661
28. Yetgin S, Tunc B, Koc A, Toksoy HB, Ceyhan M, Kanra G (2001) Two booster dose hepatitis virus vaccination in patients with leukemia. Leuk Res 25:647–649
29. Brydak LB, Rokicka-Milewska R, Machala M, Jackowska T, Sikorska-Fic B (1998) Immunogenicity of subunit trivalent influenza vaccine in children with acute luymphoblastic leukemia. Pediatr Infect Dis 17:125–129
30. Chisholm JC, Devine T, Charlett A, Pinkerton CR, Zambon M (2001) Response to influenza immunization during treatment for cancer. Arch Dis Child 84:496–500
31. Hsieh YC, Lu MY, Kao CL, Chiang BL, Liln DT, Lin KS, Huang LM (2002) Response to influenza vaccine in children with leukemia undergoing chemotherapy. J Formos Med Assoc 101:700–704
32. Porter CC, Edwards KM, Zhu Y, Frangoul H (2004) Immune responses to influenza immunization in children receiving maintenance chemotherapy for acute lymphoblastic leukemia. Pediatr Blood Cancer 42:36–40
33. Gross PA, Lee H, Wolff JA, Hall CB, Minnefore AB, Lazicki ME (1978) Influenza immunization in immunosuppressed children. J Pediatr 92:30–35

34. Ortbals DW, Liebhaber H, Presant CA, Van Amburg AL, Lee JY (1977) Influenza immunization of adult patients with malignant diseases. Ann Intern Med 87: 552–557
35. Meisel R, Toschke AM, Heiligensetzer C, Dilloo D, Laws HJ, von Kries R (2007) Increased risk for invasive pneumococcal diseases in children with acute lymphoblastic leukemia. Br J Haematol 137:457–460
36. Feldman S, Malone W, Wilbur R, Schiffman G (1985) Pneumococcal vaccination in children with acute lymphocytic leukemia. Med Pediatr Oncol 13:69–72
37. Gershon AA, LaRussa P, Steinberg S, Mervish N, Lo SH, Meier P (1996) The protective effect of immunologic boosting against zoster: an analysis in leukemic children who were vaccinated against chickenpox. J Infect Dis 173:450–453
38. Butler JC, Breiman RF, Campbell JF, Lipman HB, Broome CV, Facklam RR (1993) Pneumococcal polysaccharide vaccine efficacy. An evaluation of current recommendations. JAMA 270:1826–1831
39. Shildt RA, Boyd JF, McCracken JD, Schiffman G, Gioima JP (1983) Antibody response to pneumococcal vaccine in patients with solid tumors and lymphomas. Med Pediatr Oncol 11:305–309
40. Hartkamp A, Mulder AH, Rijkers GT, van Velzen-Blad H, Biesma DH (2001) Antibody responses to pneumococcal and haemophilus vaccinations in patients with B-cell chronic lymphocytic leukemia. Vaccine 19:1671–1677
41. Rapezzi D, Sticchi L, Racchi O, Mangerini R, Ferraris AM, Gaetani GF (2003) Influenza vaccine in chronic lymphoproliferative disorders and multiple myeloma. Eur J Haematol 70:225–230
42. van der Kolk LE, Baars JW, Prins MH, van Oers MH (2002) Rituximab treatment results in impaired secondary humoral immune responsiveness. Blood 100: 2257–2259

Chapter 13

Issues in Anti-infective Management

Graeme N. Forrest and Michael Kleinberg

Abstract Early antimicrobial therapy to patients with hematologic malignancies has been shown to improve their survival and outcomes. Structured properly, an institution-wide anti-infective program can improve the efficient management of infections with minimized toxicities in a cost-effective manner. Program objectives should encompass standardized approaches to antimicrobial prescribing, systems that can predict potentially dangerous therapeutic toxicities, and monitoring to assess outcome successes. This is ever more critical with the emergence of antimicrobial resistant organisms, newer expensive antimicrobial agents, and the significant drug interactions between anti-infectives and chemotherapeutic agents. Patients with HIV-associated malignancies represent a special challenge because of the complexities involved in managing two concurrent diseases and the potential for drug interactions potentiating toxicities between highly active antiretroviral therapy (HAART) and many chemotherapy agents.

Keywords Anti-infective management • Cost-effectiveness • Drug interactions • Drug safety • Computerized support • HIV-related malignancies

1. Establishing an Infectious Diseases Program for Patients with Hematological Malignancies

The subjects of many of the preceding chapters have focused on optimizing treatments of infections in individual patients with hematological malignancies. The essence of this practice is the presence of an experienced clinician at the patient's bedside, making a timely diagnosis, prescribing treatment, and monitoring the patient for successful outcome. To achieve this objective, the clinician draws upon his/her own experience and the medical literature. However, this ideal image contrasts with the reality that clinical care to patients with hematological malignancies usually is provided by a team zists includes hematologists and other physician specialists, nurses, nurse practitioners, nursing extenders, nutritionists, pharmacists, and respiratory therapists. The clinical care team is supported, in turn, by staff in hematology, pathology, chemistry,

From: *Managing Infections in Patients With Hematological Malignancies*: Contemporary Hematology, Edited by: M. Kleinberg, DOI 10.1007/978-1-59745-415-5_12,

and microbiology laboratories and in radiology, surgical oncology, and radiation oncology departments. The objective of this section is to explore several aspects of coordinating effectively this dedicated team at an institutional level for optimal management of infections in patients with hematological malignancies. Instituting an effective infection control program has been discussed already in Chap. 11 and infection prevention through vaccination in Chap. 12.

It is an indisputable fact that antimicrobial agents, used for prevention and treatment of infections in patients with hematologic malignancies, have been a major factor in improving survival despite intensified antineoplastic therapies [1–4]. There are numerous guidelines from various worldwide societies regarding the appropriate management of febrile neutropenia with antimicrobials [5–8]. Emergence of drug resistant bacteria and fungi in patients with hematologic malignancies, and the demand for cost-containment and patient safety emphasizes the need for a formally structured program to manage infections in these patients [9–15]. Patients with hematological malignancies, who receive intensive chemotherapy or hematopoietic stem cell transplantation (HSCT), are treated in cancer centers that specialize in the complexities of these disorders. This "closed" system is well-suited to development and implementation of center-wide protocols for managing infectious diseases.

In majority of centers, inpatient physician services are provided by a limited number of hematologists who attend on leukemia/stem cell transplant services for 2–4 weeks at a time. This model is efficient for managing the inpatient population as a whole even though some individual patients with prolonged inpatient stays may be treated by several attendings. However, the numbers of clinical staff are relatively small and staff composition is stable. Therefore, it is possible within this defined group to build consensus, educate and inform, monitor implementation, assess compliance and outcomes, and update infectious disease management strategies. Ideally, a cancer center infectious diseases team should have one or more clinicians with training in infectious diseases and extensive experience in the hematological malignancies/HSCT clinical arena in leadership positions. The leader of the infectious diseases team does not need to be formally trained in infectious diseases as training in infectious diseases varies considerably in the United States, Europe, and the rest of the world. In addition, prominence of many non-formally trained experts at important academic cancer centers around the world shows clearly that the necessary expertise can be acquired by committed hematologists in the course of years of clinical practice [6–8].

Regardless of the particulars of training, familiarity with treating infections in neutropenic patients and HSCT recipients, even if extensive, is necessary but insufficient by itself. Leaders of the infectious diseases team need to have a broad and deep understanding of the pathogens that cause infections and the anti-infectives used to fight them. As will be discussed below, knowledge of "bugs and drugs" is crucial for designing optimal treatment strategies and managing toxicities, side effects, and drug interactions of anti-infectives. Establishing a team approach to management of infected patients has many benefits including development of guidelines specific for the institution, optimizing antimicrobial treatment for successful outcomes, reducing emergence of resistant pathogens, implementing a cancer center anti-infective stewardship program, and performing infection control practices. Other goals include developing mechanisms to shorten safely lengths of hospital stays, outpatient therapies, containing costs, and developing research programs [6, 16–18]. The goal is to standardize many aspects of anti-infective therapy, taking into account the hematological malignancies in the patient population, the intensities of chemotherapy and conditioning regimens, GVHD management strategies, and the prevalence and resistance patterns of pathogens in the individual institution. Several aspects of the infectious diseases guidelines may apply universally, such as initial antibiotics for neutropenic leukemia patients or HSCT recipients. Some aspects of the guidelines may be stratified by risk, such as antibacterial and antifungal prophylaxis for patients with the highest likelihood of becoming infected. Guidelines may also encompass a standard approach to ordering and interpreting diagnostic tests and setting thresholds for requesting invasive studies such as fiberoptic bronchoscopy. Guidelines are best developed from a wide range of inputs received from all clinicians drawing on broad experiences in oncology and infectious diseases. Cooperative development of agreed upon guidelines is likely to restrict the practices outside the norm by individual clinicians (except for specific circumstances), thereby simplifying the oversight of infectious diseases practice of the oncology unit [6, 16–18].

Information on viral, bacterial, and fungal infections, as well as influences of particular hematological malignancies on infections, have been discussed extensively in preceding chapters. This information can serve as the foundation on which approaches to infectious diseases management, best suited to individual institutions, are synthesized. The remainder of this section will be devoted to implementing the infectious diseases management plan.

2. Microbiology Laboratory

The importance of the effective use of the microbiology laboratory as a critical piece in the management of patients with hematologic malignancies cannot be overstated. A central theme running through the preceding chapters is the importance of anticipating the range of infections that occur in patients with hematological malignancies. Many times reacting to a report of a positive culture from the microbiology laboratory is a failure, potentially representing a delay in providing treatment. The microbiology laboratory on site is central for early diagnosis of infections, for determining cancer center-specific susceptibility patterns, and for developing methods for efficient surveillance programs [2, 19–22]. This is becoming more complicated because many hospitals have been outsourcing infrequently ordered microbiology tests to outside reference laboratories as part of cost-containment and quality control efforts. Unfortunately, these infrequently ordered microbiology tests are requested disproportionately in diagnosis of infections in patients with hematological malignancies. This outsourcing may affect clinical decision making in high risk patients, especially if there is a delay in reporting results [23].

2.1. Antibiotic Susceptibility Determinations

It would be prudent to understand the susceptibility patterns of *Enterococci*, *Staphylococcus aureus*, enteric gram-negative rods, *Pseudomonas aeruginosa*, and other select bacteria before any cancer center guidelines are developed. Susceptibility patterns are expressed in an antibiogram which tabulates percentages of bacteria that are sensitive to different antibiotics. Susceptibility patterns for pathogenic bacteria in a cancer center usually differ from hospital-wide patterns. A central, hospital-wide antibiogram may be of no benefit because it may not be driven by the same antibiotic practices as in the cancer center, and may mislead physicians into believing there is lower or higher resistance to a specific antimicrobial [24, 25]. This is particularly true if quinolone prophylaxis is used and there is an under-reporting of Gram-negative quinolone resistance in the hospital-wide antibiogram [24, 26]. Therefore, cancer center-specific antibiograms should be formulated [17, 24, 25]. The antibiogram should represent a single culture from a single site per admission and not report multiple cultures from the same site to limit multiple counting biases [18, 24, 27]. Unfortunately, most cancer centers will need to compile susceptibility data over several years to have a statistically meaning sample size. Such a cancer center-specific antibiogram will be relatively insensitive to trends in susceptibility changes over time. The antibiogram should be updated yearly, be readily available, and should reflect the formulary antibiotics actually used by the institution [18, 27]. Lastly, patterns of susceptibilities of *Candida* species to fluconazole should also be tabulated, especially with the increased use of azoles such as fluconazole in HSCT recipients and in leukemia patients [28–30].

The role of surveillance cultures for bacteria and yeasts from patients with hematological malignancies as a guide to antimicrobial selection remains controversial, with much of the data of its benefit coming from studies that are over 30 years old [14, 19, 31]. There has not been any determination of the cost-effectiveness of these cultures in guiding specific treatment of patients. However, cost-effectiveness in screening and isolating patients for vancomycin-resistant *Enterococcus* (VRE) and methicillin-resistant *Staphylococcus aureus* (MRSA) has been well established [21, 22, 32]. With increasing mandate for active surveillance of VRE and MRSA, especially with polymerase chain reaction (PCR) technology, there is likely to be increased screening in all hospital patients, including those with hematological malignancies, with an unknown clinical benefit [33, 34].

2.2. Rapid Diagnostic Testing

There has been, and continues to be, rapid progress in developing rapid testing methods to detect and identify pathogens, and determine their anti-infective susceptibilities. A thorough discussion is beyond the scope of this chapter but those who specialize in treating infections in patients with hematological malignancies will have to become well-versed in the capabilities and limitations of the new methods. *Aspergillus* galactomannan and pan-fungal β-glucan antigen detection assays have already been discussed in Chap. 4. Similarly, antigen and PCR testing for herpes viruses, influenza and other respiratory viruses, etc. has been discussed in Chap. 2. This section will cover new laboratory technologies used for early rapid identification of organisms in blood cultures. Currently, real-time PCR (RT-PCR) remains experimental but a number of peptide nucleic acid fluorescent in situ hybridization (PNA FISH) probes have been approved for use in the USA, Canada and Europe [35].

RT-PCR offers the most sensitive testing and can be performed directly from blood, potentially making a pathogen diagnosis earlier than could be detected with conventional blood cultures. However, PCR lacks specificity because the method does not distinguish between DNA from living and non-living microbes. Specific methods have been developed that can detect specific resistance genes in bacteria and yeasts, and those targeting MRSA and *P. aeruginosa* from blood cultures are closest to commercial use [35–39]. RT-PCR requires a major commitment from the microbiology laboratory, specifically a clean room space to avoid contamination by microbial DNA from the rest of the laboratory and expenses of equipment purchase and reagents [36, 40].

PNA FISH species-specific probes hybridize with 16S ribosomal RNA targets within bacteria and 26S rRNA in yeasts [35]. PNA-FISH can only be performed off positive blood cultures after the Gram-stain is reported and, therefore, has lower sensitivity (10^4 organisms) than RT-PCR. However, PNA-FISH has greater specificity as it detects living bacteria in the blood cultures, and whose retained morphological shape assists in diagnosis [35]. There are presently three FDA-approved probes available for commercial use that detect *S. aureus*, *Candida albicans/glabrata* and *Enterococci faecalis* and other enterococci. Results can be reported to physicians within 3 h of the blood culture turning positive and leads to more targeted appropriate therapy 1 or 2 days sooner compared to conventional culturing methods [41, 42]. The early detection of VRE in patients with hematologic malignancies with the *E. faecalis* and other enterococci PNA FISH test has demonstrated improved patient survival [35]. Also, distinguishing between *S. aureus* and coagulase-negative staphylococci often leads to salvaging long-term intravenous catheters with vancomycin rather than removal [43]. Future PNA FISH probes that identify other candida species, *P. aeruginosa*, and other Gram-negative bacteria are under development, and would be very useful in managing infections in patients with hematological malignancies.

3. Anti-infective Stewardship Program

Treatment of infections is unique compared to treating other diseases because the majority of anti-infective prescriptions are written by non-specialist clinicians, with sometimes minimal training in infectious diseases. Many hospitals have developed anti-infective stewardship programs to manage in real-time anti-infective prescribing practices by staff clinicians. The driving forces behind these programs is cost containment, infection control for resistant pathogens, and increasingly, adherence to best practices for sentinel infections increasingly mandated by outside advisory and governmental bodies [16, 17, 27]. Changes in anti-infective management of many infections can save substantial sums, particularly in cancer centers which treat large numbers of patients with hematological malignancies.

Most of the literature regarding anti-infective stewardship describes experiences with hospital-wide programs [16, 17, 27]. Often cancer centers are excluded from hospital-wide anti-infective stewardship programs because of the complexities of managing infections and the heavy use of antimicrobial therapies in patients with hematological malignancies. However, because mould-active antifungals and several antivirals are expensive, incorporation of the cancer center into the hospital-wide anti-infective stewardship program is required to attain meaningful cost controls [17]. Adaptation of the hospital-wide program should recognize issues unique to the cancer center such as local pathogen resistance patterns, host factors (leukemia versus lymphoma versus stem cell transplantation), and prophylaxis requirements as discussed above [17]. Administrative support for an anti-infective stewardship program is critical for success. Support should be both financial (to cover non-billable salaries) and administrative (encouraging/enforcing clinicians to accept the program and adhere to the developed guidelines) [27, 44–46]. Providing feedback on successful clinical and financial outcomes is an added incentive for clinicians to adhere to the overall infectious diseases management program [16].

The financial impact of inappropriate and ineffective antimicrobial therapy is well described [17, 27]. For patients with hematological malignancies, cost-containment becomes a consideration only after the most effective treatment strategies with the least toxicities have been determined. However, there are ways to minimize the financial impact of antimicrobial therapy. For instance, the best contract price for many anti-infectives can be negotiated if an institution restricts on its formulary only one amongst several equivalent agents, i.e., selecting one echinocandin or one lipid-formulated amphotericin B. For instance, targeting lipid amphotericin B formulations can result in tremendous reduction in costs, especially if converting to a cheaper formulation or to an echinocandin [12, 47, 48]. Another effective strategy is to implement intravenous to oral (IV-PO) switch guidelines that encourage conversion of an intravenous anti-infective to an equivalent, highly bioavailable oral alternative when there is no contraindication such as mucositis or diarrhea. The IV-PO formulary switch is probably the easiest to implement as it can be computerized and has been shown to result in significant cost-savings for quinolones and azoles [49, 50]. Cancer center anti-infective guidelines can promote efficient use of anti-infectives which also results in cost savings. For instance, guidelines can establish circumstances where anti-infectives are to be expanded in certain clinical situations, for instance, where a resistant bacterial pathogen is suspected. Standardizing the anti-infective escalation in guidelines can limit otherwise unnecessary combinations of antimicrobials, saving both cost and potential toxicity [6, 27, 51].

3.1. Role of Hospital Pharmacy

The hospital pharmacy plays a critical role in ensuring that anti-infectives necessary for treating the range of infections seen in hematological malignancies are stocked as formulary agents or readily available from outside sources [27, 52, 53]. The pharmacy may also have important financial interests in choosing between equivalent anti-infectives depending on negotiated best prices for competing agents [27, 52]. Recent trends to reduce pharmaceutical ordering and infusion errors by hospital staff has led to pharmacy changes with the removal of anti-infectives stored on inpatient floors. The intent is to ensure that every prescription is reviewed by a pharmacist for correct dosing, non-conflict with patient allergies, and advance identification of potential drug–drug interactions. As laudable as these policy changes may be, centralizing anti-infective dispensing in the main pharmacy with no or limited emergency storage on the clinical floors potentially may interpose a dangerous delay in delivering an anti-infective to a febrile, neutropenic patient. Therefore, pharmacies must develop mechanisms for identifying instantly anti-infective orders for cancer center patients, providing the agent to nursing staff, and infusing the anti-infective into the patient all within a short time interval. Pharmacies must also have quality control systems to examine the timely delivery of anti-infectives, monitor compliance with treatment guidelines, and monitor drug use for therapeutics and safety.

In most anti-infective stewardship programs, an infectious disease clinical pharmacist (IDCP) is the central figure in day-to-day operations. The role of the IDCP is to coordinate the program serving as a liaison between the hospital pharmacy, infectious disease leadership in the cancer center, and clinical hematologists and oncologists. The IDCP also is the primary educator for other clinical pharmacists, monitors formulary and non-formulary drug use, and ensures that antimicrobial use is safe and effective [18, 27, 54]. The IDCP should be involved in formulary decisions and implementation of guidelines and is an important voice for what is realistically feasible [54]. Some centers struggle with finding an acceptable method of financial support for the IDCP since cost savings associated with a successful anti-infective stewardship program may not benefit directly whoever pays (hospital pharmacy vs. cancer center) the IDCP salary. These financial decisions depend greatly on outcomes expected of the anti-infective stewardship program (cost-savings, safety, survival) and how these measures are quantified [16]. Supervision of the IDCP varies amongst hospital anti-infective stewardship programs. In general, leadership of anti-infective stewardship programs is centered in the hospital pharmacy with different levels of clinical infectious diseases supervision and participation [17].

3.2. Anti-infective Approval Approaches

Virtually all hospital anti-infective stewardship programs divide the antimicrobial formulary into restricted and non-restricted lists. This division is inadequate for cancer centers as many of the anti-infectives needed by patients with hematological malignancies will be on the hospital restricted list. Hospitals regulate the use of restricted agent by a preapproval process (where a gatekeeper pharmacist or infectious diseases clinician permits use of the restricted agent), a post-prescription review (where permission is required to continue use of the restricted agent beyond 24 h), or a combination of both [16, 17, 27]. Potential delays in rapid initiation of antibiotic therapy to patients with hematological malignancies make the preapproval process of restricted anti-infective through a hospital-wide anti-infective stewardship program a risky proposition and hard to justify [16]. For hospitals that use a preapproval process, there must either be a provision to exempt cancer center requests for restricted agents from the hospital-wide program or to maintain a separate restricted/non-restricted list for the cancer center. Preapproval processes may be as simple as proscriptive, sometimes to the point of being coercive, strict adherence to restricted anti-infective lists with no individual patient care by the gatekeeper [16]. Ideally, cancer centers benefit most when those who preapprove restricted anti-infective requests participate at some level in clinical management of infected patients. Depending on the institution, problems with the cancer center preapproval process may be minimized through computerized order entry for anti-infectives, which has been shown to control costs and direct appropriate therapy as well [55]. Unfortunately, there can be other serious problems with a preapproval system which are beyond the scope of this chapter [16].

Post-prescription monitoring, especially with computerized support, has been very effective in intensive care units as well as in the general hospital setting [51, 56]. Automated alerting systems can assist the IDCP when there is excess antimicrobial coverage, granulocyte recovery, potential for IV-PO conversion, and predefined significant drug–drug interactions [51, 56]. These interventions have been shown to improve cost-savings, decrease antimicrobial resistance, as well as reduce toxicity and improve safety for the patient [44]. Moreover, gatekeepers for post-prescription monitoring are more likely to be involved with individual patient care. A major advantage of post-prescription monitoring is to ensure appropriate antimicrobial coverage, dosing, length of therapy, and absence of drug–drug interactions with chemotherapeutic agents and immunosuppressives [57]. The importance of proper dosing of anti-infectives for patients with renal and hepatic dysfunction cannot be overemphasized, particularly since renal and hepatic dysfunction in patients with hematological malignancies is common and can change on a day-to-day basis.

4. Managing Anti-infective Toxicities and Drug–Drug Interactions

Many patients with hematological malignancies receive multiple drugs and may already have impaired renal function, and with allogeneic stem cell transplantation may also have impaired liver function. As with chemotherapy and malignancy, infections are best treated when anti-infectives are administered at optimum doses for appropriate lengths of time. Unfortunately, the toxicities and side effects of many anti-infectives potentiate those of several chemotherapy agents. Clinicians must be mindful of these additive toxicities to minimize collateral harm to patients dually treated for both infection and malignancy. These toxicities are frequently encountered and their occurrences are predictable enough such that strategies for minimizing anti-infective/chemotherapeutic side effects should be developed within the context of a cancer center-wide infection management program.

Potential anti-infective-related side effects can be divided arbitrarily into three categories: direct toxicity from the anti-infective, synergistic worsening of toxicities shared by the anti-infective and chemotherapy agent, and potentiation of chemotherapy-specific toxicities by drug–drug interactions. In practice, these distinctions are usually blurred. However, anti-infective/chemotherapy toxicities can be managed effectively with awareness and experience.

4.1. Anti-infective Toxicities

It is beyond the scope of this chapter to enumerate all side effects of all anti-infectives likely to be used in treating infections in patients with hematological malignancies. However, potential for some anti-infectives to cause nephrotoxicity (Table 13-1) and to suppress bone marrow function (Table 13-2) deserve mention. Four anti-infectives, or classes of anti-infectives, are notorious for causing renal failure in high percentages of treated patients; aminoglycosides, amphotericin B formulations, foscarnet, and cidofovir. Aminoglycosides are third-line anti-Gram-negative bacterial agents and are used primarily to treat infections resistant to first-line antibiotics. Nephrotoxicity can be minimized with once daily dosing and with serum drug monitoring [58].

Table 13-1. Anti-infectives that cause nephrotoxicity.

Agent
Amphotericin B (all formulations)
Aminoglycosides Gentamicin, amikacin, tobramycin
Cidofovir Foscarnet
Polymixins
Pentamidine
Tenofovir
Sulfa derivatives
Vancomycin

Table 13-2. Anti-infectives that suppress bone marrow function.

Agent
Ganciclovir
Zidovudine
Linezolid
Pentamidine
Flucytosine
Sulfa derivatives
Chloramphenicol

Lipid-formulations of amphotericin B are significantly less nephrotoxic than amphotericin B deoxycholate. Hydration and salt loading prior to infusion is thought by many to reduce nephrotoxicity. Amphotericin B preparations frequently also cause infusional reactions comprising fevers and chills (rarely hypotension and transient pneumonitis) which can be lessened by pre-treatment with acetaminophen, hydrocortisone, diphenhydramine, and other measures. Steps to ensure hydration and reduce infusional reactions should be incorporated into formal institutional protocols for amphotericin B use.

Hydration is also important for reducing nephrotoxicity associated with foscarnet. Toxicity associated with cidofovir can be ameliorated by coadministering probenicid or cilastatin (as part of the imipenem/cilastatin formulation). The other anti-infectives listed in Table 13-1 are less directly nephrotoxic but can produce renal dysfunction in patients with underlying renal failure or when given concomitantly with other nephrotoxic drugs. These anti-infectives should be avoided in patients with renal failure or used in appropriately reduced doses when other alternatives are not available.

Bone marrow suppression induced by several anti-infectives is a problem, particularly in infected patients with hematological malignancies (Table 13-2). Some bone marrow suppressive anti-infectives can be avoided altogether (zidovudine, pentamidine, flucytosine) since safer alternatives are readily available. For most others, toxicity can be avoided (e.g., limiting linezolid to short courses) or the anti-infectives (e.g., sulfa drugs, ganciclovir) can be used until reversible bone marrow suppression ensues then switched to alternative agents.

Anti-infectives associated with hepatotoxicity are listed in Table 13-3. Hepatotoxicity is an infrequent side effect encountered most often with azole antifungals, especially when given to allogeneic HSCT recipients who may also have some degree of hepatitis secondary to GVHD [59].

4.2. Anti-infectives with Additive Toxicities

Side effects from certain chemotherapy agents and anti-infectives can increase toxicities compared to those observed with one agent alone. Few antineoplastic agents cause nephrotoxicity. Cisplatin is the most likely to cause renal failure. Patients treated with cisplatin and amphotericin B can develop profound, long lasting renal dysfunction characterized by increased creatinine and intractable magnesium and potassium wasting that may require significant replacement.

Peripheral neuropathy and other neurological side effects are important side effects, magnified when the toxicity is shared by some coadministered anti-infectives and chemotherapy agents. Anti-infectives with frequent neurological side effects are listed in Table 13-4. Fortunately, alternatives exist such that there is no reason to use the HIV nucleoside reverse transcriptase inhibitors listed in Table 13-4. In contrast, isoniazid and ethambutol are front-line antituberculosis agents. It may be difficult to avoid using one or both of these antibiotics, especially with the serious potential drug interaction problems associated with another front-line agent, rifampin. Pyridoxine mitigates much of the neurological side effects of isoniazid. However, treating patients with lymphoid malignancies also infected with tuberculosis remains a challenge.

Table 13-3. Anti-infectives that cause hepatic dysfunction.

Agent	
Isoniazid	
Rifampin	
Azole antifungals	Fluconazole, itraconazole, voriconazole, posaconazole
Terbinafine	
Maraviroc	
Ritonavir, saquinavir, tipranavir, lopinavir	
Nevirapine, delavirdine	
Metronidazole	
Telithromycin	

Table 13-4. Anti-infectives that cause neuropathy.

Agent
Isoniazid
Ethambutol
Zidovudine
Didanosine
Stavudine
Zalcitabine
Linezolid
Metronidazole

4.3. Drug–Drug Interactions

Managing the myriad interactions between anti-infectives and chemotherapy agents is one of the most difficult problems in infectious diseases management. Mechanisms to minimize the side effects from drug–drug interactions should be articulated in institutional policies for those frequently encountered circumstances where these problems invariably occur. By far, hepatic metabolism of drugs through one or more cytochrome P-450 (CYP) isoenzymes is the major source of drug–drug interaction problems. Chemotherapy agents and anti-infectives metabolized via CYP are listed in Tables 13-5 and 13-6, respectively. The interactions can be complex. Metabolism of chemotherapeutics listed in Table 13-5 may be either accelerated or inhibited by an interacting anti-infective. Consequently, the therapeutic effect of an antineoplastic agent may

Table 13-5. Chemotherapy agents metabolized by Cytochrome P450 isoenzymes.

Agent
Anthracyclines (doxorubicin, daurorubicin, idarubicin)
Busulfan
Vincristine
Etoposide
Bortezomib
Paclitaxel
Docetaxel
Cyclophosphamide
Tritenoin (all *trans* retinoic acid)
Imatinib
Sunitinib
Leflunomide
Corticosteroids

Table 13-6. Anti-infectives metabolized by Cytochrome P450 isoenzymes.

Agent
Ketoconazole
Itraconazole
Voriconazole
Posaconazole
Quinopristin/dalfopristin
Erythromycin
Clarithromycin
HIV non-nucleoside reverse transcriptase inhibitors Nevirapine, delavirdine, efavirenz
HIV protease inhibitors Atazanavir, darunavir, fosamprenavir, indinavir, lopinavir, ritonavir, nelfinavir, sasquinavir, tipranavir
CCR5 coreceptor antagonist Maraviroc

be diminished due to enhanced degradation by the interacting anti-infective which risks suboptimal outcomes. Alternatively, inhibited metabolism may manifest as overdose with increased chemotherapy-related toxicities, such as prolonged neutropenia or severe mucositis. Similarly, interactions may reduce levels of an anti-infective leading to treatment failure or, conversely, result in overdose of the anti-infective with possible toxicity. Dosing of voriconazole and posaconazole can be modified using drug levels measured in reference laboratories.

A chemotherapy agent may have multiple metabolic pathways mediated by different CYP isoenzymes. Preferential inhibition of one CYP isoenzyme by an anti-infective may drive metabolism of the chemotherapy drug down an alternative CYP pathway with unpredictable results. For instance, itraconazole is a preferential inhibitor of CYP 3A4. Severe cyclophosphamide toxicity was observed in patients receiving itraconazole prophylaxis during cyclophosphamide therapy [60]. Enhanced toxicity resulted from accumulation of the 4-hydroxy-cyclophosphamide metabolite [61]. In contrast, patients receiving fluconazole, a preferential inhibitor of CYP 2C9, did not develop cyclophosphamide toxicity because the toxic metabolite did not accumulate [62]. Itraconazole has been implicated as well in potentiating vincristine-associated peripheral neuropathy [63, 64], presumably by vincristine overdose secondary to inhibition of the CYP-dependent metabolism of vincristine.

Adverse drug interaction events are not limited to anti-infective/antineoplastic agent interactions. Many antiepileptics (e.g., phenytoin, carbamazepine), antidepressants, hypnotics, calcium channel blocker antihypertensives, proton pump inhibitors, H2 blocker antacids, oral anticoagulants, oral hypoglycemics, and others are metabolized by CYP isoenzymes. Coadministration of any of these drugs with CYP-metabolized anti-infectives and chemotherapy agents requires awareness of potential interactions. Phenytoin, in particular, deserves special mention because phenytoin is a powerful inducer of CYP synthesis. The net effect is potential for rapid, extensive degradation of anti-infectives or chemotherapeutics in patients also taking phenytoin. Patients with hematological malignancies taking phenytoin should be transitioned to another antiepileptic before starting chemotherapy.

The most important interactions of concern for oncologists are inhibition of the immunosuppressants cyclosporin, tacrolimus, sirolimus, and corticosteroid metabolism by azole antifungals. Fluconazole induces minimal changes in immunosuppressant metabolism in contrast to itraconazole and voriconazole. Interactions between itraconazole or voriconazole with cyclosporin and tacrolimus can be managed by monitoring immunosuppressant blood levels. In contrast, it is extremely difficult to manage sirolimus dosing even with drug monitoring in patients also taking itraconazole or voriconazole. Coadministration of sirolimus with azole antifungals is contraindicated. Side effects from interactions range from cyclosporin or tacrolimus toxicity to breakthrough GVHD when a patient stops taking the azole without a compensatory modification of the immunosuppressant dose. Therefore, stem cell transplant programs should establish procedures to prevent immunosuppressant/azole interaction adverse side effects. Examples include scheduled cyclosporin/tacrolimus level monitoring and education of patients concerning the importance of stopping drugs only under supervision. Most importantly, transplant programs should establish standard protocols using principally either tacrolimus or cyclosporin and a preferred azole for GVHD and antifungal prophylaxis/treatment, respectively.

5. Antiretroviral Therapy for HIV Patients with Hematological Malignancies

Modern, highly active antiretroviral therapy (HAART) has improved the HIV viral control in infected patients dramatically. The net effect has been a partial reconstitution of viral-ravaged immune systems and decreased mortality from opportunistic infections. However, success is incomplete and there is an apparent increase in observed HIV-associated malignancies in patients with longer survival from HAART. The most common malignancies seen are T- and B-cell hematological malignancies but the rates of solid tumors, such as various lung, squamous cell, and other cancers, are also higher compared to non-HIV-infected patients [65]. Some malignancies, such as primary effusion and immunoblastic leukemias/lymphomas, are associated with very low CD4 counts. However, intermediate grade B-cell and Burkitt's lymphomas may occur with CD4 counts greater than 200. The potential of modern HAART to prolong lifespan has made a compelling argument for treating HIV-infected patients with hematological malignancies with the same potent chemotherapy strategies used in cancer patients not infected with HIV.

Serious potential drug–drug interactions complicate simultaneous HAART for HIV and chemotherapy for malignancies, particularly for lymphomas. The non-nucleoside reverse transcriptase (NNRTI) and protease (PI) inhibitors and the lone CCR5 coreceptor antagonist antiretrovirals are potent inhibitors of CYP isoenzymes as discussed above. Therefore, coadministration of NNRTI and PI antiretrovirals, in particular, may lead potentially to overdose toxicities of several anti-lymphoma chemotherapy agents as discussed above (Table 13-5). Enhanced toxicities include peripheral neuropathy, mucositis/enterocolitis [66], and prolonged neutropenia [67]. Potential for toxicities depend to some extent on the intensity of the chemotherapy regimen. Coadministration toxicity has been seen less frequently with standard CHOP for intermediate B-cell lymphomas, especially with G-CSF support [67, 68]. However, there may be greater concern with more intensive chemotherapy regimens where there is evidence for better remission rates and long-term survival with intense anti-HIV-associated lymphoma regimens such as EPOCH [69, 70]. Higher intensity regimens, with potential for HAART drug interaction-related toxicities even greater than seen in earlier CHOP trials, are likely to become the standard approach for all HIV-associated lymphomas including most intermediate and all high grade B- and T-cell lymphomas. Adjusting doses of chemotherapeutic agents to account for HAART interactions is not practical. In fact, reduced relative dose intensity, such as lower doses of chemotherapy agents or delays in starting subsequent courses while awaiting recovery from HAART/chemotherapy toxicities, correlates with poorer successful oncological response rates [71]. Alternatively, the same toxicities, such as severe mucositis/enterocolitis and protracted neutropenia, may lead to interruptions of HAART with the potential for development of HIV resistance. In addition, anti-lymphoma chemotherapy is inherently destructive to the immune system. Therefore, the potential for reconstitution of HIV-ravaged immune system function, one of the central goals of HAART, is diminished during courses of chemotherapy. All these issues conspire to increase the risk of adverse outcomes from HAART/anti-lymphoma chemotherapy.

Counterbalancing risks for adverse events associated with HAART/chemotherapy drug interactions is the potential for better outcomes in patients whose HIV burdens (assessed by serum viral mRNA copies/ml) are controlled by HAART during and after anti-lymphoma treatment. Successful responses in HIV patients with intermediate grade lymphomas are dependent on pre-chemotherapy CD4 counts [67, 68, 72]. Improved outcomes were seen in non-Hodgkin's lymphoma patients treated concurrently with both HAART and chemotherapy whose HIV loads decreased during chemotherapy and follow-up compared to patients with poor virological responses [71]. Similarly, concurrently treated patients who had strong CD4 count recovery post-chemotherapy had significantly better hematological outcomes compared to patients with poor CD4 count recovery [71]. Taken together, preserved pretreatment CD4 counts, post-chemotherapy CD4 recovery, controlled HIV burden, and ability to tolerate high relative dose intensity chemotherapy (more likely in patients on HAART [71]) correlate with improved responses and survival in patients with HIV-related lymphomas. These observations support HAART in achieving better outcomes. There remains controversy whether the correlation of HAART virological response and better outcomes with chemotherapy for non-Hodgkin's lymphoma is true "cause and effect" or whether the HAART response is simply a marker for a better risk subpopulation with perhaps more responsive tumor or a more favorable immunological environment [70]. In patients who had HAART interrupted during the 16 weeks of EPOCH treatment, CD4 counts recovered over 12 months and viral loads decreased to baseline levels over 3–6 months [70], similar to CD4 recovery and virological responses seen in patients receiving concurrent HAART [68, 71]. It is, therefore, impossible to make a definitive recommendation about HAART/chemotherapy timing in the absence of a prospective trial comparing concurrent versus interrupted HAART (which is unlikely to be performed).

Some general comments can be made regarding HIV treatment. In the absence of data supporting a benefit to concurrent versus interrupted HAART/chemotherapy, a conservative approach is justified when considering HAART for individual patients with lymphoma. First, drug interactions, potential or real, should be avoided. Adverse effects include not just additive toxicities but also potential for reduced relative dose intensities of chemotherapeutic agents with risks for poorer hematological outcomes. Antiretrovirals with overlapping side effect profiles should be avoided (Table 13-7). Secondly, it is important to avoid risks for inducing resistance mutations in HIV such as can occur with poor compliance with HAART secondary to nausea, vomiting, and other toxicities. All antiretrovirals in a combination HAART regimen must be started and stopped together if complications lead to an interruption of HAART.

It may be helpful to consider several scenarios where concurrent HAART and anti-lymphoma chemotherapy may be contemplated. The HIV patient already receiving HAART with pre-chemotherapy undetectable viral loads and CD4 >200 may do best by withholding HAART throughout the entire sequence of chemotherapy cycles. There is a reasonable expectation that CD4 counts will rebound and HIV burden will decrease post-chemotherapy after

HAART is restarted. For many HIV patients, the HIV-associated lymphoma is an AIDS defining event and these patients are, by definition, HAART naïve. HAART naïve patients may present with a range of CD4 counts from profound depression to counts >200. Those HAART naïve with preserved immunological function and low HIV loads may also be best treated by waiting until the entire cycle of chemotherapy is complete before starting HAART.

A better argument can be made that ART-naïve patients with high viral loads and HIV patients failing HAART regimens with poorly suppressed viral loads should be treated with HAART during chemotherapy in the hope that control of HIV may improve overall outcomes. Unfortunately, three major classes of antiretrovirals are potent inhibitors of CYP isoenzymes and are likely to interfere with metabolism of chemotherapy agents (Table 13-6). For standard intensity chemotherapy, HAART has been coadministered successfully with mild to moderate toxicities [67, 68]. However, current preference for high intensity anti-lymphoma regimens significantly increases the likelihood of drug interaction-associated toxicities compared to past experience with CHOP-based treatment strategies. These realities complicate the design of effective but safe antiretroviral regimens (Table 13-7).

Intermittent HAART, where antiretrovirals are held during chemotherapy infusions and then restarted following completion, may be the preferred mechanism to administer HAART in patients with a compelling need for suppression of HIV concurrent with anti-lymphoma chemotherapy. Intermittent ART raises the danger of inducing resistance by HIV exposed to off and on retrovirals. An intermittent ART strategy precludes use of antiretrovirals with long half-lives such as NNRTI. Examples of theoretically feasible, potent HAART may include a PI plus one or more NRTI or a double PI regimen. PI antiretrovirals have a low potential for inducing resistance mutations in HIV if used in an intermittent pattern. It should be emphasized that all HAART must be started and stopped together, not just the interacting antiretrovirals. Once the courses of chemotherapy have been completed, patients can be switched to more conventional and convenient HAART regimens. Raltegravir, the first of class HIV integrase inhibitor, is effective when used in salvage HAART regimens for patients with HIV resistant to other antiretrovirals. Raltegravir is not

Table 13-7. Antiretroviral agents: recommendations for treatment with chemotherapy.

Agent	Comments
Agents to avoid	
Zidovudine	Neutropenia, neuropathy
Didanosine, stavudine, zalcitabine	Pancreatitis, neuropathy
Indinavir	Nephrolithiasis
Delavirdine, nevirapine, efavirenz	CYP inhibitors with long half life
Preferred agents	
Lamivudine, emtracitabine	
Tenofovir	
Abacavir	
Protease inhibitors	
Raltegravir	

a CYP substrate or inhibitor, and is unlikely to interfere with the metabolism of chemotherapy agents by CYP. Experience is limited with raltegravir as a component of first-line HAART treatment. However, raltegravir used in conjunction with tenofovir or abacavir may become the HAART therapy of choice for patients with lymphoma as this regimen can be given with chemotherapy with little risk of drug–drug interactions.

Monitoring HIV loads may be helpful in gauging the efficacy of intermittent HAART. Effects of chemotherapy will make monitoring CD4 counts useless during chemotherapy. Consultation with HIV experts is recommended strongly for patients in whom concurrent HAART and anti-lymphoma chemotherapy is contemplated.

Prophylaxis against *Pneumocystis* pneumonia should be maintained throughout the course of chemotherapy, regardless of pre-treatment CD4 counts. Bone marrow suppression by the combination of chemotherapy and trimethoprim/sulfamethoxazole is a problem in HIV patients with malignancies. Alternative prophylaxis with dapsone, atovaquone, and even inhaled pentamidine may be required in many patients until all chemotherapy has been completed. Prophylaxis with azithromycin against *Mycobacterium avium* complex is usually well-tolerated. Patients with histories of recurrent HSV or VZV infections should be considered for acyclovir prophylaxis during chemotherapy.

References

1. Prentice HG (1983) Use of acyclovir for prophylaxis of herpes infections in severely immunocompromised patients. J Antimicrob Chemother 12(Suppl B):153–159
2. Rolston KV (2005) Challenges in the treatment of infections caused by gram-positive and gram-negative bacteria in patients with cancer and neutropenia. Clin Infect Dis 40(Suppl 4):S246–S252
3. Rolston KV, Bodey GP (2006) Comment on: empirical antibiotic monotherapy for febrile neutropenia: systematic review and meta-analysis of randomized controlled trials. J Antimicrob Chemother 58(2):478–480
4. Segal BH, Almyroudis NG, Battiwalla M, Herbrecht R, Perfect JR, Walsh TJ et al (2007) Prevention and early treatment of invasive fungal infection in patients with cancer and neutropenia and in stem cell transplant recipients in the era of newer broad-spectrum antifungal agents and diagnostic adjuncts. Clin Infect Dis 44(3):402–409
5. Feld R, Paesmans M, Freifeld AG, Klastersky J, Pizzo PA, Rolston KV et al (2002) Methodology for clinical trials involving patients with cancer who have febrile neutropenia: updated guidelines of the Immunocompromised Host Society/Multinational Association for Supportive Care in Cancer, with emphasis on outpatient studies. Clin Infect Dis 35(12):1463–1468
6. Hughes WT, Armstrong D, Bodey GP, Bow EJ, Brown AE, Calandra T et al (2002) 2002 guidelines for the use of antimicrobial agents in neutropenic patients with cancer. Clin Infect Dis 34(6):730–751
7. Jun HX, Zhixiang S, Chun W, Reksodiputro AH, Ranuhardy D, Tamura K et al (2005) Clinical guidelines for the management of cancer patients with neutropenia and unexplained fever. Int J Antimicrob Agents 26(Suppl 2):S128–S132
8. Tamura K (2005) Clinical guidelines for the management of neutropenic patients with unexplained fever in Japan: validation by the Japan Febrile Neutropenia Study Group. Int J Antimicrob Agents 26(Suppl 2):S123–S127
9. Albrecht SJ, Fishman NO, Kitchen J, Nachamkin I, Bilker WB, Hoegg C et al (2006) Reemergence of gram-negative health care-associated bloodstream infections. Arch Intern Med 166(12):1289–1294

10. Bratu S, Quale J, Cebular S, Heddurshetti R, Landman D (2005) Multidrug-resistant Pseudomonas aeruginosa in Brooklyn, New York: molecular epidemiology and in vitro activity of polymyxin B. Eur J Clin Microbiol Infect Dis 24(3):196–201
11. Bratu S, Landman D, Haag R, Recco R, Eramo A, Alam M et al (2005) Rapid spread of carbapenem-resistant Klebsiella pneumoniae in New York City: a new threat to our antibiotic armamentarium. Arch Intern Med 165(12):1430–1435
12. Cagnoni PJ, Walsh TJ, Prendergast MM, Bodensteiner D, Hiemenz S, Greenberg RN et al (2000) Pharmacoeconomic analysis of liposomal amphotericin B versus conventional amphotericin B in the empirical treatment of persistently febrile neutropenic patients. J Clin Oncol 18(12):2476–2483
13. Garey KW, Pai MP, Suda KJ, Turpin RS, Rege MD, Mingo DE et al (2007) Inadequacy of fluconazole dosing in patients with candidemia based on Infectious Diseases Society of America (IDSA) guidelines. Pharmacoepidemiol Drug Saf 16(8):919–927
14. Marr KA (2004) Invasive Candida infections: the changing epidemiology. Oncology (Williston Park) 18(14 Suppl 13):9–14
15. Paterson DL, Lipman J (2007) Returning to the pre-antibiotic era in the critically ill: the XDR problem. Crit Care Med 35(7):1789–1791
16. Cosgrove SE, Patel A, Song X, Miller RE, Speck K, Banowetz A et al (2007) Impact of different methods of feedback to clinicians after postprescription antimicrobial review based on the Centers for Disease Control and Prevention's 12 Steps to Prevent Antimicrobial Resistance Among Hospitalized Adults. Infect Control Hosp Epidemiol 28(6):641–646
17. Fishman N (2006) Antimicrobial stewardship. Am J Infect Control 34(5 Suppl 1):S55–S63
18. Forrest GN (2007) Is there a role for antimicrobial management in organ transplantation? Curr Opin Organ Transplant 12:604–609
19. Schimpff SC, Moody M, Young VM (1970) Relationship of colonization with Pseudomonas aeruginosa to development of Pseudomonas bacteremia in cancer patients. Antimicrobial Agents Chemother (Bethesda) 10:240–244
20. Siddiqui AH, Harris AD, Hebden J, Wilson PD, Morris JG Jr, Roghmann MC (2002) The effect of active surveillance for vancomycin-resistant enterococci in high-risk units on vancomycin-resistant enterococci incidence hospital-wide. Am J Infect Control 30(1):40–43
21. Muto CA, Giannetta ET, Durbin LJ, Simonton BM, Farr BM (2002) Cost-effectiveness of perirectal surveillance cultures for controlling vancomycin-resistant Enterococcus. Infect Control Hosp Epidemiol 23(8):429–435
22. Shadel BN, Puzniak LA, Gillespie KN, Lawrence SJ, Kollef M, Mundy LM (2006) Surveillance for vancomycin-resistant enterococci: type, rates, costs, and implications. Infect Control Hosp Epidemiol 27(10):1068–1075
23. Procop GW, Winn W (2003) Outsourcing microbiology and offsite laboratories. Implications on patient care, cost savings, and graduate medical education. Arch Pathol Lab Med 127(5):623–624
24. Binkley S, Fishman NO, LaRosa LA, Marr AM, Nachamkin I, Wordell D et al (2006) Comparison of unit-specific and hospital-wide antibiograms: potential implications for selection of empirical antimicrobial therapy. Infect Control Hosp Epidemiol 27(7):682–687
25. Burke JP, Pestotnik SL (1999) Antibiotic use and microbial resistance in intensive care units: impact of computer-assisted decision support. J Chemother 11(6): 530–535
26. Paterson DL (2006) The epidemiological profile of infections with multidrug-resistant Pseudomonas aeruginosa and Acinetobacter species. Clin Infect Dis 43(Suppl 2):S43–S48
27. Dellit TH, Owens RC, McGowan JE Jr, Gerding DN, Weinstein RA, Burke JP et al (2007) Infectious Diseases Society of America and the Society for Healthcare

Epidemiology of America guidelines for developing an institutional program to enhance antimicrobial stewardship. Clin Infect Dis 44(2):159–177
28. Forrest G (2006) Role of antifungal susceptibility testing in patient management. Curr Opin Infect Dis 19(6):538–543
29. Pfaller MA, Diekema DJ, Sheehan DJ (2006) Interpretive breakpoints for fluconazole and Candida revisited: a blueprint for the future of antifungal susceptibility testing. Clin Microbiol Rev 19(2):435–447
30. Pfaller MA, Messer SA, Boyken L, Rice C, Tendolkar S, Hollis RJ et al (2007) Use of fluconazole as a surrogate marker to predict susceptibility and resistance to voriconazole among 13, 338 clinical isolates of Candida spp. Tested by clinical and laboratory standards institute-recommended broth microdilution methods. J Clin Microbiol 45(1):70–75
31. Bodey GP (1981) Antibiotic prophylaxis in cancer patients: regimens of oral, non-absorbable antibiotics for prevention of infection during induction of remission. Rev Infect Dis 3(suppl):S259–S268
32. Weinstock DM, Conlon M, Iovino C, Aubrey T, Gudiol C, Riedel E et al (2007) Colonization, bloodstream infection, and mortality caused by vancomycin-resistant enterococcus early after allogeneic hematopoietic stem cell transplant. Biol Blood Marrow Transplant 13(5):615–621
33. Diekema DJ, Edmond MB (2007) Look before you leap: active surveillance for multidrug-resistant organisms. Clin Infect Dis 44(8):1101–1107
34. Weber SG, Huang SS, Oriola S, Huskins WC, Noskin GA, Harriman K et al (2007) Legislative mandates for use of active surveillance cultures to screen for methicillin-resistant Staphylococcus aureus and vancomycin-resistant enterococci: position statement from the Joint SHEA and APIC Task Force. Am J Infect Control 35(2):73–85
35. Forrest GN (2007) PNA FISH: present and future impact on patient management. Expert Rev Mol Diagn 7(3):231–236
36. Peters RP, Mohammadi T, Vandenbroucke-Grauls CM, Danner SA, van Agtmael MA, Savelkoul PH (2004) Detection of bacterial DNA in blood samples from febrile patients: underestimated infection or emerging contamination? FEMS Immunol Med Microbiol 42(2):249–253
37. Carroll KC (2008) Rapid diagnostics for methicillin-resistant Staphylococcus aureus: current status. Mol Diagn Ther 12(1):15–24
38. Stamper PD, Cai M, Lema C, Eskey K, Carroll KC (2007) Comparison of the BD GeneOhm VanR assay to culture for identification of vancomycin-resistant enterococci in rectal and stool specimens. J Clin Microbiol 45(10):3360–3365
39. Stamper PD, Cai M, Howard T, Speser S, Carroll KC (2007) Clinical validation of the molecular BD GeneOhm StaphSR assay for direct detection of Staphylococcus aureus and methicillin-resistant Staphylococcus aureus in positive blood cultures. J Clin Microbiol 45(7):2191–2196
40. Espy MJ, Uhl JR, Sloan LM, Buckwalter SP, Jones MF, Vetter EA et al (2006) Real-time PCR in clinical microbiology: applications for routine laboratory testing. Clin Microbiol Rev 19(1):165–256
41. Forrest GN, Mankes K, Jabra-Rizk MA, Weekes E, Johnson JK, Lincalis DP et al (2006) Peptide nucleic acid fluorescence in situ hybridization-based identification of Candida albicans and its impact on mortality and antifungal therapy costs. J Clin Microbiol 44(9):3381–3383
42. Forrest GN, Mehta S, Weekes E, Lincalis DP, Johnson JK, Venezia RA (2006) Impact of rapid in situ hybridization testing on coagulase-negative staphylococci positive blood cultures. J Antimicrob Chemother 58(1):154–158
43. Safdar N, Maki DG (2006) Use of vancomycin-containing lock or flush solutions for prevention of bloodstream infection associated with central venous access devices: a meta-analysis of prospective, randomized trials. Clin Infect Dis 43(4):474–484

44. Gross R, Morgan AS, Kinky DE, Weiner M, Gibson GA, Fishman NO (2001) Impact of a hospital-based antimicrobial management program on clinical and economic outcomes. Clin Infect Dis 33(3):289–295
45. Itokazu GS, Schwartz DN, Garey KW, Rodvold KA, Danziger LH, Weinstein RA (2006) Pharmacists' perceptions of the effectiveness of antimicrobial control programs. Am J Health Syst Pharm 63(24):2504–2508
46. MacDougall C, Polk RE (2005) Antimicrobial stewardship programs in health care systems. Clin Microbiol Rev 18(4):638–656
47. Jansen JP, Kern WV, Cornely OA, Karthaus M, Ruhnke M, Ullmann AJ et al (2006) Economic evaluation of voriconazole versus conventional amphotericin B in the treatment of invasive aspergillosis in Germany. Value Health 9(1):12–23
48. Wingard JR, Leather HL, Wood CA, Gerth WC, Lupinacci RJ, Berger ML et al (2007) Pharmacoeconomic analysis of caspofungin versus liposomal amphotericin B as empirical antifungal therapy for neutropenic fever. Am J Health Syst Pharm 64(6):637–643
49. Cornely OA, Maertens J, Winston DJ, Perfect J, Ullmann AJ, Walsh TJ et al (2007) Posaconazole vs. fluconazole or itraconazole prophylaxis in patients with neutropenia. N Engl J Med 356(4):348–359
50. Fischer MA, Solomon DH, Teich JM, Avorn J (2003) Conversion from intravenous to oral medications: assessment of a computerized intervention for hospitalized patients. Arch Intern Med 163(21):2585–2589
51. McGregor JC, Weekes E, Forrest GN, Standiford HC, Perencevich EN, Furuno JP et al (2006) Impact of a computerized clinical decision support system on reducing inappropriate antimicrobial use: a randomized controlled trial. J Am Med Inform Assoc 13(4):378–384
52. Mutnick AH, Ross MB (1997) Formulary management at a tertiary care teaching hospital. Pharm Pract Manag Q 17(1):63–87
53. Mutnick AH, Sterba KJ, Szymusiak-Mutnick BA (1998) The integration of quality assessment and a patient-specific intervention/outcomes program. Pharm Pract Manag Q 17(4):25–36
54. Knox K, Lawson W, Dean B, Holmes A (2003) Multidisciplinary antimicrobial management and the role of the infectious diseases pharmacist – a UK perspective. J Hosp Infect 53(2):85–90
55. Evans RS, Pestotnik SL, Classen DC, Clemmer TP, Weaver LK, Orme JF Jr et al (1998) A computer-assisted management program for antibiotics and other antiinfective agents. N Engl J Med 338(4):232–238
56. Pestotnik SL (2005) Expert clinical decision support systems to enhance antimicrobial stewardship programs: insights from the society of infectious diseases pharmacists. Pharmacotherapy 25(8):1116–1125
57. Paterson DL (2006) The role of antimicrobial management programs in optimizing antibiotic prescribing within hospitals. Clin Infect Dis 42(Suppl 2):S90–S95
58. Schimpff SC (1986) Empiric antibiotic therapy for granulocytopenic cancer patients. Am J Med 80(5C):13–20
59. Wingard JR, Leather H (2005) Hepatotoxicity associated with antifungal therapy after bone marrow transplantation. Clin Infect Dis 41(3):308–310
60. Marr KA, Crippa F, Leisenring W, Hoyle M, Boeckh M, Balajee SA et al (2004) Itraconazole versus fluconazole for prevention of fungal infections in patients receiving allogeneic stem cell transplants. Blood 103(4):1527–1533
61. Marr KA, Leisenring W, Crippa F, Slattery JT, Corey L, Boeckh M, McDonald GB (2004) Cyclophosphamide metabolism is affected by azole antifungals. Blood 103(4):1557–1559
62. Upton A, McCune JS, Kirby KA, Leisenring W, McDonald G, Batchelder A, Marr KA (2007) Fluconazole coadministration concurrent with cyclophosphamide conditioning may reduce regimen-related toxicity postmyeloablative hematopoietic cell transplantation. Biol Blood Marrow Transplant 13(7):760–764

63. Bohme A, Ganser A, Hoelzer D (1995) Aggravation of vincristine-induced neurotoxicity by itraconazole in the treatment of adult ALL. Ann Hematol 71(6): 311–312
64. Sathiapaian RK, El-Solh H (2001) Enhanced vincristine neurotoxicity from drug interactions: case report and review of literature. Pediatr Hematol Oncol 18(8):543–546
65. Patel P, Hanson DL, Sullivan PS, Novak RM, Moorman AC, Tong TC, Holmberg SD, Brooks JT (2008) Incidence of types of cancer among HIV-infected persons compared with the general population in the United States, 1992–2003. Ann Intern Med 148(10):728–736
66. Sparano JA, Wiernik PH, Hu X, Sarta C, Henry DH, Ratech H (1998) Saquinavir enhances the mucosal toxicity of infusional cyclophosphamide, doxorubicin, and etoposide in patients with HIV-associated non-hodgkin's lymphoma. Med Oncol 15(1):50–57
67. Sparano JA, Lee S, Chen MG, Nazeer T, Einzig A, Ambinder RF, Henry DH, Manalo J, Li T, Von Roenn JH (2004) Phase II trial of infusional cyclophosphamide, doxorubicin, and etoposide in patients with HIV-associated non-Hodgkin's lymphoma: an Eastern Cooperative Oncology Group trial (E1494). J Clin Oncol 22(8):1491–1500
68. Ratner L, Lee J, Tang S, Redden D, Hamzeh F, Herndier B, Scadden D, Kaplan L, Ambinder R, Levine A, Harrington W, Grochow L, Flexner C, Tan B, Straus D (2001) Chemotherapy for human immunodeficiency virus-associated non-Hodgkin's lymphoma in combination with highly active antiretroviral therapy. J Clin Oncol 19(8):2171–2178
69. Bower M, Powles T, Stebbing J, Thirlwell C (2005) Potential antiretroviral drug interactions with cyclophosphamide, doxorubicin, and etoposide. J Clin Oncol 23(6):1329–1330
70. Little RF, Pittaluga S, Grant N, Steinberg SM, Kavlick MF, Mitsuya H, Franchini G, Gutierrez M, Raffeld M, Jaffe ES, Shearer G, Yarchoan R, Wilson WH (2003) Highly effective treatment of acquired immunodeficiency syndrome-related lymphoma with dose-adjusted EPOCH: impact of antiretroviral therapy suspension and tumor biology. Blood 101(12):4653–4659
71. Antinori A, Cingolani A, Alba L, Ammassari A, Serraino D, Ciancio BC, Palmieri F, De Luca A, Larocca LM, Ruco L, Ippolito G, Cauda R (2001) Better response to chemotherapy and prolonged survival in AIDS-related lymphomas responding to highly active antiretroviral therapy. AIDS 15(12):1483–1491
72. Bower M, Gazzard B, Mandall S, Newsom-Davis T, Thirlwell C, Dhillon T, Young AM, Powles T, Gaya A, Nelson M, Stebbing J (2005) A prognostic index for systematic AIDS-related non-Hodgkin's lymphoma treated in the era of highly active antiretroviral therapy. Ann Intern Med 143(4):265–273

Index

GPSR Compliance

The European Union's (EU) General Product Safety Regulation (GPSR) is a set of rules that requires consumer products to be safe and our obligations to ensure this.

If you have any concerns about our products, you can contact us on ProductSafety@springernature.com

In case Publisher is established outside the EU, the EU authorized representative is:

Springer Nature Customer Service Center GmbH
Europaplatz 3
69115 Heidelberg, Germany

Batch number: 10607204

Printed by Printforce, the Netherlands